D1084985

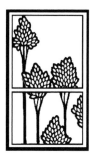

PHARMACOTHERAPY FOR MOOD, ANXIETY, AND COGNITIVE DISORDERS

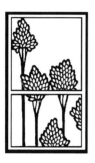

PHARMACOTHERAPY FOR MOOD, ANXIETY, AND COGNITIVE DISORDERS

EDITED BY

Uriel Halbreich, M.D.

Stuart A. Montgomery, M.D.

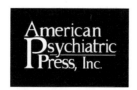

Washington, DC
London, England

Manufactured in the United States of America on acid-free paper
03 02 01 00   4 3 2 1
First Edition

American Psychiatric Press, Inc.
1400 K Street, N.W., Washington, DC   20005
www.appi.org

Library of Congress Cataloging-in-Publication Data
Pharmacotherapy for mood, anxiety, and cognitive disorders / edited by
  Uriel Halbreich, Stuart Montgomery.
       p.   cm.
  Includes bibliographical references and index.
  ISBN 0-88048-885-9
  1. Affective disorders—Chemotherapy.   2. Cognition disorders—
  Chemotherapy.   I. Halbreich, Uriel, 1943– . II. Montgomery, S.
  A.
     [DNLM: 1. Mood Disorders—drug therapy.   2. Cognition
  Disorders—drug therapy.   3. Antidepressive Agents—therapeutic use.   4. Anti-
  Anxiety Agents—therapeutic use.   WM 171 P5355 1999]
  RC537.P456   1999
  616.85′ 27061—dc21
  DNLM/DLC
  for Library of Congress   99-13399
                                                                  CIP

British Library Cataloguing in Publication Data
A CIP record is available from the British Library.

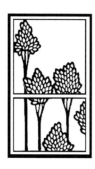

CONTENTS

SECTION II

Mood Stabilizers
Robert M. Post, M.D., Section Editor

SECTION III

Antidepressants
Alan F. Schatzberg, M.D., Section Editor

SECTION IV

Anxiolytics
Stephen M. Stahl, M.D., Ph.D., Section Editor

SECTION V

Cognition and Dementia
Juan J. López-Ibor Jr., M.D., Section Editor

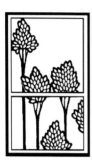

CONTRIBUTORS

JAY D. AMSTERDAM, M.D.
Professor of Psychiatry and Director of Depression Research Unit, University of Pennsylvania Medical Center, Philadelphia, Pennsylvania

DAVID BAKISH, M.D., F.R.C.P.C.
Associate Professor, Department of Psychiatry, University of Ottawa; and Head, Psychopharmacology Unit, Royal Ottawa Hospital and Institute of Mental Health Research, Ottawa, Canada

YORAM BARAK, M.D.
Clinical Investigator, Ministry of Health Mental Health Center, Faculty of Health Sciences, Ben-Gurion University of the Negev, Beersheba, Israel

JOSEPH K. BELANOFF, M.D.
Department of Psychiatry and Behavioral Sciences, Stanford University School of Medicine, Stanford, California

CAROLINE BELL, M.R.C.PSYCH.
Carey Coombs Fellow, Psychopharmacology Unit, University of Bristol School of Medical Sciences, Bristol, England

ROBERT H. BELMAKER, M.D.
Professor of Psychiatry and Director, Division of Psychiatry, Ministry of Health Mental Health Center, Faculty of Health Sciences, Ben-Gurion University of the Negev, Beersheba, Israel

JONATHAN BENJAMIN, M.D.
Clinical Investigator, Ministry of Health Mental Health Center, Faculty of Health Sciences, Ben-Gurion University of the Negev, Beersheba, Israel

JOANNE D. BERGIANNAKI, M.D.
Assistant Professor of Psychiatry, Sleep Research Unit, Department of Psychiatry, University of Athens, Eginition Hospital, Athens, Greece

YULY BERSUDSKY, M.D.
Clinical Investigator, Ministry of Health Mental Health Center, Faculty of Health Sciences, Ben-Gurion University of the Negev, Beersheba, Israel

CARLO BERTI, M.B., M.F.P.M.
Research Fellow, Department of Psychological Medicine, St. Bartholomew's Hospital, London, England

JACQUES BRADWEJN, M.D., F.R.C.P.C.
Professor and Chair of Psychiatry, University of Ottawa; and Psychiatrist-in-Chief, Royal Hospital of Ottawa, Ottawa, Canada

MATTHEW BYERLY, M.D.
Department of Psychiatry, University of Florida College of Medicine, Gainesville, Florida

ALFREDO CALCEDO-BARBA JR.
Professor of Psychiatry, Department of Psychiatry, Universidad Complutense de Madrid, Madrid, Spain

DE-MAW CHUANG, PH.D.
Chief, Section on Molecular Neurobiology, Biological Psychiatry Branch, National Institute of Mental Health, Bethesda, Maryland

KATHERINE M. CONNOR, M.D.
Professor of Psychiatry, Duke University Medical Center, Durham, North Carolina

JEREMY D. COPLAN, M.D.
Assistant Professor of Psychiatry, New York State Psychiatric Institute, New York, New York

BRENDA COSTALL, M.D.
Head of School, The School of Pharmacy, University of Bradford, Bradford, England

PINHAS N. DANNON, M.D.
Attending Physician, Psychiatric Division, Sheba Medical Center, Tel Hashomer, Israel

JONATHAN R. T. DAVIDSON, M.D.
Professor of Psychiatry, Duke University Medical Center, Durham, North Carolina

CHARLES DEBATTISTA, D.M.H., M.D.
Assistant Professor and Chief of Depression Clinic, Department of Psychiatry and Behavioral Sciences, Stanford University School of Medicine, Stanford, California

JOHAN A. DEN BOER, M.D.
Associate Professor of Biological Psychiatry, University Hospital Utrecht, Utrecht, The Netherlands

KIRK DENICOFF, M.D.
Chief, Unit on Outpatient Bipolar Studies, Biological Psychiatry Branch, National Institute of Mental Health, Bethesda, Maryland

DAVANGERE P. DEVANAND, M.D.
Associate Professor of Clinical Psychiatry, College of Physicians and Surgeons, Columbia University, New York State Psychiatric Institute, New York, New York

TIMOTHY G. DINAN, M.D., PH.D., F.R.C.P.I., F.R.C.PSYCH.
Professor and Chairman, Department of Psychological Medicine, St. Bartholomew's Hospital, London, England

ORNAH T. DOLBERG, M.D.
Attending Physician, Psychiatric Division, Sheba Medical Center, Tel Hashomer, Israel

AMOS FLEISCHMANN, PH.D.
Ministry of Health Mental Health Center, Faculty of Health Sciences, Ben-Gurion University of the Negev, Beersheba, Israel

MARK FRYE, M.D.
Biological Psychiatry Branch, National Institute of Mental Health,
Bethesda, Maryland

WAYNE K. GOODMAN, M.D.
Professor and Chairman, Department of Psychiatry, University of
Florida College of Medicine, Gainesville, Florida

JACK M. GORMAN, M.D.
Professor of Clinical Psychiatry, New York State Psychiatric Institute,
New York, New York

JOHN F. GREDEN, M.D.
Professor and Chair, Department of Psychiatry, University of Michigan
Medical Center; and Research Scientist, Mental Health Research
Institute, Ann Arbor, Michigan

PEDRO GIL GREGORIO
Associate Professor of Geriatric Medicine, Universidad Complutense de
Madrid; and Staff Geriatrician, Service of Geriatric Medicine, Hospital
Universitario de San Carlos, Madrid, Spain

URIEL HALBREICH, M.D.
Professor of Psychiatry, Research Professor of Gynecology/Obstetrics,
Director of Biobehavioral Research, State University of New York at
Buffalo, Buffalo, New York

JEAN A. HAMILTON, M.D.
Betty A. Cohen Professor of Women's Health, Medical College of
Pennsylvania, Philadelphia, Pennsylvania

ISABELLA HEUSER, M.D.
Professor of Psychiatry, Central Institute of Mental Health, Mannheim,
Germany

FLORIAN HOLSBOER, M.D., PH.D.
Professor of Psychiatry and Director, Max Planck Institute of Psychiatry,
Munich, Germany

CYNTHIA L. HOOPER, M.A.
Research Associate, Royal Ottawa Hospital and Institute of Mental
Health Research, Ottawa, Canada

CHRIS HOUGH, PH.D.
Assistant Professor, Department of Psychiatry, Uniformed Services University of the Health Sciences, Bethesda, Maryland

IULIAN IANCU, M.D.
Attending Physician, Psychiatric Division, Sheba Medical Center, Tel Hashomer, Israel

LEWIS L. JUDD, M.D.
Professor and Chairman, Department of Psychiatry, University of California, San Diego, San Diego, California

JUDY C. KANDO, PHARM.D.
Department of Psychiatry, Southwestern Medical Center, University of Texas, Dallas, Texas

PAUL E. KECK JR., M.D.
Associate Professor of Psychiatry and Co-Director, Biological Psychiatry and the Clinical Trials Programs, Department of Psychiatry, University of Cincinnati College of Medicine, Cincinnati, Ohio

TERENCE A. KETTER, M.D.
Biological Psychiatry Branch, National Institute of Mental Health, Bethesda, Maryland

ORA KOFMAN, PH.D.
Associate Professor, Ministry of Health Mental Health Center, Faculty of Health Sciences, Ben-Gurion University of the Negev, Beersheba, Israel

DIANA KOSZYCKI, PH.D.
Research Psychologist, Psychobiology and Clinical Trial Research Unit in Anxiety, Clarke Institute of Psychiatry; and Assistant Professor of Psychiatry, University of Toronto, Toronto, Canada

JELENA L. KUNOVAC, M.D.
Psychiatry Resident, Clinical Neuroscience Research Center and Department of Psychiatry, University of California, San Diego, San Diego, California

YVON D. LAPIERRE, M.D., F.R.C.P.C.
Professor and Chairman, Department of Psychiatry, University of Ottawa; Psychiatrist-in-Chief, Royal Ottawa Hospital; And Director General, Institute of Mental Health Research, Ottawa, Canada

ROBERT H. LENOX, M.D.
Professor of Psychiatry and Neuroscience, Molecular
Neuropsychopharmacology Program, Departments of Psychiatry,
Pharmacology, and Neuroscience, University of Florida College of
Medicine, Gainesville, Florida

JOSEPH LEVINE, M.D.
Clinical Investigator, Ministry of Health Mental Health Center, Faculty
of Health Sciences, Ben-Gurion University of the Negev, Beersheba,
Israel

JUAN J. LÓPEZ-IBOR JR., M.D.
Professor of Psychiatry. Department of Psychiatry, Universidad
Complutense de Madrid; and Head of the Department of Psychiatry,
Hospital Universitario de San Carlos, Madrid, Spain

HUSSEINI K. MANJI, M.D.
Director, Laboratory of Molecular Pathophysiology, Departments of
Psychiatry and Behavioral Neurosciences, Wayne State University
School of Medicine, Detroit, Michigan

CHRISTOPHER J. MCDOUGLE, M.D.
Department of Psychiatry, University of Florida College of Medicine,
Gainesville, Florida; and Department of Psychiatry and Child Study
Center, Yale University School of Medicine, New Haven, Connecticut

SUSAN L. MCELROY, M.D.
Professor of Psychiatry and Director, Biological Psychiatry Program,
Department of Psychiatry, University of Cincinnati College of Medicine,
Cincinnati, Ohio

ROBERT K. MCNAMARA, PH.D.
Molecular Neuropsychopharmacology Program, Departments of
Psychiatry, Pharmacology, and Neuroscience, University of Florida
College of Medicine, Gainesville, Florida

CHERRI M. MINER, M.D., M.B.A.
Medical Director, Behavioral Health Division, Winter Haven Hospital,
Winter Haven, Florida

STUART A. MONTGOMERY, M.D.
Professor of Psychiatry, Department of Pharmacology, Imperial College
of Medicine, St. Mary's Hospital, London, England

TANYA MURPHY, M.D.
Assistant Professor of Child and Adolescent Psychiatry, Department of Psychiatry, University of Florida College of Medicine, Gainesville, Florida

ROBERT J. NAYLOR, M.D.
Professor of Pharmacology, The School of Pharmacy, University of Bradford, Bradford, England

PAUL NEWHOUSE, M.D.
Professor of Psychiatry, Clinical Neuroscience Research Unit, Department of Psychiatry, University of Vermont College of Medicine, Burlington, Vermont

MITCHELL S. NOBLER, M.D.
Assistant Professor of Clinical Psychiatry, College of Physicians and Surgeons, Columbia University, Department of Biological Psychiatry, New York State Psychiatric Institute, New York, New York

DAVID J. NUTT, D.M., M.R.C.P., F.R.C.PSYCH.
Professor of Psychiatry, University of Bristol School of Medical Sciences, Bristol, England

JOHN P. O'REARDON, M.D.
Associate Professor, Depression Research Unit, University of Pennsylvania Medical School, Philadelphia, Pennsylvania

ROBERTA PALMOUR, PH.D.
Associate Professor, Department of Psychiatry, McGill University, Montreal, Quebec, Canada

LASZLO A. PAPP, M.D.
Associate Professor of Psychiatry, Columbia University; and Director, Biological Studies Unit, New York State Psychiatric Institute, New York, New York

PEGGY J. PAZZAGLIA, M.D.
Biological Psychiatry Branch, National Institute of Mental Health, Bethesda, Maryland

ROGER M. PINDER, PH.D., D.SC.
International Medical Director, CNS and Cardiovascular Medical Services, Akzo Nobel Pharmaceuticals, West Orange, New Jersey

DANIEL S. PINE, M.D.
Associate Professor of Child Psychiatry, Columbia University, New York State Psychiatric Institute, New York, New York

ROBERT M. POST, M.D.
Chief, Biological Psychiatry Branch, National Institute of Mental Health, Bethesda, Maryland

JOHN POTOKAR, M.R.C.PSYCH.
Lecturer, Psychopharmacology Unit, University of Bristol School of Medical Sciences, Bristol, England

WILLIAM Z. POTTER, M.D., PH.D.
Senior Research Fellow, Eli Lilly Clinical Research, Indianapolis, Indiana

HAROLD A. SACKEIM, PH.D.
Professor of Clinical Psychology in Psychiatry and Chief of Department of Biological Psychiatry, College of Physicians and Surgeons, Columbia University, New York State Psychiatric Institute, New York, New York

ALAN F. SCHATZBERG, M.D.
Professor and Chairman, Department of Psychiatry and Behavioral Sciences, Stanford University School of Medicine, Stanford, California

MARK E. SCHMIDT, M.D.
Clinical Research Physician, Eli Lilly Clinical Research, Indianapolis, Indiana

KLAUDIUS R. SIEGFRIED, PH.D.
Associate Professor of Human Psychopharmacology and Clinical Neuropsychology, Johann Wolfgang Goethe University; and Head, European Clinical Development Neuroscience, Corporate Clinical Development, Clinical Research, Hoechst AG, Frankfurt am Main, Germany

DANIEL SILVERBERG, M.D.
Faculty of Health Sciences, Ben-Gurion University of the Negev, Beersheba, Israel

CONSTANTIN R. SOLDATOS, M.D.
Professor of Psychiatry, and Director, Sleep Research Unit, Department of Psychiatry, University of Athens, Eginition Hospital, Athens, Greece

STEPHEN M. STAHL, M.D., PH.D.
Adjunct Professor of Psychiatry and Director of Clinical Neuroscience Research Center, Department of Psychiatry, University of California, San Diego, San Diego, California

ROBYN STEIN, M.D.
Biological Psychiatry Branch, National Institute of Mental Health, Bethesda, Maryland

STEPHEN M. STRAKOWSKI, M.D.
Associate Professor of Psychiatry and Director of Division of Psychotic Disorders Research, Department of Psychiatry, University of Cincinnati College of Medicine, Cincinnati, Ohio

JOGIN H. THAKORE, PH.D., M.R.C.PSYCH.
Lecturer, Department of Psychological Medicine, St. Bartholomew's Hospital, London, England

GARY D. TOLLEFSON, M.D., PH.D.
Vice President, Eli Lilly Research Laboratories, Indianapolis, Indiana

FRANCO VACCARINO, PH.D.
Senior Research Consultant, Clarke Institute of Psychiatry; and Professor, Departments of Psychiatry and Psychology, University of Toronto, Toronto, Canada

HERMAN M. VAN PRAAG, M.D., PH.D.
Professor and Chairman, Department of Psychiatry and Neuropsychiatry, University of Limburg Maastricht, Maastricht, The Netherlands

EERO VASAR, M.D., PH.D.
Head, Institute of Physiology; and Professor, Faculty of Medicine, University of Tartu, Tartu, Estonia

HERBERT E. WARD, M.D.
Associate Professor and Director, Psychiatry Specialty Clinic, Department of Psychiatry, University of Florida College of Medicine, Gainesville, Florida

SUSAN R. B. WEISS, PH.D.
Chief, Unit of Behavioral Biology, Biological Psychiatry Branch, National Institute of Mental Health, Bethesda, Maryland

HERMAN G. M. WESTENBERG, PH.D.
Professor of Psychopharmacology, Department of Psychiatry, University Hospital Utrecht, Utrecht, The Netherlands

KIMBERLY A. YONKERS, M.D.
Associate Professor of Psychiatry, Department of Psychiatry, Yale University Medical School, New Haven, Connecticut

JOSEPH ZOHAR, M.D.
Professor of Psychiatry and Director of Psychiatric Division, Sheba Medical Center, Tel Hashomer, Israel

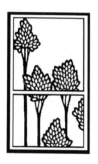

SECTION I

Overviews

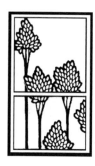

CHAPTER 1

Pharmacotherapy for Mood, Anxiety, and Cognitive Disorders: An Overview

Uriel Halbreich, M.D.

We are currently witnessing an explosion of new antidepressant and anxiolytic medications, as well as mood stabilizers and compounds that are aimed at improving cognition. One of the most significant characteristics of the new wave of psychotropic drug development is that it is hypothesis driven. Discovery, research, and development teams in the pharmaceutical industry as well as in academia are searching for and developing compounds that are custom made for a specific neuropharmacological action and not only for specific descriptive phenomena or syndromes.

We believe that we are at a point in time when there is a need to take a critical look at the inventory of available mood and cognition drugs, their relevance to pathobiology and underlying mechanisms, their limitations, and their unfulfilled promises. This objective evaluation can be conducted from a comfortable position of strength and relative satisfaction. This book demonstrates that pharmacotherapy of mood and cognition is quite effective and is improving. The efficacy of therapeutic options is as good as, and sometimes even better than, many treatments of chronic nonbehavioral physical conditions. However, our treatment success is still not optimal, and with current antidepressants it appears to hit a threshold. Most antidepressants have been shown to be effective in about 60% of patients in double-blind, placebo-controlled studies. This consistent percentage might be of interest considering the diverse modes of action of these medications. The different actions of effective antidepressants are part of the rationale for theories on the pathophysiology of mood disorders; however, there are multiple theories (see Holsboer, Chapter 2, in this volume) and they are not always consistent with one another or with treatment response. Are all of these models correct? Do we need an integrative pathophysiological model of depression? Or is it possible that several pathobiological pathways might lead to similar syndromal manifestations?

Differential treatment response might be one of the ways to refine, validate, or refute diagnostic entities (see Lapierre et al., Chapter 3, in this volume). However, treatment response might also demonstrate common denominators among descriptive entities and might lead to unifying some current subgroups under a common umbrella, replacing some subgroups with behavioral and mood dimensions, or further dissecting other subgroups into smaller, narrowly defined subgroups.

Accurate diagnosis is important for optimization of treatment response. It is apparent that especially the serotonin reuptake inhibitors (SRIs) are effective in a broad spectrum of affective and anxiety disorders. It is arguable that alternative diagnostic approaches should be considered and tested. Some of the arguments for reexamining our current system and some tentative solutions are reviewed by Van Praag in Chapter 4.

Even in people with the same diagnosis and the same inclusion and exclusion criteria, there are different treatment responses based on individual variability. The most important individual variables are probably sex and age. It is unfortunate that even though affective disorders and some anxiety disorders are more prevalent in women than in men, until recently results of clinical trials did not take into consideration sex differences and variables unique to women (e.g., reproductive status and menstrual cycle). As is demonstrated by Yonkers et al. (see Chapter 5, in this volume), there are substantial sex differences in the pharmacokinetics and pharmacodynamics of most antidepressants and anxiolytics, which influence treatment response. Attention to these variables will indeed improve the efficacy of treatment.

MOOD STABILIZERS

One of the advances in descriptive diagnosis is the increasingly clear distinction between unipolar and bipolar illnesses. In bipolar illness there is primarily a disordered stabilization of mood, whereas monopolar illnesses are mostly characterized by the development of acute or stabile depressions. The distinction between the two groups is supported by the distinction between mood stabilizers and mood elevators or antidepressants. From the therapeutic and practical as well as the heuristic perspective it is important to note that the stabilizing and homeostatic effect can be achieved by multiple, diverse mechanisms and points of action. Lithium was the first effective mood stabilizer and is still the most widely used. It has also been the most widely studied compound for the elucidation of mood-stabilizing mechanisms (see Manji et al., Chapter 7, in this volume). Despite this extensive research, the underlying biological basis for the therapeutic efficacy of this drug remains unknown. Lithium affects multiple neurotransmitter-related functions as well as postsynaptic signal transduction. There are also suggestions for alterations at the genomic level. The drug actions are probably region- and structure-specific. The wealth of data calls for an integrative approach not only to the mode of action of lithium but also to the biological processes in the brain that are responsible for the episodic dysphoric states. These states might be caused by an inability to mount the appropriate compensatory responses necessary to maintain homeostatic regulation, thereby resulting in sudden oscillations beyond immediate adaptive control (see Manji et al., Chapter 7, in this volume).

More recently, several alternatives to lithium have been introduced to the clinical armamentarium of mood stabilizers. Valproate may constitute a viable alternative (see Strakowski et al., Chapter 8, in this volume), especially for patients with mixed affective states, comorbid substance abuse, and histories of rapid cycling and failed treatment with lithium. Its response time is shorter than that of lithium, a fact that might provide an additional advantage, especially in manic patients and in situations where time and length of hospitalization are of essence. As it is demonstrated by Post and colleagues (see Chapter 6 in this volume), other alternative mood stabilizers such as carbamazepine and calcium channel blockers (such as nimodipine) might exert their therapeutic effect in different ways. It is not yet clear (although it is suggested by some evidence) whether there are different baseline processes in responders to each of these medications, or whether they truly have an augmenting complementary effect in cases of nonresponses to one of them.

Lithium inhibits inositol monophosphate and decreases brain levels of inositol. Belmaker's group (see Levine et al., Chapter 9, in this volume) showed a selective therapeutic effect of inositol in patients with either depression or panic disorder. Because of the possible importance of the second-messenger system of the phosphatidylinositol (PI) cycle in mood regulation, and because of its influence by lithium, it would be of future interest to elucidate the role of exogenous inositol in mood stabilization.

Electroconvulsive therapy (ECT) is mostly used for severe depression. However, a balanced, extensive review of the literature by Sackeim's group (see Nobler et al., Chapter 10, in this volume) reveals not only the remarkable potency and safety of this politically controversial mode of treatment, but also the multiplicity of its biological influence and impact on a diversified gamut of brain functions. ECT is probably also effective in acute manic states and might be viewed as a "mood stabilizer." Whether or not maintenance ECT acts as a mood stabilizer is still unknown. It might be viewed as an antidepressant with a broad stabilizing effect.

Transcranial magnetic stimulation (TMS) is a very promising new technique that is quite similar to ECT but shows the advantage of depolarizing neurons located deep in the brain without inducing seizures. The Israeli group (see Fleischmann et al., Chapter 11, in this volume) are among the pioneers in the application of this noninvasive technique, which may well be found to have antidepressant and mood-stabilizing effects.

In the context of an updated comprehensive evaluation of mood stabilizers, it is worthwhile to mention the recent studies showing a beneficial effect of thyroid hormones and melatonin in rapid-cycling patients. A detailed account of these hormones appears elsewhere in this book series and is briefly described by Halbreich in Chapter 17.

ANTIDEPRESSANTS

Serotonergic agonists are the current antidepressants of choice (see Montgomery, Chapter 12, in this volume). This is a result of a combined impact of efficacy that is comparable to that of the tricyclic antidepressants, with a more favorable side-effect profile. Efficient marketing certainly adds to their success. The use of current serotonergic antidepressants is being refined, and a wave of new, mostly more selective ones are being introduced (see Thakore et al., Chapter 13, in this volume). The new wave of antidepressants also involves those with targeted combined action (e.g., norepinephrine [NE] and serotonergic reuptake inhibition). These medications remind us that until recently the main hypothesis on the pathobiology of depression was the NE one. Drugs based on that hypothesis are being suggested and developed in more refined and specific modes than the earlier tricyclic antidepressants (see Potter and Schmidt, Chapter 15, in this volume). The selectivity of these drugs, as well as that of the SRIs, is nonetheless questionable because of the complex interactions between the various neurotransmitter systems.

The current fashion to focus on NE and serotonin has left aside the other catecholamine—dopamine (DA). A compelling case can be presented (see Pinder, Chapter 14, in this volume) that DA should not be ignored in this context. It does play a role in the pathobiology of depressive symptomology and the homeostatic maintenance of euthymic mood. It is quite possible that new drugs directed primarily, or initially, at dopaminergic processes will find their way into the antidepressant market.

An emerging group of antidepressant interventions comprises several hormones that have been shown to have mood-elevating or mood-modulating effects (see Halbreich, Chapter 17, in this volume). This group includes mostly cortisol suppressors, thyroid hormones, estrogen, and other steroids. However, more recently several other hormones, such as melatonin and oxytocin, were proclaimed as players in the field, but their place is still to be claimed.

It is quite intriguing that the efficacy of almost all antidepressants (probably with the exception of ECT) does not exceed two-thirds of patients involved in double-blind controlled trials. Besides the heuristic significance of this "ceiling," it creates an important problem of management of the one-third of depressive patients who are resistant to treatment. Nonresponse to seemingly adequate antidepressant treatment (see O'Reardon and Amsterdam, Chapter 18, in this volume) might be due to a broad spectrum of unrecognized medical problems that might be manifested as (or be associated with) depression. It might also be attributed to a suggested comorbidity with other mental syndromes or disorders. A series of treatment algorithms for treatment-resistant depression have been developed for optimization, augmentation, and combined treatment efforts to minimize treatment resistance. Nonetheless, probably up to 10% of depressed patients still will not respond to any current treatment.

One of the reasons for initial nonresponse may be a psychotic subtype of depression (see DeBattista et al., Chapter 19, in this volume). The pathophysiology of this subtype of depression is intriguing; it might involve the dopaminergic system and glucocorticoids. Treatment of patients with psychotic major depression may call for combined treatment with antidepressants and neuroleptics, use of cortisol suppressors, or treatment with single compounds that produce combined serotonergic reuptake inhibition, serotonin downregulation, and probably also dopaminergic blockade.

The length of continuation of pharmacotherapy once a euthymic state has been achieved—as well as what antidepressants and in what dosages should be applied—is still uncertain (see Greden, Chapter 20, in this volume). It has been shown that the rate of relapse is substantially reduced if adequate doses are taken for at least 5 years. The efficacy of longer-term maintenance therapy is still unknown.

ANXIOLYTICS

Anxiety disorders can be viewed as resulting from interactions among physiological, hormonal, and environmental factors with strong vulnerability, genetic, and developmental components (see Pine et al., Chapter 22, in this volume). Advances in the study of the pathobiology of anxiety led to the development of anxiolytic medications that act on brain systems that are putatively involved in these processes. These medications currently include primarily benzodiazepines acting as agonists on the γ-aminobutyric acid (GABA) system and the benzodiazepine receptors (see Stahl et al., Chapter 21). Selective serotonergic agonists, neurosteroids, cholecystokinin octapeptide (CCK-8) receptor antagonists, corticotropin-releasing hormone (CRH) receptor antagonists, neuropeptide Y, and antagonists at the N-methyl-D-aspartate (NMDA) receptor channel complex. Recently, specific serotonergic agonists have been very widely used as anxiolytics (see Kunovac and Stahl, Chapter 23). The emphasis on the possible uniqueness and action specificity of serotonergic receptor subtypes is also manifested in the growing efforts for increasingly specific medications. The near future will tell if this strategy is justified.

SRIs are currently the most prevalent pharmacological treatment used for panic disorder (see Westenberg and Den Boer, Chapter 24, in this volume), even though tricyclic antidepressants, monoamine oxidase inhibitors (MAOIs), and benzodiazepines are also effective. The efficacy of the SRI antidepressants and the observation that initially they may induce deterioration of symptoms (which is usually not the case with treatment of depressed patients with the same medications) raise issues related to the pathobiology of anxiety and its comorbidity with depression.

The distinction among the anxiety disorders brought social phobia to the limelight. It has been documented (see Miner et al., Chapter 25, in this volume) that benzodiazepines are also highly effective as treatment for this disorder. However, because of dependency and other undesirable side effects of the benzodiazepines, MAOIs (especially selective reversible MAOIs), β-blockers, and especially SRIs have been introduced as treatment modalities with quite promising efficacy.

The complexity of the pathobiology of anxiety disorders and the diversified treatment choices are further emphasized by the examination of the role of neuropeptides (NPs) in anxiety and their possible application as treatment modalities (see Tollefson, Chapter 26, in this volume). More than 50 NPs have been identified; many of them interact with conventional neurotransmitter systems as well as with each other. Some of them or their mimetics have already been tested as anxiolytics and are therapeutically and heuristically promising. CCK antagonists have received some of the most advanced study among NP interventions. Cholecystokinin tetrapeptide (CCK-4) was demonstrated to be anxiogenic and panicogenic. The detailed description of this representative of NPs shows that it is abundant in brain regions implicated in anxiety (see Bradwejn et al., Chapter 27, in this volume). It meets the criteria for a neurotransmitter, it interacts with multiple other neurotransmitters, and its antagonism has an anxiolytic effect.

Similarly to the NPs, the discovery of neurosteroids was a major step toward the understanding of depressive and anxiety disorders (see Heuser, Chapter 28, in this volume). High-affinity intercellular steroid hormone receptors were demonstrated at several mood-related regions of the brain. Several progestins were shown to be anxiolytic, whereas others are anxiogenic via interaction with $GABA_A$ receptors. Progestins have also been shown to influence memory, pain, mood, and seizure activity. Indeed, medications to intervene in these processes have been and are being developed. The importance of the $GABA_A$ receptor as a target for anxiolytic action is further recognized by Nutt's group (see Bell et al., Chapter 29, in this volume), who also stress the role of neurosteroids in this system but place them in perspective with the multitude of different compounds whose common denominator is being anxiolytics with partial or full GABA agonism. This list includes alcohols, barbiturates, benzodiazepines and their derivatives, carbolines, imidazopyridines, and a variety of other compounds. The symptom specificity of some of these medications is still under investigation.

Compared with patients with other syndromes that are considered to be anxiety disorders, patients with obsessive-compulsive disorder (OCD) show a propensity to respond well to serotonergic agonists (mostly SRIs or clomipramine) and less well to other medications that are effective for treatment of anxiety disorders (see Iancu et al., Chapter 30, in this volume). This phenomenon is important for the elucidation of the pathobiology of OCD, but it also poses a challenge in cases of nonresponse to initial treatment with an SRI (see Goodman et al., Chapter 31, in this volume). Combinations of several serotonergic agonists—SRIs with neuroleptics or SRIs with lithium or benzodiazepines—have been reported, as well as brain surgery, intravenous administration of serotonergic agonists, clonidine (an α_2 NE agonist) treatment, ECT, bromocriptine (a DA agonist), oxytocin and other NPs, addition of aminoglutethimide (steroid suppressant) and immunosuppressors, and some other treatment modalities have also been attempted for helping OCD nonresponders—all with limited success. This is a challenge and is still awaiting an answer.

COGNITION AND DEMENTIA

Aging populations in many countries bring to the forefront dementia and other age-related cognitive impairments. This is in addition to the many other reasons for impaired cognition (see López-Ibor et al., Chapter 32, in this volume). Based on putative pathobiological mechanisms, several treatment approaches have been developed. Some are based on intervention in neurotransmitter systems (e.g., cholinergic, serotonergic, or nicotinic), and some are based on presumed neurostructural processes (e.g., amyloid formation) or neurotropic factors associated with neural growth, survival, and loss (e.g., nerve growth factor [NGF] or free radicals). In this context it is worthwhile to mention nootropic drugs that facilitate brain metabolism, drugs that increase cerebral blood flow and membrane permeability, as well as hormones like estrogen, which have been shown to selectively improve cognition in a mechanism that is still awaiting clarification. Here again, the multitude of treatment modalities is promising to an eventual solution to this problem. It also points to the multifaceted complexity of the mechanisms that might lead to impairment in cognitive functions.

One of the better-developed examples of a neurotransmitter approach to cognitive impairment is the cholinergic hypothesis of geriatric memory dysfunction and dementia of the Alzheimer's type (see Siegfried, Chapter 33, in this volume). Associations between anatomical and biochemical cholinergic abnormalities on one side, and cognitive (mostly memory) impairment on the other have been quite convincingly established. This has been followed by precursor therapy with choline or lecithin, treatment with cholinesterase inhibitors (e.g., tacrine), and treatment with muscarinic and nicotinic agonists, as well as some other cholinergic modulations. A focus on nicotinic receptors (see Newhouse, Chapter 35, in this volume) reveals that nicotinic antagonists can produce selective cognitive impairment, whereas nicotine and nicotine mimetics improve several cognitive tasks, especially when acutely administered intravenously. Like other previous examples, the nicotinic systems probably modulate the release of other neurotransmitters (such as catecholamines, serotonin, and acetylcholine) and interact with several other systems. Therefore, this system should not be evaluated with a narrow vision or in a vacuum. The loss of nicotinic receptors or increased levels of nicotine might influence degrees of control of cognitive processes rather than underlying basic functions.

Serotonin (5-HT) is involved in a multitude of mood and behavior processes. It may also modify cognitive processes (see Costall and Naylor, Chapter 34, in this volume). The agonists of some serotonin receptors (e.g., 5-HT$_{1A}$) might impair performance, whereas 5-HT$_3$ receptor antagonists can restore impaired performance. Therefore, agonists and antagonists of selective serotonin receptor subtypes might be developed as modulators of selective cognitive functions. This will probably be in a multidimensional interactive system and probably as one of a system of neuromodulators of cellular changes induced by excitatory amino acids and other neurotransmitters.

CONCLUSION— FUTURE DRUG DEVELOPMENT

An overview of current pharmacotherapy for mood and cognitive disorders emphasizes neurotransmitters and other extraneuronal processes, with a focus on the synapse and its immediate environment. It also draws attention to the multitude of processes by which mood and cognition might be manipulated. By implication it emphasizes the multitude of underlying pathobiological processes that lead to affective disorder, anxiety, and impaired cognition. These processes cannot be viewed in isolation. They interact with each other, influence each other, and constitute a state of homeostasis or imbalance that might be associated with symptoms or syndromes. The fact that some medications (e.g., SRIs) are effective for a diversity of descriptive diagnostic entities suggests common underlying mechanisms for these entities or other common denominators that call for reexamination of current theories.

The progress in molecular biology allows for clarification of the signal transduction from the neuronal synapse inside to the intracellular effectors, genes, and other functions. As is demonstrated by Lesch and Manji (1992), by directing the magnitude and duration of postsynaptic receptor-mediated signaling, the carrier-facilitated transport of serotonin (and other neurotransmitters) into and release from the presynaptic neuron plays a pivotal role in the integration and fine-tuning of neurotransmission. The development of drugs that specifically affect neurotransporters or genes related to neurotransporters' function, and neurotransporter gene transcription, would affect pharmacotherapy for mood and cognitive disorders. The development of manipulations of genetic expression and of other intracellular processes seems promising not only for mood stabilization. Intracellular abnormalities might be a common denominator or a common end-pathway of several neurotransmitter systems—a possibility that might at least partially explain similar results achieved with different synaptic manipulations. Drugs that act on intraneuronal signal transduction are currently being developed, and their introduction to the clinical arena is around the corner. Drugs that act on the genetic vulnerability for developing affective disorders are hopefully not far behind.

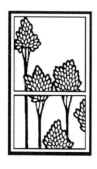

CHAPTER 2

Current Theories on the Pathophysiology of Mood Disorders

Florian Holsboer, M.D., Ph.D.

Our lack of knowledge about the pathophysiology underlying mood disorders contrasts sharply with the efficacy of the treatment modalities developed by clinical scientists over the past decades. Initiated by the pharmacology of certain drugs that affect mood such as reserpine, a *Rauwolfia* alkaloid antihypertensive that depletes biogenic amines and often produces depressive symptoms, the catecholamine hypothesis was originated by pioneers such as Schildkraut (1965), Bunney and Davis (1965), and Matussek (1968). This early work was enhanced by the discovery of drugs that enhance catecholaminergic neurotransmission either through blockade of presynaptic reuptake (e.g., imipramine) or through inhibition of catecholamine degradation by monoamine oxidase inhibitors (MAOIs) (e.g., tranylcypromine). In parallel, Coppen (1968) and Lapin and Oxenkrug (1969) hypothesized that defective serotonin (5-hydroxytryptamine [5-HT]) neurotransmission produces depressive symptoms, a concept that was supported by the observations of Åsberg and colleagues (1976), who found that patients with depression, particularly those at increased risk for suicide or suicide attempts, had lowered cerebrospinal fluid (CSF) concentrations of 5-hydroxyindoleacetic acid (5-HIAA), the major metabolite of 5-HT. Clearly, these neurotransmitter systems should not be considered in isolation. Work by the laboratories of Sulser and Fuxe emphasized a functional link between noradrenergic and serotonergic systems, because noradrenergic neurons, whether projecting from the locus coeruleus or other brain stem regions, receive input from the dorsal raphe nucleus, the main source of central serotonergic fibers (Dahlström and Fuxe 1964; Manier et al. 1989).

Independent from the biogenic amine hypothesis, the observation that endocrine diseases, particularly those affecting secretion of adrenocortical and thyroid hormones, are often associated with severe depression led to the formulation of a neuroendocrine hypothesis of mood disorders (Holsboer 1995). This concept was bolstered by the highly reproducible finding of altered regulation of the hypothalamic-pituitary-adrenocortical (HPA) system in the vast majority of patients with depression and by the close association between normalization of the HPA system and resolution of depressive psychopathology. Because certain neurotransmitters whose release and degradation are altered by antidepressants also regulate central hypothalamic neurons that drive peripheral hormone secretion, an integrative hypothesis must take into account neurotransmitter systems and their receptors. Focusing on the interaction between neurotransmitter receptor function, neuroendocrine regulation, and subsequent intracellular signaling appears to be the most promising approach to a unifying and testable hypothesis of the causality of mood disorders.

In this brief overview, I attempt to highlight several selected examples to demonstrate how this area has developed and also how new tools and technologies can be used to develop a navigational chart through the intimidating number of complex findings.

NEUROENDOCRINE HYPOTHESES

Hypothalamic-Pituitary-Adrenocortical System: Clinical Studies

The most highly recognizable neuroendocrine symptom of depression is altered HPA regulation (Table 2–1). At baseline, signs of increased cortisol production can be observed in more than 50% of patients (Carroll et al. 1976b, 1976c; Halbreich et al. 1985a, 1985b; Rubin et al. 1987; Sachar et al. 1973). If more sophisticated function tests such as the combined dexamethasone–corticotropin-releasing hormone (CRH) test are administered, the possibility of detecting altered HPA system regulation increases—depending on the age of the cohort—to approximately 90% (Heuser et al. 1994).

TABLE 2–1.   Abnormalities of the hypothalamic-pituitary-adrenocortical system

Plasma cortisol and corticotropin (ACTH) concentrations are elevated as a result of increased hormone release per secretory pulse

Urinary-free cortisol concentrations are elevated

Nocturnal plasma cortisol levels increase earlier (i.e., HPA activity is active at night and time span between sleep onset and cortisol secretion nadir is shortened)

Pituitary and adrenal glands are enlarged

Density of CRH receptors in frontal cortex is decreased

CRH and vasopressin-generating neurons in hypothalamic parvocellular neurons are hyperactive

CRH concentrations in cerebrospinal fluid are elevated

Plasma ACTH and corticosteroid concentrations are not adequately suppressed by dexamethasone

Plasma ACTH but not plasma cortisol levels are blunted in response to CRH

Plasma ACTH and cortisol secretion is enhanced in response to a combined dexamethasone-CRH challenge

Note.   ACTH = adrenocorticotropic hormone; CRH = corticotropin-releasing hormone; HPA = hypothalamic-pituitary-adrenocortical.

Whatever the measure used to assess HPA activity, it has been replicated consistently that at some early part of a depressive episode HPA hyperactivity gradually normalizes along with successful treatment (Gerken et al. 1985; Greden et al. 1983; Heuser et al. 1996; Holsboer et al. 1982, 1987; Holsboer-Trachsler et al. 1991, 1994; Nemeroff and Evans 1984). Moreover, indirect signs of HPA hyperactivity such as adrenal gland hypertrophy have proven to be state-dependent (Rubin et al. 1995). Studies using the dexamethasone suppression test or the combined dexamethasone-CRH test not only agree that normalization of an initial aberrancy predicts favorable treatment response, but also corroborate that persistent HPA abnormality correlates with chronicity or relapse (Heuser et al. 1996; Holsboer et al. 1982; Holsboer-Trachsler 1994). The close relationship between the time of HPA normalization and the subsequent resolution of psychic symptoms and, vice versa, the finding that emergence of HPA abnormality precedes recurrence of depressive psychopathology pose the intriguing question of the possible causal relationship between the mechanisms driving the HPA system and those producing depression (Barden et al. 1995). The findings of blunted adrenocorticotropic hormone (ACTH) response to human CRH (Holsboer et al. 1984, 1986) and to ovine CRH (P. W. Gold et al. 1986), the elevated levels of CRH in the CSF (Nemeroff et al. 1984), the decreased number of

CRH binding sites in the frontal cortex of patients with depression who have committed suicide (Nemeroff et al. 1988), the increased number of CRH-expressing neurons in the hypothalamic paraventricular nucleus of patients with depression (Raadsheer et al. 1994), and the finding that CRH concentrations in the spinal fluid decrease during long-term treatment with fluoxetine or amitriptyline (De Bellis et al. 1993) support the idea that CRH is the key neurohormone responsible for HPA alterations in depression. To clarify this point, two questions must be resolved: 1) Are all HPA alterations explained by the supposed CRH hypersecretion? and 2) Is CRH hypersecretion responsible for the behavioral changes seen in depression?

We addressed the first question in a study in which increasing dosages of either CRH or vasopressin were administered to dexamethasone-pretreated control subjects. This did not result in ACTH and cortisol concentrations comparable to those found in dexamethasone nonsuppressed subjects with depression (von Bardeleben et al. 1985). Only when both neuropeptides, CRH and vasopressin, were infused concurrently were plasma ACTH and cortisol levels achieved that were comparable to those found in dexamethasone-pretreated subjects with depression who received CRH alone (von Bardeleben and Holsboer 1989; von Bardeleben et al. 1985). These findings led us to hypothesize that hypersecretion of both neuropeptides, CRH and vasopressin, account for the apparent HPA hyperdrive in depression (von Bardeleben and Holsboer 1989). The group led by Swaab recently corroborated this hypothesis by showing that the number of not only CRH-immunoreactive neurons but also vasopressin-immunoreactive neurons in the paraventricular nucleus of the hypothalamus is increased in patients with depression (Purba et al. 1996).

Another line of evidence for an HPA role in the causality of depression emerged from studies of control subjects without depression but with a high genetic risk for depression, in whom studies of sleep electroencephalography (EEG) and neuroendocrinology resulted in changes that were—although less pronounced—comparable to those seen in patients acutely depressed (Holsboer et al. 1995; Lauer et al. 1995). In the dexamethasone-CRH test specifically, these subjects had hormonal response patterns that fell among those of subjects with depression, whereas patients with depression and control subjects without a family history of psychiatric disorder had hormonal responses that were indistinguishable from those of control subjects (Figure 2–1).

The questions of whether psychological signs and symptoms of depression are also related to hypersecretion of CRH and vasopressin and how antidepressants work to remedy both the neuroendocrine and the behavioral aspect of this dysregulation have been the subject of intense preclinical research.

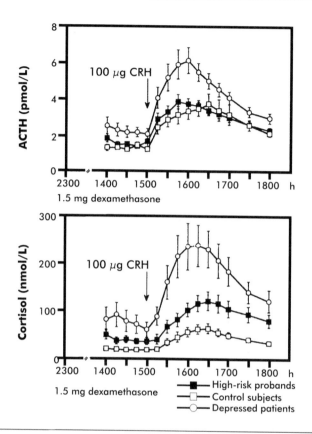

FIGURE 2–1. Plasma adrenocorticotropic hormone (ACTH) and cortisol concentrations (mean ± SEM) in dexamethasone-pretreated subjects before and after intravenous corticotropin-releasing hormone (CRH) injection. ACTH response curves were higher in 18 patients with major depression (open circles) than in 47 probands at high familial risk for depression (closed squares) and 20 control subjects without depression and with no psychiatric family history (open squares). The plasma cortisol response curves were different in all three groups, with the high-risk probands showing response curves that were higher than those in control subjects, but lower than those in patients with depression. The higher plasma cortisol values in high-risk probands despite normal plasma ACTH levels indicate that long-term stimulation of the adrenal cortex by ACTH has rendered this gland hypersensitive to ACTH.

Source. Reprinted from Holsboer F, Lauer CJ, Schreiber W, et al: "Altered Hypothalamic-Pituitary-Adrenocortical Regulation in Healthy Subjects at High Familial Risk for Affective Disorders." *Neuroendocrinology* 62:340–347, 1995. Copyright 1995, S. Karger AG. Used with permission.

Hypothalamic-Pituitary-Adrenocortical System: Preclinical Studies

Since the isolation, cloning, and characterization of CRH by Vale et al. (1981), many studies have emerged that consistently show that CRH plays a key role not only in the neurohumoral adaptation to stress, but also in the co-ordination of behavioral responses (A. J. Dunn and Berridge 1990; Holsboer et al. 1992; Owens and Nemeroff 1991). Specifically, the groups led by Koob and by Nemeroff showed that CRH is critically involved in producing symptoms that are prevalent in depression, such as increased anxiety, anorexia, and decreased sexual activity (Butler et al. 1990; Heinrichs et al. 1992; Swerdlow et al. 1989). In addition, vegetative signs and sleep EEG alterations typical for stress and depression are likely to be mediated by CRH (Ehlers et al. 1986; Holsboer et al. 1988).

Recently, these studies were enhanced by studies using antisense probes directed against the messenger ribonucleic acid of CRH (CRH mRNA), which resulted in anxiolytic effects similar to those observed with CRH antagonists (Skutella et al. 1994). Also recently, a transgenic mouse was generated that overexpressed CRH and showed increases in anxiety-related behavior as assessed by the elevated plus-maze experiment (Stenzel-Poore et al. 1994). The possibility that this anxiogenic effect of CRH overexpression was not mediated primarily by CRH, but rather by developmental compensation of the transgene, had been ruled out by the effect of α-helical CRH-(9-41), which is a CRH antagonist that was able to reduce anxiety-related behavior in these mice.

A new dimension was introduced into the CRH hyperdrive hypothesis when the groups of both Vale and de Souza showed the presence of two different CRH receptors with a distinct pharmacology and tissue localization (Lovenberg et al. 1995; Perrin et al. 1993). In addition to these two receptors, CRH_1 and CRH_2, a CRH-binding protein (CRH-BP) has been identified and found to be present in abundance in the brain, mainly in the neocortex, the dentate gyrus, the olfactory bulb, the amygdala complex (excluding the medial nucleus), the raphe nucleus, and the reticular formation. Localization at the pituitary is limited to corticotropic cells. This distribution pattern strongly suggests that CRH-BP contributes to neuroendocrine and behavioral functions (E. Potter et al. 1992). Both the anatomical distribution and the pharmacology of CRH receptors in the brain point to distinct functional properties. Analysis of CRH_1 and CRH_2 receptor mRNA expression in the rat brain showed that CRH_1 receptors are abundant in neocortical, cerebellar, and sensory systems as well as at pituitary corticotrophs. In contrast, the distribution of CRH_2 receptors appears to be more specific, with higher concentrations at subcortical structures, including the lateral septum and various hypothalamic nuclei. It is noteworthy that both receptors are expressed in the hypothalamus and hippocampus.

In a preliminary attempt to sort out which of these two receptors might mediate anxiogenic effects of CRH, we conducted a number of behavioral studies in rats pretreated with intracerebroventricularly administered antisense probes targeted against either the CRH_1 or the CRH_2 receptor (Liebsch et al. 1995). As illustrated in Figure 2–2, only an antisense-generated "knock-down" against CRH_1 receptors, not CRH_2, was able to reduce anxiety-related behavior in rats. Based on this finding, we concluded that the CRH_1 receptor is a prime candidate for pharmaceutical interventions to decrease disorders related to stress, particularly anxiety, that may ultimately

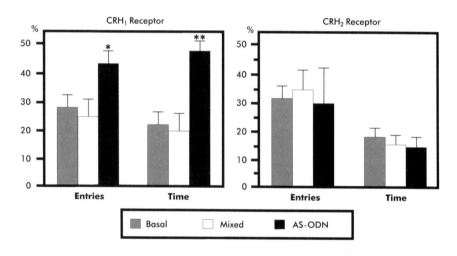

FIGURE 2–2. Intracerebral infusion of antisense oligonucleotides (AS-ODN) that were targeted to the cloned CRH_1 and CRH_2 receptor mRNA prevent translation into the receptor protein. Only a "knock-down" of the CRH_1 receptor, but not of the CRH_2 receptor, reduces anxiety-related behavior in rats that were exposed to the elevated plus-maze test after central corticotropin-releasing hormone (CRH) administration. *$P < .05$, **$P < .01$.

Source. Adapted from Liebsch G, Landgraf R, Gerstberger R, et al: "Chronic Infusion of a CRH_1 Receptor Antisense Oligodeoxynucleotide Into the Central Nucleus of the Amygdala Reduced Anxiety-Related Behavior in Socially Defeated Rats." *Regulatory Peptides* 59:229–239, 1995. Copyright 1995, Elsevier Science – NL. Used with permission. Data also from Skutella et al. 1994.

result in the development of a mood disorder.

CRH probably does not act alone. According to clinical neuro-endocrinology, vasopressin is a prime candidate for the synergy of CRH effects at pituitary CRH_1 receptors, and it also has behavioral effects that are compatible with a role in depression. Chronic psychosocial stress enhances vasopressin expression and increases the number of hypothalamic neurons coexpressing CRH and vasopressin. Infusion of an antisense oligodeoxy-nucleotide, which corresponds to the mRNA of vasopressin type I receptor, into the septum led to reduced anxiety-related behavior that parallels decreases in vasopressin receptor binding (Landgraf et al. 1995).

Yet another peptide candidate possibly involved in mood disorder–related behaviors has been identified only recently by the laboratory of Vale. These researchers characterized a member of the CRH family that has sequence identity of 64% with urotensin I (mainly occurring in the suckerfish) and of 45% with human CRH, and they named it urocortin (Vaughan et al. 1995). This peptide is of interest, as it is 10-fold more potent than CRH in accumulating cyclic adenosine monophosphate (cAMP) in cells transfected transiently with CRH_2 receptors. This is consistent with the view that urocortin is the preferred mammalian ligand for the CRH_2 receptor, particularly the $CRH_{2\beta}$ splice variant. However, urocortin also acts powerfully at CHR_1 receptors, as evidenced by its 7-fold higher potential to induce secretion of ACTH from pituitary cells. Urocortin appears to be much more potent than CRH in suppressing feeding behavior, as shown by abolishment of food consumption in fasting rats, whereas, in contrast to CRH, urocortin has no anxiogenic effects (Koog and Spina, personal communication, cited in Vaughan et al. 1995). Finally, urocortin binds strongly to CRH-BP, which underscores how intricately these neuropeptide systems are intertwined (Figure 2–3).

Corticosteroid Receptors and Antidepressants

Whereas it is conceivable that a CRH/vasopressin hyperdrive contributes to behavioral, emotional, and hormonal symptoms of mood disorders, the question remains which mechanisms mediate this hyperactivity of CRH and vasopressin-secreting neurons. The gene expression of both neuropeptides is suppressed by ligand-activated glucocorticoid receptors. The efficiency of this negative feedback action of circulating corticosteroids depends on the number of corticosteroid receptors, their affinity, and the degree of interaction with other factors (e.g., heat shock protein) involved in the transcription machinery.

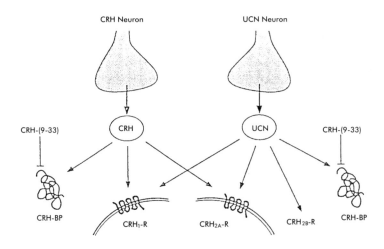

FIGURE 2-3. Corticotropin-releasing hormone (CRH) synthesized and released from parvocellular neurons of the paraventricular nucleus binds to CRH_1 receptors at the pituitary corticotrophs to elicit expression of the pro-opiomelanocortin (POMC) gene via a G-protein–coupled signaling step enhancing cyclic adenosine monophosphate (cAMP) formation. CRH has a much lower affinity to CRH_{2A} receptors, which are less widely distributed over the brain and mainly expressed in the lateral septal, ventromedial hypothalamic, and medial amygdaloid nuclei. Urocortin (UCN), which has a 63% sequence identity with urotensin and a 45% sequence identity with CRH, also binds at CRH_1 receptors to evoke POMC and subsequent adrenocorticotropic hormone (ACTH) release. In addition, UCN is much more potent than CRH at binding and activating CRH_{2A} receptors, indicating that UCN is an endogenous ligand for the CRH_{2A} receptors. Both neuropeptides (CRH and UCN) bind to CRH-binding protein (UCN: $K_i = 0.1$ nM; CRH: 0.21 nM).
Source. Adapted from Vaughan J, Donaldson C, Bittencourt J, et al: "Urocortin, a Mammalian Neuropeptide Related to Fish Urotensin I and to Corticotropin-Releasing Factor." *Nature* 378:287–292, 1995. Copyright 1995, Macmillan Magazines Limited. Used with permission.

Corticosteroids act in the brain mainly through regulation of genes by binding to intracellular receptors, which then bind to specific response elements at promoter regions of steroid-regulated genes. Two different receptors mediate corticosteroid effects at the nucleus as dimers, the high-affinity ($K_D = 0.3$ nM for corticosterone in the rat) mineralocorticoid receptor (MR) and the low-affinity (K_D = 3.0 nM) glucocorticoid receptor (GR) (DeKloet and Reul 1987). The highest expression of these receptors is in the hippocampus, in which many neurons colocalize MR and GR to act as homodimers or heterodimers (Trapp et al. 1994). The occurrence of high- and low-affinity receptors that have distinct DNA-binding properties after homodimerization or heterodimerization keeps the cellular response to corticosteroids at a high level of flexibility, which is important if one considers the large circulating corticosteroid concentration range (Trapp and Holsboer 1996).

Defective negative feedback of the HPA system is the most common neuroendocrine symptom of mood disorders (Holsboer 1995). As documented for the combined dexamethasone-CRH test in control subjects, increasing dosages of dexamethasone suppress the releasable amount of ACTH and cortisol in response to CRH (Heuser et al. 1994). Modell et al. (unpublished observations) established a dose-response curve and showed that patients with depression needed higher dexamethasone dosages than control subjects to suppress CRH-induced ACTH and cortisol release. This finding and the observation that probands without depression but at genetic risk for it also have signs of negative feedback disturbance (Holsboer et al. 1995) led us to hypothesize that the pathogenesis of mood disorders involves impaired corticosteroid receptor function (Holsboer and Barden 1996).

Our view is supported by the actions of antidepressants that increase the capacity of corticosteroid receptors and subsequently reduce basal and stress-stimulated levels of ACTH and corticosterone when administered to rats (Reul et al. 1993, 1994a). This finding in rats would explain the gradual normalization of negative feedback disturbance in patients with depression during treatment with antidepressants and would also explain the findings by Checkley, who demonstrated in patients with depression that metyrapone (a drug that inhibits hydroxylation at the C-11 position of the steroid molecule and thus reduces cortisol synthesis) not only diminished cortisol hypersecretion, but also ameliorated depressive symptomatology (O'Dwyer et al. 1995). Finally, transgenic mice that express antisense directed to GR mRNA proved to be severely impaired in their cognitive function as well as showed exaggerated HPA activity when stressed. After long-term treatment with antidepressants, both cognitive and neuroendocrine disturbances gradually disappeared (Montkowski et al. 1995). This transgenic mouse appears to be well suited as a test model for several signs and symptoms of depression and their response to drug treatment (Holsboer and Barden 1996).

Animal studies have also provided insights into the mechanisms underlying the preeminent role of stressors in early life. Plotsky and Meaney (1993) showed that daily handling and maternal separation of rat pups produces increased hypothalamic CRH mRNA and CRH concentrations at baseline and increased CRH depletion and plasma corticosterone levels in response to restraint stress. Ladd et al. (1996) studied the long-term effects of early stress on the development of CRH neural systems in the rat brain. They showed that early environmental stressors can lead to changes in CRH pathways that are manifested by enhanced basal and stress-induced plasma ACTH concentrations, which—if extrapolated to humans traumatized early—can increase the vulnerability to stress-related mood disorders. Likewise, adverse early rearing of nonhuman primates may lead to long-term overactivity of CRH-producing neurons, as reflected by elevated cisternal CSF content (Coplan et al. 1996).

Given that disturbed regulation of CRH neuronal circuitries plays a causative role in producing cardinal signs and symptoms of depression, these studies demonstrate that early trauma may increase the vulnerability to developing a mood disorder in later life. Reul et al. (1994b) showed that an immune challenge with human red blood cells in pregnant rats changes fetal brain development in a way that results in decreased hippocampal MR and GR concentrations in adults. These long-term effects render the adult animals more susceptible to stressors as they show higher stress-elicited ACTH and corticosterone levels throughout their lifetime than control animals.

In summary, these clinical and preclinical findings support the view that mood disorders can be seen as stress system disorders, in which impairment of GR and MR action plays a causal role. The impairments may be genetically determined or acquired through a variety of early stressors, or both. It is possible that antidepressants exert their clinical efficacy through reinstatement of complete corticosteroid receptor function. Of course, other important actions of these drugs also need careful consideration.

Thyroid Hormones

It has long been established that patients with thyroid disease usually have a variety of psychiatric problems. Hypothyroid patients are frequently dysphoric and complain of anxiety, fatigue, and irritability. In hypothyroid patients, depression and impairment of cognitive function are common mental sequelae. These observations and the original findings of Prange et al. (1972), who showed that a small dose of thyroid hormone may enhance the effects of antidepressants in many patients with depression who are euthyroid according to usual criteria, have led to the hypothesis that changes in hypothalamic-pituitary-thyroid (HPT) regulation are also involved in the pathogenesis of depression (Bauer and Whybrow 1990; Bauer et al. 1990).

Neuroendocrine testing of the HPT system in depression leaves us with an unclear picture as 25% of patients have a blunted thyroid-stimulating hormone (TSH) response to thyrotropin-releasing hormone (TRH), a hypothalamic tripeptide released from the median eminence into the portal vessels to stimulate TSH at pituitary thyrotrophs. As argued by Nemeroff et al. (1980), the blunted TSH response is probably secondary to enhanced TRH secretion, which reduces the number of pituitary TRH receptors and makes the thyrotropic cells insensitive to exogenous TRH. What remains unexplained is why approximately 15% of patients with depression have an exaggerated TSH response to TRH despite normal baseline plasma triiodothyronine (T_3), thyroxine (T_4), and TSH levels (grade III hypothyroidism). Patients with depression also have an increased occurrence of symptomless autoimmune thyroiditis, as defined by the abnormal presence of circulating antimicrosomal thyroid and/or antithyroglobulin antibodies (M. S. Gold et al. 1982b), without any other changes of basal or stimulated HPT hormones, and thus may be categorized as having grade IV hypothyroidism. Interestingly, these patients present more often than others with inadequately suppressed plasma cortisol concentration after dexamethasone administration. In addition, other findings support an interaction between the HPA and HPT system. For example, CRH-induced ACTH release was found to correlate with the TRH-elicited amount of TSH in patients with depression and control subjects (Holsboer et al. 1986).

It cannot yet be ruled out that the mechanism driving the HPA system is also responsible for the blunted TSH response to TRH. In this context, the recent finding by Redei et al. (1995) is remarkable. These authors showed that TRH precursor prepro TRH(178–199) can inhibit the CRH-induced release of ACTH in vitro and in vivo.

BIOGENIC AMINE AND AMINO ACID HYPOTHESES

As outlined previously, initial biological hypotheses of mood disorders were derived from the pharmacological actions of antidepressant drugs, which increase synaptic concentrations of noradrenaline (NA) and/or serotonin. Consequently, the biogenic amine hypothesis was formulated, but it lacks consistent proof that NA and/or serotonin release is indeed diminished. This failure is in part a result of the limited access to relevant brain areas. Measurements of NA and serotonin and their metabolites in blood, urine, and CSF failed to provide any consistent evidence for decreased neurotransmitter release in depression. Moreover, antidepressants that block the reuptake transporter do so immediately, thus a neurotransmitter synaptic deficit would be compensated quickly, whereas the clinical efficacy would take much longer. The lack of immediate clinical effects and the absence of recognizable laboratory signs of neurotransmitter deficiency led to a modification of the amine deficiency hypothesis into a "receptor sensitivity hypothesis" (Charney et al. 1981) and a "dysregulation hypothesis" (Siever and Davis 1985).

Serotonin

Although no specific evidence for a primary defect in central nervous system function is available, two series of clinical studies support the view that an enhancement of serotonin neurotransmission might be the basis for the treatment response to several antidepressants. First, all selected serotonin reuptake inhibitors are effective regardless of their chemical structure. Second, many patients with depression experience a rapid relapse when serotonin is depleted either by administration of *p*-chlorophenylalanine (PCPA, an inhibitor of tryptophan hydroxylase) or through dietary methods. The latter series of studies, by the group led by Charney, is of particular interest. Based on the fact that neurons need tryptophan to synthesize serotonin, these investigators administered a low-tryptophan diet and then a tryptophan-free diet on successive days to patients with depression who had recently improved on antidepressant medication. Two-thirds of the patients experienced a transient relapse of depressive symptoms. Interestingly, the proportion of relapse was much higher in those patients who responded more favorably to serotonin reuptake inhibitors and MAOIs than to NA reuptake inhibitors. These observations support the idea that a functioning serotonin system is necessary for maintenance of response to those antidepressants that primarily affect the serotonin system. Findings by the same group of investigators showing that acute tryptophan depletion did not worsen depressive mood in drug-free patients with depression are quite surprising. However, the day after serotonin depletion and return to unrestricted food, some patients (37%) improved (decrease in Hamilton Depression Scale score > 10 points [M. Hamilton 1960]), whereas other patients (23%) experienced only a transient improvement (increase in Hamilton Depression Scale score >10 points). The following questions arise from these studies: 1) Are central serotonin systems involved in only the mode of antidepressant action and not the pathophysiology of depression? and 2) Does short-term improvement or worsening of depressive symptomatology predict response to antidepressants with specific pharmacological actions? With the development of selective ligands for a vast number of serotonin receptors (Figure 2–4), more specific questions can be addressed. Most importantly, with the recent availability of tianeptine, a new serotonin reuptake enhancer that produces antidepressant effects according to preliminary studies (Wilde and Benfield 1995), the unanswered

Serotoninergic neurotransmission

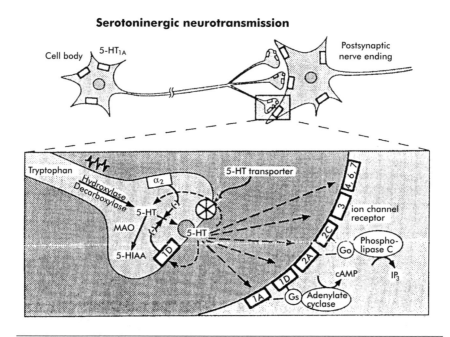

FIGURE 2–4.   G-protein–coupled serotonin (5-HT) receptors that inhibit adenylyl cyclase constitute the 5-HT$_1$ family, including the 5-HT$_{1A}$, 5-HT$_{1B}$, 5-HT$_{1D}$, 5-HT$_{1E}$, and 5-HT$_{1F}$ receptors. G-protein–coupled 5-HT receptors that stimulate adenylyl cyclase include 5-HT$_4$, 5-HT$_6$, and 5-HT$_7$ receptors. Three 5-HT receptors, 5-HT$_{2A}$, 5-HT$_{2B}$, and 5-HT$_{2C}$, stimulate the phospholipase C second messenger system. For two receptors, which are also G-protein coupled, 5-HT$_{5A}$ and 5-HT$_{5B}$, no coupling to any known transduction mechanism has yet been found. The only family of ligand-gated channel receptors are 5-HT$_3$ receptors, which are permeable to monovalent cations. MAO = monoamine oxidase; 5-HIAA = 5-hydroxyindoleacetic acid; IP$_3$ = inositol triphosphate.

Source.   Adapted from Bockaert J: "Serotonin Receptors: From Genes to Pathology," in *Critical Issues in the Treatment of Affective Disorders.* Edited by Langer SZ, Brunello N, Racagni G, et al. Basel, Switzerland, S. Karger AG Basel, 1994, pp. 1–8. Copyright 1994, S. Karger AG Basel. Used with permission.

question of in which direction the serotonin system must be driven to remedy depression can be addressed.

Noradrenaline

Measurements of NA and 3-methoxy-4-hydroxyphenylglycol (MHPG, the primary metabolite of NA) in the CSF, plasma, and urine of patients with depression failed to produce patterns that would allow conclusions to be drawn about alterations in neurotransmitter bioavailability and turnover. In a study by Charney's group, it was determined whether a rapid reduction in catecholamines in the brain induced a transient relapse in patients with depression who had recently undergone remission and were being maintained on antidepressant drugs (H. L. Miller et al. 1996a, 1996b). These authors administered α-methyl-*p*-tyrosine (AMPT), which inhibits tyrosine hydroxylase (the key enzyme for catecholamine biosynthesis), to patients who have undergone remission and were treated either with desipramine, an NA reuptake inhibitor, or with the serotonin reuptake inhibitor fluoxetine or sertraline. In response to AMPT-induced catecholamine depletion, eight of nine patients maintained remission on NA reuptake inhibitors, but none of the 10 patients maintained on serotonin reuptake inhibitors met the criteria for relapse (Figure 2–5). In contrast to patients receiving antidepressant treatment, drug-free patients with depression did not experience worsening of depressive symptoms after catecholamine depletion with AMPT.

These data and findings from serotonin depletion studies show that, in patients treated successfully, NA and serotonin systems are involved in maintenance of drug-induced remission. However, the absence of an increased severity in depressive symptoms in drug-free patients with depression suggests that alterations in serotonin and catecholamine release may not be causally involved in the pathophysiology of mood disorders.

This conclusion does not dispute the heuristic value of a large number of studies that either used neuroendocrine probes or platelet-binding studies, which in aggregate point to functional alterations of the adrenoceptors under study (Table 2–2). It remains unresolved whether these changes are related to changes in receptor number and/or affinity, which are the primary defects in depression, or are secondary to other humoral events, for example, neuroendocrine alterations that interfere strongly with aminergic receptor function. For example, β-adrenoceptor downregulation by antidepressants is counteracted by an elevation of corticosteroids, and through this mechanism HPA overactivity may oppose the effects of antidepressants on β-adrenoceptors.

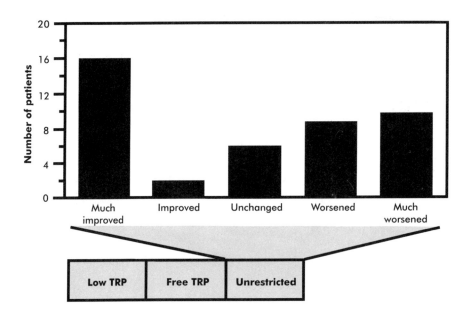

FIGURE 2–5.   Patients received a diet containing only a low level (160 mg/day) of tryptophan (TRP) (low TRP) on day 1 and a TRP-free, 15–amino acid drink on day 2. For the control condition, the patients received a diet containing normal amounts of TRP on day 1 and a 16–amino acid drink containing 2.3 g of TRP on day 2. On day 3, food was unrestricted under both conditions. The change in score on the Hamilton Depression Scale (HAM-D) at the 420-minute time point from day 2 to day 3 during the TRP depletion test, minus the HAM-D score on the control test, was calculated. Patients are grouped as much improved (≥10 point decrease in total HAM-D score), improved (5- to 9-point decrease), unchanged (0.4-point change), worsened (5- to 9-point increase), or much worsened (≥10-point increase).

Source.   Adapted from Delgado PL, Price LH, Miller HL, et al: "Rapid Serotonin Depletion as a Provocative Challenge Test for Patients With Major Depression: Relevance to Antidepressant Action and the Neurobiology of Depression." *Psychopharmacology Bulletin* 27:321–330, 1991. Used with permission.

Dopamine

Drugs, such as amphetamine or cocaine, that enhance dopaminergic neurotransmission produce massive behavioral and psychomotor activation and

TABLE 2-2. Abnormalities of noradrenaline function

Probe	Type of change
cAMP response to β-adrenoceptor agonists in platelets	Decreased
β-Adrenoceptors in brains of suicide victims	Increased
Growth hormone release in response to clonidine or desmethylimipramine, thought to reflect postsynaptic α_2-adrenoceptor sensitivity	Decreased
MHPG release after desmethylimipramine, thought to reflect presynaptic α_2-adrenoceptor sensitivity	Increased

Note.   cAMP = cyclic adenosine monophosphate; MHPG = 3-methoxy-4-hydroxy-phenylglycol.

continue to have a place in the treatment of refractory depression. Cocaine action involves blockade of the dopamine transporter that controls temporal and spatial activity of dopamine through presynaptic reuptake. Disruption of the dopamine transporter gene in transgenic mice produces enhanced dopamine concentration in the extracellular space together with hyperlocomotion and no response to cocaine administration (Giros et al. 1996). Whereas these clinical and preclinical findings would support a role for dopaminergic neurotransmission as a target for drug intervention in depression, particularly the retarded subtype, neither direct nor circumstantial evidence for such a possibility exists. Studies that have measured decreased homovanillic acid (HVA), the main metabolite of dopamine in the CSF of patients with depression, are likely confounded by psychomotor retardation (Post et al. 1973). A. Roy et al. (1992), however, found that patients with depression who have attempted suicide have lower HVA titers in their CSF than those who never were suicidal. The connection between the midbrain ventral tegmentum and the nucleus accumbens in the striatum is crucially involved in motivational and reward processes that are the current focus of drug abuse research.

After long-term administration, antidepressants may enhance dopaminergic neurotransmission, even if direct acute effects are absent (Serra et al. 1990b). For example, the stress-induced decrease in the binding of quinpirole, an agonist of D_2 and D_3 receptors, can be reversed by chronic imipramine treatment (Papp et al. 1994). These and related data, however, do not allow the formulation of a dopamine hypothesis of depression, but rather point to a role for decreased dopaminergic neurotransmission in specific neuronal circuits that are responsible for those depressive syndromes associated with motivational loss, psychomotor retardation, and anhedonia (Willner 1995).

The Cholinergic System

Some cholinomimetic drugs such as physostigmine, which interferes with acetylcholinesterase (the acetylcholine-degrading enzyme), or the non-selective muscarinic agonist arecoline can produce depressive symptoms in control subjects and may aggravate these symptoms in patients with depression (Janowski et al. 1972). To what extent altered cholinergic neurotransmission is involved in the pathophysiology of mood disorders has been studied only tangentially. The most convincing results have been those that used the cholinergic M_1 receptor agonist RS-86. M. Berger et al. (1989) administered RS-86 to patients with depression and control subjects and found that the latency between sleep onset and the occurrence of the first rapid eye movement (REM) sleep period was shortened significantly in patients with depression. This finding agrees with the view that there is an increased sensitivity of cholinergic receptors in depression. Such a possibility is supported by a study from Schreiber et al. (1992), who administered RS-86 to control subjects without depression who were recruited from families with a high genetic load for depression. This study showed that, in probands at risk for depression, RS-86 may induce a more pronounced shortening of REM latency than in control subjects from unaffected families. This lends support to the existence of a premorbid muscarinic receptor hypersensitivity in probands at risk for depression. Studies showing that patients with depression have an exaggerated ACTH and cortisol response after a physostigmine challenge (Risch 1982) and that physostigmine can also elevate cortisol in dexamethasone-pretreated control subjects without depression (Doerr and Berger 1983) agree with this view.

γ-Aminobutyric Acid

After the initial report by Emrich et al. (1980), who found that the γ-aminobutyric acid (GABA) agonist valproate may ameliorate manic symptoms, a large amount of data has been accumulated supporting the idea that decreased GABA-ergic neurotransmission is responsible for the genetic vulnerability of mood disorder (Petty 1995). Studies in support of such a GABA hypothesis include those by B. I. Gold et al. (1980), who showed that patients with depression had lower CSF GABA concentrations than control subjects, and those by Petty (1995), who found that GABA levels were decreased in the plasma of patients with depression. Finally, Honig et al. (1989) found decreased GABA concentrations in the cortices of patients with severe depression. In animals, blockade of $GABA_A$ receptors produces a learned helplessness, an animal model of depression that can be reversed by antidepressants concomitantly with desensitized $GABA_A$ receptors, most likely through increased GABA levels (A. D. Sherman and Petty 1982). In contrast, $GABA_B$ receptors are upregulated by antidepressants in parallel with desensitization of β-adrenoceptors. Virtually every neuron is responsive to the action of GABA and GABA-ergic activity. Thus, GABA also modulates noradrenergic synaptic activity, as shown by the increase in NA turnover induced by the GABA agonists fengabine and progabide. These two drugs have been claimed to be equally as effective as imipramine and nortriptyline; however, they have not yet entered clinical use. Because GABA levels in various tissues are altered by factors such as exercise, hormonal fluctuations, and diurnal rhythms, the potential use of GABA to establish a GABA hypothesis requires the execution of further studies that take into account the psychomotor, neuroendocrine, and diurnal disturbances that are common in mood disorders.

N-Methyl-D-Aspartate Receptor

The *N*-methyl-D-aspartate (NMDA) receptor subtype of the glutamate receptor is one of several mediating excitatory amino acid synaptic transmissions and is constituted as a hetero-oligomer similar to other ligand-gated ion channels (Kutsuwada et al. 1992; Meguro et al. 1992). This receptor complex has multiple allosterically coupled recognition sites for glutamate, glycine, polyamines, and use-dependent channel blockers. Unlike other ligand-gated channels, activation of the NMDA receptor requires binding of an agonist (e.g., glutamate) to its transmitter recognition site and binding of glycine to a strychnine-insensitive receptor. The findings of Trullas and Skolnick (1990) showed that a partial agonist at strychnine-insensitive glycine receptors (1-aminocyclopropane-1-carboxylic acid [ACPC]) produced behavioral changes that are usually produced by antidepressants when given to mice that were submitted to the forced swim test (Porsolt et al. 1977). In this test, animals swim in a basin from which there is no escape, and having concluded this they start floating as a sign of behavioral despair. Antidepressants reduce the floating time and the immobility. Not only ACPC but also dizocilpine (MK-801), a noncompetitive NMDA antagonist, and AP-7, a competitive NMDA antagonist, reduced immobility in the forced swim test without altering motor activity. Some of these treatments produced desensitization of cortical β-adrenoceptors in a way similar to that firmly established for prototypic tricyclic antidepressants (I. A. Paul et al. 1992). Intrigued by this finding, these investigators studied whether antidepressants may act through alterations of NMDA receptor characteristics. In summary, chronic but not acute treatment with a large variety of structurally and pharmacologically different antidepressants altered the radioligand-binding properties of the NMDA receptor. Therefore, these authors concluded that NMDA receptor adaptations are a final common pathway of antidepressant action, and they further suggested that glutamatergic pathways may be involved in the pathophysiology of mood disorders (I. A. Paul et al. 1993). In line with this suggestion are recent studies by Altamura et al. (1995), who found significantly higher plasma glutamate levels in subjects with affective disorders, although it is unclear to what extent these measures had been affected by other humoral changes, such as neuroendocrine alterations, in these patients. Although the NMDA receptor hypothesis is attractive, it needs to be tested by the use of more specific drugs targeted to individual NMDA receptors.

NEUROTROPHIC FACTORS

Neurotrophins not only contribute to the survival and growth of neurons, but they are also involved in generating and maintaining neuronal plasticity (Korte et al. 1995; Lo 1995; Thoenen 1995). The neurotrophin family includes nerve growth factor (NGF), brain-derived neurotrophic factor (BDNF), and neurotrophin 3 (NT-3), which bind to receptors with tyrosine kinase activity (trkA, NGF; trkB, BDNF; and trkC, NT-3). M. A. Smith et al. (1995) found that chronic stress decreases levels of BDNF mRNA in the hippocampus (dentate gyrus, CA_1, CA_3), whereas NT-3 mRNA is increased in the dentate gyrus and CA_1. The expression of the respective receptors (trkB and trkC) remains unchanged, which points to a compensatory role of NT-3 if BDNF is decreased by stress-associated mechanisms. Glucocorticoids have a modulatory effect on neurotrophin expression, and the hippocampus is richly endowed with corticosteroid receptors. The stress-induced change in the expression ratio of BDNF/NT-3 is secondary to stress-induced glucocorticoid excess. BDNF decreased slightly and NT-3 levels remained unchanged in adrenalectomized rats treated with high dosages of glucocorticoids. This finding may be taken as an indication that corticosteroids do not cause the stress-related change in neurotrophin expression. However, these studies do not fully account for the differential effects that corticosteroids exert in the brain through MR and GR. These differences depend critically on the extent to which GR homodimers and GR-MR heterodimers are formed (Trapp and Holsboer 1996). Only ligand-activated homodimers increase neuronal vulnerability to noxious conditions such as hypoglycemia and hypoxia. An excess of naturally occurring corticosteroids is much less dangerous in this regard and may even protect neurons from GR-specific synthetic corticosteroids (Hassan et al. 1996). The stress-induced decrease of BDNF is of interest for depression research because this neurotrophic factor possibly mediates the stress-induced decrease in long-term potentiation, a cellular model of memory. One may speculate that the impaired cognitive function of patients with depression is related to stress-elicited decreases in hippocampal BDNF expression. To what extent one may extrapolate from long-term potentiation to memory and cognition is still subject to speculation. Whereas increased expression of BDNF mRNA in rat hippocampus was found to be associated with improved spatial memory (Falkenburg et al. 1992), transgenic mice, which are heterozygous for BDNF gene disruption, performed indistinguishably from control mice in various tests for memory and cognition, including the Morris water maze test (Montkowski and Holsboer, in press). This apparent absence of memory deficit is of interest because these transgenic mice show reduced long-term potentiation in the hippocampus (Korte et al. 1995).

Antidepressants such as tranylcypromine, sertraline, and desipramine, with different acute pharmacological effects, all increase expression of BDNF and its cognate receptor trkB in the frontal cortex and hippocampus (Nibuya et al. 1994). The primary role of BDNF and other neurotrophins in the pathogenesis of depression and their function as antidepressant targets can be evaluated only if studies of the stress- and antidepressant-induced changes in neurotrophin expression consider the role of stress hormone-activated corticosteroid receptor homodimers and heterodimers on expression of transcription factors that induce BDNF expression after phosphorylation. One such factor is cAMP response element–binding protein (CREB). If CREB mRNA translation into protein is impaired by antisense treatment, BDNF also decreases (Nibuya et al. 1994). Duman et al. (1994) showed that the CREB and cAMP system plays a role in the enhanced expression of BDNF and trkB after antidepressant treatment. It is of note in this context that the CRH gene promoter contains a CREB response element (D. Spengler et al. 1992), which underscores how neurotrophins, antidepressants, and stress hormones are intrinsically intertwined.

INTRACELLULAR SIGNALING

After a neurotransmitter's release and binding to its cognate membranous receptor, a cascade of intracellular processes is induced that coordinate the incoming information. Guanine nucleotide–binding proteins (G proteins) are composed of subunits (α, β, and γ) that convey information from the cell surface to intracellular effectors, such as adenylyl cyclase, that are needed to form cAMP-activating protein kinases for gene transcription. The most obvious biochemical effect of long-term antidepressant treatment is a decrease in the β-adrenergic agonist–stimulated production of cAMP. This change can be explained by increased ligand exposure secondary to antidepressant effects at the reuptake transporter (Sulser 1984). However, direct antidepressant effects on cell signaling have also been reported by Rasenick's group, who showed that chronic antidepressant treatment of rats promotes increased activation of adenylyl cyclase by a stimulatory G protein ($G_S\alpha$ subtype) without changing the intracellular content of individual G-protein subtypes (J. Chen and Rasenick 1995). These investigators further suggested that antidepressants act at an element of the synaptic membrane or cytoskeleton in which structural changes result in enhancement of $G_S\alpha$ protein coupling to adenylyl cyclase. In addition, Nestler's group showed that chronic antidepressant treatment activates the adenylyl cyclase system, which then further activates protein kinase A (Nestler et al. 1989). Whereas Rasenick reported that antidepressant-activated adenylyl cyclase results from enhanced functional coupling with a $G_S\alpha$ protein whose concentration remains unaltered, Lesch and Manji (1992) found that antidepressants decrease $G_S\alpha$ protein concentration, at least in the hippocampus.

The relevance of these findings for the pathophysiology of mood disorders has not yet been established. A study by L. T. Young et al. (1991) found elevated $G_S\alpha$ subunit levels in the cerebral cortex of patients with bipolar affective disorder. The significance of this finding is difficult to gauge because corticosteroids, which are elevated in this disorder, were reported to increase this particular G-protein subunit in rat cerebral cortex (Saito et al. 1989).

CONCLUSION

The enormous investments in neuroscience research have led to a dramatic expansion of our knowledge of how neuronal systems work. Surprisingly, little progress has been made in understanding the pathophysiology underlying mood disorders and the mechanisms by which antidepressants exert their clinical effect. The common strategy of extrapolation from the pharmacological effects of drugs to the pathogenesis of the disease they remedy is useful to only a limited extent. This became clear in studies challenging the biogenic amine hypothesis, for which a primary role in the causality of depression is still not clearly indicated. The likelihood of a major defect at the receptor level has also been ruled out by pharmacological as well as genetic studies.

Other concepts, particularly those focusing on intracellular signaling, are evolving and have only recently become accessible for research by refined technology.

In my admittedly biased view, the most coherent approach is that of a profoundly disturbed stress system that under specific conditions paves the way to development of mood disorders. These stress-system alterations can be genetic or acquired through trauma in early life or even in utero. Consistent with this neuroendocrine hypothesis are findings that centrally released neuropeptides that drive the HPA system also have behavioral effects that are similar to affective symptoms. This view is further supported by the documented ability of various antidepressants to enhance corticosteroid receptor synthesis and efficacy. Moreover, the stress system, particularly the corticosteroids and their receptors, interferes with all of the neurotransmitter receptor systems, including intracellular signaling, that have been considered in the context of mood disorders. New drugs targeted directly to various elements of the stress system will constitute a major step forward.

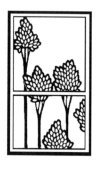

CHAPTER 3

Pharmacological Validity of Diagnostic Separation

Yvon D. Lapierre, M.D., F.R.C.P.C.,
David Bakish, M.D., F.R.C.P.C., and
Cynthia L. Hooper, M.A.

Physicians have tended to relate physiognomy to physiology and pathophysiology since the Hippocratic era. Individual personality styles were related to pathological reactions: the bilious character was more prone to depression, body and environmental functions were associated with disease, and treatment was often directed at correcting these "pathogenic humors." With the passage of time, this mind-set continued in psychiatry with the sheldonian approach of body structure being associated with a predisposition to certain disorders. The pyknic body type was considered to predispose one to manic-depressive and other mood disorders, whereas the asthenic body type was thought to render one more susceptible to schizophrenia.

The advent of somatic treatments and more particularly the advent of effective psychopharmacology gave an impetus to a conceptual change in the approach to psychiatric illness, focusing on a more medical model. This resulted from the discovery of improved and more efficacious treatments. These gave more credibility to the approach and served as instrumentation for further progress.

Initially, psychotropic drugs had focused mechanisms of action on levels of arousal and vigilance. Those drugs that depressed arousal levels were considered for states of anxiety, agitation, neuroses, psychoses, and situational or reactional states. Historically, the first of all anxiolytics was alcohol. It was followed by the barbiturates. Toward the end of the 1940s, the propanediols, especially meprobamate, became the tranquilizers par excellence. Following that came the discovery of the benzodiazepines. Simultaneously, for states of depressed arousal, psychostimulants, such as the amphetamines, were the treatment of choice.

It became obvious, however, that psychostimulants were not effective in situations of lowered arousal resulting from mood depression. In the 1950s, antidepressants such as the monoamine oxidase inhibitors (MAOIs) and tricyclic antidepressants (TCAs) became recognized as more effective in treating depression. The differentiation between arousal and mood thus became clearer. It is through the action of drugs that sedate and thus reduce anxiety versus those drugs that do not sedate but are anxiolytic that the basic concepts of anxiety have forcibly to be reconsidered. This inevitably led to the need for a reconceptualization of psychotropic modes of action in relation to psychiatric disorders.

The conceptualization of psychopathology simultaneously followed nearly parallel lines of developments. The modern period started with Kraepelin who developed detailed descriptions of phenomenology and syndromal classifications of disorders based on close clinical observation of symptoms. Kraepelin's observations were transversal and longitudinal, leading to improved diagnostic precision. Unfortunately, this diagnostic precision was not accompanied by a comparable and matching therapeutic armamentarium. The lack of effective somatic therapies led to the adoption of psychodynamic or psychological treatments. These evolved and led to a more psychodynamic approach to diagnostic concepts and philosophy. This is well illustrated in DSM-II (American Psychiatric Association 1968), in which the underlying philosophy is one of "psychodynamic reaction," where a diagnosis-based psychopathological phenomenology is secondary to the psychodynamic formulation.

As therapeutics advanced, so did psychopathological conceptualization. This well illustrates the circularity of the wheel of progress where available treatments inevitably lead to greater diagnostic precision. This in turn depends on the understanding of the concepts of pathophysiology, which itself relies on the knowledge surrounding the newly available treatment.

The effect of psychopharmacology on psychiatry has essentially been a return to the medical model where clinical history and examination lead to the formulation of a diagnosis. The diagnosis thus allows the development of prognosis, course of illness, and prediction of ultimate outcome. Most important, a diagnosis should theoretically lead to a specific treatment for a specific condition. The early psychopharmacological agents addressed broad-based, nonspecific mechanisms in a similarly broad-based, nonspecific manner. These treatments, in their lack of specificity, were accompanied by side effects that decreased the quality of life, impeded recovery, or even created additional problems or conditions that then had to be addressed. In fact, these treatments were often rejected by practitioners and not used for therapy.

To overcome these difficulties, pharmacological developments strived to identify the key mechanisms of drug action that could be related to the therapeutic outcome of a treatment. Technological advances, particularly in molecular biology, have greatly contributed to these advances in the search for specificity. Initially, the mechanisms of identifying the cause of side effects led to the development of neurotransmitter-specific drugs. This was followed by the more receptor-specific treatments. Examples such as serotonin-1a partial agonists and serotonin-2 antagonists illustrate this trend toward receptor specificity in pharmacotherapy.

Psychiatric diagnosis continued to lag behind these advances in pharmacology and molecular biology. Nevertheless, there has been a significant effort to bring about more specificity and precision to psychiatric diagnosis. It is possible to identify two phases in this development. As a first phase, the class of drugs (i.e., tranquilizers in the generic sense) could be applied to broadly treat a class "diagnosis" of hyperarousal or the behavior derived from the hyperarousal. In the second phase, a more specific diagnostic category could lead to a more specific drug entity being applied in treatment. At the present time, diagnostic categorization is still at a syndromal level, but the direction is to more specific subgroupings.

Earlier attempts at arriving at a syndromal profile of drugs were the European efforts surrounding the clinical physiognomy of psychotropic agents (Bobon and Gottfries 1974). This approach consisted of mapping the individual psychopharmacotherapeutic pattern of action of a drug, based on six effects: ataraxic, antimanic, antiautistic, antidelusional, extrapyramidal, and adrenolytic. The drug's relative intensity on each effect was identified and then mapped. This primarily applied to neuroleptics and had as an ultimate objective the close matching of the symptom configuration therapeutic profile of a compound to the symptom profile of a patient. Thus, individual presentation of a clinical syndrome could be addressed more specifically by matching the templates.

Thus, there is a long and successful history of using pharmacological effects to validate psychiatric diagnosis. Examination of the individual areas of diagnosis demonstrates these specific validation efforts.

ANXIETY DISORDERS

The treatment of anxiety disorders has made remarkable progress with the advent of psychopharmacological treatment. Anxiety was traditionally conceptualized as being a state of hyperarousal. This led to treatments that were essentially focused on sedation. For a number of years, benzodiazepines were the treatment of choice for generic anxiety. The observations of D. F. Klein (1964, 1980) led to the identification of panic disorder as a major subgrouping of the anxiety disorders. Patients with panic disorder were not as responsive to the low-potency benzodiazepines such as chlordiazepoxide and diazepam (Dunner et al. 1986). However, patients with panic disorder were observed to respond prophylactically to TCAs such as imipramine (D. V. Sheehan et al. 1980; Zitrin et al. 1983). Patients with panic disorder were also later found to be responsive to the high-potency benzodiazepines (Ballenger et al. 1988). The degree of response, side-effect profile, and tolerance to therapeutic effects found with benzodiazepines led to a focus on treatment with the newer, more tolerable selective serotonin reuptake inhibitors (SSRIs) (Gorman et al. 1988; Schneier et al. 1990).

The separation of panic disorder with or without agoraphobia was validated by the psychopharmacological variation in responsiveness. The avoidance behavior characteristic of agoraphobia is generally unresponsive to both TCAs and MAOIs. Thus, there is the added requirement of behavior modification. The initial findings with brofaromine, a reversible inhibitor of monoamine oxidase A (RIMA), suggest that the avoidance behavior of agoraphobia is corrected with this drug without any necessary psychotherapeutic intervention (Bakish 1994; Bakish et al. 1993a).

Social phobia also has a component of avoidance and has been successfully treated with the RIMAs brofaromine and moclobemide (Keck and McElroy 1997). However, the SSRIs and venlafaxine have also shown efficacy in social phobia (Gorman and Kent 1999; Keck and McElroy 1997), suggesting that further divisions of anxiety diagnostic categories may result from future pharmacological research.

GENERALIZED ANXIETY DISORDER

Generalized anxiety disorder is still considered the gold standard indication for benzodiazepines (P. J. Perry et al. 1990). However, buspirone, a serotonin-1a partial agonist, has been demonstrated as effective in this disorder

(Goa and Ward 1986; Pecknold et al. 1989; Rickels et al. 1982). In contradistinction to benzodiazepines, the therapeutic effect of buspirone has a lag period similar to that of antidepressants in depression, suggesting that its therapeutic benefits derive from receptor modulation. In addition, buspirone seems to act preferentially in those patients who are not responsive to benzodiazepines, suggesting a possible subgrouping of generalized anxiety disorders.

Several preliminary lines of research have started to suggest that antidepressants, once considered ineffective in generalized anxiety disorder, may be very efficacious (Gorman and Kent 1999). In particular, venlafaxine has been effective in treating generalized anxiety disorder in both open-label and double-blind trials, and imipramine and paroxetine were as effective as a benzodiazepine in the long-term treatment of generalized anxiety disorder.

The findings derived from psychopharmacotherapy of the anxiety disorders have led to the identification of a number of subgroupings that are determined by such pharmacological dissection of a generic group of disorders. Thus, generalized anxiety disorder may eventually be subject to further dissection through pharmacological probes.

OBSESSIVE-COMPULSIVE DISORDER

Obsessive-compulsive disorder (OCD) is traditionally considered in the same grouping as the anxiety disorders. However, it has certain characteristics that lead to it being identified as a discrete entity. This has been supported further with pharmacotherapy. In an earlier period of treatment with psychotherapeutic drugs, OCD was treated with tranquilizing medications. It later became clear that this form of treatment addressed only the epiphenomenon of anxiety found in these patients. The observations of Ananth et al. (1979, 1981) and others (Barr et al. 1993; R. Fontaine and Chouinard 1985; W. K. Goodman et al. 1990b; López-Ibor 1992) have identified the role of serotonin in OCD. Initial findings indicated that these patients responded to serotonin reuptake inhibiting drugs such as clomipramine, and this serotonin relationship was subsequently confirmed more specifically through treatment with SSRIs. This observation solidified the separation of OCD from anxiety disorders as a unique diagnostic entity.

MOOD DISORDERS

Psychopharmacology has contributed to bringing mood disorders under one diagnostic entity instead of creating multiple subgroupings. Prior to the availability of effective antidepressant and mood-stabilizing medications, mood disorders were considered to be either affective psychosis (which was a group considered as treatable with pharmacological means) or nonpsychotic mood disorders (which were generally treated with psychotherapy). It is now apparent that all mood disturbances may be modulated and corrected through pharmacotherapy without in any way discounting the added benefit of psychotherapeutic interventions.

Mood disorders as a whole may thus be separated as those demonstrating bipolarity versus those that tend toward the direction of depression. Thus, the bipolar group may be addressed pharmacologically with mood stabilizers as the baseline therapeutic approach. Lithium was originally observed to control manic behavior (Cade 1949). Along these initial observations, it was subsequently demonstrated by Schou et al. (1954) that lithium was not only effective in the control of the manic phase of bipolar illness, but it also prevented relapse in a prophylactic manner over many years. Unfortunately, approximately only 70% of patients with bipolar disorder do benefit from relapse prevention. This indicates a subgroup of patients with bipolar disorder who do not respond to lithium. These patients may be genetically different from the patients who respond to lithium (P. Grof et al. 1993). As well, the pharmacological dissection suggests that a number of patients with bipolar disorder are responsive to anticonvulsive treatments such as carbamazepine, sodium valproate, or clonazepam. This subgroup has yet to be clearly identified and delineated. It does suggest, however, the potential for further diagnostic subgrouping.

The treatment of the major depressive disorders such as unipolar and bipolar depressions was initially considered to be uniform. However, with psychopharmacological advances, it has been demonstrated that the patients with bipolar depression may be partially responsive, at least prophylactically responsive, to lithium therapy, whereas the patients with unipolar depression are not as responsive (Abou-Saleh 1992). In addition, the treatment of depression may contribute through serendipity to the confirmation of a subgroup of patients with a bipolar disorder referred to as *bipolar II*. These patients, following treatment with antidepressants, will switch over to a hypomanic or fully manic phase resulting from pharmacological mechanisms. Thus, another subgroup of the bipolar disorder may be identified in the future.

Another subgrouping of patients with depression who have a differential pharmacological response are those diagnosed with depression with psychotic features, previously referred to as psychotic depression. These patients generally do not respond well to antidepressant therapy alone but require the addition of antipsychotic medications such as neuroleptics (Frances and Hall 1991). The patients of this subgroup were at one time considered potential candidates for the use of amoxapine, an antidepressant that has as its metabolite a neuroleptic derivative.

The so-called minor depressive disorders have now been regrouped as dysthymia. Prior to the recognition of the treatability of this condition with antidepressants, patients with this condition were relegated to long-term psychotherapy with variable degrees of success. The work of Akiskal (1983; Akiskal et al. 1980) and Kocsis and Frances (1987) demonstrated the responsiveness of patients with this condition to antidepressant medication. This has been extended to the serotonergic drugs such as ritanserin (Bakish et al. 1993b) and the SSRIs (Bakish et al. 1994; Lapierre 1994; Lapierre et al. 1993; Ravindran et al. 1994c). The evidence for this subgroup of patients with depression has been supported clinically and also biochemically (Ravindran et al. 1994a, 1994b, 1994d).

Those patients presenting with atypical symptoms of depression (i.e., rejection-sensitivity, hypersomnia, hyperphagia, and hysteroid personality types) were confirmed as a unique subgroup responsive to MAOIs including phenelzine (Liebowitz et al. 1988). There are indications that atypical symptomatology may also be responsive to the RIMAs such as moclobemide (Lonnqvist et al. 1994; Paykel 1995); however, results are preliminary.

Through the use of psychopharmacotherapy, it thus appears that bipolar, unipolar, and atypical depressions are discrete entities. They are also separate from dysthymia, which may be the bridging condition to the anxiety disorders.

OUTLOOK

As the specificity of psychotherapeutic compounds increases and as our knowledge of molecular biology advances, it appears that the diagnostic categories we recognize today are but generic groupings of conditions that will be eventually considered as broad categories to be further dissected. It also appears that certain categories of receptors of different neurotransmitter groups may be the intervening biological substrate controlling these conditions. For example, agonists of serotonin-1a receptors are indicated in the treatment of anxiety disorders—specifically, generalized anxiety disorder. The serotonin-2 receptors are a point of entry to the treatment of depressive disorders. Dopamine neurotransmission may be a link to the effective treatment of psychotic disorders. This does not imply the etiological relationship of these neurotransmitter systems, but certainly indicates a point of entry to the underlying pathophysiology. As the steps leading to the underlying psychopathology become identified through pharmacological probe, this will be followed closely by advances in molecular biology and neurochemistry that will eventually undoubtedly lead to the biochemical or neurochemical identification of several uniquely specific disorders.

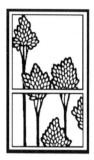

CHAPTER 4

Signal Amplification in Psychiatric Diagnosis: A Quintessential Challenge for Biological Psychiatry

Herman M. Van Praag, M.D., Ph.D.

To study the biological underpinnings of a given psycho-pathological state, its precise phenomenological definition and clear differentiation from bordering psychopathological states is essential, especially for replication studies in which there should be no queries as to the kind of syndrome one has to look for. Thus, in studying a particular syndrome one should include only those patients who show all the required features and no or only few others. This procedure probably will result in many false-negative diagnoses, and its application will certainly slow down biological psychiatric research. This disadvantage, however, is amply compensated by the fact that the test group is symptomatologically homogeneous and recognizable. Terminological clearness is a basic prerequisite for biological psychiatric research.

After sufficient data have been collected on the pathophysiology of a given syndrome in its pure form, one might consider studying patients with heterologous symptoms or incomplete syndromes. The problem of cosyndromality forms part of the larger issue of comorbidity, which is further discussed.

MULTIAXIAL DIAGNOSES ARE NOT TO BE EQUATED WITH CATEGORICAL DIAGNOSES

A particular psychopathological condition should of course be scrutinized as to symptomatology and a variety of nonsymptomatological variables, such as duration, severity, cyclicity, premorbid personality pathology, family loading, preceding life events, and others. These nonsymptomatological variables should be assessed independent of the syndrome and independent of each other until predictable mutual relationships have been established.

The current prevailing taxonomy, based on nosological principles as it is, recognizes discrete disorders, to be defined on various axes. As such, the multiaxial manner of diagnosing psychiatric disorders, introduced by DSM-III (American Psychiatric Association 1980), was a valuable contribution, but it was used to prematurely authorize "disorders," before predictable relationships between the syndrome and the various nonsymptomatological variables had been convincingly demonstrated. As a result, psychiatry was flooded with disease entities carrying the official DSM imprimatur but of unproven validity (Van Praag 1992a).

I interpolate a few instances to demonstrate this point. According to DSM-III and DSM-IV (American Psychiatric Association 1994) criteria, dysthymia is a chronic, low-grade form of depression, accompanied by premorbid personality pathology. Major depression, on the other hand, is a more severe form of depression, with intermittent course and, at least in the melancholic subtype, undisturbed premorbid personality structure. Our studies, however, led us to the conclusion that no predictable relationship exists between the phenomenology of a depression and its severity (Van Praag 1989). In other words, depressive syndromes, whatever their symptomatological composition, do occur in all degrees of severity, from very mild to severe. Moreover, duration and premorbid personality characteristics predict little about syndromal depression type. Those variables vary independently of the prevailing syndrome. The same holds for the schizophrenic syndromes. Type of syndrome predicts little about variables such as future course, family loading, treatment response, and premorbid personality structure (Berrios 1995; Kendall and Nahorski 1987; Lindenmayer et al. 1994; Moller et al. 1988; M. A. Roy and Crowe 1994; Tsuang et al. 1990; Wolkowitz et al. 1990).

CAUTION WITH THE
ACCEPTANCE OF NOVEL DISORDERS

DSM-I (American Psychiatric Association 1952) contained 106 diagnoses; DSM-II (American Psychiatric Association 1968) contained 182. In DSM-III-R (American Psychiatric Association 1987), 292 diagnostic categories were recorded. In DSM-IV, 13 categories have been added and 8 were deleted (J. Cooper 1995).

A typical example of diagnostic splintering provides the group of mood disorders. One reads about major depression, minor depression, double depression, dysthymia, unipolar and bipolar depression, depressive personality, depression not otherwise specified, brief recurrent depression, subsyndromal symptomatic depression, mixed anxiety depression disorder, seasonal depression, and adjustment disorder with depressive mood.

The validity of many of those novel diagnostic concepts is unproven, uncertain, or even questionable. If one day they would be shown to lack validity, our persistent efforts to find biological markers of such a disorder, to elucidate its genetics and its epidemiology, and to unravel the differential therapeutic effects of the various biological and psychological interventions would have been largely futile. Validity studies should have taken precedence over all others. Research of nonvalidated concepts runs the risk of generating nonvalid results, however great its methodological sophistication.

LANDMARKS BETWEEN THE
STILL NORMAL AND THE JUST ABNORMAL
MUST BE ESTABLISHED

Cutoff points have to be established between mental distress and mental disorder. If, for instance, one is interested in the pathogenesis of major depression, one is well-advised to develop clear criteria to distinguish that condition from states of apprehension, demoralization, and sorrow.

So far, however, boundaries have not been established and, even worse, no systematic attempts to do so are noticed. This hampers biological psychiatry and may well be among the reasons that the search for biological markers of psychiatric disorders over the past 35 years has been remarkably unsuccessful. A concrete example may illustrate this point: a score of at least 16–18 on the Hamilton Depression Scale (M. Hamilton 1960) is generally accepted as a criterion to include someone in a depression study. One could, however, easily obtain such a score with low ratings on items referring to mood, anxiety, guilt feelings, and suicidal ideation and high ratings on items such as sleep disturbances, anxiety equivalents, somatic symptoms, weight loss, and hypochondriasis. By using this criterion, the test group could well consist of a mixture of distressed and depressed people, reducing the chance of finding markers of depression.

How could one approximate a meaningful demarcation between distress and disorder, between the point where normality comes to an end and pathology commences? It is hard to imagine absolute criteria, but even in hard-core somatic medicine those are rare. There is nothing absolute in the agreement that a blood pressure of 120 over 80 is normal, and one of 160 over 110 is pathological. Pathology in this case is defined in terms of diminished life expectancy, that is, an increased risk of being struck by brain, cardiac, and some other disorders.

In the same vein, the transition of mental distress to mental disorder could be defined and operationalized on the basis of prognostic criteria, that is, the risk that a particular behavior or experiential state will lead to vocational or social disability or to a significant and sustained drop in quality of life.

COMPLETENESS OF PSYCHIATRIC DIAGNOSES

Current diagnoses are preferably *based* on phenomena in observable behavior, which may be diagnosed independent of verbal communication and on symptoms unambiguously agreed to upon direct questioning. Diagnoses are preferably *anchored* to etiological variables that leave little room for doubt, such as definite family loading, demonstrable brain lesions, and life events with "absolute" valence, that is, with traumatic impact for the average individual. Diagnoses are preferably *assessed* with so-called objective instruments, that is, instruments that are minimally influenced either by the patient who exhibits the symptoms or by the investigator who registers them.

On the one hand, the move toward greater objectivity in psychiatric diagnosing has been wholesome, contributing as it did to scientification of the diagnostic process. On the other hand, it is responsible for a profound reductionism and coarsening in characterizing psychiatric conditions. The preoccupation with the objective led to neglect of the subjective constituents of the psychopathological spectrum (Van Praag 1992b), such as those that are confined to the patient's experiential world and are not expressed in observable behavior.

Symptoms of this kind escape today's psychometric methods; they are not easily ascertained and measured. Consequently, they are considered to be "soft" and hardly worthy of scientific efforts. This, however, is a prejudice because it is simply not known how diagnostically important subjective psychopathology actually is. Hence, sustained attempts should be made to develop the appropriate psychometric instruments. It seems a priori unlikely that extensive psychopathological domains can be ignored with impunity. Our preliminary data suggest that subjective phenomena might indeed contain significant prognostic and therapeutic information (Van Praag 1992b).

A comprehensive diagnosis of a psychiatric condition requires, furthermore, an assessment of the main etiological determinants. For biological research in psychiatry, this information is indispensable because the pathogenesis of a particular condition might vary with the etiological conditions under which it has emerged. The concept of *pathogenesis* is defined as the complex of cerebral dysfunctions underlying a given psychopathological syndrome, whereas the concept of *etiology* encompasses all variables—biological, psychological, and environmental in nature—that have contributed to that dysfunctional cerebral state.

Particularly the evaluation of life events is unsatisfactory. Axis IV provides an opportunity to assess the pathogenic valence of a psychosocial stressor. According to DSM-III-R, however, the rating should be based on the clinician's assessment of the stress an "average" person in similar circumstances and with similar sociocultural values would experience from the particular psychosocial "stressor" (American Psychiatric Association 1987, p. 19). But the factor personality vulnerability is ignored and only "absolute" events are recorded.

In the future, research in psychiatry will probably be increasingly focused on the sequence: traumatic life events, disruption of brain development and/or brain functioning, then behavioral and experiential disturbances. For such truly psychobiobehavioral research programs, scientific scrutiny of the factor psychogenesis will be indispensable.

HIERARCHICAL ORDERING OF MENTAL DISORDERS IS INCOMPATIBLE WITH EXPERIMENTAL PSYCHIATRY

Psychiatric patients frequently qualify for a number of diagnoses; two or three Axis I and the same number of Axis II diagnoses in the same patient are the rule rather than the exception. How, then, should one interpret a biological disturbance observed in a diagnostically multiform patient? This dilemma is the most fundamental of problems encountered in biological psychiatry today and the principal factor restraining progress in the field. Yet, it does not get the attention it deserves. The three latest editions of the DSM do provide a solution of sorts. The hierarchical principle is adopted. Psychiatric disorders, at least some of them, are rank-ordered according to severity. According to the hierarchical principle, a disorder considered to be more severe takes precedence over one considered to be less severe. For the diagnosis of major depression, psychotic and organic conditions have to be ruled out. The diagnosis of generalized anxiety disorder cannot be made in the presence of a mood disorder.

This principle is not applicable in biological psychiatry. One can and should not simply discard the possibility that a biological variable observed in a psychotic condition is linked to a concurrent depression or that one found in depression is in fact related to a comorbid anxiety disorder. The hierarchical principle is a deus ex machina that resolves the problem of comorbidity only in appearance. *Comorbidity* in itself is merely a descriptive, not an explanatory, term. The multiplicity of psychiatric disorders, as they are presently defined, in so many patients permits a variety of explanations (Van Praag 1996), and thus the term *comorbidity* conceals more than it discloses.

The comorbidity problem may be clarified according to two approaches. The first is restriction of biological studies to those patients who show the syndrome to be studied in a pure form, that is, without admixture of extraneous features. Though we can strive toward that ideal, it is hard to achieve. For that reason, the second approach, complementary to the first, is all-important. It might be called *functional approach* (Van Praag 1990; Van Praag and Leijnse 1965; Van Praag et al. 1975, 1987, 1990). The psychopathological state presented by a given patient is dissected in its component parts, being the various psychological dysfunctions, and biological variables are studied as to linkage to the various dysfunctioning psychological domains. The morass of comorbidly occurring syndromes is thus avoided by relinquishing the concept of discrete and separable disease entities and syndromes. Functional psychopathology has merits more fundamental than the opportunistic one of avoiding the comorbidity labyrinth. Those are discussed in the next two sections.

THREE-TIER DIAGNOSING IN PSYCHIATRY

Diagnosing in psychiatry is generally confined to two tiers: a characterization of the prevailing syndrome(s) and a decision on the best-fitting diagnosis or diagnoses. The third diagnostic level is underdeveloped and mostly disregarded. This tier is arrived at by dissecting the syndrome to its elementary units of psychopathology, that is, the psychological dysfunctions, such as in case of a depression; disturbances in mood, anxiety, and aggression regulation; motoricity; information processing; memory; hedonic functioning; and concentration. Psychiatric symptoms are the manifestation forms of psychological dysfunctions. Functional analysis of a psychiatric syndrome, thus, is fundamentally different from symptom analysis. "Functionalization" of psychiatric diagnoses is important for several reasons. The first is to bypass the comorbidity problem. Second, this approach provides insight in the functional abilities of the patient, that is, which psychological domains are deranged and which are still functioning within normal limits. Functionalization of psychiatric diagnoses, systematically carried out, will ultimately lead to the equivalent of what pathophysiology is for somatic medicine: the discipline providing an understanding of what the deflections in the psychological apparatus are that underlie a particular psychiatric disorder. A third reason of principle to include a third, that is, functional, tier in diagnosing mental disorders is that psychological dysfunctions are measurable, many of them quantitatively. This is not the case with psychiatric syndromes or disorders; they permit at best a qualitative estimate of presence and severity. Functionalism is the obvious way to make psychiatric diagnosing more scientific.

There is a fourth reason to introduce functional analysis as a basic procedure in psychiatric diagnosing, particularly for biological psychiatric research (i.e., it provides the tools to study the scientific merits of the reaction-form model of psychiatric disorders). Nosology has dominated psychiatry since its founding as a scientific discipline by Kraepelin. Psychiatric disorders are regarded as true diseases, that is, discrete entities, each with their own causation, symptomatology, course, and outcome and thus are clearly identifiable. Biological research is aimed at uncovering markers and, ultimately, causes of such diseases.

Mental disorders, however, can be conceived of in a different way, that is, as reaction patterns to noxious stimuli, with considerable interindividual variability and little consistency, rather than as discrete and separable entities (Van Praag 1996). Adolph Meyer (1957), of course, first proposed an outline of such a diagnostic model. The noxious stimulus might be of a biological or psychological nature, could come from within or without, and might be genetically transmitted or acquired during life. Noxious stimuli have in common that an individual cannot cope with them, physically and/or psychologically.

In this model, the symptomatological variability of psychiatric conditions within and between individuals could be understood in the following manner. Noxious stimuli, that is, stimuli an individual is unable to assimilate, will perturb a variety of neuronal circuits and hence a variety of psychological systems. The extent to which the various neuronal circuits will be involved varies individually, and, consequently, psychiatric conditions will lack symptomatological consistency and predictability. For instance, mood lowering is blended with fluctuating measures of anxiety, anger, obsessional thoughts, addictive behavior, cognitive impairment, and psychotic features. The components these psychopathological clusters consist of will vary in intensity and prominence between subjects and, over time, within subjects, so that their appearance is highly variable. According to the reaction-form model, the co-occurrence of various discrete mental disorders is mainly appearance. In fact, we deal with ever-changing composites of psychopathological features. The measure of neuronal disruption a noxious stimulus will induce is, as said, variable, contingent as it is on a number of factors. Most important are the intrinsic qualities of the stimulus and the resilience of the brain. Preexistent neuronal defects may cause certain brain circuits to function marginally. An equilibrium just maintained under normal conditions could fail if demands are increased. Increased vulnerability can also be conceptualized on a psychological level in that imperfections in personality makeup make stimuli the average person can cope with psychologically disruptive.

The reaction-form model, if valid, would have profound consequences for biological psychiatry. The search for markers and, eventually, causes of discrete mental disorders would be largely futile. The furthest one could go is to group the multitude of reaction patterns in a limited number of diagnostic "basins," such as the group of the psychotic, the dementing, and the affective reaction forms, each of which, however, would show considerable heterogeneity. As much as it is futile to search for the antecedents and characteristics of, for instance, the group of abdominal disorders, it would equally lack wisdom to hope for the discovery of, for instance, the pathogenesis of the basin of affective reaction forms. Within the scope of this model, the focus of biological psychiatric research has to shift from the alleged mental "disorders" to disordered psychological domains. Adopting the three-tier diagnostic approach in psychiatry would offer the opportunity to explore the relative merits of both diagnostic viewpoints—the nosological and reaction-form models—for experimental psychiatry.

Two ways, then, could make biological research in psychiatry more diagnostically meaningful: precise definition of the syndromes to be studied and their systematic functional analysis. Methods to carry out such analyses in a sophisticated way should be developed in collaboration with experimental clinical psychologists.

"VERTICALIZATION" OF PSYCHIATRIC DIAGNOSES

A mental disorder is a composite of psychological dysfunctions, mutually interacting in a complex way. The diagnostic weight of the various components is presumably unequal. Some of them are primary, that is, the direct consequence of the underlying cerebral substratum; others are secondary, that is, derivatives of the pathogenetic process. Primary symptoms, as compared with secondary symptoms, are the diagnostically more important. They should be the aim of therapeutic interventions and the target of research into the biology of the disorder.

Since the times of Emil Kraepelin, Eugen Bleuler, and Kurt Schneider, the fundamental distinction between primary and secondary symptoms has received hardly any attention. The reason is not difficult to guess: for want of methods to study the brain, it was virtually impossible to validate the primary/secondary distinction. Thanks to advances in biological psychiatry and psychopathology, that argument is no longer valid. Our studies in mood disorders are a case in point. They led us to the conclusion that a subgroup of depression exists in which serotonergic functioning is demonstrably disturbed and in which anxiety and/or aggression dysregulation are the primary psychopathological features, and mood lowering is a subsidiary. If true, the proper treatment of such depressions, what we have called serotonin-related, anxiety/aggression-driven depressions, would be an anxiolytic and/or "serenic" that ameliorates anxiety and/or aggression via regulation of serotonergic circuits (Van Praag 1992b, 1996). Verticalization of psychiatric diagnoses could fundamentally change the strategy in developing novel psychopharmacological principles. Instead of categorical entities, dysfunctioning psychological domains with a primary channeler would become the focus of attention. I have called this approach *functional psychopharmacology* (Van Praag 1992a).

Attempts to distinguish primary from secondary psychopathological symptoms are an essential exercise for biological psychiatry because only the former are pointers to the biology of a given syndrome, while pathogenetic processes in their turn guide the search for novel therapeutic principles. In present-day psychiatry, the trend is the other way around. We tend to group symptoms horizontally, as if they were all of equal diagnostic weight. It is a priori unlikely that all components of a syndrome are of equal diagnostic importance. It follows that psychiatric diagnosing should once more develop a vertical momentum, and attempts to weigh psychiatric symptoms should be reinstated as a rightful endeavor in scientific psychiatry. Studies of that kind presuppose careful dissection of the prevailing syndrome in its component parts: the psychological dysfunctions. This is another reason that the functional approach should be an integral part of psychiatric diagnosing.

DISCUSSION

Progress in biological psychiatry is contingent on advances in the two founding disciplines, neurobiology and psychopathology. Neurobiology is advancing rapidly, and in this respect the future of biological psychiatry seems assured. At first sight, the bearing power of the second pilar seems also to be on the increase. For, since 1980, with DSM-III, diagnoses are standardized and operationalized, and the impact of this taxonomy on the diagnostic process in psychiatry is tremendous. Diagnosing in psychiatry oftentimes translates into data collection with the objective to meet the DSM-dictated directives. Since 1980, two revised editions of the DSM have appeared; so it seems that we are moving from good to better. The appearance, however, is deceptive. Research into the biological determinants of abnormal behavior exacts particular standards on psychiatric diagnosing and, in this, the present diagnostic philosophy and methodology falls short in many respects. What are the principal shortcomings?

1. Research into the biological determinants of abnormal behavior gets off the track, if the object of study is not precisely defined in terms of manifestation form and not demarcated carefully from related syndromes. The present diagnostic system represents just the opposite, in that most of the diagnostic labels cover a variety of syndromes, only vaguely distinguished from bordering diagnoses.
2. Biological psychiatry, today, aims at elucidation of the biology of disease entities. This intention presumes the validity of those entities, but this premise is disputable. Many of the disease entities presently distinguished seem to represent, at best, basins of a variety of more or less comparable, but in many ways dissimilar, disorders. It is hard to believe that the search for particular brain dysfunctions underlying a diagnostic construct, representing in point of fact a diversity of disorders, stands much chance to score a success.

3. The neo-nosological Zeitgeist permits the authorization of ever more psychiatric disorders, often without sufficient legitimization. Yet they are being studied, as if we deal with genuine disease entities. Not their validity is under scrutiny but, for instance, their biology. Soon sight is lost that the construct actually is hypothetical and that convincing validity data are still to be awaited. The same has happened in psychiatry before. Psychoanalytical theory was raised on a number of brilliant hypotheses, before those were properly substantiated. Edifices thus erected cannot be else than shaky. Validity studies should take precedence above all others in experimental psychiatry.

4. Another urgent requirement for biological psychiatry is that the border between mental illness and mental distress needs to be clearly marked. As an analogy, the distinction between the common cold and tuberculosis is crucial if one set oneself to elucidate the pathogenesis of the latter. In the same vein is the distinction between sorrow and depression crucial in biological studies of depression. Modern psychiatry, however, has shown little interest in this problem.

5. Psychiatric diagnosing cannot afford blind spots. Equal allowance should be made for objective symptoms (those manifest in observable behavior and easily assessable by direct questioning) and for subjective phenomena (symptoms largely confined to the patient's experiential world). In biological psychiatry, the subjective domain has often been minimized as scientifically soft and of marginal diagnostic importance. Neither the one nor the other has been demonstrated. Beforehand, it seems unlikely that substantial domains of psychopathology could be ignored with impunity. Disregard for subjective psychopathology could thus easily diminish the relevance of biological psychiatric research. Methods to incorporate subjective psychopathology within experimental psychiatry are urgently needed (Delespaul 1995).

6. Most psychiatric patients do not meet the criteria of one particular disorder as presently defined, but show signs and symptoms of a multitude of disorders, or rather they display a patchwork of parts of different disorders. This situation faces biological psychiatry with insurmountable problems in determining which of the disorders in a given patient is the behavioral correlate of a particular biological disturbance. The hierarchical principle as applied in the later DSM editions—albeit inconsistently—provides no more than an ostrich solution. The problems of comorbidity do not disappear by concealing them.

   Until the time comes that this thorniest of all problems psychiatry is faced with has been resolved (and attempts to do so should be granted high priority), one cannot do better than to bypass it by adopting a three-tier diagnostic approach: The disorder(s) established in a given patient is (are) characterized; next the syndrome(s) is (are) identified; and finally, the syndrome(s) is (are) dissected in its (their) component parts, that is, the psychological dysfunctions. The latter are being assessed, measured, and studied as to possible relationships with biological variables.

This, what I have called, *functional psychopathological approach* has merits over and above the opportunistic ones I mentioned. Because many psychological dysfunctions are measurable, in contrast to disorders and syndromes, this approach will provide psychopathology with a scientific foundation. Moreover, this psychological "spectral analysis" provides a map of functions still operating within normal limits and those that deviate from the norm.

The third reason to add a third tier to the diagnostic process is that it provides insight in the fundamental abilities of the patients. The fourth reason is the most important. From its inception as a scientific discipline, the nosological model has been, and still is, taken for granted in psychiatry. Psychiatric disorders are viewed as discrete entities, with a fixed and predictable set of attributes and distinguishable from adjacent disorders. Within the framework of this model, biological psychiatry searches for markers and, eventually, causes of true disease entities.

It is possible, however, to view mental pathology from a different angle, that is, as reaction forms to noxious stimuli. The number of reaction forms is limited, but the syndromal variability within each psychopathological basin is large. Much as it seems illogical to hope to once find the pathogenesis of the group of abdominal disorders, it seems promising to search for the biological roots of, for instance, the basin of affective disorders. With the reaction-form model as a starting point, biological research would not be focused on the inherently heterogenous reaction forms, but on the biology of the main psychological domains being perturbed within that basin.

Adopting the three-tier diagnostic system would open the possibility to study the merits of both disease models, the nosological and the reaction-form models, for psychiatry in general and for experimental psychiatry in particular.

7. Finally, in diagnosing psychiatric disorders, systematic attempts should be made to "verticalize" psychopathological symptoms. It is a priori unlikely that all symptoms of a particular syndrome have equal diagnostic weight. It is much more plausible that some are primary, that is, the direct consequences of the brain dysfunctions underlying that syndrome,

whereas others are secondary, that is, derivatives of the pathogenetic processes. Biological psychiatry should target its efforts on the primary phenomena. Attempts to verticalize symptomatology are necessarily preceded by functional analysis of the syndrome. This is another reason why functionalization of psychopathology is so important. The present diagnostic philosophy, however, is attuned otherwise. It favors a horizontal, not a vertical, approach. Symptoms are not weighted but simply displayed on a horizontal plane. This approach reduces the chance of finding meaningful relationships between abnormal brain functions and abnormal behavior.

In short, there are reasons to be concerned about the philosophy and practice of psychiatric diagnosing. In many ways, developments over the past two decades run counter to what I believe to be the diagnostic prerequisites for fruitful biological psychiatric research. I presume this to be a major reason that, so far, biology has made no significant contributions to diagnosing mental disorders.

One edition of the DSM follows the other. Revisions, however, are made within the adopted system. The underlying premises are hardly being discussed. Our diagnostic approach is in danger of becoming prematurely sanctified. This attitude seriously endangers the prospect of biological psychiatry.

SUMMARY

Progress in biological psychiatry is contingent on progress in neurobiology and on research into proper characterization and assessment of abnormal behavior. Advances in neurobiology are rapid and steady; diagnostic research does not keep pace. On the contrary, the diagnostic approach seems solidified, as today's basic premises are uncritically accepted. The diagnostic requirements for meaningful biological psychiatric research are discussed and contrasted with modern diagnostic practices. Psychiatric diagnosis is in need of serious scrutiny.

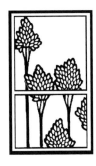

CHAPTER 5

Gender Differences in Treatment of Depression and Anxiety

Kimberly A. Yonkers, M.D.,
Judy C. Kando, Pharm.D.,
Jean A. Hamilton, M.D., and
Uriel Halbreich, M.D.

Depressive and anxiety disorders are common medical illnesses that induce profound personal distress as well as substantial economic costs. The economic burden of depression alone was estimated to be $44 billion in 1990 (Greenberg et al. 1993a). A poorly understood feature of depressive illnesses and selected anxiety disorders is the disproportionate expression of these maladies in women. Thus, not only do depression and anxiety lead to substantial personal morbidity but they disproportionately affect women's health. The most recent estimates of major depression find that approximately 21% of women and 13% of men will experience an episode during their lifetime (Kessler et al. 1994). Although the rates of individual entities of anxiety disorders are less than those of depression for both men and women, the rate for the overall group of anxiety disorders is more substantial. The National Comorbidity Study (NCS) estimates that 20% of men and 30% women are at risk for developing an anxiety disorder (Kessler et al. 1994).

Optimal treatments for both men and women are needed to help ameliorate the personal and community burden of depressive and anxiety disorders. Unfortunately, most available data on the pharmacokinetics of psychotropic agents depended on a male model because women with childbearing capacity were excluded from the early stages of drug testing. In part this occurred because of concerns about the teratogenic potential of drugs, but an additional reason was the desire to increase homogeneity and decrease variance in study samples. This missed opportunity for studying gender differences in the pharmacological treatment of psychiatric disorders should be reversed by recent changes in U.S. Food and Drug Administration regulations that now mandate that all new compounds must be evaluated in various subgroups of the target population (i.e., men, women, and the elderly). Reviews of what is known regarding gender differences in the pharmacokinetics, pharmacodynamics, and efficacy of antidepressants and anxiolytics can help guide future research and analyses in these areas. Given the limitations in data currently available, in this chapter we review the existing literature on gender differences in the pharmacokinetics, pharmacodynamics, and therapeutic efficacy of various antidepressants and anxiolytics.

The pharmacology of a psychotropic drug can be divided into two components: pharmacokinetic parameters and pharmacodynamic properties. Pharmacokinetic parameters quantify factors that lead to the delivery of a drug to its site of action and include aspects of absorption, bioavailability, distribution, metabolism, and elimination. The pharmacodynamic properties of a drug describe its mechanism of action, or in other words, the compound's activity at its receptor site. Pharmacodynamics may also include drug-drug interactions and the behavioral impact of drug administration. It is likely that both the pharmacokinetic and the pharmacodynamic properties contribute to a drug's efficacy. Gender differences in the pharmacodynamic effects of medications may be at least as meaningful as pharmacokinetic effects, especially if therapeutic compounds interact with testosterone, estrogen, or progesterone.

PHARMACOKINETIC PRINCIPLES

A brief review of pharmacokinetic principles will place the available data on gender differences in context. Bioavailability, which refers to the amount of drug eventually reaching the systemic circulation, is influenced by absorption, metabolism in the gastrointestinal tract, and the hepatic first-pass effect. The impact of the first-pass effect is greater for drugs that have high hepatic extractability. After the compound has entered systemic circulation, it is distributed and the degree of distribution is referred to as the volume of distribution. Lipophilic compounds are likely to be disbursed widely, including into the central nervous system (CNS). The compound is then metabolized and eliminated. The greatest degree of metabolism occurs in the liver, although metabolism also occurs in the small intestine, kidneys, and brain. An individual's gender may affect a number of the pharmacokinetic variables mentioned above. This has been addressed in detail by J. A. Hamilton and Yonkers (1996) and in earlier reviews by J. Hamilton and Parry (1983), Skett (1988), K. Wilson (1984), and Yonkers and colleagues (1992) and is summarized in Table 5–1.

Absorption

The degree of a drug's absorption is a component of bioavailability. Most commonly, psychotropic medications are orally ingested and absorbed through the intestinal villus border, where they may undergo a minor degree of metabolism (P. B. Watkins 1992). The delivery of a drug to its site of absorption and the period of time the compound is extant in the intestine can affect the rate and degree of absorption. For example, slower gastric emptying may lead to higher residual gastric volume and slower intestinal absorption (Sellers 1985). On the other hand, slowed motility in the small intestine can facilitate overall drug absorption. At least 10 different studies have evaluated gender differences in the rate of gastric emptying (J. A. Hamilton and Yonkers 1996). It appears that, for solid compounds, gastric emptying is 29%–55% slower in women, and for solids, emptying is 25%–78% slower in

TABLE 5–1. Factors influencing sex-related differences in pharmacokinetics

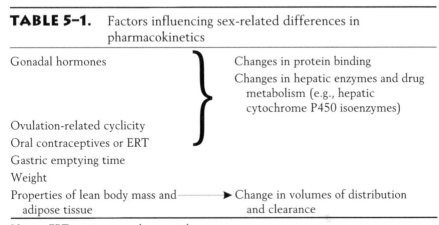

Gonadal hormones	Changes in protein binding
Ovulation-related cyclicity	Changes in hepatic enzymes and drug metabolism (e.g., hepatic cytochrome P450 isoenzymes)
Oral contraceptives or ERT	
Gastric emptying time	
Weight	
Properties of lean body mass and adipose tissue	→ Change in volumes of distribution and clearance

Note. ERT = estrogen replacement therapy.

women (J. A. Hamilton and Yonkers 1996). Less is known about gender differences in intestinal motility. It does appear, however, that oral contraceptives (OCs) lessen the gender difference in gastric emptying at least for liquids (Wedmann et al. 1991).

Gastric acidity will also affect the absorption of medication. An acidic environment increases the absorption of weak acids, whereas the absorption of weak bases is facilitated by a less acidic environment. Many psychotropic agents such as tricyclic antidepressants (TCAs) and benzodiazepines are weak bases. Older studies of gastric acid secretion found that women have approximately 33%–40% lower basal gastric acid secretion than do men (Yonkers and Hamilton 1995). Gastric acid secretion may be further decreased in the luteal phase of the menstrual cycle (Booth et al. 1957).

After the drug is absorbed, it may be taken up by hepatocytes and metabolized, a process that is referred to as the *hepatic first-pass effect*. If the compound is highly extractable, then the amount of drug removed is high and the degree of available drug is lowered. It is not known whether there are gender differences in hepatic blood flow that can influence the extraction rate of some medications.

Antidepressants are generally well absorbed (60%–100%), with the serotonin reuptake inhibitors (SRIs) undergoing more complete absorption (70%–90%) (DeVane 1994), so it is likely that the overall effects resulting from gender differences are relatively small.

Volume of Distribution

The volume of distribution (V_d) is the theoretical volume assumed if the drug concentration is homogeneous throughout the body with the blood concentration (DeVane 1994; Sellers 1985). This assumption is rarely met with psychotropic agents, which tend to be lipophilic, and thus, the V_d is frequently greater than 5 L, the actual volume of blood. Gender differences in the V_d of a medication may arise from the different average size of men and women and the dissimilar percents of lean body mass. The lower percent of lean body mass in women confers higher V_d for lipophilic compounds. Also important are gender differences in blood flow and protein binding. Of concern in psychiatry is the distribution of drug to the CNS. This is higher for more lipophilic compounds, but it is also greater if blood flow to the CNS is more rapid. Some researchers find that blood flow is approximately 15% higher in women than men (Gur et al. 1982), particularly during the second and third decades (M. V. Seeman 1989).

The degree of protein binding is important because this comprises the percentage of unbound drug that is available for pharmacological action. For medications (e.g., TCAs) that are highly protein bound (e.g., 98%–99%) and have a narrow therapeutic index, even a small increase in free drug can lead to a substantial increase in drug effect. Importantly, research suggests that OCs influence drug binding by altering the concentration of a number of binding proteins, including plasma albumin (K. Wilson 1984) and lipoproteins. This effect appears to be more robust with older OCs because chronic use of the lower hormone concentration pills are not associated with alterations in protein binding (Abernethy et al. 1982).

Metabolism and elimination are critical in determining medication blood level and longevity of action. Two main categories of metabolic reactions are phase I reactions and phase II reactions. Phase I reactions are oxidative reactions that involve the cytochrome P450 system, and phase II reactions are conjugative reactions. The rate-limiting step for most compounds occurs through phase I metabolism.

Although a number of important gender differences in the activity of P450 enzymes have been found in animals (Skett 1988), only a few investigations in humans identify reactions that are influenced by an individual's gender or hormonal status. The activity of hepatic P450 IIIA3 and IIIA4 (which share substantial homology and are difficult to differentiate from each other) is higher in women (Hunt et al. 1992). It is not known whether this difference also occurs in the P450 IIIA3/4 enzymes at the intestinal border or in the kidney (P. B. Watkins 1992). On the other hand, P450 IA1 and IA2 are less active in women (Eugster et al. 1993; Guerciolini et al. 1991), and their activity changes across the menstrual cycle (Bruguerolle et al. 1990). The activity of P450 IIC19, which is involved in the metabolism of diazepam as well as the desmethylation of TCAs, and P450 IID6, which metabolizes a number of psychotropics, are inhibited by progestogens (Pollock 1994; P. B. Watkins 1992). A number of these gender-related effects are summarized in Table 5–2.

As mentioned above, oxidative reactions will be rate-limiting in most instances. However, some medications are simply metabolized through conjugation. For example, benzodiazepines such as lorazepam are conjugated and excreted. The rate of conjugative reactions may be increased by OCs accelerating the elimination of these compounds because this reaction is rate-limiting (Yonkers and Hamilton 1995; Stoehr et al. 1984).

Effects of Pregnancy

Ovarian hormones may influence pharmacokinetic parameters, and the physiological state of pregnancy can affect a drug's distribution and metabolism.

TABLE 5–2.   Selected effects of gender and exogenous hormones on hepatic enzyme activity

Enzyme	Women vs men	In vitro effect of exogenous hormones	Substrate	Inhibitor
P450 IA2	↓ in women	Inhibited by β-estradiol, progesterone, and OCs	Caffeine, theophylline, demethylation of TCAs	Fluvoxamine
P450 IIC19	↑ in women	Inhibited by OCs	Diazepam, desmethyl/diazepam, TCAs	Fluoxetine
P450 IID6	↓ in women	Inhibited by OCs	Hydroxylation of nortriptyline and desipramine, haloperidol, clozapine, risperidone, venlafaxine	Fluoxetine, fluvoxamine, paroxetine, sertraline
P450 IIIA3/4	↑ in women	Inhibited by OCs	Demethylation of TCAs, alprazolam, midazolam, triazolam, sertraline	Fluoxetine, sertraline
Glucuronidation conjugation/ sulfation	↑ in women	Accelerated by OCs	Oxazepam, lorazepam, temazepam	Not available

Note.   OCs = oral contraceptives; TCAs = tricyclic antidepressants.

When a woman is pregnant, her plasma volume increases to approximately 6–7 L (approximately 50% over the pregravid state), potentially lowering plasma blood levels. Additionally, there is an increase in cardiac output, which will facilitate the delivery of drug to the kidneys and the ultimate elimination of drug. Elimination is further facilitated by changes in plasma protein binding and an increase in available free drug for renal excretion. On the other hand, there is a suggestion that hepatic metabolic activity is lowered during pregnancy (Mortola 1989). The half-life of caffeine progressively increases during pregnancy, suggesting that the activity of P450 IA2 is being inhibited (Knutti et al. 1981).

PHARMACODYNAMICS

Although little is written about gender differences in the pharmacokinetics of psychopharmacological agents, even less attention has been devoted to the pharmacodynamic aspects of psychotropic medications. A small amount of research using animal models supports the existence of meaningful interactions between sex hormones and antidepressant and anxiolytic activity (Maggi and Perez 1985; K. Wilson 1984). This is probably related to the effect of hormones on neurotransmitter receptors. It has been shown that estrogen decreases the number of 5-hydroxytryptamine subtype 1 (5-HT_1) and β-adrenergic receptors but increases 5-HT_2 receptors in the cortex of rats (Biegon et al. 1983). The effects of ovarian hormones may be important for the downregulation of postsynaptic 5-HT_2 receptors in the cortex of rats because this decline is abolished with castration (Kendall et al. 1981). The influence of ovarian hormones is likely site-specific, depends on the concentration of hormone, and may vary if progesterone is available with estradiol (Maggi and Perez 1985; M. A. Wilson et al. 1989). An interaction between antidepressants and either estradiol or progesterone has been shown in an animal model of depression (Bernardi et al. 1989).

Strong associations between progesterone and its metabolites and anxiolysis have been found (Crawley et al. 1986). Progesterone is metabolized to two anxiolytic compounds, allopregnanolone and deoxycorticosterone, which bind to the γ-aminobutyric acid (GABA)-benzodiazepine receptor site (MacDonald et al. 1991). In studies of animal models, it was found that allopregnanolone increases exploration in the plus-maze test, a measure of anxiolysis (D. Bitran et al. 1993). After exogenous administration in humans, the level of plasma progesterone and its metabolites are correlated with measures of fatigue and immediate recall (E. W. Freeman et al.

1993). Exogenous progesterone and benzodiazepines may have important pharmacodynamic interactions in that cognitive impairment to benzodiazepines may be enhanced with exogenous progesterone (Kroboth et al. 1985; McAuley et al. 1995).

GENDER DIFFERENCES IN ANXIOLYTIC TREATMENTS

Benzodiazepines: Pharmacokinetics

Benzodiazepines are the most commonly used treatment for anxiety disorders. A gender difference in metabolic rates (Table 5–3) has been shown for the metabolism of both chlordiazepoxide and diazepam. The clearance is lower and elimination half-life longer in women compared with men given intravenous chlordiazepoxide (D. J. Greenblatt et al. 1977; R. K. Roberts et al. 1979). When gender differences are evaluated for diazepam metabolism, the total clearance is equivalent in men and women, but the elimination half-life is significantly longer in women. As can be seen in Table 5–4, when women are concurrently given OCs, the elimination half-life for those compounds is extended and clearance is generally decreased.

The pharmacokinetics of benzodiazepines that are hydroxylated, including alprazolam, triazolam, and midazolam, do not differ greatly in young men and young women. However, as can be seen in Table 5–5, the elimination half-life of all three compounds increases if the woman is concurrently using OC agents (Holazo et al. 1988; Scavone et al. 1988; Stoehr et al. 1984). This effect would be predicted because progestogens inhibit P450 IIIA3/4 (Holazo et al. 1988; Kirkwood et al. 1991; R. B. Smith et al. 1983).

Both temazepam and lorazepam undergo glucuronidation. The clearance rates for these compounds are lower in women (Divoll et al. 1981; D. J. Greenblatt et al. 1980; R. B. Smith et al. 1983). This is the direction predicted based on animal models (Skett 1988). OCs have been shown to increase the rate of these reactions, and one would expect the elimination half-lives to be briefer in women who are using OCs. In fact, the elimination half-life does decrease in women who take OCs (Patwardhan et al. 1983; Stoehr et al. 1984).

Benzodiazepines: Pharmacodynamics

There is a suggestion that cognitive impairment resulting from concurrent administration of OCs and benzodiazepines is not simply the result of a

TABLE 5–3. Sex-related effects on the 2-keto subgroup of anxiolytics

Study	Total clearance (mL/min/kg)		Elimination half-life (hour)		Volume of distribution (L/kg)	
	Female	Male	Female	Male	Female	Male
Chlordiazepoxide						
D. J. Greenblatt et al. 1977						
(N = 11 women and 11 men)						
Mean	.37	.59	13.0	7.9	.34	.34
(SD)	(.07)	(.14)	(3.5)	(1.1)	(.04)	(.05)
R. K. Roberts et al. 1979						
(N = 7 women and 7 men)						
Mean	.35	.43	14.8	8.9*	.40	.33
(SD)	(.17)	(.12)	(5.9)	(2.5)	(.14)	(.12)
Diazepam						
D. J. Greenblatt et al. 1980						
(N = 11 women and 11 men)						
Mean	.39	.39	42.4	36	1.73	1.1
(SD)	(.28)	(.18)	(13.5)	(14.5)	(.28)	(2.9)

*Significant to at least $P < .05$.

TABLE 5–4.   Effect of oral contraceptives on chlordiazepoxide and diazepam

Study	Total clearance (mL/min/kg)		Elimination half-life (hour)		Volume of distribution (L/kg)	
	OCs (−)	OCs (+)	OCs (−)	OCs (+)	OCs (−)	OCs (+)
Chlordiazepoxide						
R. K. Roberts et al. 1979						
(N = 11 women and 7 men)						
Mean	.35	.34	14.8	24.3	.4	.62
(SD)	(.17)	(.12)	(5.9)	(12.0)	(.14)	(.23)
Diazepam						
H. G. Giles et al. 1981						
(N = 10 (−) OCs and 5 (+) OCs)						
Mean	.52	.21	40.3	73.8	1.69	1.44
(SD)	(.17)	(.07)	(11.9)	(49.3)	(.28)	(.92)
Abernethy et al. 1982						
(N = 8 (−) OCs and 8 (+) OCs)						
Mean	.45*	.27*	47.0	69.0*	1.57	1.73
(SD)	(.11)	(.06)	(11.3)	(25.5)	(.56)	(.28)

Note. This includes a secondary analysis of published data. (−) OCs = not using oral contraceptives; (+) OCs = using oral contraceptives.
*Significantly different to at least $P = .05$.

TABLE 5–5. Elimination half-life of benzodiazepines undergoing hydroxylation

Study	(–) OCs	(+) OCs
Alprazolam		
Stoehr et al. 1984	9.6	12.4
Scavone et al. 1988	11.9	12.3
Triazolam		
Stoehr et al. 1984	1.9	2.2
Midazolam		
Holazo et al. 1988	1.8	2.9
Lorazepam		
Abernethy et al. 1983	13.1	12.2
Patwardhan et al. 1983	16.5	12.8
Stoehr et al. 1984	14.0	6.0
Temazepam		
Stoehr et al. 1984	13.3	8.0
Oxazepam		
Abernethy et al. 1983	12.1	7.7
Patwardhan et al. 1983	7.6	7.2

Note. (–) OCs = not using oral contraceptives; (+) OCs = using oral contraceptives.

pharmacokinetic effect (Kroboth et al. 1985). Psychomotor impairment is increased in OC users who are administered alprazolam, lorazepam, and triazolam. Of note, changes in plasma concentration do not correlate with performance differences, suggesting that this is not an effect of plasma levels. On the other hand, women who are administered both OCs and temazepam show no increase in psychomotor impairment (Kroboth et al. 1985). It may be that the psychodynamic effect of progesterone on benzodiazepine receptors accounts for at least part of this effect. In a later paper, this same group finds that the oral administration of progesterone worsens performance on memory and psychomotor tasks in women who are also given triazolam (McAuley et al. 1995). Further, the levels of the progesterone metabolite allopregnelalone correlate with the performance impairment.

Anxiolytics: Treatment Efficacy

The results of 40 panic treatment trials conducted between 1975 and 1995 were reviewed. This included studies evaluating TCAs, SRIs, benzodiazepines, anticonvulsants, and propranolol. Three studies report efficacy rates by gender, and two of these reports are case reports of fewer than 15 patients. Because one case series include only one male, results by gender cannot be compared. In an open study of 15 patients treated with desipramine, improvement occurred in 63% of women and 50% of men (Lydiard 1987). An open trial of 50 patients with panic disorder who were treated with clonazepam reported response in 74% of women and 91% of men (Spier et al. 1986). Given the paucity of data on outcome by gender, little can be said about how an individual's gender influences efficacy.

Anxiolytics: Summary

There appear to be gender differences in the pharmacokinetics of selective benzodiazepines such as chlordiazepoxide and diazepam. As would be predicted from studies evaluating the effect of OCs on various P450 enzymes, the levels of hydroxylated and demethylated benzodiazepines are increased in OC users, and the levels of conjugated benzodiazepines are decreased in OC users. Importantly, however, the pharmacokinetic effect may not always predict the impairment on psychomotor and cognitive tasks seen in women who are concurrently given OCs and benzodiazepines.

There is a paucity of data on the efficacy of psychopharmacological treatment by gender. Given the pharmacokinetic differences among men and women found for selected benzodiazepines, this should be evaluated further.

GENDER DIFFERENCES IN ANTIDEPRESSANT TREATMENTS

Tricyclic Antidepressants: Pharmacokinetics

As noted above, the hepatic metabolism of a number of medications shows gender differences in animals. The major pathway for imipramine (IMI) metabolism is demethylation to desipramine (DMI) with inactivation through hydroxylation. The drug is then conjugated and excreted (L. S. Goodman and Gilman 1985). As reviewed by Yonkers and Hamilton (1996), the first step is more rapid in male rodents, but then the second step is less rapid, leading to greater accumulation of desipramine in both plasma and the central nervous system (Skett 1988; M. A. Wilson and Roy 1986). This coincides with evidence that the hydroxylation reaction is more rapid in females (Roskos and Boudinot 1990).

A single study in humans reports clearance and elimination by gender for

IMI (Gram and Christiansen 1975). Unfortunately, this study is limited in that there are only two subjects in each group. Results are consistent with predictions based on animal studies: the half-life for females is 13% higher and the clearance 38% lower than the corresponding results for males. J. A. Hamilton and Grant (1993) tested whether plasma levels are higher in women by applying meta-analysis to all IMI trials ($N = 13$) that include gender-relevant data. In this study, IMI and DMI levels were higher in women by 18% and 12%, respectively. This difference is significant at the $P < .05$ level.

Amitriptyline (AMI) is also demethylated, and this metabolite, nortriptyline, is hydroxylated to one of two enantiomers. It would be expected that AMI would share some of the gender differences found for IMI. Although not all studies found an association (Ziegler and Biggs 1977), one study found that gender differences yield higher plasma levels for older women (Preskorn and Mac 1985). A report evaluating cerebral spinal fluid levels of nortriptyline and height found an association for men but not for women. Interestingly, female gender is a determinant of higher 10-hydroxynortriptyline levels but not nortriptyline levels (Nordin 1993). These findings are consistent with a study that shows that the amitriptyline/nortriptyline ratio is .76 in women and 1.3 in men (Edelbroek et al. 1986).

Several (Gex-Fabry et al. 1990; Nagy and Johansson 1977), but not all (Vazquez-Rodriguez et al. 1991), research groups found that women achieve higher plasma levels of clomipramine. Some evidence shows that the apparent clearance of the hydroxylated metabolites of clomipramine is slower in women (Gex-Fabry et al. 1990).

As with benzodiazepines, some antidepressants interact with OCs. The combination of IMI and OCs increases absolute bioavailability of IMI (Abernethy et al. 1984). Some case reports also support OC-induced changes (Gram and Christiansen 1975). This is likely to be clinically relevant for older, higher dose OCs, which have higher hormonal content. It is important to emphasize that the above review pertains to plasma levels of drug rather than CNS drug levels. However, animal models show a high degree of correlation between brain and plasma levels (M. A. Wilson and Roy 1984).

Nontricyclic Antidepressants: Pharmacokinetics

Gender-related effects have been evaluated for trazodone, and clearance is lower for elderly men compared with elderly women (D. J. Greenblatt et al. 1987). Differences exist in the metabolic rate of the SRI sertraline (Warrington 1991). The effect of OCs on the pharmacokinetics of SRIs or other new agents has not been examined. Differences in plasma levels have little clinical relevancy for this group of compounds because these differences are not related to efficacy.

Antidepressants: Pharmacodynamics and Treatment Efficacy

Only a few small studies evaluate what might be considered gender-related pharmacodynamic responses to antidepressant agents. In one study, the effects of a monoamine oxidase inhibitor (MAOI) were compared with those of an amphetamine in men and women (J. A. Hamilton et al. 1984). Men showed a negative correlation between changes in anxiety and changes in activation with clorgiline. When amphetamine was administered, only women experienced an increase in anxiety correlating with an increase in dysphoria. Another study found that postmenopausal women experience dysphoria when administered amphetamine, whereas young men become euphoric (Halbreich et al. 1981).

Possible psychodynamic effects are inferred by studies comparing men to women in their response to psychopharmacological treatments. In an older study, the efficacy of TCAs was compared with that of MAOIs in depressed men and women. Women with panic attacks had a more favorable response to MAOIs, whereas men who were depressed and had panic preferentially responded to TCAs (Davidson and Pelton 1986). In partial support of this is a reanalysis by Raskin (1974), who investigated gender-related effects in antidepressant treatment. In this reanalysis the response rate to IMI was lower in young women compared with older women and men. Thus, older data in smaller samples suggest that women have a slightly lower response to TCAs than men have.

An analysis investigating gender differences in treatment response to paroxetine was conducted from pooled results of six multicenter placebo-controlled clinical trials. IMI was the comparator drug in this analysis. Both men and women treated with IMI were more likely to show 50% improvement on the Hamilton Rating Scale for Depression (HRS-D; M. Hamilton 1960) compared with men and women given placebo. When the authors analyzed the change in HRS-D scores, they found that the change was greatest for women treated with paroxetine, and the change was significantly greater than the change found with either placebo or IMI. In addition, the change secondary to paroxetine was greater for women than for men.

A recently conducted study compared the efficacy of IMI to that of sertraline in patients with double depression and chronic depression. After

12 weeks of treatment, 73% of men responded either fully or partially to IMI. The corresponding rate in women was 55%. When the response rates for both men and women who were treated with sertraline were compared, they were found to be nearly equivalent, with 59% of men and 61% of women responding to sertraline (Kornstein et al. 1995). Data from the study were also analyzed with reference to premenopausal versus postmenopausal status. There was a trend for postmenopausal women to have a superior response compared with the response of premenopausal women when the treatment was IMI (Schatzberg et al. 1995).

Results from two large multicenter trials evaluating SRIs for the treatment of dysthymia were similar to those found above (M. Steiner, personal communication, December 1995; Halbreich et al., in press). In a study evaluating the efficacy of sertraline versus that of IMI and placebo for the treatment of dysthymia, women were again found more likely to respond to sertraline than to either IMI or placebo. Similarly, dysthymic women treated with paroxetine were more likely to respond using a definition of 50% decrease in the HRS-D. In this latter case, 54% of women treated with paroxetine responded compared with 21% of women treated with placebo, whereas 30% of men in either treatment cell responded (M. Steiner, personal communication, December 1995).

Antidepressants: Summary

Among the various antidepressants, TCAs appear to have a different metabolic profile in women compared with that in men. This is potentially clinically important because TCA levels are linked with response and toxicity. OCs have been shown to inhibit selected P450 isoenzymes and may further increase TCA levels. This is more meaningful for the older, higher-dose OCs rather than the newer agents.

Accumulating data comparing response rates in men and women given either SRIs or TCAs show that women preferentially respond to SRIs. Although it is possible that this is a pharmacokinetic effect, one would argue that it is more likely to be a pharmacodynamic effect because plasma blood levels of SRIs are not linked to response.

SUMMARY

Evaluations of gender differences in the pharmacokinetics, pharmacodynamics, and response to treatment for anxiolytics and antidepressants are sparse. Although a number of factors contribute to this, a small amount of data supports the existence of meaningful clinical differences. The new data suggesting a superior response among women to SRIs are exciting. Further investigations may allow us to optimize pharmacotherapy for both men and women and may help us to discover some of the biological sources underlying gender differences in the prevalence of these illnesses.

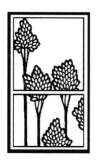

SECTION II

Mood Stabilizers

Robert M. Post, M.D., Section Editor

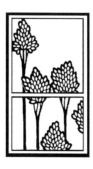

CHAPTER 6

Carbamazepine and Nimodipine in Refractory Bipolar Illness: Efficacy and Mechanisms

Robert M. Post, M.D.,
Peggy J. Pazzaglia, M.D.,
Terence A. Ketter, M.D.,
Kirk Denicoff, M.D.,
Susan R. B. Weiss, Ph.D.,
Chris Hough, Ph.D.,
De-Maw Chuang, Ph.D.,
Robyn Stein, M.D., and
Mark Frye, M.D.

Carbamazepine is increasingly recognized as an effective treatment for bipolar affective illness, whereas the data on nimodipine and related calcium channel blockers (CCBs) are much more preliminary. In this chapter, we review data on the efficacy and putative mechanisms of action of carbamazepine and nimodipine in the recurrent affective disorders.

EFFICACY AND MECHANISMS OF CARBAMAZEPINE

Carbamazepine and Mania

Considerable evidence supports the acute antimanic efficacy of carbamazepine as summarized in Tables 6–1A and 6–1B. At least 19 double-blind trials using a variety of methodologies have documented therapeutic response in some 60% or more of patients with mania. Four of these 19 studies indicate a comparable time course of carbamazepine antimanic responsivity compared with that of neuroleptics, with two studies (D. Brown et al. 1989; Emrich 1990) reporting slightly faster onset for neuroleptics. In our study (Post et al. 1987), responses were often reconfirmed on a blind basis following placebo discontinuation with good initial responders reresponding to reinstitution of carbamazepine treatment ($n = 8$) (Figure 6–1). Overall, the magnitude, incidence, and general time frame of response were comparable in most studies, and several (Emrich 1990; Okuma et al. 1979) reported that carbamazepine (or oxcarbazepine) was better tolerated than neuroleptics.

These findings are of considerable interest given that carbamazepine, unlike neuroleptics, does not block dopamine receptors (Post et al. 1986b). However, carbamazepine is capable of blocking dopamine turnover (Post et al. 1986b; Waldmeier 1987); decreasing cocaine-induced dopamine overflow in the nucleus accumbens, as measured by in vivo dialysis (Baptista et al. 1993); and affecting dopaminergic mechanisms in the frontal cortex (Baf et al. 1994; Elphick 1989b). Whatever the contribution of these dopaminergic mechanisms is to the psychotropic profile of carbamazepine, it is clear that carbamazepine does not block D_2 receptors in the striatum, which have been closely linked to the development of extrapyramidal side effects and tardive dyskinesia with typical neuroleptics.

As such, carbamazepine, along with the other mood-stabilizing anticonvulsant valproate, may play an important role as an alternative to neuroleptic augmentation for patients breaking through lithium therapy. This is of great clinical importance from several different perspectives. Neuroleptics may be dysphorogenic and are associated with their own range of acute and long-term neurological side effects such as akathisia, which many patients find uncomfortable. Moreover, Sernyak et al. (1994) described a dependency in which patients acutely treated with neuroleptics continued to use them on long-term maintenance. This possibility, together with the loss of an opportunity to evaluate acute responsivity with an alternative mood-stabilizing agent (if a neuroleptic is chosen as the initial augmentation therapy), leaves the patient at a disadvantage for finding optimal adjunctive mood-stabilizing treatment for long-term prophylaxis, should the patient continue to have breakthrough episodes on lithium.

Long-Term Efficacy of Carbamazepine

The data supporting the long-term efficacy of carbamazepine are strong and substantial in some respects, but controversial and lacking definitive confirmation in others. As outlined in Table 6–2, a group of studies present data on carbamazepine prophylaxis with some degree of control in terms of randomization or blindness. With a few exceptions (Bellaire et al. 1990; Elphick et al. 1988; Placidi et al. 1986), most studies reported carbamazepine to be of equal efficacy compared with that of lithium. The response rate in these double-blind or partially controlled studies is also similar to the rate reported in the larger open literature.

These studies are further supplemented by a variety of other methodologies, including on-off-on (A-B-A) designs, which confirm response in individual patients with a considerable degree of certainty. The mirror-image design approach provides evidence that patients who were showing a substantial, if not accelerating, illness morbidity have been adequately treated with carbamazepine alone or as an augmentation strategy (Post et al. 1990) (Figure 6–2). These design strategies, which augment the more traditional parallel-group designs, have been cited by Prien and Gelenberg (1989) in their review as the most convincing, as many other parallel design studies were noted to have methodological flaws.

Loss of Efficacy of Carbamazepine

In some instances, responses to carbamazepine have persisted for long periods of time. Particularly with deterioration of illness, as evidenced by an accelerating course of illness before treatment, there is some tendency for loss of efficacy (perhaps via tolerance) to occur (Post 1990a, 1990b) (Figure 6–3, top). Loss of efficacy has also been observed during lithium (M. Maj et al. 1989; Post et al. 1993b) and valproate (Post et al. 1993a) administration and appears to be a general problem requiring systematic clinical study into the precipitating factors, underlying mechanisms, treatment approaches, and algorithms associated with its occurrence. In refractory affective illness, we conceptualize that the development of treatment resistance to initially effective long-term prophylactic treatments may be subject to systematic clinical and molecular exploration similar to the development of multidrug resistance in the cancer chemotherapies. Some of the molecular events involved in

TABLE 6-1A.   Controlled studies of carbamazepine and oxcarbazepine

Study	N[a]	Diagnosis	Design	Daily dose (blood level)
Ballenger and Post 1978; Post et al. 1984, 1987	19 CBZ, 19 placebo	Manic	DB (B-A-B-A) randomized	600–2,000 mg CBZ (8–12 µg/mL)
Okuma et al. 1979	30 CBZ, 25 CPZ	Manic	DB vs CPZ randomized	300–900 mg CBZ (2.7–11.7 µg/mL [mean, 7.2 ± 3.4]) 150–450 mg CPZ (3.6–311.4 µg/mL)
Grossi et al. 1984	15 CBZ, 17 CPZ	Manic	DB vs CPZ randomized	200–1,200 mg CBZ [mean, 655.5 ± 295.5] 200–800 mg CPZ [mean, 362.5 ± 166.83]
E. Klein et al. 1984a	23 CBZ, 20 placebo	Manic/ excited S/SA	DB vs placebo addition to HAL randomized	600–1,200 mg CBZ (8–12 µg/mL)
A. A. Muller and Stoll 1984	10 OXCBZ, 10 HAL	Manic	DB vs HAL randomized	900–1,200 mg OXCBZ 15–20 mg HAL
Goncalves and Stoll 1985	6 CBZ, 6 placebo	Manic SA	DB vs placebo randomized	200–1,200 mg CBZ
Emrich et al. 1985	7 OXCBZ, 5 placebo	Manic psychosis	DB (B-A-B)	1,800–2,100 mg [max dosage range] OXCBZ
Lenzi et al. 1986	11 CBZ, 11 Li	Excitation psychosis	DB vs Li randomized	400–1,600 mg CBZ (7–12 µg/mL) 300–900 mg Li (0.6–1.2 mEq/L)
K. D. Stoll et al. 1986	14 CBZ, 18 HAL	Manic	Randomized vs HAL	600–1,200 mg CBZ 5–30 mg HAL

Note.   B-A-B = off-on-off; BMS = Bipolar Manic Scale; BPRS = Brief Psychiatric Rating Scale (Overall and Gorham 1962); BRMS = Bech-Raefelson Mania Scale (Bech et al. 1979); Bunney-Hamburg = Bunney-Hamburg Rating Scale (Bunney and Hamburg 1963); CBZ = carbamazepine; CGI = Clinical Global Impressions scale (Guy 1976); CPRG = Clinical Psychopharmacology Group rating scale for mania (R. Takahashi et al. 1975); CPZ = chlorpromazine; DB = double-blind; EPS = extrapyramidal side effect; GMS = Global Mania Scale; HAL = haloperidol; HS = at night (for sleep);

in acute mania

Other drugs	Duration	Outcome measures	Results
None	11–56 days	Bunney-Hamburg BPRS	12/19 (63%) improved time-course similar to neuroleptics; frequent relapses on placebo substitution
Bedtime hypnotics	3–5 weeks	CPRG	21/30 (70%) improved on CBZ 15/25 (60%) improved on CPZ (moderate to marked) Fewer side effects on CBZ Slightly faster onset with CBZ
Bedtime hypnotics	3 weeks	MSRS BMS	10/15 (67%) improved on CBZ 10/17 (59%) improved on CPZ (moderate to marked) Fewer side effects with CBZ than with CPZ Slightly faster onset with CBZ
HAL, 15–45 mg, all patients	5 weeks	BPRS CGI	13/23 (57%) showed BPRS improvement on CBZ + HAL 11/20 (55%) showed BPRS improvement on placebo + HAL Improvement in CGI in both groups
HAL and hypnotics	2 weeks	BRMS	BRMS scores decreased in both groups Onset faster with OXCBZ
HAL and hypnotics	3 weeks	MS-M	6/6 CBZ better than placebo ($P < .01$)
None	Variable	IMPS	6/7 (86%) improved with OXCBZ (> 25% improvement on IMPS)
CPZ, all patients	19 days average	BPRS CGI	Significant improvement with CBZ and Li on CGI and BPRS CBZ group required less CPZ CBZ produced less paranoia and fewer EPSs
Neuroleptics and hypnotics	3 weeks	MS-M	12/14 (86%) improved on CBZ 12/18 (67%) improved on HAL (good to very good)

Note (continued). IMPS = Inpatient Multidimension Rating Scale (Lorr et al. 1962); Li = lithium; MS-M = Murphy Scale for Mania (D. L. Murphy et al. 1974a); MSRS = Beigel-Murphy State Rating Scale (Beigel and Murphy 1971); OXCBZ = oxcarbazepine; PMS = Petterson Mania Scale (Petterson et al. 1973); S = schizophrenic; SA = schizoaffective; SDMS-D&M = Manic subsection of the Depression & Mania Scale (Raskin et al. 1969); YMS = Young Mania Scale (Young et al. 1978). [a]Total number of subjects who completed study and were used for analysis.

(continued)

TABLE 6-1A. Controlled studies of carbamazepine and oxcarbazepine

Study	N^a	Diagnosis	Design	Daily dose (blood level)
Desai et al. 1987	5 CBZ, 5 placebo	Manic	DB vs placebo addition to Li randomized	400 mg fixed dose CBZ
Lerer et al. 1987	14 CBZ, 14 Li	Manic	DB vs Li randomized	600–2,600 mg CBZ (3.2–14 µg/mL) 900–3,900 mg Li (0.2–2.0 mEq/L)
Lusznat et al. 1988	22 CBZ, 22 Li	Manic/ hypo- manic	DB vs Li randomized	200 mg CBZ until serum level reached (6–12 µg/mL) 400 mg Li until serum level reached (0.6–1.4 mmol/L)
Okuma et al. 1988	72 CBZ, 75 placebo	Manic/ excited S/ SA	DB vs placebo	600 mg CBZ (mean ±SD = 586 ±178 mg)
D. Brown et al. 1989	8 CBZ, 9 HAL	Manic	DB vs HAL randomized	400–1,600 mg CBZ 20–80 mg HAL
Moller et al. 1989	11 CBZ, 9 placebo	Manic or SA	DB vs placebo	600 mg CBZ
Emrich 1990	19 OXCBZ, 19 HAL	Manic	DB vs HAL	2,400 mg mean dose OXCBZ 42 mg mean dose HAL
Emrich 1990	28 OXCBZ, 24 Li	Manic	DB vs Li	1,400 mg mean dose OXCBZ

Note. B-A-B = off-on-off; BMS = Bipolar Manic Scale; BPRS = Brief Psychiatric Rating Scale (Overall and Gorham 1962); BRMS = Bech-Raefelson Mania Scale (Bech et al. 1979); Bunney-Hamburg = Bunney-Hamburg Rating Scale (Bunney and Hamburg 1963); CBZ = carbamazepine; CGI = Clinical Global Impressions scale (Guy 1976); CPRG = Clinical Psychopharmacology Group rating scale for mania (R. Takahashi et al. 1975); CPZ = chlorpromazine; DB = double-blind; EPS = extrapyramidal side effect; GMS = Global Mania Scale; HAL = haloperidol; HS = at night (for sleep);

in acute mania *(continued)*

Other drugs	Duration	Outcome measures	Results
Li, all patients (0.5–1.7 mEq/L)	4 weeks	BRMS GMS	CBZ + Li produced better BRMS and GMS scores than Li alone ($P < .05$)
Chloral hydrate Barbiturates HS	4 weeks	CGI BPRS MSRS	4/14 (29%) improved CGI score on CBZ ($P < .05$) 11/14 (79%) improved CGI score on Li BPRS and MSRS scores improved with both CBZ and Li, nonsignificantly
CPZ, HAL, neuro-leptics	6 weeks	BRMS	No significant differences
Neuro-leptics	4 weeks	Global improve-ment rate	48% global improvement rate on CBZ 30% global improvement rate on placebo (moderate to marked)
CPZ	4 weeks	YMS PMS	6/8 (75%) showed marked improvement on CBZ 3/9 (33%) showed marked improvement on HAL CBZ had slower onset, higher completion rate (75% vs 22%), fewer EPS
HAL 24 mg, all patients Levomepro-mazine	3 weeks	BRMS BPRS MS-M	Both groups showed highly significant antimanic effect on all scales No significant difference between groups CBZ group needed less levomepromazine
Unknown	15 days	BRMS	Both groups had significantly lowered BRMS score Side effects were $3\frac{1}{2}$ times greater in HAL group
Unknown	15 days	BRMS	Both groups had significantly lowered BRMS score Side effects slightly higher in OXCBZ group

Note (continued). IMPS = Inpatient Multidimension Rating Scale (Lorr et al. 1962); Li = lithium; MS-M = Murphy Scale for Mania (D. L. Murphy et al. 1974a); MSRS = Beigel-Murphy State Rating Scale (Beigel and Murphy 1971); OXCBZ = oxcarbazepine; PMS = Petterson Mania Scale (Petterson et al. 1973); S = schizophrenic; SA = schizoaffective; SDMS-D&M = Manic subsection of the Depression & Mania Scale (Raskin et al. 1969); YMS = Young Mania Scale (Young et al. 1978).
[a]Total number of subjects who completed study and were used for analysis.

(continued)

TABLE 6–1A.   Controlled studies of carbamazepine and oxcarbazepine

Study	N[a]	Diagnosis	Design	Daily dose (blood level)
Okuma et al. 1990	50 CBZ, 51 Li	Manic	DB vs Li	400–1,200 mg CBZ [mean, 7.3 µg/mL] 400–1,200 mg Li [mean, 0.46 mEq/L]
J. G. Small et al. 1991	24 CBZ, 24 Li	Manic	DB vs Li randomized	700–1,036 mg CBZ [30–37 µmol/L] 1,035–1,278 mg Li [0.6–0.9 mmol/L]
Total of all 19 studies	324 patients on CBZ 64 patients on OXCBZ 146 patients on Li 98 patients on neuroleptics 139 patients on placebo			

Note.   B-A-B = off-on-off; BMS = Bipolar Manic Scale; BPRS = Brief Psychiatric Rating Scale (Overall and Gorham 1962); BRMS = Bech-Raefelson Mania Scale (Bech et al. 1979); Bunney-Hamburg = Bunney-Hamburg Rating Scale (Bunney and Hamburg 1963); CBZ = carbamazepine; CGI = Clinical Global Impressions scale (Guy 1976); CPRG = Clinical Psychopharmacology Group rating scale for mania (R. Takahashi et al. 1975); CPZ = chlorpromazine; DB = double-blind; EPS = extrapyramidal side effect; GMS = Global Mania Scale; HAL = haloperidol; HS = at night (for sleep);

multidrug resistance have now been identified, such as the induction of the P-glycoprotein (Kiwit et al. 1994), and various techniques (using CCBs and more direct molecular targeting) have been used in attempting to suppress resistance (T. P. Miller et al. 1991).

Mechanism of tolerance.   The molecular events involved in the development of tolerance to carbamazepine have not been clearly identified. However, in a preclinical animal model using amygdala-kindled seizures, S. R. B. Weiss and colleagues (1995) in our laboratory have found that the variety of seizure-induced adaptive changes that usually emerge following seizures fail to do so with development of tolerance to the anticonvulsant effects of carbamazepine. The loss of these adaptive changes, such as increases in in acute mania *(continued)*

Other drugs	Duration	Outcome measures	Results
Neuroleptics, bedtime hypnotics	4 weeks	CPRG	31/50 (62%) improved on CBZ 30/51 (59%) improved on Li No significant difference between groups CBZ had earlier onset, more EPS
Hypnotics	6–8 weeks	SDMS-D&M YMS BPRS CGI	8/24 (33%) improved on CBZ 8/24 (33%) improved on Li No significant difference between groups after 8 weeks 123/203 (61%) improved on CBZ 6/7 (86%) improved on OXCBZ 49/89 (55%) improved on Li 51/89 (57%) improved on neuroleptics

Note (continued).   IMPS = Inpatient Multidimension Rating Scale (Lorr et al. 1962); Li = lithium; MS-M = Murphy Scale for Mania (D. L. Murphy et al. 1974a); MSRS = Beigel-Murphy State Rating Scale (Beigel and Murphy 1971); OXCBZ = oxcarbazepine; PMS = Petterson Mania Scale (Petterson et al. 1973); S = schizophrenic; SA = schizoaffective; SDMS-D&M = Manic subsection of the Depression & Mania Scale (Raskin et al. 1969); YMS = Young Mania Scale (Young et al. 1978).
[a]Total number of subjects who completed study and were used for analysis.

thyrotropin-releasing hormone (TRH) (J. B. Rosen et al. 1994), neuropeptide Y, and γ-aminobutyric acid $(GABA)_A$ receptors (M. Clark et al. 1994), which could be conceptualized as inhibitory endogenous anticonvulsant principles or processes, could be important to the loss of efficacy of carbamazepine, at least in the preclinical animal model (Figure 6–3, bottom). If animals are taken off the drug, or even if they are continued on the drug but the drug is administered after each seizure has occurred, that is, the seizures occur in the absence of drug, the adaptive changes may be reinduced, and there is an associated renewal of anticonvulsant efficacy (S. R. B. Weiss et al. 1995).

Approaches to treatment resistance via tolerance.   Whether similar principles could be used in the treatment of the development of treatment resis-

TABLE 6–1B.   Carbamazepine and oxcarbazepine in acute mania: 19 double-blind studies

Placebo–active placebo
  Ballenger and Post et al. 1978; Post et al. 1987
  Emrich et al. 1985 (OXCBZ)
vs placebo
  Okuma et al. 1988
  Goncalves and Stoll 1985
vs placebo as adjunct
  E. Klein et al. 1984a (+ HAL)
  Desai et al. 1987 (+ Li)
  Moller et al. 1989 (+ HAL)
vs neuroleptics
  Okuma et al. 1979 (CPZ)
  A. A. Muller and Stoll 1984 (OXCBZ vs HAL)
  Grossi et al. 1984 (CPZ)
  K. D. Stoll et al. 1986 (HAL)
  D. Brown et al. 1989 (HAL)
  Emrich 1990 (OXCBZ vs HAL)
vs lithium
  Lenzi et al. 1986
  Lerer et al. 1987
  Lusznat et al. 1988
  Okuma et al. 1990
  J. G. Small et al. 1991
  Emrich 1990 (OXCBZ)

Summary: > 355 patients on CBZ; marked to excellent response in 123/203 (61%)

Note.   CBZ = carbamazepine; CPZ = chlorpromazine; HAL = haloperidol; Li = lithium; OXCBZ = oxcarbazepine.

tance to carbamazepine in the long-term prophylaxis of bipolar disorder remains to be discerned in systematic clinical trials. However, it is of interest that several clinical studies support the proposition that a period of time off medications in the face of treatment resistance development may be associated with the renewal of responsivity (Pazzaglia and Post 1992; Post et al. 1993c). Possible illness emergence before renewal of responsivity may occur during the medication-free period and might be avoided by switching from one class of drugs to another class that does not demonstrate cross-tolerance as a preferential alternative.

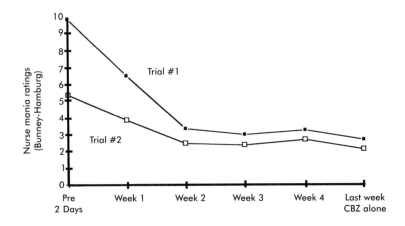

FIGURE 6-1.   Graph showing reconfirmation of antimanic response to carbamazepine (CBZ) in two trials following placebo discontinuation. Patients were less severely ill at baseline in the second trial because active treatment was reinstituted more rapidly. Mania ratings on the Bunney-Hamburg Scale (Bunney and Hamburg 1963) were reduced in each of the two trials (*N* = 8).

Cross-tolerance between carbamazepine and valproate has been observed in the contingent tolerance model to anticonvulsant effects on amygdala-kindled seizures (S. R. B. Weiss et al. 1993). In this instance, the loss of $GABA_A$ receptors, which is selective for the α-4 subunit of the $GABA_A$ receptor (M. Clark et al. 1994), may be sufficient to render valproate ineffective in light of its putative actions on this system (Higuchi et al. 1986; Nagaki et al. 1990). However, cross-tolerance may or may not occur between these drugs in bipolar disorder, as they may cross-adapt some mechanisms (e.g., GABA) but not others (adenosine and peripheral-type benzodiazepine receptors). There is a lack of cross-tolerance between carbamazepine and drugs such as diazepam and clonazepam that are active at central-type benzodiazepine receptors (C. K. Kim et al. 1992; S. R. B. Weiss et al. 1995), suggesting their possible use as an augmentation strategy.

The use of combination therapy with carbamazepine and valproate (Keck et al. 1992b; Ketter et al. 1992) may also be helpful in avoiding or delaying the development of episodic breakthroughs progressing toward tolerance. We have observed that many animals show cyclic response to the anticonvulsants while they are progressing toward the development of complete loss of efficacy via tolerance (Post and Weiss 1996). If doses of

TABLE 6–2.   Controlled and partially controlled studies of carbamazepine and oxcarbazepine prophylaxis in affective illness

Investigators	Design	Placebo	CBZ		Lithium	
			Responders	% Response	Responders	% Response
Ballenger and Post 1978	DB, M		6/7	86	—	—
Post et al. 1983						
Okuma et al. 1981	DB	2/9	6/10	60	—	—
Svestka et al. 1985	R		14/24	62	12/24	50
A. Kishimoto and Okuma 1986	C		?/18	↓ # hosp vs Li	—	—
Cabrera et al. 1986[a]	R		2/4	50	3/6	50
Placidi et al. 1986	DB, R		21/29	72	20/27	74
S. E. Watkins et al. 1987	DB, R		16/19	84	15/18	83
Elphick et al. 1988	DB, R		3/8	37	8/11	73
Lusznat et al. 1988	DB, R		?/9	Fewer depressions	?/5	—
Bellaire et al. 1990	R		34/40	85	42/49	86
Di Costanzo and Schifano 1991	R[b]		?/16	Li + CBZ fewer episodes than Li alone	?/16	—
Mosolov 1991	R		?/30	Episodes ↓58%	?/30	Episodes ↓54%
Coxhead et al. 1992	DB, R		7/15	47	7/16	44
Denicoff et al. 1997	DB, R		11/35	31	14/42	33
Greil et al. 1997a	R		23/43	53	43/60	72
Greil et al. 1997b	R		15/32	47	16/37	43
Wolf et al. 1997	DB, R		59/84	70	59/84	70
All controlled studies			217/350	62	239/374	64

Note.   C = crossover; CBZ = carbamazepine; DB = double-blind; Li = lithium; M = mirror image; R = randomized; — = not applicable;
? = unknown. [a]Oxcarbazepine. [b]Pseudorandomized to Li versus CBZ and Li; greater antimanic and antidepressant efficacy in first year versus Li alone.

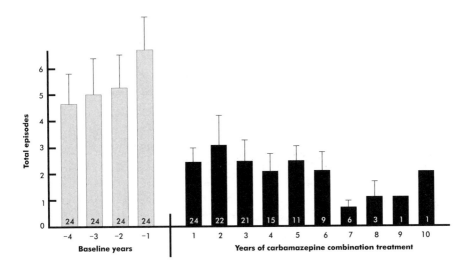

FIGURE 6-2. Graph showing sustained prophylactic efficacy of carbamazepine combination treatment in patients ($N = 24$) with increasing primary affective illness morbidity before institution of treatment. Numbers within bars are numbers of patients.

carbamazepine and valproate (each of which is associated with the loss of efficacy via tolerance within a relatively rapid time course) are used in combination, the development of tolerance is markedly slowed (X. L. Li et al., unpublished observations, September 1987). Again, whether this would be the case in clinical situations remains to be delineated.

L-TYPE CALCIUM CHANNEL BLOCKERS

Controlled and uncontrolled or open studies of the CCBs in affective illness are reviewed in Table 6–3. Initial open and blind studies of the phenylalkylamine L-type CCB verapamil were positive in the affective disorders, particularly in the treatment of acute mania. However, some preliminary controlled data are negative (Janicak et al. 1998); these data are highly subject to a type II error with the design used, the relatively small numbers of patients randomly selected for verapamil and placebo, and the associated relatively high placebo response rate in acute mania observed in many controlled studies

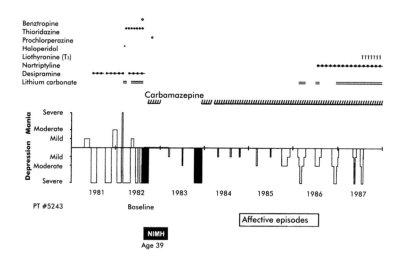

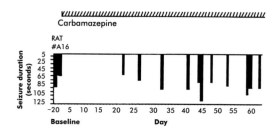

FIGURE 6-3.   *(Top)* Life chart of a patient with affective disorder showing a progressive loss of efficacy of carbamazepine. *(Bottom)* Preclinical data showing progressive loss of efficacy of carbamazepine in an amygdala-kindled rat.

of this type (Bowden et al. 1994b). Bowden et al. (1994b) had to use substantial sample sizes to demonstrate significant effects of valproate compared with those of placebo. Also, in this analysis (Bowden et al. 1994b), the effect of lithium versus placebo on the manic syndrome was nonsignificant, presumably because of the smaller number of patients randomly selected to that arm compared with the other groups. Thus, this largest controlled study of lithium in acute mania to date illustrates the perils of the use of this type of parallel design in initial or exploratory studies of the potential efficacy of psychotropic agents in acute mania or depressive syndromes.

To help avoid these study design confounds, we have used other statistical designs such as mirror-image strategies and B-A-B-A (off-on-off-on) designs. These designs are subject to statistical verification within individual subjects and reconfirmation of responsivity by the appropriate mood assessments in different phases of active treatment. Thus, once efficacy has been established in a subgroup of patients, clinical focus can shift rapidly from demonstration of acute efficacy to determination of whether a subgroup of patients with specific clinical or biological markers predicts this response. Although these strategies are not widely used in the psychiatric community, and have been criticized, they would appear to markedly accelerate the potential development of new agents, bringing them into a focus for clinical therapeutics. That is, once efficacy has been unequivocally established in a small group of well-characterized individuals studied with systematic blind designs, the percentage response rate and identification of potential clinical and biological markers of response can then be ascertained in other designs:

> Once a true process or effect has been established as having occurred in one person it can reasonably be assumed, or inferred, that there will be other persons as well in which the process or effect will occur. (Chassen 1992, p. 177)

Moreover, for patients who show a wide range of cycle frequencies (as is typical for bipolar illness), this strategy is likely to avoid many of the pitfalls associated with a high rate of "placebo" response, actually attributable to the natural course of illness and highly predictable on the basis of systematic retrospective and prospective life charting (Post et al. 1988; Squillace et al. 1984).

We have adopted such a strategy in the exploration of the psychotropic and antimanic effects of the dihydropyridine L-type CCB nimodipine in patients with rapid, ultrarapid, and ultra-ultrarapid (or *ultradian*) cycling bipolar illness. Nimodipine has important differences from verapamil and diltiazem in pharmacokinetics (better central nervous system [CNS] entry [D. D. Freedman and Waters 1987] and fewer drug interactions [Ketter et al. 1995]) and a host of biochemical and pharmacological differences (Table 6–4). In the initial work of Pazzaglia et al. (1993), response in five of nine patients in the group evaluated was, in many instances, reconfirmed in a B-A-B-A design. A total of 10 of 30 (30%) patients responded to blind nimodipine monotherapy (Pazzaglia et al. 1998). P. J. Goodnick (1995) has also reported positive nimodipine response with open trials in two patients with ultradian cycling bipolar illness.

TABLE 6–3.   Calcium channel blockers in affective illness

Open studies	Results	Blind studies	Results
Verapamil		Verapamil	
Gitlin and Weiss 1984	1/1 BP	Dubovsky et al. 1982	1/1 M
Brotman et al. 1986	6/6 M	Dubovsky and Franks 1983	2/2 M
Solomon and Williamson 1986	2/2 M	Giannini et al. 1984	10 M equal to Li, better than placebo
Barton and Gitlin 1987	0/8 M (acute) 1/4 M (prophyl) 2/2 M[a]	Giannini et al. 1987	20 M equal to Li
Patterson 1987	1/1 M	Giannini et al. 1989	10 M equal to Li, better than valproate
Pollack and Rosenbaum 1987	1/1 UP	Dubovsky et al. 1985	1/1 M[a]
Deicken 1990	1/1 BP	Dose et al. 1986	7/8 M
Hoschl et al. 1992	?/4 BP-Dep ?/7 UP	Dubovsky et al. 1986	5/7 M vs 1/7 Li
	Verapamil more effective than anti-depressants and neuro-leptics	Dubovsky and Franks 1987	1/2 M using Li-verapamil combination
		Hoschl and Kozeny 1989	12 M significantly improved over neuroleptics or neuroleptics + Li
		Garza-Trevino 1990	17 M equal to Li
		Garza-Trevino et al. 1992	12 M equal to Li
		Hoschl 1983	1/1 Dep
		Walton et al. 1996	Less effective than Li in mania
		Janicak et al. 1998	3/17 vs 2/15 placebo
Nimodipine		Nimodipine	
Brunet et al. 1990	6/6 M	Pazzaglia et al. 1993, 1998	7/23 BP
Manna 1991	12 M[b]		0/4 UP

(continued)

TABLE 6-3. Calcium channel blockers in affective illness *(continued)*

Open studies	Results	Blind studies	Results
Nimodipine		**Nimodipine**	
P. J. Goodnick 1995	2/2 BP	McDermut et al. 1995	3/3 RBD
Grunze et al. 1996	1/1 BP (Li + Nimod-ipine)	F. Eckman 1985 F. Eckman 1985	27/30 Dep vs 11/30 on placebo 29/30 Dep vs 16/30 on placebo
Walden et al. 1995a	9/10 UP	Montenegro et al. 1985	22/37 able to D/C with amitriptyline or nimodipine vs. 1/38 able to D/C with placebo
		Ban et al. 1990	87 on nimodipine 88 on placebo In elderly patients with cognitive decline, significantly more favorable changes in depressive symptomatology with nimodipine.
Flunarizine		**Flunarizine**	
Lindelius and Nilsson 1992	1/1 M	Eckmann 1985	14/17
Diltiazem		**Isradipine**	
Caillard 1985	5/5 M	Pazzaglia et al. 1993, 1998 McDermutt et al. 1995	2/2 BP nimodipine responders
Nifedipine			
Eccleston and Cole 1990	0/1 UP		
Moderate to marked responders	44/58 (76%)		125/185 (68%)

Note. BP = bipolar disorder; D/C = discontinue; Dep = depression; Li = lithium; M = mania; SA = schizoaffective; RBD = recurrent brief depression; UP = unipolar.
[a]Drug-induced hypomania.
[b]Lithium and nimodipine combination in prophylaxis is better than either drug alone.

TABLE 6–4.   Differential effects of dihydropyridine L-type calcium channel blockers versus verapamil

Effect	Dihydropyridine Nimodipine/ isradipine	Phenylalkylamine Verapamil	Reference(s)
Lipid soluble	+ +	±	D. D. Freedman and Waters 1987
Anticonvulsant Animals:			
a. Kindling	+ +	±	Wurpel and Iyer 1994 Vezzani et al. 1988
b. Reperfusion	+ +	0	F. B. Meyer et al. 1986
c. Kainic	+	0	Vezzani et al. 1988 Paczynski et al. 1990
Patients	+ +	NA	Brandt et al. 1988 Larkin et al. 1991 de Falco et al. 1992
Block cocaine-induced:			
a. Hyperactivity	+ +	0	Pani et al. 1990 Rossetti et al. 1990
b. Sensitization	+ +	NA	S. R. B. Weiss et al., unpublished data, June 1996
c. Dopamine overflow	+ +	0	Pani et al. 1990 Rossetti et al. 1990
Positive in forced swim model	+ +	0	Czyrak et al. 1989 de Jonge et al. 1993 Mogilnicka et al. 1987, 1988
Positive in learned helplessness model	+ +	0	Geoffroy et al. 1988 P. Martin et al. 1989 de Jonge et al. 1993
Like antidepressants:			
↓Glycine inhibition of ^{3}[H] 5,7-DCKA binding	+ +	NA	Nowak et al. 1993
Rapid-cycling affective illness	+ +	0, ±	Pazzaglia et al. 1993, 1998

Much more detailed analysis of the statistical methodology used with this design was reported in the study of McDermut et al. (1995), again documenting the unequivocal statistically and clinically significant effects of nimodipine monotherapy in a patient with refractory depression and previous ultrarapid cycling (Figures 6–4A to 6–4C). This ultrarapid cycling course reemerged during the period of placebo administration and was again suppressed with active nimodipine therapy. Remarkably, when a blind crossover to the maximal tolerated daily dose of 320 mg of phenylalkylamine CCB verapamil was attempted, mood instability rapidly reemerged. Even at maximally tolerated doses, this patient was unable to maintain her former degree of clinical improvement. When verapamil was replaced with nimodipine on a third double-blind trial, response was evident. In an attempt to see whether this type of response to the dihydropyridine L-type CCB would show cross-responsivity to another dihydropyridine CCB, the patient was switched in a blind fashion to isradipine (21 mg/day), a successful transition that resulted in discharge on monotherapy.

This case report (Figures 6–4A to 6–4C) (McDermut et al. 1995) of selective response to dihydropyridine CCBs but not a phenylalkylamine CCB is of considerable interest in relationship to the patient's history of nonresponsivity to multiple tricyclic antidepressants, the selective serotonin reuptake inhibitors, lithium, carbamazepine (the patient developed drug-induced hepatitis on carbamazepine and was unable to be evaluated), alprazolam, trazodone, and phenelzine. This suggests that patients with refractory mood disorders may have differential responses to various CCBs and that nonresponse to one CCB does not preclude response to another CCB, particularly if the other CCB is from a different category (Table 6–3).

Brunet et al. (1990), in an open study, reported positive antimanic effects of nimodipine in six patients with acute mania. Our results showed a much lower response rate. However, our patients were much more refractory by history, were treated in a tertiary referral research center, and generally showed a higher incidence of rapid, ultrarapid, and ultradian cycling patterns than in more traditional studies. Our results, however, are consistent with those of Manna (1991), who reported equal long-term efficacy of nimodipine and lithium monotherapy and greater efficacy on a combination of the two drugs than on either drug alone.

Although to date we have studied only 30 patients in a double-blind fashion on nimodipine (Pazzaglia et al. 1998), given the methodology involved and the consistency of clinical response observed in the small subgroup (*n* = 10) of refractory patients, together with the larger double-blind literature on verapamil and other CCBs, it would appear that CCB therapy should

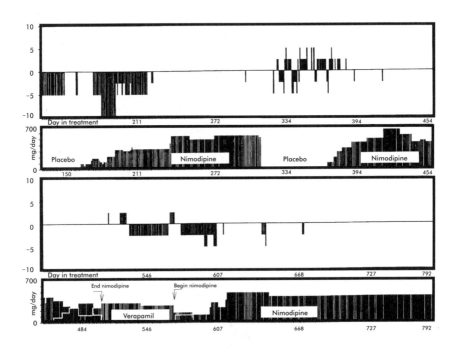

FIGURE 6-4A. Prospective daily life chart ratings of a patient's mood as determined by nurses blind to medication status. Boxes above the horizontal line (euthymia) represent mild, moderate, or severe mania. Boxes below the line represent mild, moderate, or severe depression. A complete record of all the patient's medications for each day of the study is presented below each life chart line. Numbers indicating the day of the patient's hospitalization are in 2-month intervals.

receive greater systematic study and clinical experimentation, particularly in treatment-responsive and -refractory patient subgroups. Other data support this view, such as Dubovsky and Franks' (1987) observations that nonresponders to lithium predict nonresponders to verapamil. Most of the responders to nimodipine in our study were lithium-nonresponsive in the past, however, and the relationship of these two different L-type CCBs to ultimately responsive clinical subtypes remains to be further delineated. Dubovsky (1995), moreover, noted that the CCBs show relatively greater safety in pregnancy, thus offering another potential alternative to lithium and the teratogenic mood-stabilizing anticonvulsants valproate and carbamazepine. Furthermore, in light of the adjunctive role for nimodipine described by Manna (1991) and in our studies of the combination of

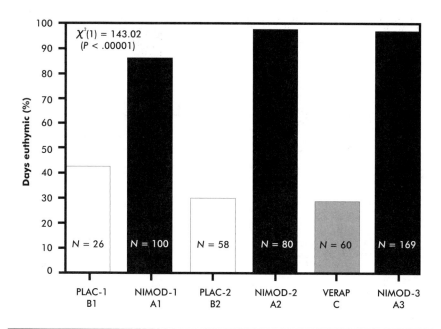

FIGURE 6-4B. Graph depicting the efficacy of nimodipine in a woman with bipolar II disorder in a B-A-B-A-C-A trial. The number in each bar is the number of days during that phase of the study that were included in data analyses. For example, medication phases did not include periods of titration or overlap with another psychotropic medication. The statistic represents the percentage of days euthymic during the three nimodipine (NIMOD) phases compared with the percentage of days euthymic during the two placebo (PLAC) phases plus the verapamil (VERAP) phase.

nimodipine and carbamazepine, the use of nimodipine and related agents in augmentation therapy remains a promising area for clinical exploration.

CARBAMAZEPINE AND NIMODIPINE COMBINATION THERAPY

Clinical Efficacy

Although the subgroup of patients described above showed good responses to nimodipine in double-blind conditions (Pazzaglia et al. 1993, 1998) and, in one instance, documented and redocumented in the B-A-B-A design (McDermut et al. 1995), some patients showed insufficient magnitude of

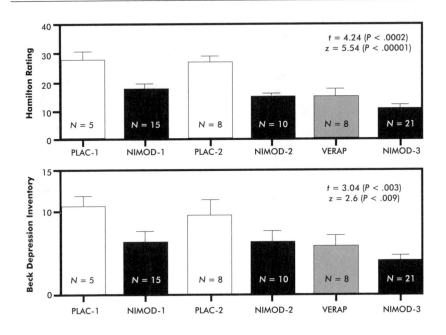

FIGURE 6–4C.   Graph showing that nimodipine (NIMOD) alleviates depressive symptoms as determined by two different scales (Hamilton Rating Scale for Depression [M. Hamilton 1960] and Beck Depression Inventory [Beck et al. 1961]) in a single patient. The number in each bar is the number of days during that phase of the study that were included in data analyses. PLAC = placebo; VERAP = verapamil.

clinical response to be discharged on monotherapy with this dihydropyridine L-type CCB. Accordingly, we began augmentation studies of nimodipine with the mood-stabilizing anticonvulsant carbamazepine.

This augmentation was initiated based on both clinical and theoretical rationales. Clinically, we hoped to provide additional therapeutic response with carbamazepine, in a manner similar to that observed when combining this agent with lithium (Post et al. 1990a), and valproate (Ketter et al. 1992). We hypothesized that such a response might occur through carbamazepine's actions on non–L-type calcium channels or on other mechanisms of action that would converge with those of the L-type CCBs to produce a greater therapeutic effect. This effect had been demonstrated in other branches of medicine, and data from calcium-related seizure models showed that a potentiation of effect occurred with carbamazepine and verapamil (Walden et al. 1992, 1995b). Walden et al. (1992, 1995b) observed that doses of either drug that were insufficient in blocking calcium-related spiking events in hippocampal preparations were able to completely suppress these events when the two drugs were used in combination. The molecular mechanisms for this combination effect, however, were not precisely identified.

In our study of carbamazepine augmentation of nimodipine (Pazzaglia et al. 1998), 4 of 14 patients treated with the combination showed evidence of clinical improvement, and in two cases improvement was of sufficient magnitude that patients were discharged on the combination. One such patient' course is illustrated in Figures 6–5A to 6–5D. The patient's life chart is illustrated (Figure 6–5A), showing a long history of intermittent bipolar II illness and incomplete and inadequate response to a variety of agents following the induction of ultradian cycling during the phase of treatment with the selective serotonin reuptake inhibitor fluoxetine. This patient showed remarkable degrees of mood instability, with profound mood switches three to six times per day. These fluctuations were captured by both nurse ratings and patient self-ratings completed at 2-hour intervals, as illustrated in Figure 6–5B. The unequivocal response to nimodipine was documented in a B-A-B-A design

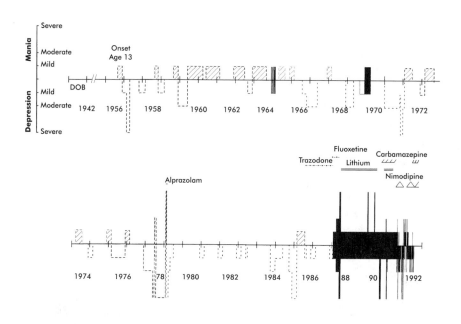

FIGURE 6–5A.   Life chart depicting a woman's long history of periodic bipolar II illness and progression to ultra-ultrarapid cycling following treatment with fluoxetine.

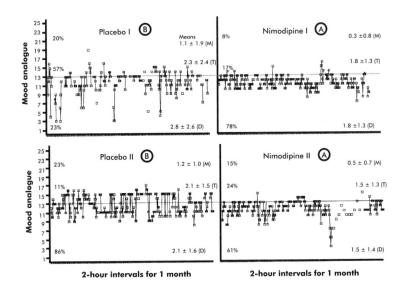

FIGURE 6-5B.   Mood analogue ratings showing unequivocal response to nimodipine after placebo substitution in a patient with bipolar II disorder with ul-tra-ultrarapid cycling. Mean deviation above 13 for the entire treatment phase (not just the 1 month illustrated). M = mania; D = depression; T = euthymia.

showing statistically significant improvement in both the depressed and the manic phases (Figures 6–5B and 6–5C). Although depressive fluctuations re-mained clinically problematic, fluctuations in the manic phase were almost completely ameliorated. When carbamazepine was added on a double-blind basis, there was a further statistically significant improvement in depressive ratings (Figure 6–5D), such that the patient's life chart ratings (Post et al. 1988; Squillace et al. 1984) and nurses' blind ratings were in the euthymic range for an extended period for the first time in more than 4 years.

In an attempt to switch the patient to the less expensive L-type CCB verapamil for discharge, she was introduced slowly to the transition on a blind basis and was also unable to maintain her previous degree of clinical im-provement with carbamazepine and nimodipine (Figure 6–5C). Maximally tolerated daily doses were 320 mg of verapamil and 600 mg of carba-mazepine. In light of this recrudescence of clinical symptomatology, the pa-tient was introduced to the transition on a blind basis back to nimodipine, and substantial recapturing of her clinical responsivity was again observed. After a slowly tapered transition to the less expensive dihydropyridine CCB

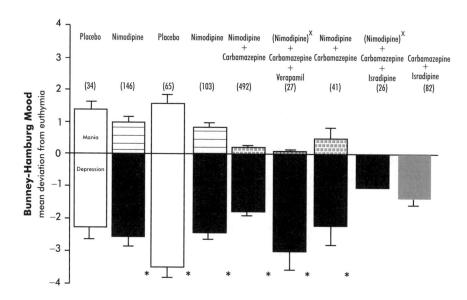

FIGURE 6–5C.   Efficacy of dihydropyridine L-type calcium channel blockers. Mean deviation from euthymia ratings (number of days in parentheses) in a patient with bipolar II disorder with ultra-ultrarapid cycling showing the following: efficacy of nimodipine monotherapy; efficacy of nimodipine-carbamazepine combination therapy; unsuccessful transition from nimodipine to verapamil; successful reinstitution of nimodipine-carbamazepine combination therapy; and, finally, successful transition to isradipine-carbamazepine combination therapy. *$P < .05$; ^xnimodipine slowly tapered to zero.

isradipine (Figure 6–5C), she remained stabilized, was discharged on carbamazepine-isradipine combination therapy, and has continued to do well for 2 years. It is notable from her life chart (Figure 6–5A) that she had formerly been nonresponsive to alprazolam, trazodone, fluoxetine, lithium, carbamazepine, and lithium and carbamazepine in combination.

Another patient in this series, as reported by Pazzaglia et al. (1998), has shown a good response to the combination of carbamazepine and nimodipine and has been discharged on the combination. Two additional patients failed to show a good response in a crossover from nimodipine to verapamil (for a total of four patients) but did make the transition to isradipine. These preliminary data, although using only four subjects, begin to demonstrate a pattern of responsivity to dihydropyridine L-type CCBs (nimodipine and isradipine) in patients with rapid and ultradian cycling patterns and lack of

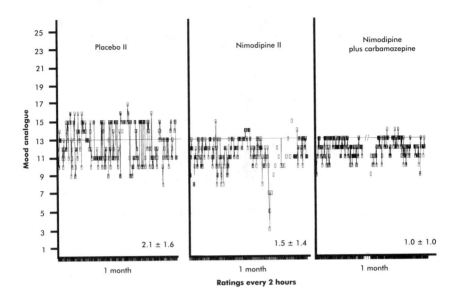

FIGURE 6–5D.   Mood analogue ratings comparing the efficacy of the nimodipine-carbamazepine combination with second placebo and nimodipine trials in a patient with bipolar II disorder and ultra-ultrarapid cycling.

responsivity to the phenylalkylamine CCB verapamil. Several patients with recurrent brief depressions (RBDs) did, however, sustain their nimodipine response on verapamil, suggesting the possibility, which needs further exploration, that cross-response among the L-type CCBs may vary across different affective syndromes.

Theoretical Perspective

What could be the molecular basis for the differential effects of the L-type CCBs in recurrent affective illness? The more lipophilic dihydropyridine CCBs appear to act at a site within the L-type calcium channel, whereas verapamil and related phenylalkylamine CCBs appear to act on a site at the outer membranous edge of the channel (as reviewed by Janis and Triggle 1991; Triggle 1992). Our initial clinical observations suggest the possibility that this differential biochemical mechanism of action could have differential behavioral and clinical effects. This possibility is supported by a variety of data indicating that the two classes of L-type CCBs have very different effects on biochemistry and behavior in other systems (Table 6–4), most notably nimodipine's ability to block cocaine-induced hyperactivity and associated dopamine overflow measured by in vivo dialysis in the nucleus accumbens. Other drug classes in the L-type category either do not possess this effect or may actually potentiate cocaine hyperactivity (Pani et al. 1990). Thus, it appears that all of the L-type CCBs are not equivalent in their biobehavioral reactivity; this characteristic appears to extend beyond issues of lipid solubility or pharmacokinetics. In addition, considerable clinical advantage may exist in using dihydropyridine CCBs, as these agents have fewer interactions with a variety of drugs (including carbamazepine) than the phenylalkylamine verapamil or benzothiazepine diltiazem (Ketter et al. 1995).

Certainly, further clinical trials might determine whether this distinction is retained in a larger patient population, or whether this distinction applies only to a subgroup of psychiatric patients. For example, we have observed several patients with RBD who showed unequivocal response to nimodipine and good response with double-blind transition to verapamil and were able to be maintained on long-term treatment (Pazzaglia et al. 1998). It may be, therefore, that patients with ultrarapid cycling bipolar disorder require some of the properties inherent in the dihydropyridine CCB class, whereas patients with RBD may be more responsive to both dihydropyridine and phenylalkylamine CCBs. This postulate would be convergent with the data in Table 6–3 that many patients with traditional cycle frequencies do, in fact, show good response to verapamil. Whether nimodipine would be equally or more effective in this subgroup of patients, as appears to be the case in our preliminary refractory group, remains for further clinical delineation.

POTENTIAL NEUROBIOLOGICAL MECHANISMS IN THE CARBAMAZEPINE-NIMODIPINE COMBINATION

Carbamazepine produces complex effects in a variety of neurotransmitters, receptors, and second messenger and neuropeptide systems (Post et al. 1992, 1994a). Determining which of these effects is most closely associated with its psychotropic properties in bipolar disorder and which of these or other effects may be responsible for the augmentation response in combination therapy with dihydropyridine L-type CCBs remains to be further evaluated. However, discussion of two possibilities might be beneficial. One possibility, of course, is that actions of carbamazepine unrelated to calcium dynamics account for its augmenting effects with nimodipine. The plethora of these other possibilities and candidate mechanisms are described in detail elsewhere (Elphick 1989a; Maitre et al. 1984; Olpe et al. 1991; Post and Chuang 1991; Post et al. 1992, 1994b). Preliminary data suggest that differential baseline (medication-free) cerebral metabolic topographies may be associated with differential response to carbamazepine and nimodipine (Ketter et al. 1996). Patients with basal hypometabolism (the traditional pattern in unipolar depressed patients) appear to respond to nimodipine, whereas those with basal temporal lobe hypermetabolism (a pattern more associated with the bipolar depression) respond to carbamazepine, consistent with the possibility that these agents have complementary mechanisms. Ascertaining how these differential profiles link to the biological effects of these agents will be of considerable clinical and theoretical interest.

A particularly intriguing possibility is that carbamazepine may exert effects on different calcium-related mechanisms to augment the CCB effects (Figure 6–6). This possibility is strengthened by the recent observations of Hough et al. (1996) and others that carbamazepine may block calcium influx, not through L-type voltage-dependent calcium channels but through the receptor-mediated N-methyl-D-aspartate (NMDA) glutamate receptor channel (Table 6–5). Although carbamazepine is highly potent in blocking this influx in cerebellar granule cells or hippocampal cells in culture, the ED_{50} approaches values that are involved in the clinical therapeutics of carbamazepine. Moreover, the recent data of Hough and colleagues suggest that carbamazepine is particularly effective in blocking a putative type or form of glutamate receptor that may have been induced following prolonged depolarizations in cell culture. Carbamazepine tends to gain access to glutamate channels only when channels are in the open condition associated with depolarization. This access could provide a mechanism for increased efficacy of carbamazepine at phases of high neuronal firing, such as those found in the seizure disorders or, hypothetically, in the paroxysmal pain disorders as well. Should prolonged seizures and depolarization events be associated with the induction of a new type of receptor, as postulated by Hough and colleagues, carbamazepine's particular potency in blocking calcium influx through this receptor could be of even greater clinical interest and value.

Calcium dysregulation has long been implicated in the potential pathophysiology of different phases of affective disorders (Carman et al. 1984; Dubovsky and Franks 1983; Dubovsky et al. 1992b, 1994; Jimerson et al. 1979; H. L. Meltzer 1990). This is based on a combination of data suggesting that 1) calcium-related endocrinopathies are associated with mood disorders; 2) abnormal levels of calcium have been found in blood and spinal fluid in association with mood dysregulation; 3) abnormalities in intracellular cal-

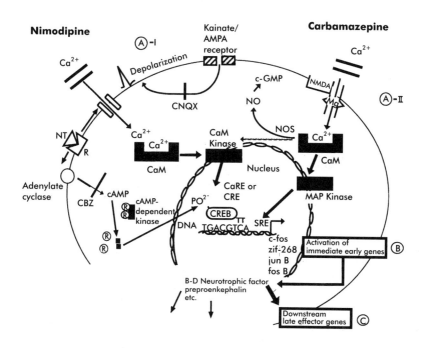

FIGURE 6–6.   Differential targets of carbamazepine (CBZ) and nimodipine on intracellular calcium. AMPA = α-amino-3-hydroxy-5-methyl-isoxazolepropionate; B-D = brain-derived; CaM = calmodulin; CaRE = calcium-response element; cGMP = cyclic guanosine monophosphate; CNQX = 6-cyano-7-nitroquinoxaline-2,3-dione; CRE = cyclic adenosine monophosphate (cAMP)–response element; CREB = cAMP response element–binding protein; MAP = mitogen-activated protein; NMDA = *N*-methyl-D-aspartate; NO = nitric oxide; NOS = nitric oxide synthase; NT = neurotrophin; R = receptor; SRE = serum response element. *Source.*   Adapted from B. Cheng et al. 1993, T. H. Murphy et al. 1991, Chuang et al. 1992, Fukunaga and Soderling 1990, Bading et al. 1993, and J. Patel et al. 1991.

cium have now been overwhelmingly documented in studies of blood elements of patients with unipolar and bipolar mood disorders compared with control subjects (Table 6–6); and 4) preliminary data reviewed above indicate that calcium-active treatments may be therapeutically effective.

Multiple molecular sites of calcium regulation are necessary for normal neuronal excitability, synaptic plasticity, and learning and memory in the

TABLE 6–5.   Evidence that carbamazepine inhibits glutamate receptors

Carbamazepine acutely
  Displaces MK 801 binding; $IC_{50} = 28 \mu M$
  Inhibits NMDA $\rightarrow$ PI turnover
  Inhibits NMDA $\rightarrow$ Ca^{2+} influx
Carbamazepine chronically
  Upregulates [^{3}H]-NMDA binding
  Upregulates NMDA $\rightarrow$ release [^{3}H]aspartate
  Upregulates NMDA $\rightarrow$ PI turnover
NMDA protects against carbamazepine toxicity

Note. IC_{50} = concentration that inhibits 50%; NMDA = N-methyl-D-aspartate;
PI = phosphoinositide.

models of long-term potentiation and kindling, and even in the balance of neurotrophic versus apoptotic processes (Gao et al. 1995; Hough et al. 1996; Marangos et al. 1990). As this balance is apparently necessary for the normal integration of so many cellular functions, it is not unlikely that there would be multiple and highly regulated systems to buffer its level and maintain homeostasis (Figure 6–7). Therefore, it would be of considerable interest to ascertain whether the blockade of voltage-dependent L-type CCBs by nimodipine, as supplemented by a blockade of calcium influx selectively through the NMDA receptor, would contribute to the augmenting effects of these agents in the affective disorders (Figure 6–6). That is, both drugs would putatively block intracellular calcium excesses and associated neuronal excitability, but the differential and dual impact of each drug acting at different regulatory sites could produce greater effects than either drug alone.

Convergent with this argument are the data of Walden et al. (1995a, 1995b), indicating that carbamazepine can be used in combination, not only with the L-type CCBs, but also with the partial serotonin 1A (5-HT$_{1A}$) receptor agonists buspirone and ipsapirone to produce clinically relevant effects in calcium-related disorder models of neuronal excitability. Of course, as noted above, it remains possible that many of carbamazepine's actions could account for this potentiation, and calcium-related effects are not necessary. However, it is noteworthy that many of carbamazepine's other actions directly involve the regulation of calcium at other molecular sites of action. For example, as illustrated in Figure 6–7, calcium regulation is affected by carbamazepine's 1) actions at adenosine-A$_1$ receptors; 2) putative indirect effects on GABA$_B$ mechanisms (Bernasconi 1982; Schmutz et al. 1986); 3) ability to increase TRH in cerebrospinal fluid (Marangell et al.

TABLE 6-6.   Evidence of intracellular calcium in blood elements of bipolar patients

Investigator	Preparation/Stimulation	Baseline	Stimulated
Bowden et al. 1988	Platelets/RBCs	**	
Dubovsky et al. 1989	Platelets/Thrombin, PAF	***	*
Tan et al. 1990	Platelets/Thrombin	***	**
Dubovsky et al. 1991a	Platelets/Thrombin	**	**
Dubovsky et al. 1992a	Platelets/Lymphocytes	*** ***	
Kusumi et al. 1992	Platelets/Thrombin		*
Berk et al. 1994	Platelets/Thrombin/ dopamine	*	***
Dubovsky et al. 1994	Platelets/Lymphocytes	***	
Förstner et al. 1994	Neutrophils/fMLP		*
Okamoto et al. 1995	Platelets/5-HT	NS	**
Berk et al. 1996	Platelets/5-HT	***	**
Emamghoreishi et al. 1997	B-lymphoblasts/PHA		*

Note.   fMLP = formylmethionylleucylphenylalanin; 5-HT = serotonin; NS = not significant; PAF = platelet activating factor; PHA = phytohemagglutinin; RBCs = red blood cells.
*$P < .05$. **$P < .01$. ***$P < .001$.

1994); and 4) ability to decrease somatostatin (Rubinow 1986; Steardo et al. 1986). Nevertheless, other systems unrelated to calcium actions cannot yet be ruled out as related to this apparent augmentation effect.

The clinically therapeutic time-course of action of both agents in bipolar disorder suggests a relatively slow onset, with a typical lag of several weeks before achieving maximal efficacy. This time-course suggests that the differential effects of these agents on gene expression could ultimately be related to maintenance of therapeutic effectiveness. For example, Figure 6–6 shows that regulation of calcium influx through the L-type calcium channels and NMDA receptor maintains a differential impact on gene expression (Bading et al. 1993); the effect of the combination could thus exert maximally greater effects on a single downstream target effector site than either drug alone. Of these two pathways, both could invoke differential long-term alterations in gene expression. The first possibility could be directly assessed by combining nimodipine with other, more specific blockers of NMDA receptors to determine if carbamazepine's efficacy could be replicated. Some of these agents are being used in clinical trials and should be forthcoming in the near future.

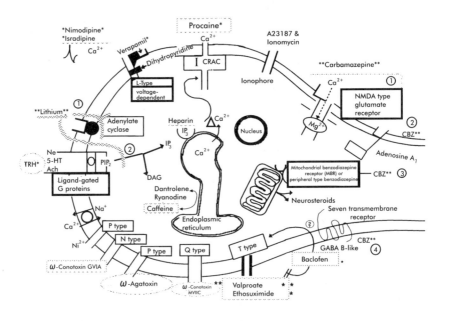

FIGURE 6-7.   Schematic diagram outlining the multiple extracellular and intracellular membrane effects of different agents (** = commonly used drugs; * = drugs explored in some psychiatric patients) and the diversity of other calcium channel regulatory sites that could be amenable to new drug development. Carbamazepine (CBZ) is shown to have four putative actions on different aspects of cellular biochemistry; two of lithium's many actions are highlighted, including adenylate cyclase and phosphoinositide turnover. ACh = acetylcholine; CRAC = Ca^{2+} release-activated Ca^{2+} current; DAG = diacylglycerol; GABA = γ-aminobutyric acid; GVIA = omega-conotoxin GVIA; 5-HT = 5-hydroxytryptamine; IP_3 = 1,4,5-inositol triphosphate; MVIIC = omega-conotoxin; NMDA = N-methyl-D-aspartate; PIP_2 = phosphatidylinositol-4,5-biphosphate; TRH = thyrotropin-releasing hormone.

   Manna's data (1991) of the efficacy of a nimodipine and lithium combination are of particular interest in reference to the above hypotheses related to combined effects on calcium-related mechanisms. Lithium obviously exerts complex effects on a variety of systems in brain, but its effects on phosphoinositide turnover and cyclic adenosine monophosphate and downstream effects on 1,4,5-inositol triphosphate (IP_3) metabolism in calcium-related processes (as reviewed by Berridge 1989; H. L. Meltzer 1990; and

Post et al. 1992) are also worthy of consideration. Effects on the IP_3 receptor-mediated calcium release have also been shown to affect ultrarapid neuronal and cellular calcium oscillations in several different types of preparations, raising the possibility that IP_3 modulation, either directly or indirectly through effects on phosphoinositide turnover, could be important to some elements of lithium's and related agents' mood-stabilizing effects (Berridge 1989; Dixon et al. 1992; Lupu-Meiri et al. 1994; Varney et al. 1994). Differential effects of the three major mood stabilizers on phosphatase activity have been reported: lithium blocks activity, carbamazepine increases activity, and valproate has no effect (Vadnal and Parthasarathy 1995).

Thus, hypothetically, in a partial but unequivocal responder to nimodipine, one could systematically examine the ability to alter calcium mechanics through different subtypes to determine which mechanism might potentially be the most efficacious (Figure 6–7): calcium and related NMDA antagonists for the NMDA receptor; lithium, heparin, and related drugs at the adenylate cyclase and IP_3-mediated receptors; procaine and related ligands through the Ca^{2+} release-activated Ca^{2+} current (I_{CRAC}) channel; and valproate and ethosuximide through T-type calcium channels. A multiplicity of other types of calcium channels have been identified, and their differential effects, as well as the effects of psychoactive peptides such as TRH and somatostatin on calcium dynamics, and their potential for therapeutics remain for further systematic preclinical and clinical experimentation (Table 6–7).

CONCLUSION

Carbamazepine (or its keto congener oxcarbazepine) is approved for use in bipolar illness in almost 90 countries throughout the world. Although carbamazepine is not likely to be approved by the U.S. Food and Drug Administration for use in bipolar illness in the near future because of lack of commercial pharmaceutical support, it is widely recognized that this agent, along with lithium and valproate, plays a major role in the therapeutics of bipolar illness. It is now time to more precisely identify clinical and biological markers of carbamazepine response that may be useful in optimizing treatment decisions. A major therapeutic problem with carbamazepine (and to some extent with lithium and valproate) concerns the progressive loss of efficacy during long-term prophylaxis. Thus, considerable clinical trial work must be undertaken to optimally assess the degree of this problem in the clinical therapeutics of bipolar affective illness.

TABLE 6-7.   Differential biochemical and physiological effects of carbamazepine versus nimodipine

	CBZ	Nimodipine
Somatostatin	↓ ↓	↑ ↑
TRH	↑	↓
NPY	↓	↓
NMDA Ca²⁺	↓	–
L-type Ca²⁺	—	↓
Hypofrontality response	– –	+ +
Temporal hypermetabolism response	+ +	(–)

Note.   CBZ = carbamazepine; NMDA = N-methyl-D-aspartate; NPY = neuropeptide Y; TRH = thyrotropin-releasing hormone; (–) = equivocal.

Although clinical trials with the L-type CCBs are preliminary, initial data are highly promising. Traditional studies with verapamil are largely positive, with the exception of the study of Janicak et al. (1998), the statistical problems of which have been previously addressed. Even more promising are the preliminary studies of the dihydropyridine class of L-type CCBs nimodipine, isradipine, and potentially amlodipine. Patients with typical bipolar affective illness, as well as those with refractory forms of the illness, deserve the benefit of further clinical trials and experimentation with this drug class to optimally determine its role in the clinical therapeutics of mood disorders. Initial clinical studies in small series are highly promising, as well as the demonstration of unequivocal responsiveness in some individual patients (McDermut et al. 1995; Pazzaglia et al. 1993, 1998). Based on the statement of Chassen (1992) that these kinds of case-controlled studies provide an alternative methodology to the widely recognized randomized parallel-group design, the inability to conduct large, systematic, parallel-group design studies of the CCBs in patients with affective disorders (because of a lack of funding, organizational structure, or impetus) should no longer serve as a rationale for failing to investigate this promising research area. The work reviewed in this chapter and elsewhere (Dubovsky 1995) suggests a wealth of new targets for clinical trials using the L-type CCBs and augmentation with the mood-stabilizing anticonvulsants and lithium.

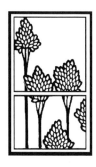

CHAPTER 7

Mechanisms of Action of Lithium in Bipolar Disorder

Husseini K. Manji, M.D.,
Robert K. McNamara, Ph.D., and
Robert H. Lenox, M.D.

Although the symptoms of bipolar disorder have been recognized and recorded for more than 2,000 years, the element lithium was discovered in 1817 and has been used as a medication for approximately 150 years. Following early observations of Alexander Ure in the 1840s, Sir Alexander Garrod was the first to introduce the oral use of lithia salts as a treatment for gout or "uric acid diathesis," which was believed to encompass affective symptoms of both mania and depression (Garrod 1859; Trousseau 1868; Ure 1844/1845). However, it was not until the observations of the American physician John Aulde and the Danish internist Carl Lange in the 1880s that lithium was considered to be a treatment of recurrent symptoms associated with depression independent of gout (Aulde 1887; Lange 1886). After falling into disrepute as a medication because of serious toxicity associated with its widespread use in elixirs and tonics as well as a salt substitute, it was the rediscovery by John Cade 45 years ago and seminal clinical studies by Schou in the 1950s that positioned lithium as an effective antimanic treatment and prophylactic therapy for bipolar disorder (Cade 1949; Schou 1979).

MEMBRANE TRANSPORT AND BIOLOGICAL RHYTHMS

Lithium shares many of the physiochemical properties of the group IA elements in the periodic table. It is the smallest member among these alkali metals, yet it has the highest electrical field density and largest energy of hydration. These characteristics permit it ready access to sodium ion channels while conferring properties similar to that of divalent cations such as calcium and magnesium (G. Johnson et al. 1971). The physiological role of lithium in events associated with the transport and cofactor activities of these monovalent and divalent cations in cells throughout the body, especially the brain, has remained a focus of investigations over the years.

Numerous studies have characterized the membrane transport of lithium and its interaction with other cations in both the brain and the peripheral cells in an effort to examine the mechanism of action of lithium in the treatment of bipolar disorder (reviewed in Bach and Gallicchio 1990; Mota de Freitas et al. 1991; and Riddell 1991). Accumulated evidence suggests that in excitable cells, lithium influx occurs primarily through the voltage-sensitive Na^+ channel (Carmiliet 1964; El-Mallakh 1990; Keynes and Swan 1959). Upon activation of the cell during depolarization, lithium is ushered through the Na^+ channel preferentially. Extrusion of lithium from the cells appears to depend on the gradient-dependent Na^+-Li^+ exchange process (Hitzemann et al. 1989; Sarkadi et al. 1978).

The balance of resting lithium conductance and net transport-efflux mechanisms regulates steady-state lithium homeostasis, but the gating of lithium through ion channels will alter this homeostasis to varying degrees. Modeling calculations reveal that the flux of lithium through voltage-dependent Na^+ channels is unlikely to be of much importance in the regulation of lithium homeostasis throughout the neuron, even on a short-term basis or as a consequence of high levels of neuronal activity. However, in the local environment of a dendritic spine, the surface area–to–volume ratio becomes relatively large, such that the lithium component of a synaptic current can cause very significant increases in the local lithium concentration, as much as a 5- to 10-fold increase in intracellular lithium following a train of synaptic stimuli (Kabakov et al. 1998). Such an activity-dependent mechanism for creating focal increases of intracellular lithium at sites of high synaptic activity may be crucial for lithium's therapeutic specificity and ability to regulate synaptic function in the brain.

Clinical studies over the years have provided evidence that Na^+K^+-ATPase may be decreased especially in the depressed phase of both unipolar and bipolar disorder associated with an increase in Na^+ retention (Coppen and Shaw 1963; Coppen et al. 1966; Hokin-Neaverson and Jefferson 1989a, 1989b; Naylor and Smith 1981; Naylor et al. 1970, 1971, 1980; Nurnberger et al. 1982). Long-term lithium treatment has been observed to result in an increased accumulation of lithium and a reduction of intraerythrocyte Na^+ and calcium in patients with bipolar disorder (Dubovsky et al. 1991b; Mullins and Brinley 1977; Riddell 1991; Torok 1989). Because free calcium ion concentration tends to parallel free sodium concentration, this may account for the action of lithium as well as observations that intracellular calcium is increased in patients with bipolar disorder (Dubovsky et al. 1991a, 1992a). Clinical studies of erythrocytes of patients with bipolar disorder treated with lithium have revealed evidence for an increased activity of Na^+K^+-ATPase (Bunney and Garland-Bunney 1987; D. A. T. Dick et al. 1978; Hokin-Neaverson et al. 1976; B. B. Johnson et al. 1980; Mallinger et al. 1987; Naylor et al. 1974, 1980; Reddy et al. 1989; Swann 1988; A. J. Wood et al. 1989), which may be accounted for by a lithium-induced activation of protein kinase C (PKC) activity as described below under "Signal Transduction, Phosphoproteins, and Gene Expression."

Long-term lithium treatment has also been reported to increase intraerythrocyte concentrations of choline by more than 10-fold (Jope et al. 1978, 1980; G. Lee et al. 1974; Lingsch and Martin 1976; H. L. Meltzer et al. 1982; Rybakowski et al. 1978; A. L. Stoll et al. 1991; Uney et al. 1985). This appears to be the result of not only inhibition of choline transport but also enhanced phospholipase D–mediated degradation of phospholipids, which may also be mediated via PKC activation (Ehrlich et al. 1983). Long-term lithium treatment may induce an evolving change in membrane structure or interaction with membrane-bound enzymes, consistent with the observations noted above. Furthermore, it is of interest that lithium has been shown to slow circadian oscillators in a wide variety of living organisms from plants to humans. Herein it has been suggested that lithium may exert its chronotropic effects by virtue of an as yet undefined action on membrane processes, which may be particularly evident in discrete areas of the brain such as the suprachiasmatic nucleus (reviewed in Klemfuss and Kripke 1989; and Lenox and Manji 1995).

CLASSICAL NEUROTRANSMITTER AND NEUROPEPTIDE SYSTEMS

Considerable effort over the years has been expended to identify specific neurotransmitter systems that might mediate the therapeutic action of lithium in the treatment of patients with bipolar disorder. As we critically review the evidence from these studies, it will be evident that lithium can affect a variety of neurotransmitter systems, but these effects may be secondary to more fundamental modulation of signal transduction responsible for regulating the balance of signaling in critical regions of the brain.

Norepinephrine

In view of the long-standing interest in the role(s) of the catecholamine systems in affective disorders (Schildkraut 1965), it is not surprising that extensive research has been conducted on the nonadrenergic system, and overall, lithium's effects on norepinephrine (NE) appear to be temporally and brain-region specific (reviewed in Bunney and Garland-Bunney 1987; P. J. Goodnick and Gershon 1985; F. K. Goodwin and Jamison 1990b; and Lenox and Manji 1995). Both short- and long-term lithium treatment have been reported to increase (Schildkraut et al. 1966, 1969) or not to change (Ahluwalia and Singhal 1980; Ho et al. 1970) the turnover of NE in some but not all regions of the brain. As is the case with the other neurotransmitters (see below), effects of lithium on NE receptor binding studies in rodent brain have been generally inconclusive (Maggi and Enna 1980; Schultz et al. 1981; Treiser and Kellar 1979). However, significant effects have been consistently observed on β-adrenergic receptor (βAR)–mediated cyclic adenosine monophosphate (cAMP) accumulation, with lithium inhibiting the response both in vivo and in vitro (discussed in detail below). Lithium is unable to block antidepressant-induced βAR downregulation (Rosenblatt et al. 1979) and in fact produces a greater subsensitivity (cAMP response) (Mork et al. 1990), but prevented reserpine or 6-hydroxydopamine-induced βAR supersensitivity (Hermoni et al. 1980; C. B. Pert et al. 1979; Treiser and Kellar 1979). Additional data from preclinical and clinical studies suggest that lithium treatment results in subsensitive α_2 receptors (Catalano et al. 1984; P. J. Goodnick and Meltzer 1984; G. M. Goodwin et al. 1986b; Huey et al. 1981; D. L. Murphy et al. 1974b). In preclinical studies, long-term lithium attenuates α_2-adrenergic-mediated behavioral effects (G. M. Goodwin et al. 1986b; D. F. Smith 1988) and presynaptic α_2 inhibition of NE release (R. N. Spengler et al. 1986), while enhancing K^+-evoked NE release (Ebstein et al. 1983). Although lithium has been reported to reduce high-affinity platelet [^{3}H]clonidine binding (Garcia-Sevilla et al. 1986; Pandey et al. 1989; K. Wood and Coppen 1983), compatible with a functional "uncoupling" of the receptor from the G protein (M. H. Kim and Neubig 1987; Neubig et al. 1988), interpretation of these data is confounded by the coexistence of a newly discovered imidazoline binding site.

In clinical investigations, both increases and decreases in plasma and urinary NE metabolite levels have been reported after lithium treatment (Beckmann et al. 1975; Corona et al. 1982; P. Goodnick 1990; Greenspan et al. 1970; E. Grof et al. 1986; Linnoila et al. 1983; D. L. Murphy et al. 1979; Schildkraut 1973, 1974; Swann et al. 1987). Lithium has been reported to reduce excretion of NE and metabolites in patients with mania, while increasing excretion in patients with depression associated with higher plasma NE concentrations in some cases (Beckmann et al. 1975; Bowers and Heninger 1977; Greenspan et al. 1970; Schildkraut 1973). However, there is also evidence that urinary excretion of 3-methoxy-4-hydroxyphenylglycol is low during bipolar depression and elevated during mania-hypomania (Bond et al. 1972; F. D. Jones et al. 1973; Post et al. 1977; Schildkraut et al. 1973; Wehr 1977). In part, these inconsistencies may be related to the inability to adequately control for state-dependent changes in affective states, with associated changes in activity level, arousal, and sympathetic outflow. Studies have demonstrated that 2 weeks of lithium administration in psychiatrically healthy subjects resulted in increases of urinary NE, normetanephrine, and fractional NE release and a trend toward significantly increased plasma NE, suggesting an enhanced neuronal release of NE (Manji et al. 1991b). These data are compatible with a similar observation of increased plasma dihydroxyphenylglycol (a major extraneuronal NE metabolite) levels (Poirier-Littre et al. 1993). Thus, current evidence supports an action of lithium in facilitating the release of NE, possibly via effects on the presynaptic α_2 "autoreceptor," and reducing the β-adrenergic–stimulated adenylyl cyclase (AC) response, which may contribute to lithium's attenuation of the euphorigenic effects of amphetamine.

Dopamine

The effect of lithium on dopamine (DA) synthesis and transmission has been investigated extensively in preclinical studies by directly determining changes in DA or homovanillic acid and indirectly examining lithium-induced changes in DA-linked behaviors (Bunney and Garland 1984; Bunney and Garland-

Bunney 1987; P. J. Goodnick and Gershon 1985). Lithium administration has also been found to cause a dose-dependent decrease of DA formation (Ahluwalia and Singhal 1980, 1981; Engel and Berggren 1980; Eroglu et al. 1981; Frances et al. 1981; E. Friedman and Gershon 1973; Hesketh et al. 1978), which occurs at 25% lower doses in the striatum than in the limbic forebrain (Laakso and Oja 1979; Poitou and Bohuon 1975; Segal et al. 1975). Based on the heuristic hypothesis that supersensitive DA receptors underlie the development of manic episodes, it has been postulated that lithium would prevent DA receptor supersensitivity (Bunney and Garland 1984; Bunney and Garland-Bunney 1987; P. J. Goodnick and Gershon 1985). In a series of studies, it was found that lithium prevented haloperidol-induced DA receptor upregulation (Bunney 1981; Rosenblatt et al. 1980; Verimer et al. 1980) and supersensitivity to iontophoretically applied DA or intravenous apomorphine (Gallager et al. 1978). Indeed, lithium appears to be effective in blocking both the behavioral and the biochemical manifestations of supersensitive DA receptors induced by receptor blockade. A proposed site of action for lithium's ability to block behavioral supersensitivity is the postsynaptic receptor, and lithium also prevents haloperidol-induced increases in DA receptors. Despite significant evidence for lithium's effect on receptor-mediated function, DA receptor–binding studies have contributed only inconclusive evidence. These data suggest a possible site for lithium action at receptor-effector coupling. Interestingly, a number of studies have reported a lack of effect if lithium is administered *after* the induction of DA supersensitivity (Bloom et al. 1983; Klawans et al. 1976; Staunton et al. 1982a, 1982b), suggesting that in this model lithium exerts its greatest effects prophylactically.

Among the numerous behavioral effects of lithium in animals, perhaps the best studied are those on stimulant-induced activity. Lithium's ability to antagonize increases in locomotor activity produced by amphetamine have gained much attention, perhaps because this model has been postulated to be a better representation of lithium's effects on manic behavior (Allikmets et al. 1979; Bunney and Garland-Bunney 1987; P. J. Goodnick and Gershon 1985; Klawans et al. 1976; A. Pert et al. 1978; Staunton et al. 1982a). It is also of interest that lithium has been reported to attenuate the euphoriant and motor-activating effects of oral amphetamine in depressed patients, although equivocal results have been observed on methylphenidate challenge (Huey et al. 1981; van Kammen et al. 1985). Results of studies of DA and its metabolites in patients' cerebrospinal fluid (CSF) before and after lithium treatment have been conflicting (Berrettini et al. 1985a; Bowers and Heninger 1977; Fyro et al. 1975; P. J. Goodnick and Gershon 1985; Linnoila et al. 1983; Swann et al. 1987). A longitudinal study of one woman with unipolar disorder and seven women with bipolar disorder found that lithium reduced the levels of DA, dihydrophenylacetic acid, and homovanillic acid in all of the patients (Linnoila et al. 1983), but the possible role of alterations in mood state and motor activity remained a confounding variable, as it does for all clinical investigations using this research strategy. Overall, although the data from human investigations are sparse, lithium's postulated ability to reduce both presynaptic and postsynaptic aspects of DA transmission represents an attractive mechanism for its antimanic therapeutic action.

Serotonin

Preclinical studies show that lithium's effects on serotonin (5-hydroxytryptamine [5-HT]) function may occur at a variety of levels including precursor uptake, synthesis, storage, catabolism, release, receptors, and receptor-effector interaction (reviewed in Bunney and Garland-Bunney 1987; P. J. Goodnick and Gershon 1985; L. H. Price et al. 1990). Overall, there is reasonable evidence from preclinical studies that lithium enhances serotonergic neurotransmission, although its effects on serotonin appear to vary depending on brain region, length of treatment, and serotonin receptor subtype (Bunney and Garland 1984; Bunney and Garland-Bunney 1987; P. J. Goodnick and Gershon 1985; L. H. Price et al. 1990). In contrast to short-term studies, most long-term studies tend to show that serotonin and 5-hydroxyindoleacetic acid (5-HIAA) levels decrease with lithium administration (Ahluwalia and Singhal 1980; Bunney and Garland 1984; Collard 1978; Collard and Roberts 1977; Shukla 1985; Treiser et al. 1981). Treiser et al. (1981) found that long-term lithium use increased basal and K^+-stimulated serotonin release in the hippocampus, but not in the cortex. Another study also reported that lithium increased serotonin release in the parietal cortex, hypothalamus, and hippocampus after 2–3 weeks, but not after a single injection or 1 week of treatment (E. Friedman and Wang 1988).

Receptor-binding studies have shown complex, regionally specific effects of short- or long-term lithium treatment on the density of 5-HT_1 or 5-HT_2 receptors, although most studies suggest decreases in both sites, at least in the hippocampus (Godfrey et al. 1989; P. J. Goodnick and Gershon 1985; G. M. Goodwin et al. 1986a; Hotta and Yamawaki 1988; Maggi and Enna 1980; Mizuta and Segawa 1989; M. E. Newman et al. 1990; Odagaki et al. 1990; Tanimoto et al. 1983; Treiser and Kellar 1980; Treiser et al. 1981). Similarly, the reported effects of both short-term and long-term lithium treatment on 5-HT_2-mediated head-twitch behavior as well as hyperactivity responses to the serotonin precursor hydroxytryptophan have been inconsistent (E. Friedman et al. 1979; G. M. Goodwin et al. 1986a; Grahame-Smith and Green 1974; Harrison-Read 1979). The prolactin response to serotonin is, however, more consistently reported to be increased after short-term lithium treatment (Koenig et al. 1984; H. Y. Meltzer and Lowy 1987; H. Y. Meltzer et al. 1981). Investigators using a variety of methodologies have provided evidence that lithium produces a subsensitivity of presynaptic inhibitory 5-HT$_{1A}$ receptors (E. Friedman and Wang 1988; G. M. Goodwin et al. 1986b; Hotta and Yamawaki 1988; Mork and Geisler 1989a; M. E. Newman et al. 1990; Wang and Friedman 1988), which might result in a net increase of the amount of serotonin released per impulse. In a series of important preclinical investigations, de Montigny used electrophysiological recordings to measure the effects of lithium on the serotonin system. Short-term lithium treatment did not affect the responsiveness of the postsynaptic neuron to serotonin nor the electrical activity of the serotonin neurons, but enhanced the efficacy of the ascending (presynaptic) serotonin system (Blier and de Montigny 1985; Blier et al. 1987). These observations led de Montigny and colleagues to propose that lithium might increase the efficacy of antidepressant action (Blier and de Montigny 1985; Blier et al. 1987). Several open and double-blind clinical investigations have now demonstrated that approximately 50% of nonresponders to traditional antidepressants are converted to responders upon lithium administration within 2 weeks (de Montigny et al. 1981, 1983; Heninger et al. 1983).

Many early CSF studies in humans are difficult to interpret because of the methodology and study design and are most often confounded by concomitant alterations in mood state and neurovegetative symptomatology. Small increases in CSF 5-HIAA levels have been reported after subchronic lithium treatment in patients with bipolar disorder (Berrettini et al. 1985a; Bowers and Heninger 1977; Fyro et al. 1975; P. Goodnick 1990; P. J. Goodnick and Gershon 1985; Linnoila et al. 1984; L. H. Price et al. 1990; Swann et al. 1987). Several studies have suggested that long-term lithium treatment "normalizes" a previously low platelet serotonin uptake in patients with bipolar disorder, which may persist for several weeks after discontinuation (Born et al. 1980; Coppen et al. 1980; H. Y. Meltzer et al. 1983; Poirer et al. 1988). The effects of lithium treatment on [^{3}H]imipramine binding in platelets remain inconclusive (H. Y. Meltzer and Lowy 1987; Poirer et al. 1988; L. H. Price et al. 1990; K. Wood and Coppen 1983). Neuroendocrine studies in patients have been more consistent, showing that short-term or moderate-term lithium treatment results in augmented prolactin and/or cortisol responses to various challenges (fenfluramine, tryptophan, hydroxytryptophan) in affectively ill patients (Cowen et al. 1989; Glue et al. 1986; McCance et al. 1989; H. Y. Meltzer et al. 1984; Muhlbauer 1984; Muhlbauer and Muller-Oerlinghausen 1985; L. H. Price et al. 1989). However, studies of volunteers without affective disorders do not reveal increased neuroendocrine responses after 2 weeks of "therapeutic" lithium, suggesting that lithium's effect on the serotonergic system may depend on its underlying activity (Manji et al. 1991b).

Overall, current evidence from both preclinical and clinical studies supports a role for lithium in enhancing presynaptic activity in the serotonergic system in the brain. Direct studies in the past of lithium's effects on serotonergic neurotransmission in humans have been limited by the complexity of the widespread distribution of different types of serotonergic fibers throughout the brain, the only recently recognized multiple receptor subtypes, the relative lack of serotonin-specific pharmacological agents and outcome variables reflecting selective serotonergic responses, and inadequate attention to effects dependent on duration of treatment and affective/physiological state of the patient. With our current understanding of the molecular neurobiology of both receptor subtypes and the transporter in the serotonergic system, we anticipate newer, more specific pharmacological probes for future preclinical and clinical investigations.

Acetylcholine

Neurochemical, behavioral, and physiological studies have all suggested that the cholinergic system is involved in affective illness (Dilsaver and Coffman 1989) and that lithium alters the synaptic processing of acetylcholine (ACh) in rat brain. Addition of up to 1 mM lithium in vitro has no effect on ACh synthesis or release, but long-term in vivo lithium treatment appears to increase ACh synthesis, choline transport, and ACh release in rat brain (Jope 1979; Simon and Kuhar 1976). Although some investigators have reported reductions in ACh levels in rat brain following subchronic administration (Ho and Tsai 1975; Krell and Goldberg 1973; Ronai and Vizi 1975), Jope has reported increased synthesis of ACh in cortex, hippocampus, and striatum following 10 days of lithium administration (Jope 1979). With respect to the density of muscarinic receptors, long-term lithium treatment has been reported to increase (Kafka et al. 1982; Lerer and Stanley 1985; Levy et al. 1983), decrease (Tollefson and Senogles 1982), or not to change (Maggi and Enna 1980) the binding of [^{3}H]quinuclidinyl benzilate (QNB) in various areas of rat brain. However, in human caudate nucleus, lithium has been reported to reduce the affinity of [^{3}H]QNB binding. The effects of lithium on both upregulation and downregulation of muscarinic receptors in brain have also been investigated. Although there have been reports that lithium is able to abolish the increase in [^{3}H]QNB binding produced by atropine but is without effect on the downregulation induced by the cholinesterase inhibitor diisopropylfluorophosphonate, these data are variable and inconclusive (Lerer and Stanley 1985; Levy et al. 1983). Ellis and Lenox (1990) have examined both receptor binding and muscarinic receptor–coupled phosphoinositide (PI) response in rat hippocampus during atropine-induced upregulation. These investigators found that long-term treatment with atropine results in an upregulation of muscarinic receptors and a supersensitivity of the PI response in the hippocampus. Long-term coadministration of lithium prevented the development of the supersensitivity of the muscarinic receptor PI response, without significantly affecting the extent of upregulation of receptor binding sites. These findings suggest that lithium's actions are exerted at a point beyond the receptor binding site, possibly affecting the coupling of the newly upregulated receptors at the level of the signal-transducing G proteins. Thus, similar to the case for dopaminergic receptors and βARs, it has been suggested that lithium can block the development of cholinergic receptor supersensitivity.

In behavioral studies, long-term lithium treatment has been reported to enhance a number of cholinergically mediated responses, including catalepsy and hypothermia. The effect of lithium on pilocarpine-induced catalepsy and hypothermia was of the same order of magnitude as the enhancement induced by long-term scopolamine pretreatment; combined administration of both pretreatments resulted in additive effects, suggesting that different mechanisms may be involved (Dilsaver and Hariharan 1988; Lerer and Stanley 1985; R. W. Russell et al. 1981). Of interest in this regard is a study by Dilsaver and Hariharan (1989) reporting that long-term lithium treatment results in a supersensitivity of nicotine-induced hypothermia in rats. Perhaps the most striking example of lithium's ability to potentiate muscarinic responses comes from the lithium-pilocarpine seizure model (Hirvonen et al. 1990; Honchar et al. 1983; Jope et al. 1986; Ormandy and Jope 1991; Persinger et al. 1988; J. B. Terry et al. 1990). In large doses, pilocarpine and other muscarinic agonists cause prolonged, usually lethal seizures in rats. Although lithium alone is not a convulsant, pretreatment with lithium increases the sensitivity of pilocarpine almost 20-fold (Hirvonen et al. 1990; Honchar et al. 1983; Jope et al. 1986; Ormandy and Jope 1991; Persinger et al. 1988; J. B. Terry et al. 1990). Interestingly, this behavioral effect of lithium is markedly attenuated by intracerebroventricular administration of *myo*-inositol in both rats and mice (Kofman et al. 1991; Tricklebank et al. 1991), representing perhaps the best correlation between a biochemical and behavioral effect of lithium (see section "Phosphoinositide Cycle" later in this chapter). A synergism with the cholinergic system also occurs in electrophysiological studies of hippocampal slices, in which pilocarpine and lithium together, but not alone, produce spontaneous epileptiform bursting (Jope et al. 1986; Ormandy and Jope 1991). Elegant studies in rat hippocampus have demonstrated that lithium can reverse muscarinic agonist-induced desensitization, an effect that is mediated through PI hydrolysis and can be reversed by inositol (Pontzer and Crews 1990). Studies by M. S. Evans and colleagues (1990) suggested that lithium's role in lithium-pilocarpine seizures is to increase excitatory transmission via a presynaptic facilitatory effect. Lithium alone also augmented synaptic responses, and this effect of lithium could be blocked by a PKC inhibitor. These results suggest that lithium's effects in this model may occur via a PKC-mediated presynaptic facilitation of neurotransmitter release (discussed later). Biochemical, electrophysiological, and behavioral data suggest that long-term lithium administration stimulates ACh synthesis and release in rat brain and potentiates some cholinergic-mediated physiological events. Interestingly, similar to the situation observed with the catecholaminergic system, pharmacological studies indicate that long-term lithium treatment prevents muscarinic receptor supersensitivity, most likely via postreceptor mechanisms.

Amino Acids and Neuropeptides

In contrast to the abundant literature on lithium's effects on monoamine neurotransmitters, much less work has been conducted on amino acid neurotransmitters and neuropeptides (Bernasconi 1982; Lloyd et al. 1987; Nemeroff 1991b). Studies have suggested that previously low levels of plasma and CSF γ-aminobutyric acid (GABA) are normalized in patients with bipolar disorder who are being treated with lithium (Berrettini et al. 1983, 1986), paralleling reported GABA changes observed in several regions of rat brain (Ahluwalia and Singhal 1981; Gottesfeld et al. 1971; Maggi and Enna 1980). Interestingly, following withdrawal of lithium after long-term treatment, GABA levels return to normal in striatum and midbrain but remain elevated in the pons and medulla (Ahluwalia and Singhal 1981), possibly resulting from reportedly elevated levels of the GABA-synthesizing enzyme, glutamic acid decarboxylase. Lithium has also been postulated to prevent GABA uptake, and long-term lithium treatment was shown to significantly decrease low-affinity [^{3}H]GABA sites in corpus striatum and hypothalamus (Maggi and Enna 1980). Because lithium has no effect on in vitro [^{3}H]GABA binding, these receptor changes have been interpreted as downregulation secondary to activation of the GABA-ergic system (Maggi and Enna 1980). Although the clinical relevance of these findings remains unclear, it is noteworthy that decreases in CSF GABA have been reported in patients with depression (Berrettini et al. 1982; Post et al. 1980).

The effect of lithium on glutamate, a major excitatory neurotransmitter in the brain, has been studied using monkey cerebral cortical slices, in which it stimulates glutamate release at doses ranging from 1.5 to 25 mM (Dixon et al. 1994). Lithium-induced glutamate release is associated with an increased inositol trisphosphate accumulation, which is prevented by prior treatment with N-methyl-D-aspartate (NMDA) receptor antagonists, but not by non-NMDA, muscarinic, α_1-adrenergic, serotonergic (5-HT$_2$), or histaminergic (H$_1$) receptor antagonists. Blockade of glutamate release with carbetapentane also prevented basal and lithium-induced inositol trisphosphate accumulation (Dixon et al. 1994).

Among the peptides, the opioid system has been the most extensively studied. Lithium administration has been reported to produce time- and dose-dependent increases in metenkephalin and leuenkephalin levels in the basal ganglia and nucleus accumbens and to increase dynorphin A(1–8) levels in the striatum (Sivam et al. 1986, 1988). The lithium-induced increase in dynorphin was accompanied by an increase in the abundance of prodynorphin messenger ribonucleic acid (mRNA) (Sivam et al. 1988), suggesting that the effects on the levels are mediated, at least in part, through increased transcription and translation. Studies of short-term lithium treatment have demonstrated enhanced release of a number of opioid peptides from hypothalamic slices and have suggested an effect at the inhibitory presynaptic opioid autoreceptor (Burns et al. 1990). Long-term lithium treatment did not affect the basal hypothalamic release of any of the opioids, but prevented the naloxone-stimulated release of the peptides in vitro, compatible with lithium-induced autoreceptor subsensitivity (Burns et al. 1990). Lithium is reported to decrease the affinity of opiate receptors in vitro, whereas subchronic lithium administration is reported to decrease the number of opioid binding sites in rat forebrain structures in some, but not all, studies (P. J. Goodnick and Gershon 1985). Additional support for effects on the opioidergic system comes from the behavioral studies in which lithium produces aversive states in rats that can be blocked by the depletion of central pools of β-endorphin or by the blockade of μ-opioid receptors; additionally it has been demonstrated that long-term lithium treatment abolishes both the secondary reinforcing effects of morphine and the aversive effects of the opioid antagonist naloxone (Blancquaert et al. 1987; Lieblich and Yirmiya 1987; Mucha and Herz 1985; Shippenberg and Herz 1991; Shippenberg et al. 1988).

Lithium has been shown to increase the substance P content of striatum when administered long term to rats, effects that are antagonized by the concurrent administration of haloperidol (J. S. Hong et al. 1983). Other studies have demonstrated a lithium-induced increase in tachykinin levels that appears to be associated with an increase in transcription of the rat pre-protachykinin gene (Sivam et al. 1989). Studies of the effects of subchronic lithium treatment on regional brain concentrations of substance P, neurokinin A, calcitonin gene–related peptide, and neuropeptide Y have demonstrated a regionally specific increase in the immunoreactivity of all the peptides except calcitonin gene–related peptide, which was significantly decreased in the pituitary gland (Mathe et al. 1990). In one of the few applicable clinical studies, CSF levels of various pro-opiomelanocortin peptides were examined in euthymic patients with bipolar disorder before and during lithium treatment; no significant effects of lithium on the CSF levels of any of the peptides were observed (Berrettini et al. 1985b, 1987).

Similar to carbamazepine and valproic acid, lithium may facilitate certain aspects of GABA-ergic neurotransmission via several mechanisms. The clinical relevance of these findings at this point remains largely unknown; however, as one of the few systems affected in a similar manner by the other commonly used mood stabilizers, the GABA-ergic system is worthy of further, more carefully controlled investigation. With respect to the peptides, only the opioidergic system has been studied to any extent, and the bulk of the evidence suggests that lithium facilitates presynaptic opioidergic function, while antagonizing certain opioid-mediated effects. The preliminary reports of effects of alterations in the levels of tachykinins in the striatum may be intriguing in view of the commonly observed lithium-induced side effect of tremor.

SIGNAL TRANSDUCTION, PHOSPHOPROTEINS, AND GENE EXPRESSION

Phosphoinositide Cycle

In recent years, research on the molecular mechanisms underlying lithium's therapeutic effects has focused on intracellular second messenger generating systems and, in particular, receptor-coupled hydrolysis of phosphoinositide 4,5-biphosphate (PIP_2) (Baraban et al. 1989). Lithium, at therapeutically relevant concentrations in the brain, is a potent inhibitor of the intracellular enzyme, inositol monophosphatase ($K_i = 0.8$ mM), which plays a major role in the recycling of inositol phosphates (J. H. Allison and Stewart 1971; Hallcher and Sherman 1980). Because the brain has limited access to inositol other than that derived from recycling of inositol phosphates, the ability of a cell to maintain sufficient supplies of *myo*-inositol can be crucial to the resynthesis of the PIs and the maintenance and efficiency of signaling (W. R. Sherman 1991). Furthermore, because the mode of enzyme inhibition is *uncompetitive* (Nahorski et al. 1991), lithium's effects have been postulated to be most pronounced in systems undergoing the highest rate of PIP_2 hydrolysis (reviewed in Nahorski 1991, 1992). Thus, Berridge and associates (1982, 1989) first proposed that the physiological consequence of lithium's action is derived through a depletion of free inositol and that its selectivity could be attributed to its preferential action (as a result of the *uncompetitive* nature of the inhibition) on the most overactive receptor-mediated neuronal pathways. Because several subtypes of adrenergic, cholinergic, and serotonergic receptors are coupled to PIP_2 turnover in the central nervous system (Chuang 1989; S. K. Fisher et al. 1992; Rana and Hopkin 1990), such a hypothesis offers a plausible explanation for lithium's therapeutic efficacy in treating multiple aspects of bipolar illness.

Numerous studies have examined the effects of lithium on receptor-mediated PI responses, and although some report a reduction in agonist-stimulated PIP_2 hydrolysis in rat brain slices following short- or long-term lithium treatment, these findings have often been small and inconsistent and subject to numerous methodological differences (Casebolt and Jope 1989; Ellis and Lenox 1990; Godfrey 1989; Kennedy et al. 1989; L. Song and Jope 1992; Whitworth and Kendall 1988, 1989). Additionally, several lines of evidence suggest that the action of lithium, in the long term, may not simply be directly manifest in receptor-mediated PI turnover. Although investigators have observed that levels of inositol in brain remain reduced in rats receiving long-term lithium administration (W. R. Sherman 1991; W. R. Sherman et al. 1985), it has been difficult to demonstrate that this results in a reduction in the resynthesis of PIP_2, which is the substrate for agonist-induced PI turnover. This, however, may be the result of the methodological difficulties in accurately measuring alterations in a rapidly turning over, small, signal-related pool of PIP_2 and/or recent evidence that resynthesis of inositol phospholipids may also occur through base exchange reactions from other larger pools of phospholipids such as phosphatidylcholine (Manji and Lenox 1994; Nishizuka 1992). Interestingly, some (Kennedy et al. 1990; Varney et al. 1992), but not all (Kendall and Nahorski 1987), studies have demonstrated that the addition of high concentrations of exogenous inositol can attenuate some of lithium's effects on the PI cycle. However, although pharmacological concentrations of extracellular inositol appear to attenuate some of lithium's effects, in animal studies the addition of inositol *prevented* but did not *reverse* the effects of lithium on the PI system (Kennedy et al. 1990; Kofman and Belmaker 1993; Maslanski et al. 1992; Tricklebank et al. 1991), suggesting that lithium may induce long-term changes beyond simple inositol depletion.

Investigators have also examined lithium's effects on the PI system distal to the receptor because, as noted above, experimental evidence has shown that lithium may alter receptor coupling to PI turnover. Because a fluoride ion will directly activate G protein–coupled second messenger response, efforts have been made to examine the effect of lithium on sodium fluoride–stimulated PI response in brain. Although Godfrey et al. (1989) reported a reduction of fluoride-stimulated PI response in cortical membranes of rats treated with lithium for 3 days, no change in response was observed in cortical slices from rats administered lithium for 30 days. More recently, using labeled PI as a substrate (which should bypass any putative inositol depletion), L. Song and Jope (1992) reported an attenuation of PI turnover in response to guanosine triphosphate (GTP) analogues. Taken together, these results suggest that, although long-term lithium administration may affect receptor-mediated phosphoinositide signaling, these effects are unlikely to be simply the result of an inositol depletion in the central nervous system (Lenox and Manji 1995; Manji and Lenox 1994; L. Song and Jope 1992). Most importantly, the therapeutic actions of lithium occur only after long-term treatment and remain in evidence long after discontinuation, actions that cannot be attributed only to inositol reductions evident in the presence of lithium. Thus, although the preponderance of the data suggests that the initial actions of lithium may occur with a relative depletion of inositol and thereby alterations in receptor-coupled PI response, the effects of long-term lithium treatment (and likely those representing the therapeutically relevant ones) are more likely to be mediated by resultant changes at different levels of the signal transduction process (Jope and Williams 1994; Manji and Lenox 1994; Manji et al. 1995), including at the level of G proteins and PKC isozymes (see below).

Adenylate Cyclase

The other major receptor-coupled second messenger system on which lithium exerts significant effects is the cAMP generating system. Forn and Valdecasas (1971) were the first to report that lithium in vitro attenuated NE-stimulated cAMP accumulation; since then, numerous studies have clearly demonstrated that cAMP accumulation by various neurotransmitters and hormones is inhibited by lithium at therapeutic concentrations both in vivo and in vitro (Belmaker 1981; Dousa and Hechter 1970a, 1970b; Ebstein et al. 1976, 1980, 1987; Geisler et al. 1985; Gelfand et al. 1979; Mork and Geisler 1989a, 1989b, 1989c; Mork et al. 1992; M. E. Newman and Belmaker 1987; Risby et al. 1991; Singer 1981; Singer et al. 1972). NE- and adenosine-stimulated cAMP accumulation in rat cortical slices are inhibited significantly by 1–2 mM lithium, although generalizability of this to human brain tissue has not yet been fully determined (M. Newman et al. 1983). Studies in humans have demonstrated that lithium treatment at therapeutic levels results in an attenuation of the plasma cAMP increase in response to epinephrine (Belmaker et al. 1980; Ebstein et al. 1983; E. Friedman et al. 1979) as well as shown evidence for an attenuation of receptor coupling to AC in peripheral cells (Ebstein et al. 1976, 1987; Gelfand 1979; Lonati-Galligani et al. 1989; M. E. Newman et al. 1992; Risby et al. 1991). In fact, lithium inhibition of vasopressin-sensitive or thyroid-stimulating-hormone–sensitive AC is generally believed to underlie two of lithium's more common side effects, namely nephrogenic diabetes insipidus and hypothyroidism (Dousa 1974; Goldberg et al. 1988; F. Y. Tseng et al. 1989; Urabe et al. 1991).

Lithium attenuation of β-adrenoceptor-stimulated AC activity has been shown in membrane, slice, and synaptosomal preparations from rat cerebral cortices (Andersen and Geisler 1984; Geisler et al. 1985; Mork and Geisler 1987, 1989a; M. E. Newman and Belmaker 1987), and several studies have also revealed lithium-induced increases in basal cAMP (Ebstein et al. 1980; Masana et al. 1991; M. E. Newman and Belmaker 1987). Lithium in vitro inhibits the stimulation of AC by the poorly hydrolyzable analogue of GTP, Gpp(NH)p, and also by Ca^{2+}/calmodulin, suggesting that lithium in vitro is directly able to inhibit the catalytic unit of AC. Because these inhibitory effects of lithium in vitro can be overcome by Mg^{2+} (Andersen and Geisler 1984; Geisler et al. 1985; Mork and Geisler 1987, 1989a; Mork et al. 1992; M. E. Newman and Belmaker 1987), they appear to be mediated (at least in part) by a direct competition with Mg^{2+} (whose hydrated ionic radius is similar to that of lithium) for a binding site on the catalytic unit of AC (Andersen and Geisler 1984; Mork and Geisler 1989a; Mork et al. 1992; M. E. Newman and Belmaker 1987). However, the inhibitory effects of *long-term* lithium treatment on rat brain AC are not reversed by Mg^{2+} and persist after washing of the membranes, but are reversed by increasing concentrations of GTP (Mork and Geisler 1989a; Mork et al. 1992). These results suggest that the therapeutically relevant effects of lithium (i.e., those seen on long-term drug administration and not reversed immediately on drug discontinuation) may be exerted at the level of signal-transducing G proteins at a GTP responsive step.

G Proteins

As noted above, abundant experimental evidence has shown that lithium attenuates receptor-mediated adenylyl cyclase activity and PI turnover in rodents and in humans in the absence of consistent changes in the density of the receptors themselves. The first direct evidence that G proteins may be the targets of lithium's actions was provided by Avissar and colleagues (1988), who reported that lithium dramatically *eliminated* isoproterenol- and carbachol-induced increases in [^{3}H]GTP binding to various G proteins in rat cerebral cortical membranes. These effects were reported to occur both in vitro in the presence of 0.6 mM LiCl and in washed cortical membranes from rats treated with lithium carbonate for 2–3 weeks, suggesting that the function of several G proteins (e.g., G_s, G_i, G_o) might be modified by this mood-stabilizing drug. In animals withdrawn from lithium for 2 days, agonist-stimulated response ([^{3}H]GTP binding) returned. Although these studies have been of considerable heuristic interest and the preponderance of data *does* suggest an action of long-term lithium at the level of G proteins, such a *direct* action of lithium on G protein function has been difficult to replicate in light of a number of methodological problems (Ellis and Lenox 1991; Manji et al. 1995); moreover, the fact that routine assays of agonist-stimulated PI hydrolysis in brain slices are conducted in the presence of 10 mM LiCl suggests that the lithium ion does not *directly* exert any major effects on Gq/11 protein function.

However, considerable evidence indicates that *long-term* lithium administration affects G protein function; numerous investigations have addressed the role of G proteins in the attenuated receptor-mediated AC activity and PI responses observed after long-term lithium administration in rodents and in humans (Casebolt and Jope 1989; Ebstein et al. 1976, 1987; Jope and Williams 1994; Manji 1992; M. E. Newman and Belmaker 1987; M. E. Newman et al. 1990; Risby et al. 1991; L. Song and Jope 1992). Using in vivo microdialysis measurements of cAMP, Masana and associates (1991, 1992) found that long-term lithium treatment produced a significant increase in basal and post-receptor-stimulated (cholera toxin or forskolin) AC activity, while attenuating the β-adrenergic-mediated effect in rat frontal cortex. Interestingly, long-term lithium treatment resulted in an almost absent cAMP response to pertussis toxin (Masana et al. 1991, 1992); taken together, these results suggest a lithium-induced attenuation of G_i function and of the

$\beta AR/G_s$ interaction. These researchers did not observe alterations in the amounts of α_s, α_{i1-3}, or α_o, but observed a significant increase in pertussis toxin–catalyzed $[^{32}P]$adenosine diphosphate (ADP)-ribosylation in both frontal cortex and hippocampus. Because pertussis toxin selectively ADP-ribosylates the undissociated, inactive $\alpha\beta\gamma$ heterotrimeric form of G_i (Hsiao et al. 1993; Ui 1990), these results suggest that lithium inactivates G_i via a stabilization of the inactive conformation (discussed in detail below). Long-term lithium administration also produces an alteration in measures of high-affinity binding to the βAR (thought to reflect its coupling to the G protein). Because the effects of long-term lithium administration on rat brain adenylyl cyclase activity are reversed by increasing concentrations of GTP (Mork and Geisler 1989a), these results suggest that lithium's effects may be exerted at a GTP responsive step and may result in an alteration in the conformational state (active/inactive) of the G protein.

At present, the possible effects of long-term lithium on the absolute *levels* of $G\alpha_s$ and $G\alpha_i$ remain unclear—two independent laboratories have not observed any alterations (Hsiao et al. 1993; Li et al. 1991; Masana et al. 1992), whereas another one has reported small but significant decreases in the levels of the α_s, α_{i1}, and α_{i2} in rat frontal cortex (Colin et al. 1991). However, long-term lithium administration reduces the mRNA levels of a number of G proteins in rat brain, including α_s, α_{i1}, and α_{i2} (Colin et al. 1991; Li et al. 1991), suggesting that lithium produces complex transcriptional and posttranscriptional effects after long-term administration (see below).

Studies have also examined the effects of long-term lithium treatment on G protein function in humans and have generally found reduced receptor/ G protein coupling (Ebstein et al. 1976, 1987; Garcia-Sevilla et al. 1986; Hsiao et al. 1992; Lonati-Galligani et al. 1989; M. E. Newman et al. 1992; Risby et al. 1991). The effects of 2 weeks of lithium administration on G protein measures has also been examined (Manji et al. 1991a; Risby et al. 1991) in psychiatrically healthy volunteers (which overcomes the potentially confounding, significant effects of alterations in mood–state-dependent biochemical and neuroendocrine parameters). Long-term lithium administration resulted in an increase in both basal and post-receptor- stimulated platelet AC activity, most compatible with an attenuation of G_i function (Manji et al. 1991a; Risby et al. 1991). Similar to the findings in rat brain, lithium did not affect the levels of platelet G protein α subunits, but produced a significant 40% increase in pertussis toxin–catalyzed $[^{32}P]$ADP-ribosylation, once again suggesting a stabilization of the inactive undissociated $\alpha\beta\gamma$ heterotrimeric form of G_i (Hsiao et al. 1993; Masana et al. 1992; Ui 1990).

Overall, the preponderance of the evidence from cell cultures and from rodent and human studies argues for an effect of *long-term* lithium on the G protein function in both humans and rodents. Interestingly, for both G_s and G_i, lithium's major effects appear to be a stabilization of the hetero-trimeric, undissociated ($\alpha\beta\gamma$) conformation of the G protein. This might produce a built-in temporal and spatial selectivity to lithium's actions, be-cause lithium would exert its major effects on those neurotransmitter sys-tems/ neuronal pathways undergoing the greatest activation and thus the highest rate of guanine nucleotide exchange. Such allosteric modulation of G proteins might also serve to explain the long-term prophylactic efficacy of the cation in protecting susceptible individuals from spontaneous and stress- and drug- (e.g., antidepressant, stimulants) induced cyclic affective episodes.

At present, the molecular mechanism(s) underlying lithium's effects on G proteins remains to be fully established. Although data indicate that com-petition with magnesium accounts for some of lithium's in vitro effects on G proteins, and speculation that an interaction with GTP binding might be relevant to the long-term effects of lithium (Avissar et al. 1988; Mork and Geisler 1989a), a *direct* effect of lithium on guanine nucleotide activation of G protein remains at this time unsubstantiated. Long-term effects (and argu-ably the therapeutically relevant effects) of long-term lithium on G protein may more likely be attributable to an indirect posttranslational modification of the G protein(s) and a relative change in the dynamic equilibrium of the active/inactive states of protein conformation, potentially resulting in modu-lation of receptor-mediated signaling in critical regions of the brain. Because G protein function is known to be regulated by phosphorylation (Garcia-Sainz and Gutierrez 1989; Halenda et al. 1986; Houslay 1991; Sagi-Eisenberg 1989), one potential mechanistic explanation for lithium's effects on G protein subunit dissociation is phosphorylation by PKC, an enzyme re-sponsible for considerable convergence and "cross-talk" between multiple second messenger systems (Houslay 1991; Manji 1992; Nishizuka 1992). Thus, in addition to exerting a negative feedback on receptors coupled to PIP_2 hydrolysis, activation of PKC also desensitizes several receptors coupled both positively and negatively to adenylyl cyclase, by affecting the coupling to the G proteins (Houslay 1991; Huganir and Greengard 1990; Manji 1992; Nishizuka 1992). Additionally, in a number of cell types, including platelets and striatal membranes, evidence suggests that PKC (similar to lithium) may enhance basal AC activity by attenuating the tonic inhibitory influence of G_i (Houslay 1991; Katada et al. 1985; Olianas and Onali 1986). Because accu-mulating evidence has demonstrated an effect of lithium on PKC isozymes (discussed below), and as PKC activation can affect both the PI and the AC transmembrane signaling pathways, PKC represents an attractive mechanism by which long-term lithium treatment modulates G protein function. It is also possible that the effects of lithium on G protein mRNA are mediated via PKC, because studies have demonstrated that PKC activation produces a similar decrease in $G\alpha_s$ mRNA and $G\alpha_{i2}$ mRNA levels in cells in vitro (Thiele and Eipper 1990). Such a contention receives additional support from the recent study demonstrating that daily coadministration of *myo*-inositol (administered intracerebroventricularly) markedly attenuates lithium-induced increases in pertussis toxin–catalyzed [^{32}P]ADP-ribosylation in rat brain (Manji et al. 1996). We now discuss the evidence for an effect of lithium on PKC isozymes.

Protein Kinase C and Phosphoprotein Substrates

Calcium-activated, phospholipid-dependent PKC is a ubiquitous enzyme, highly enriched in the brain, where it plays a major role in regulating presynaptic and postsynaptic aspects of neurotransmission (K. P. Huang 1989; Nishizuka 1992; Stabel and Parker 1991). PKC is one of the major intracellular mediators of signals generated upon external stimulation of cells via a variety of neurotransmitter receptor subtypes that induce the hydrolysis of membrane phospholipids. PKC is now known to exist as a family of closely related subspecies, has a heterogeneous distribution in the brain (with particularly high levels in presynaptic nerve terminals), and, together with other kinases, appears to play a crucial role in the regulation of synaptic plasticity. Molecular cloning has revealed the presence of multiple, closely related PKC isoforms; the differential tissue distribution of PKC isozymes, as well as the fact that several isoforms are expressed within a single cell type, suggests that each isozyme may exert distinct cellular functions (K. P. Huang 1989; Nishizuka 1992; Stabel and Parker 1991). At rest, the PKC isozymes exist in both cytosolic and membrane-bound forms, but with partitioning predominantly in the cytosolic form. Activation of PKC-coupled receptors (which results in the production of diacylglycerol [DAG]) facilitates the translocation of cytosolic PKC to the membrane and PKC's activation.

Evidence accumulating from various laboratories points to a role for PKC in mediating the action of lithium in a number of cell systems and the brain (Manji and Lenox 1994, in press). Currently available data suggest that short-term lithium exposure facilitates a number of PKC-mediated responses, whereas longer-term exposure results in an attenuation of phorbol ester–mediated responses, which may be accompanied by a downregulation of PKC (S. M. P. Anderson et al. 1988; J. A. Bitran et al. 1990; M. S. Evans et al. 1990; Lenox et al. 1992; Manji and Lenox 1994; Manji et al. 1993; Reisine and Zatz 1987; Sharp et al. 1991; Wang and Friedman 1989; Zatz and Reisine 1985). Interestingly, this pattern of effects is seen both in cultured cells in vitro and in brain in vivo. Biochemical studies have revealed biphasic effects of lithium on PKC-mediated events in rat hippocampus: short-term (3-day) lithium administration augments serotonin release, whereas longer-term (3-week) lithium administration at "therapeutic" levels attenuates both the phorbol ester–induced cytosol to membrane PKC translocation and the ^{3}H-labeled serotonin release in hippocampus (S. M. P. Anderson et al. 1988; Sharp et al. 1991; Wang and Friedman 1989). Using [^{3}H]phorbol ester dibutrate quantitative autoradiography, Manji and associates (1993) demonstrated that long-term (5-week) lithium administration results in a significant decrease in membrane-associated PKC in several hippocampal regions, most notably the subiculum and CA1 region, in the absence of any significant changes in the various other cortical and subcortical structures examined. Furthermore, immunoblotting using monoclonal anti-PKC antibodies revealed an isozyme-specific decrease in PKC α and ε in the absence of significant alterations in the β, γ, δ, or ζ isozymes following lithium treatment (Manji et al. 1993, in press). The mechanism(s) by which lithium, presumably via an elevation of DAG levels (Brami et al. 1991a, 1991b; Drummond and Raeburn 1984; S. P. Watson et al. 1990), produces the intriguing, isozyme-selective decrease of PKC α and ε is unclear, although the subspecies of PKC do exhibit subtle differences in their biochemical characteristics and intracellular and intercellular locations. Because PKC activation is often followed by its rapid proteolytic degradation (K. P. Huang 1989; Nishizuka 1992; Stabel and Parker 1991; S. Young et al. 1987), a prolonged increase in DAG levels by lithium may lead to an increased membrane translocation and subsequent degradation of PKC. This suggestion receives support from the recent study demonstrating that daily coadministration of *myo*-inositol (administered intracerebroventricularly) markedly attenuates lithium-induced decreases in PKC α and ε (Manji et al. 1996). Such a mechanism would also be consistent with the accumulating evidence that lithium acutely activates PKC, whereas prolonged treatment is associated with decreased PKC-mediated responses, including neurotransmitter release (Manji and Lenox 1994).

PKC activation results in phosphorylation of a number of membrane-associated substrates. Prominent PKC substrates include the growth-associated protein GAP-43 (also known as F1, P57, pp46, B-50, neuromodulin, 43–57 kDa), myristoylated alanine-rich C-kinase substrate (MARCKS, 80–87 kDa), and neurogranin (also known as RC3, BICKS, and 17 kDa). Each of these proteins shares a PKC phosphorylation domain and a calmodulin-binding domain. Preliminary studies investigating the effects of long-term lithium administration in vivo on in vitro PKC substrate phosphorylation indicate increased phosphorylation of four endogenous proteins in the soluble fraction (16, 17, 30, and 22 kDa) and reduced phosphorylation of three endogenous proteins in the particulate fraction (18, 19, and 87 kDa) in the rat hippocampus (Casebolt and Jope 1991). The identity and functional significance of these proteins remains to be determined. In a second study, lithium administered long-term in vivo reduced PKC- mediated in vitro phosphorylation of two endogenous PKC substrates (45 and 83 kDa) while having no effect on three other PKC (105-, 170-, and >200-kDa) and two non-PKC (54- and >250-kDa) substrates in the soluble fraction in rat hippocampus (Lenox et al. 1992). Although the 43-kDa protein was not identified, the 83-kDa protein was determined to be MARCKS by Western blot analysis. Animal studies found that MARCKS was reduced in both soluble and particulate fractions of the hippocampus following long-term (but not short-term) lithium administration and remained decreased 40 hours following lithium withdrawal (Lenox and Watson 1994; Lenox et al. 1992). Studies in neuronal and nonneuronal cell populations indicate that phorbol ester–induced PKC activation will downregulate MARCKS protein and mRNA levels (Broocks et al. 1992; D. G. Watson et al. 1994). Additional studies in immortalized hippocampal cells strongly support a role for PKC in the downregulation of MARCKS following long-term lithium administration and its dependency on the level of receptor-coupled PI hydrolysis and inositol recycling (D. G. Watson and Lenox 1996). It appears that both chronic valproate and lithium share the property of regulating the expression of MARCKS in immortalized hippocampal cells at clinically relevant concentrations to the exclusion of the other psychotropic agents examined (D. G. Watson et al. 1998). MARCKS cross-links filamentous actin and has been implicated in cellular processes including cytoskeletal restructuring, transmembrane signaling, and neurotransmitter release (Blackshear 1993). MARCKS is enriched in neuronal growth cones, is developmentally regulated, and is necessary for normal brain development (McNamara and Lenox 1998; Stumpo et al. 1995; Swierczynski et al. 1996). MARCKS expression remains elevated in restricted neuronal populations in the adult rat (McNamara and Lenox 1997) and human brain (McNamara et al. 1999), and its expression is induced in the mature central nervous system during axonal regeneration (Schnizer et al. 1997). Adult mutant mice expressing MARCKS at 50%, but with no apparent morphological abnormalities in brain, show significant spatial learning deficits that are transgenically "rescued" (McNamara et al. 1998). Finally, the induction of long-term potentiation, a physiological model of activity-dependent synaptic plasticity, elevates MARCKS phosphorylation (Ramakers et al., in press). Collectively, these data reveal that MARCKS plays an important role in the mediation of neuroplastic processes in the developing and mature CNS. Its reduction following long-term lithium administration may therefore play a role in altering pre- and postsynaptic membrane structure to stabilize aberrant neuronal activity in key brain regions (Lenox and Watson 1994).

Gene Expression

As discussed, there has been a growing appreciation that any relevant biochemical model of lithium's actions must account for the observation that its prophylactic efficacy generally requires weeks to develop (F. K. Goodwin and Jamison 1990b; Jope and Williams 1994; Manji and Lenox 1994); biochemical changes requiring such prolonged administration of a drug suggest alterations at the genomic level. In this context, it is noteworthy that increasing evidence suggests that lithium affects gene expression, possibly via PKC-induced alterations in nuclear transcription regulatory factors responsible for modulating the expression of specific genes (Bohmann 1990; Hunter and Karin 1992). Several studies have demonstrated that lithium alters the expression of the early response gene c-*fos* in different cell systems including the brain through a PKC-mediated mechanism (reviewed in Manji and Lenox 1994). For example, preincubation of cultured PC12 cells (a rat pheochromocytoma cell line) with lithium for 16 hours markedly potentiates *fos* expression in response to the muscarinic agonist carbachol. Lithium pretreatment in these cells also potentiates *fos* expression in response to phorbol esters, which directly activates PKC and thus bypasses PI turnover (Divish et al. 1991; Kalasapudi et al. 1990). Moreover, lithium's effects show a selectivity for the PKC signal transduction pathway and do not appear to be a result of a nonspecific alteration in mRNA stability, because the *fos* expression in response to AC activation is unaffected under identical conditions (Divish et al. 1991; Kalasapudi et al. 1990). Paralleling the results observed in cell culture, a single intraperitoneal injection of lithium results in an augmentation of pilocarpine-induced *fos* gene expression in rat brain, which can be antagonized by the M_1 muscarinic antagonist pirenzepine (E. D. Weiner et al. 1991). These lithium-induced effects on the expression of *fos* mRNA, generally thought to represent a "master switch" to turn on a "second wave" of specific neuronal genes of functional importance, offer a mechanism for affecting long-term events in the brain. In this regard, incubation of cerebellar granule cells with 1.5 mM lithium has been shown to result in biphasic effects on the levels of both *fos* mRNA and muscarinic M_3 receptor mRNA, consistent with the previously noted short-term versus long-term effects of lithium on PKC-mediated responses (Gao et al. 1993). Long-term "therapeutic" in vivo administration of lithium also significantly changes the expression of a number of genes in rat brain, several of which are known neuromodulatory peptide hormones (prodynorphin, preprotachykinin) and their receptors (glucocorticoid type II), and are known to contain PKC-responsive elements (neuropeptide Y) (Kislauskis and Dobner 1990; Pfeiffer et al. 1991; Sivam et al. 1988, 1989; Weiner et al. 1991). In view of lithium's proposed actions on synaptic function and signal transducing systems, it is also noteworthy that *long-term* lithium administration (3–4 weeks) has been reported to alter the *expression* of various components of second messenger generating systems including $G\alpha_{i1}$, $G\alpha_{i2}$, and $G\alpha_s$ mRNA and AC type I and type II mRNA in rat brain (Colin et al. 1991; Li et al. 1991).

It has been demonstrated recently that lithium, at therapeutically relevant concentrations, regulates AP-1 DNA binding activity in vitro (G. Chen et al. 1997, 1999; Jope, in press; Ozaki and Chuang 1997; Yuan et al. 1998). A luciferase reporter gene system known to be regulated by AP-1 has been used to confirm that these effects on AP-1 DNA binding activity do, in fact, translate into changes at the gene expression level in vitro (G. Chen et al. 1999; Yuan et al. 1998). Lithium exposure results in a time- and concentration-dependent increase in the expression of a luciferase reporter gene driven by an SV40 promoter/enhancer that contains transcription regulatory factors (TREs) (G. Chen et al. 1997, 1999; Yuan et al. 1998). Furthermore, mutations in the TRE sites of the reporter gene promoter markedly attenuated these effects. These data indicate that lithium may stimulate gene expression (at least in part) through the AP-1 transcription factor pathway, and these effects may play an important role in its long-term clinical actions. However, to ascribe any potential therapeutic relevance to the above biochemical findings, it is obviously necessary to show that they *do*, in fact, also occur in critical regions of the central nervous system in vivo. We have therefore investigated the effects of chronic lithium on AP-1 DNA binding activity in rat frontal cortex and hippocampus. Similar to what has been seen in rat and human cells in vitro, lithium markedly increased the DNA binding activity of the AP-1 family of transcription factors (Manji and Lenox, in press). It is of interest that valproate has had similar effects on AP-1 DNA binding activity both in vitro and in vivo. In view of the key roles of these nuclear transcription regulatory factors in long-term neuronal plasticity and cellular responsiveness, and the potential to regulate patterns of gene expression in critical neuronal circuits (Boyle et al. 1991; Lin et al. 1993), these effects may play a major role in lithium's and valproate's long-term beneficial effects.

The demonstration of the long-term modulation of the genetic expression of critical proteins involved in the regulation of synaptic and transmembrane signaling in the brain is of considerable heuristic importance and offers new strategies for unraveling the complex physiological effects of long-term lithium treatment in the prophylaxis of recurrent episodes of affective illness in patients with bipolar disorder.

NEUROANATOMICAL SITE OF ACTION

Neuroimaging and lesion studies have provided important information as to the neuroanatomical basis of bipolar illness (reviewed in Bolwig 1993; Nasrallah et al. 1989). Examination of whole brain metabolic rates indicates significantly lower rates in drug-free patients with bipolar depression relative to rates in patients with bipolar mania or unipolar depression or subjects who are psychiatrically healthy (L. R. Baxter et al. 1985; Phelps et al. 1984 [but see Buchsbaum et al. 1986]), which normalized when subjects shifted to a euthymic or manic state (L. R. Baxter et al. 1985). Other studies indicate that patients with bipolar mania exhibit higher global glucose metabolism (H. Kishimoto et al. 1987) and significantly higher global cerebral blood flow (Rush et al. 1982 [but see Delvenne et al. 1990]) relative to that of psychiatrically healthy subjects. Anteroposterior differences have not been observed (L. R. Baxter et al. 1985; Devous et al. 1984), although a relative hypofrontality was found in subjects with bipolar disorder when a series of painful stimuli were administered during tracer uptake (Buchsbaum et al. 1986). Moreover, no consistent hemispheric differences in metabolism have been observed in subjects with bipolar disorder (L. R. Baxter et al. 1985; Buchsbaum et al. 1986; Phelps et al. 1984), but lesion studies indicate that damage to right hemisphere structures is more commonly associated with the development of secondary mania (M. R. Cohen and Niska 1980; Cummings and Mendez 1984; Forrest 1982; R. G. Robinson et al. 1988; Starkstein et al. 1990).

Several studies have demonstrated an enlargement of third and lateral ventricle volume in patients with bipolar disorder (Dewan et al. 1988; Pearlson et al. 1984; Rieder et al. 1983; Schlegel and Kretzschmar 1987; Strakowski et al. 1993b; Swayze et al. 1992), although the lateral ventricle enlargement is not consistently observed (Johnstone et al. 1986; Swayze et al. 1990). Ventricular enlargement would be expected to affect the functional integrity of structures that line the ventricles. Indeed, caudate and thalamic nuclei, two paraventricular structures, exhibit an increased density bilaterally in bipolar patients (Dewan et al. 1988), and lesions of the right head of the caudate and right thalamus are associated with the development of secondary mania (Starkstein et al. 1991). However, other studies have found no difference in metabolic and blood flow rates in caudate or thalamus in patients with bipolar disorder (L. R. Baxter et al. 1985), and caudate and thalamus volume did not differ in patients with first-episode mania (Strakowski et al. 1993b) or in patients with bipolar disorder (Swayze et al. 1992).

Several converging lines of evidence indicate that abnormalities in the temporal lobe contribute to bipolar illness. First, temporal lobe epilepsy in the right hemisphere has been associated with the onset of bipolar symptomatology (Barczak et al. 1988; Drake 1988; Flor-Henry 1969; Gillig et al. 1988). Second, significantly lower regional cerebral blood flow is observed in the basal portion of the right temporal cortex of subjects with mania (Migliorelli et al. 1993), whereas higher blood flow is observed in the left temporal lobes of subjects with bipolar disorder who are depressed (Devous et al. 1984) relative to control subjects. Third, temporal lobe volume is smaller bilaterally (Altshuler et al. 1991) or larger in the right hemisphere of subjects with bipolar disorder (Dewan et al. 1988), although another study found right temporal lobe volume to be larger in both psychiatrically healthy subjects and subjects with bipolar disorder (Swayze et al. 1992). Finally, lesions of the basotemporal cortex are significantly correlated with the development of secondary mania (Jorge et al. 1993; Starkstein et al. 1991). Importantly, the volume of the right hippocampus, a structure located within the temporal lobe, has been reported to be significantly reduced in patients with bipolar disorder (Swayze et al. 1992).

Lithium-induced depletion of inositol via the *un*competitive inhibition of *myo*-inositol-1-phosphatase has been proposed to account for the physiological consequences of lithium and predicts that lithium will have the greatest impact on cells undergoing the greatest receptor-mediated PIP_2 hydrolysis (e.g., Nahorski et al. 1991). Studies assessing regional changes in PI turnover indicate no consistent change in PI levels following long-term in vivo lithium treatment in either cortex or caudate/putamen (Honchar et al. 1989) or a comparable reduction of PI turnover in cortical, hippocampal, and striatal membranes (L. Song and Jope 1992). However, other studies have demonstrated that lithium-induced depletion of inositol is similar in magnitude among hypothalamus, hippocampus, and caudate, but unchanged in cerebellum (see W. R. Sherman et al. 1986); and K^+- or agonist-stimulated $[^3H]IP$ accumulation is highest in cortex, thalamus, hippocampus, and striatum, moderate in hypothalamus, pons, and medulla, but low to absent in cerebellum in the presence of lithium in vitro (5–10 mM) (R. D. Johnson and Minneman 1985; Rooney and Nahorski 1986). Hence, lithium appears to have its greatest impact on PI signaling in diencephalic and telencephalic regions, perhaps relating to its accumulation in these regions (see below). It is of note that PKC, which is activated by elevations of DAG in response to lithium-induced inositol depletion (reviewed in Manji and Lenox 1994), is selectively reduced in hippocampus, but not in other cortical and subcortical structures, following long-term lithium treatment (Manji et al. 1993).

Evidence from studies examining the effects of lithium on classic neurotransmitter systems in different brain regions would also indicate that lithium's actions have regional specificity. Following long-term lithium treatment, ^{3}H-labeled serotonin binding is reduced in hippocampus and striatum but not in cortex or hypothalamus (Maggi and Enna 1980; Odagaki et al. 1990). Serotonin synthesis is reduced in hypothalamus and brain stem but not in cortex or cerebellum (Ho et al. 1970), and K^+-stimulated serotonin release is enhanced in hypothalamus, hippocampus, and cortex, but spontaneous release is reduced in hypothalamus and cortex but increased in hippocampus following long-term, but not short-term, lithium treatment (E. Friedman and Wang 1988). In a related study, basal and K^+-induced serotonin release was increased in hippocampus but not in cortex following long-term lithium treatment (Treiser et al. 1981). Subchronic lithium administration reduces serotonin synaptosomal reuptake in striatum, hypothalamus, hippocampus, and midbrain but not in pons or cortex (Ahluwalia and Singhal 1985). A competitive binding assay revealed that long-term lithium treatment reduced 5-HT$_1$, 5-HT$_{1C}$, and 5-HT$_2$ in frontal cortex, hippocampus, and choroid plexus, whereas 5-HT$_{1A}$ receptors were reduced in hippocampus and choroid plexus, but not in frontal cortex (Mizuta and Segawa 1989). Short-term (5-day) lithium treatment was found to reduce tryptophan levels in limbic forebrain and striatum but reduced 5-HT synthesis only in striatum (Berggren 1987). DA content in brain following long-term lithium treatment is significantly reduced in pons and midbrain but not in hypothalamus, striatum, hippocampus, or cortex (Ahluwalia and Singhal 1980), whereas other studies indicate little variation in DA content across brain regions (Ho et al. 1970). NE binding in brain following long-term lithium treatment is significantly increased in the caudate nucleus but unchanged in brain stem, hypothalamus, or parietal cortex (O. G. Cameron and Smith 1980), and another study found no change in β-adrenergic binding in cortex, hippocampus, or striatum (Maggi and Enna 1980). NE concentrations are reduced in pons, hypothalamus, and midbrain but not in striatum or hippocampus (Ahluwalia and Singhal 1980), and NE reuptake is increased in pons, striatum, hippocampus, midbrain, and cortex but not in hypothalamus following long-term lithium treatment (Ahluwalia and Singhal 1985). ACh (muscarinic) binding in brain following long-term lithium treatment revealed no significant changes in cortex, hippocampus, or striatum (Maggi and Enna 1980), although the synthesis of ACh was observed to be increased in striatum, hippocampus, and cortex (Jope 1979). Finally, GABA receptor binding is reduced significantly in corpus striatum and hypothalamus but not in cortex, cerebellum, or hippocampus following long-term lithium treatment (Maggi and Enna 1980).

The premise that lithium exerts its therapeutic actions by acting at specific neuroanatomical sites is supported by several lines of evidence. Lithium does not distribute evenly throughout the brain following either short- or long-term administration, but accumulates in specific regions where it may exert its greatest impact on cell signaling processes. Although there is some discrepancy between individual studies in terms of the regions showing the highest levels of lithium, a general trend has emerged. Studies using atomic absorption spectrophotometry to determine regional lithium concentrations indicate high levels in the striatum, intermediate levels in the hippocampus and hypothalamus, and low levels in the spinal cord and medulla in the rat following short-term in vivo administration (Ebadi et al. 1974). Following long-term in vivo administration (2–5 weeks, 30–45 mM lithium diet), high lithium levels are detected in diencephalic structures, particularly the hypothalamus, and in telencephalic structures including the striatum and hippocampus, whereas low levels are detected in metencephalic structures such as the cerebellum (Bond et al. 1975; Edelfors 1975; Lam and Christensen 1992; Savolainen et al. 1990; D. F. Smith and Amdisen 1981; Spirtes 1976). Studies using radiographic dielectric track registration or nuclear magnetic resonance to localize lithium distribution also indicate forebrain accumulation (Heurteaux et al. 1986; S. C. Nelson et al. 1980; Ramaprasad et al. 1992; Thellier et al. 1980).

CONCLUSION

Lithium remains our most effective treatment for reducing the frequency and severity of recurrent affective episodes, but, despite extensive research, the underlying biological basis for the therapeutic efficacy of this drug remains unknown. Lithium is a monovalent cation with complex physiological and pharmacological effects within the brain. By virtue of the ionic properties it shares with other important monovalent and divalent cations such as sodium, magnesium, and calcium, its transport into cells provides ready access to a host of intracellular enzymatic events affecting short- and long-term cell processes. It may be that, in part, the therapeutic efficacy of lithium in the treatment of both poles of bipolar disorder may rely on the "dirty" characteristics of its multiple sites of pharmacological interaction.

Strategic models to further delineate the mechanism(s) of action of lithium relevant to its therapeutic effects must account for a number of critical variables in experimental design. Lithium has a relatively low therapeutic index, requiring careful attention to the tissue concentrations at which effects of the drug are being observed in light of the known toxicity of lithium within the central nervous system. Although such a poor therapeutic index may suggest a continuum between some of the biological processes underlying therapeutic efficacy and toxicity, it may also account in part for the variability of effects of lithium observed in animal and in vitro studies. The therapeutic action of lithium is delayed, requiring long-term administration to establish efficacy for both its treatment of acute mania and its prophylaxis of the recurrent affective episodes associated with bipolar disorder. Although its therapeutic effects are not reversed immediately upon abrupt discontinuation, there is accumulating evidence that abrupt withdrawal of lithium may sensitize the system to an episode of mania (E. Klein et al. 1992; Suppes et al. 1991).

In recent years, there has been dramatic progress in the identification of signal transduction pathways as targets for lithium's actions. Regulation of signal transduction within critical regions of the brain by lithium affects the "throughput" of multiple neurotransmitter systems; the ability of lithium to stabilize an underlying dysregulation of limbic and limbic-associated function is critical to our understanding of its mechanism of action. A general trend is beginning to emerge implicating right hemisphere structures, particularly the temporal lobe, caudate, thalamic nuclei, and, by implication, those regions that give and receive projections from these regions, including the hippocampus and hypothalamus, in the production of bipolar symptomatology. The biological processes in the brain responsible for the episodic clinical manifestation of mania and depression may be due to an inability to mount the appropriate compensatory responses necessary to maintain homeostatic regulation, thereby resulting in sudden oscillations beyond immediate adaptive control (Depue et al. 1987; F. K. Goodwin and Jamison 1990b; Mandell et al. 1984). The resultant clinical picture is reflected in disruption of behavior, circadian rhythms, neurophysiology of sleep, and neuroendocrine and biochemical regulation within the brain. Lithium's efficacy in treating these symptoms may be the result of its ability to target and stabilize disruptive activity in critical regions of the brain. The behavioral and physiological manifestations of the illness are complex and are mediated by a network of interconnected neurotransmitter pathways. The biogenic amines have been strongly implicated in the regulation of these physiological processes by virtue of their pharmacological actions and predominant neuroanatomical distribution within limbic-related regions of the brain. Thus, lithium's ability to modulate release of serotonin at presynaptic sites and affect DA-induced supersensitivity in the brain remains a relevant line of investigation into the respective action of lithium in altering the clinical manifestation of depression and mania in the patient with bipolar disorder.

Some of the most exciting recent advances in our understanding of the long-term therapeutic action of lithium have been the identification of the effects on PKC-mediated events, particularly the posttranslational modification of important proteins responsible for regulation of signal transduction in the brain. Biochemical changes requiring prolonged administration of a drug such as lithium also suggest alterations at the genomic level, which may be mediated in large part by the activation and inactivation of subsets of genes with temporal specificity. In this context, the complex effect of lithium on PKC isozymes represents an attractive and heuristic mechanism by which the expression of various proteins involved in long-term neuronal plasticity and cellular response is modulated, thereby compensating for as yet genetically undefined physiological abnormalities in critical regions of the brain.

Many questions remain to be answered. For example, do the effects of chronic lithium on signal transduction pathways and gene expression stem exclusively from its demonstrated efficacy as an inhibitor of inositol monophosphatase and resultant changes in the DAG pathway, or does lithium under therapeutic conditions have other, more direct effects? Studies examining the effects of other inositol monophosphatase inhibitors (with no structural similarity to lithium) may provide important clues and offer insights into new drug development. In an interesting series of studies in the *Xenopus*, in which lithium exposure significantly altered the dorsal-ventral axis of the developing embryo, inhibition of inositol monophosphatase by another inhibitor did not result in similar alterations in morphogenesis, suggesting that lithium may be acting in an alternative pathway (Kao and Elinson 1989, 1998; P. S. Klein and Melton 1996). These studies have found that lithium inhibits glycogen synthase kinase-3β (GSK-3β) activity ($K_i = 2.1$ mM), which antagonizes the *wnt* signaling pathway associated with normal dorsal-ventral axis development in the *Xenopus* embryo. Studies that used an embryo expressing a dominant negative form of GSK-3β suggested that *myo*-inositol reversal of dorsalization of the embryonic axis by lithium may be mediated by events independent of inositol monophosphatase inhibition (Hedgepeth et al. 1997). To what extent these findings relate to the therapeutic action of lithium in the brain has not yet been determined. However, it is at the molecular level that some of the most exciting advances in the understanding of the long-term therapeutic action of lithium will occur over the coming years. It would appear that the current studies of the long-term lithium-induced changes in PKC-mediated events, including gene expression and transcriptional modification of important phosphoproteins responsible for regulation of signal transduction in the brain, are a most promising avenue for future investigation. This is particularly of interest in light of converging data from studies of chronic lithium relating its therapeutic efficacy to the regulation of membrane-related events such as ion transport, neurotransmitter release, and the receptor-response complex, all of which involve some degree of cytoskeletal restructuring. Forthcoming research along these lines also may provide clues to a molecular basis for the pathophysiology of bipolar disorder.

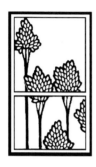

CHAPTER 8

Clinical Efficacy of Valproate in Bipolar Illness: Comparisons and Contrasts With Lithium

Stephen M. Strakowski, M.D.,
Susan L. McElroy, M.D., and
Paul E. Keck Jr., M.D.

Bipolar disorder is a common psychiatric illness, affecting up to 1%–1.6% of the general population (Kessler et al. 1994; Weissman et al. 1991). For the past 20 years, the mainstay of the pharmacological treatment for bipolar disorder has been lithium. Although lithium was identified in the 1940s as a potential antimanic agent, it was not approved for use in the United States until the early 1970s, and, until very recently, it remained the sole pharmacological compound approved for the treatment of bipolar disorder. During the past decade, however, it has become evident that the anticonvulsants valproate and carbamazepine are also effective antimanic agents. Recent well-designed, large studies of the divalproex formulation of valproate were completed and led to U.S. Food and Drug Administration (FDA) approval of this compound as an antimanic agent. In this chapter, we review the evidence supporting the efficacy of valproate and lithium in bipolar disorder, and compare and contrast each drug's effects.

EFFICACY OF LITHIUM IN ACUTE MANIA

Lithium entered psychiatry following John Cade's observations that it produced a calming effect in rodents and, ultimately, in psychiatric patients (Cade 1949). Unfortunately, as a result of severe toxic reactions following its use as a sodium substitute, the FDA approval of the drug occurred slowly. Although there is a large literature of uncontrolled lithium trials (F. K. Goodwin and Jamison 1990b), only five placebo-controlled clinical trials for the treatment of acute mania have been reported. (For detailed review, see Manji et al., Chapter 7, in this volume.)

EFFICACY OF VALPROATE IN ACUTE MANIA

Valproate, a simple branched-chain fatty acid, was first reported as a successful treatment for acute mania by Lambert and colleagues in 1966. Following this report, at least 16 uncontrolled trials consistently supported the observation that valproate has acute and long-term mood-stabilizing effects in patients with bipolar disorder (reviewed by Keck et al. 1992a). Recently, five double-blind controlled studies of valproate have been completed that provide definitive evidence of its efficacy in acute mania.

The earlier controlled studies involved small numbers of patients in which valproate was compared with placebo in crossover trial designs (Brennan et al. 1984; Emrich et al. 1981). Ten of the 13 patients (71%) in these trials were rated as having a marked response to valproate using a variety of clinical efficacy measures, but the small number of subjects in each study precluded definitive conclusions. In 1991, Pope and colleagues compared valproate (divalproex sodium) with placebo in 36 patients with acute mania meeting criteria for DSM-III-R (American Psychiatric Association 1987) bipolar disorder treated for up to 3 weeks in the first parallel-group, double-blind, placebo-controlled study of this agent. Study patients were limited to those who were either treatment refractory or lithium intolerant. Compared with the 19 patients who received placebo, the 17 patients who received valproate demonstrated significant improvement on all rating scales used by the investigators (i.e., the Young Mania Rating Scale [R. C. Young et al. 1978], the Global Assessment Scale [GAS; Endicott et al. 1976], and the Brief Psychiatric Rating Scale [BPRS; Overall and Gorham 1962]). They also required significantly less "rescue" lorazepam, which was the only other psychotropic allowed in this trial.

T. W. Freeman et al. (1992) reported the first double-blind, parallel-group comparison of valproate and lithium in acute DSM-III-R–defined mania. Response was measured at the end of the 3-week trial as a 50% reduction in scores on the Schedule for Affective Disorders and Schizophrenia, change version (SADS-C; Spitzer and Endicott 1978). Freeman and co-workers observed a response rate of 92% of patients on lithium and 64% on valproate. Additionally, significant improvement was noted on other rating scales (GAS, BPRS) for both treatment groups. These researchers stated that these results suggested that lithium was a more effective antimanic agent. However, the lithium response rate in this study was unusually high, and, in fact, the differential response did not meet statistical significance.

More recently, a large, multicenter randomized, double-blind, parallel-group study of treatment outcomes of Research Diagnostic Criteria (RDC; Spitzer et al. 1985)–defined acute mania in 179 hospitalized patients comparing valproate (in the divalproex form), lithium, and placebo was reported (Bowden et al. 1994b). Patients were entered into the 3-week treatment arms in a ratio of 2:1:2 for valproate ($n = 68$), lithium ($n = 35$), and placebo ($n = 73$), respectively. Response was defined as a 50% reduction in the Manic Syndrome Subscale of the SADS-C. Patients receiving lithium had a 49% response rate; those receiving valproate, a 48% response rate; and those receiving placebo, a 25% response rate. The dropout rate resulting from lack of efficacy was similar for that of lithium (33%) and valproate (30%), but higher for placebo (51%). Thus, the authors concluded that lithium and valproate were equally effective for the treatment of acute mania and more effective than placebo.

In total, 61 (54%) of 113 patients with acute mania treated with valproate in controlled clinical trials showed moderate or better improvement. In those trials comparing it with placebo, valproate demonstrated significant efficacy. Further, when compared with lithium, no significant differences in response rates were observed. In summary, valproate has demonstrated considerable efficacy in the treatment of acute mania, although, as with lithium, 25%–50% of the patients in these trials did not respond.

EFFICACY OF LITHIUM IN BIPOLAR DEPRESSION

In contrast with studies of the treatment of acute mania, studies of lithium in bipolar depression are less common. Initially, Cade (1949) reported that lithium had no efficacy in the treatment of depression, although this opinion was reversed by the results of several open trials and finally a controlled study by Fieve et al. in 1968. Subsequently, eight placebo-controlled trials have been reported (M. Baron et al. 1975; Donnelly et al. 1978; Fieve et al. 1968; F. K. Goodwin et al. 1969, 1972; Mendels 1976; Noyes et al. 1974; Stokes et al. 1971).

In the earliest controlled study, Fieve et al. (1968) compared lithium, imipramine, and placebo in the treatment of 29 patients clinically diagnosed with manic-depressive illness, depressed-type. Patients were treated with placebo for 2–4 weeks, then randomly assigned to receive imipramine or lithium. Both active treatments demonstrated improvement in all mean depression score ratings compared with those from the placebo period, although improvements in the imipramine-treated group were greater than those in the lithium group. However, the level of significance of these differences was not determined, nor did the authors mention whether lithium serum levels were monitored. Nonetheless, the authors concluded that lithium demonstrated antidepressant activity.

Shortly thereafter, F. K. Goodwin and colleagues (1969, 1972) studied lithium compared with placebo in the treatment of bipolar depression and observed an "unequivocal response" in only 30% of patients, although another 50% exhibited "equivocal" responses. Stokes et al. (1971) observed a 59% lithium response in 18 patients with bipolar depression compared with a 48% response to placebo, a nonsignificant difference. As noted previously, this double-blind, crossover study kept patients on lithium only 7–10 days. Nonetheless, Stokes and co-workers concluded that lithium was not a particularly effective agent for bipolar depression. More recent studies have replicated these findings, reporting response rates to lithium in bipolar depression of 44%–100% (M. Baron et al. 1975; Donnelly et al. 1978; Mendels 1976; Noyes et al. 1974). In summary, 160 patients received lithium in these crossover studies with placebo with a pooled response rate of 72%. Of note, many of these responses were only partial, and there are no parallel studies with placebo, which is an important limitation given the well-known high placebo response rate in depression (cf. Stokes et al. 1971). Nonetheless, lithium has been the most widely studied antidepressant treatment in bipolar disorder and appears to be effective without the risk of inducing mania or rapid cycling associated with other antidepressants (Zornberg and Pope 1993).

EFFICACY OF VALPROATE IN BIPOLAR DEPRESSION

In contrast with lithium, there are no controlled trials of valproate in the treatment of bipolar depression. Three uncontrolled reports (Hayes 1989;

Lambert 1984; McElroy et al. 1988b) suggested that valproate may be a much better antimanic than antidepressant agent. In a study of 78 consecutively re-cruited patients with rapid-cycling bipolar disorder treated with open-label valproate alone or in combination with other psychotropic agents, Calabrese and colleagues (Calabrese and Delucchi 1990; Calabrese et al. 1992) reported a 54% valproate response in acute mania, an 87% response in acute mixed states, and a 19% response in acute depression. However, they did observe a prophylactic antidepressant effect in patients subsequently. Additional con-trolled studies are needed to clarify valproate's antidepressant efficacy.

EFFICACY OF LITHIUM IN MAINTENANCE TREATMENT OF BIPOLAR DISORDER

Lithium has been well studied as a prophylactic agent in bipolar disorder in a number of open trials (reviewed in F. K. Goodwin and Jamison 1990b) and in at least nine placebo-controlled trials (Baastrup et al. 1970; Coppen et al. 1971, 1973; Cundall et al. 1972; Dunner et al. 1976; Fieve et al. 1976; Melia 1970; Prien et al. 1973a, 1973b; Stallone et al. 1973). In their controlled study, Baastrup and colleagues (1970) studied 50 female patients with a clini-cal diagnosis of manic-depressive illness, bipolar type, who had been stabi-lized on lithium (open-label) and were switched in a double-blind fashion to either receive placebo or continue on lithium. Patients were followed for up to 5 months and evaluated at 2- to 4-month intervals. Relapse was defined as the recurrence of either depression or mania of "sufficient severity" to require either hospitalization or home monitoring. None of the patients receiving lith-ium, but more than half of those receiving placebo, relapsed within a 5-month period. Several other smaller studies followed that provided further support for the effectiveness of lithium as a prophylactic agent (Coppen et al. 1971, 1973; Cundall et al. 1972; Melia 1970; Stallone et al. 1973).

In a large multicenter parallel-group trial prospectively evaluating the ef-fectiveness of lithium ($n = 101$) compared with that of placebo ($n = 104$) in preventing relapse, Prien et al. (1973b) observed a marked benefit for pa-tients receiving lithium. In this study, hospitalized patients with clinical diag-noses of manic-depressive illness, manic type, received standard clinical treatment until achieving "remission" of the acute manic episode. Patients were then stabilized on lithium and, at discharge, randomly assigned to con-tinue to receive lithium or placebo. Patients were followed up for up to 2 years, and outcome was defined in terms of the frequency and severity of "relapses." Outcome variables (relapse and remission) were based on clinical assessment, rather than being operationally defined. Relapses requiring hospitalization were considered "severe," and those requiring medication modification, but not hospitalization, were defined as "moderate." Eighty percent of those receiving placebo experienced relapse compared with 43% receiving lithium. These data, combined with those of prior studies, led to FDA approval of lithium for maintenance treatment in manic-depressive illness.

Following these studies, Fieve and colleagues (Dunner et al. 1976; Fieve et al. 1976) also demonstrated a significant effect for prophylactic lithium therapy in patients with bipolar type II. In summary, 248 patients treated with lithium for 5–40 months had a pooled relapse rate of 32% compared with 260 patients who received placebo and had a relapse rate of 75%.

EFFICACY OF VALPROATE IN MAINTENANCE TREATMENT OF BIPOLAR DISORDER

To our knowledge, there have been no reports of controlled clinical trials of valproate as a prophylactic agent in bipolar disorder. Results from a number of open trials suggest that perhaps half of patients treated with valproate experience prophylactic benefit (reviewed in Keck et al. 1992a). A placebo-controlled, double-blind study of the efficacy of the divalproex form of valproate is under way and may provide additional information regarding the use of this drug in the maintenance therapy of bipolar disorder.

PREDICTORS OF LITHIUM RESPONSE AND NONRESPONSE

Although studies reviewed thus far support the efficacy of lithium treatment for acute mania, the presence of concurrent depression or depressive symptoms during mania, the so-called mixed state, has been associated with poor lithium response. In 1976, Himmelhoch et al. observed that patients with mixed states were significantly less likely to demonstrate a good treatment response than were manic patients (42% vs. 81%) in a retrospective chart review of 84 consecutively referred patients with bipolar disorder. Secunda et al. (1985) reported on 18 patients with mania studied as part of the Collaborative Study of the Psychobiology of Depression and found that patients with concomitant depression and mania ($n = 8$) had a significantly lower rate of recovery (25%) than did patients with mania without depression (90%). Prien et al. (1988) studied 103 patients with mania who were initially treated by "psychiatrist's choice" in an open fashion, generally with lithium and with or without a neuroleptic or an antidepressant. Patients stabilized on lithium treatment ($n = 45$) were then randomly assigned to receive lithium alone, imipramine alone, or lithium plus imipramine in a double-blind fashion. Fifty-nine percent of the patients with pure mania completed the initial treatment and entered the double-blind prophylactic phase of the study, compared with only 36% of patients with mixed mania. Only 1 (6%) of 17 patients with pure mania treated with lithium or the combination exhibited a recurrence during the 24-month follow-up, compared with 14 (78%) of 18 patients with mixed states. All patients receiving imipramine ($n = 12$) had recurrences. Bowden (1995) reported unpublished data from Swann et al. in which 81% of 16 patients with pure mania compared with 37% of 19 patients with mixed mania had at least a 20% improvement in the manic syndrome by day 5 of treatment. However, others have suggested that mixed states simply require longer lithium trials than does mania to respond (McElroy et al. 1992), which was not reported in this study. Nonetheless, these data suggest that lithium is less effective in treating mixed than manic bipolar disorder.

The frequency and sequence of affective episodes has also been observed to predict clinical nonresponse to lithium. Dunner and Fieve (1974) studied 55 patients who had been treated with lithium carbonate for at least 6 months. Eleven of those patients (20%) had a history of rapid cycling (i.e., four or more affective episodes per year) were significantly more likely to fail lithium prophylaxis than were the remaining patients (82% vs. 41%, respectively). P. F. Goodnick et al. (1987) treated 54 patients with bipolar disorder, type I, and 27 with bipolar disorder, type II, for a mean of 45 weeks with lithium carbonate. Patients with four or more relapses per year before beginning this treatment had higher rates of interepisode depressive symptoms and manic relapses while receiving lithium. Sarantidis and Waters (1981) reviewed the charts of 46 patients with bipolar or schizoaffective disorder who had been treated with lithium carbonate for more than 2 years and found the lower the frequency of episodes before beginning lithium, the better the outcome. Finally, Faedda et al. (1991), using meta-analysis for a review of the literature, concluded that the sequence of affective episodes during the course of bipolar disorder may influence lithium response. Specifically, they found that patients with continuous or rapid cycling, or with depression preceding mania (i.e., depression-mania-euthymia), respond less well to lithium than patients who present with mania preceding depression (i.e., mania-depression-euthymia).

The presence of psychiatric comorbidity and substance abuse has also been associated with lithium treatment failure in two retrospective chart reviews of patients with mania (D. W. Black et al. 1988b; Himmelhoch et al. 1976). In the study reviewed previously, Himmelhoch et al. (1976) observed drug abuse to be strongly associated with poor outcome, and although drug abuse was also more common in mixed states, this negative effect was observed independent of affective state assignment. D. W. Black et al. (1988b) retrospectively reviewed the records of 438 patients with bipolar disorder, mania, and found that the absence of comorbidity was associated with good outcome at hospital discharge. Similarly, Strakowski et al. (1993a) prospectively studied 60 patients hospitalized with a first episode of psychotic mania and observed that patients with psychiatric comorbidity had a significantly lower rate of recovery by hospital discharge than did patients without comorbidity (36% vs. 63%). However, in this latter study, the specific treatment used was not reported.

Other factors associated with poor lithium response in mania include a history of prior lithium failure and a diagnosis of schizoaffective disorder. Bowden et al. (1994b) observed in a double-blind, placebo-controlled trial of patients with acute mania that those with a history of lithium response improved on lithium in this trial, whereas those with a history of prior lithium failure did not. Patients with a diagnosis of schizoaffective disorder may respond less well to lithium than patients with bipolar disorder, although this has not been extensively studied (Keck et al. 1994, for review).

PREDICTORS OF VALPROATE RESPONSE AND NONRESPONSE

In contrast with lithium, valproate has been associated with a good antimanic response in patients with concurrent depressive symptoms or syndromes. Calabrese and colleagues (Calabrese and Delucchi 1990; Calabrese et al. 1992, 1993a, 1993b) have reported favorable responses in patients with rapid-cycling bipolar disorder with index episodes of either mixed or pure mania who received open-label valproate alone or in combination with other psychotropic medication. For those patients who received valproate alone, 18 (95%) of 19 patients with pure mania had a moderate or better response, and 8 (80%) of 10 with mixed mania did similarly. T. W. Freeman et al. (1992) reported on 14 patients treated with valproate in a double-blind trial with lithium carbonate and found that patients responding to valproate had significantly higher depression scores than those not responding. Response was measured by changes in SADS-C mania, BPRS, and GAS scores. Moreover, all four of the patients with mixed states treated with valproate demonstrated a favorable response. In comparison, in that same study, the four patients with mixed states who were treated with lithium had a significantly less favorable response than did the remaining nine patients who received lithium. West et al. (1994) observed a marked or better antimanic response in five of six adolescents (mean age 15 years) with mixed states who had valproate added to their drug regimen in an open-label fashion. Four of five adolescents with mania showed a similar response in that study. McElroy et al. (1991b; Pope et al. 1991), in their double-blind, placebo-controlled trial of valproate in 36 patients with acute mania, reported a 71% response rate without differences in response associated with level of depressive symptoms. Finally, Bowden (1995), reporting an unpublished study by Swann et al., observed that, in contrast with lithium, as mentioned above, the response rate to valproate was essentially the same in the 43 patients with mixed states (72% response) and the 24 patients with pure mania (67% response). These data suggest that valproate, in contrast with lithium, is equally efficacious for treating pure mania and mania with concurrent depressive symptoms or syndromes.

Valproate has also been reported to be effective in the treatment of patients with rapid-cycling bipolar disorder. McElroy et al. (1988a, 1988c) reported a case series of six consecutively hospitalized patients with rapid-cycling bipolar disorder who demonstrated a moderate or better response to valproate. These patients were identified by retrospective chart review as part of a larger series of patients (McElroy et al. 1987). As reviewed previously, the large cohort ($N = 101$) of patients with rapid-cycling bipolar disorder treated by Calabrese and colleagues (Calabrese and Delucchi 1990; Calabrese et al. 1992, 1993a, 1993b) demonstrated significant short-term and prophylactic responses to valproate for mania and mixed states. Although this was an open study, these investigators showed that valproate can be used effectively in this often lithium-nonresponsive patient population. Bowden et al. (1994b), in the previously reviewed study of valproate and lithium in acute mania, identified eight patients with a history of rapid cycling (4.5% of the total sample), and all eight of these patients received valproate. Four of them had a therapeutic response that was similar to the rate of response of the remaining patients who received either valproate or lithium. Together, these studies suggest that valproate, in contrast with lithium, is as efficacious in patients with a history of rapid cycling as in those patients without such a history.

Because valproate is also an anticonvulsant, several investigators have examined whether response to valproate is related to electroencephalographic (EEG) or other neurological abnormalities. McElroy et al. (1987), in a retrospective chart review of 36 consecutively hospitalized patients who had received valproate, observed that the presence of nonspecific EEG abnormalities, neurological soft signs, and computed tomography (CT) scan abnormalities was associated with a positive valproate response. However, when the authors expanded this study to include additional patients ($N = 73$ total), these associations with neurological abnormalities were diminished (McElroy et al. 1988a). Moreover, in their double-blind, placebo-controlled trial of valproate for the treatment of acute mania (Pope et al. 1991), these authors found no association between valproate response and EEG, CT scan, or neurological abnormalities (McElroy et al. 1991b). Pope et al. (1988) reported two cases of patients with bipolar disorder that began following closed-head injury who had failed standard therapy, but demonstrated a marked valproate response. The authors then retrospectively identified, through examination of medical records, eight additional patients with bipolar disorder with a history of head injury, seven of whom responded clinically to valproate. Finally, A. L. Stoll et al. (1994) retrospectively examined the medical records of 115 consecutively hospitalized patients who received valproate treatment for bipolar or schizoaffective disorder. These researchers observed that 68% ($n = 78$) of these patients had a history of some neurological abnormality including a history of seizures, head injury, or abnormal EEG, magnetic resonance imaging, or neurological examinations. Forty-four percent of those patients with a neurological abnormality exhibited a marked valproate response, compared with only 24% of those without such an abnormality ($n = 37$). Notably, all of these studies have been performed at a single site (McLean Hospital, Belmont, MA); most have relied on retrospective chart reviews for information; and some of the same patients may have been included in different studies. Thus, these findings may not be from independent samples. Therefore, it is unclear if neurological abnormalities are associated with a valproate response.

Several studies suggest that valproate is effective in patients with a history of lithium treatment failure. In the study by Pope et al. (1991), 71% of patients receiving valproate exhibited an antimanic response, even though all of the patients had a history of lithium treatment failure or intolerance. Sixty-four percent of the patients with rapid-cycling bipolar disorder studied by Calabrese and Delucchi (1990) had a history of lithium failure, and the majority of these subsequently responded to valproate. Similarly, the six patients with rapid-cycling bipolar disorder described by McElroy et al.

(1988c) had all failed lithium treatment, but responded to valproate.

Bowden et al. (1994b) observed that a history of lithium nonresponse predicted lithium nonresponse, but not valproate nonresponse. Taken together, these studies suggest that a history of lithium nonresponse does not predict valproate nonresponse. Notably, no studies have examined whether a history of valproate treatment failure predicts future valproate or lithium response.

A single report by Brady et al. (1995) suggested that valproate may be useful in the treatment of bipolar disorder complicated by substance abuse. These investigators gave open-label valproate to nine patients with bipolar disorder and comorbid drug abuse and observed improvement in affective ratings and frequency of substance use during the (mean) 16-week trial. This study was limited by the open-label, nonblinded design in a very small patient sample but suggested that valproate may be useful in this difficult-to-treat patient population.

COMPARISON OF LITHIUM AND VALPROATE SIDE-EFFECT PROFILES

The side-effect profiles of both lithium and valproate have been well defined, as both agents have been clinically available for many years. Common side effects for lithium include tremor (27%), weight gain (19%), gastrointestinal (GI) disturbance (10%), polyuria/polydipsia (30%–35%), memory problems (28%), sedation (12%), and decreased thyroid hormone levels (5%–35%), which may progress in some patients to persistent hypothyroidism (percents in parentheses taken from review by F. K. Goodwin and Jamison 1990b). Lithium toxicity can produce marked tremor, ataxia, dysarthria, delirium, seizures, autonomic instability, coma, and death. Severe toxicity rarely occurs below 2.0 mEq/L, although symptoms of toxicity can occur in some patients even at serum levels below 1.0 mEq/L. The common side effects of valproate include sedation (19%), GI disturbance (20%–30%), and weight gain (percents in parentheses taken from Bowden et al. 1994b). Less common side effects include alopecia, thrombocytopenia, and severe hepatotoxicity, although fatal cases of the latter have been restricted to children younger than 10 years (Schatzberg and Cole 1991). Like lithium toxicity, valproate toxicity can result in ataxia, coma, and death, although generally toxicity occurs with serum levels above 150 mg/L.

Two studies have directly compared lithium and valproate (Bowden et al. 1994b; T. W. Freeman et al. 1992), which permits some comparison of relative effects of side effects in clinical samples. Bowden et al. (1994b) observed that the rate of termination resulting from intolerance of treatment was 11% for lithium and 6% for valproate. Compared with valproate, lithium caused significantly higher rates of fever (14% vs. 1%). Compared with lithium, valproate caused significantly higher rates of pain (19% vs. 3%). In the study by T. W. Freeman et al. (1992), no patients left the study because of adverse events, and the authors did not report on other side-effect experiences. Thus, there are limited data directly comparing tolerance of these two pharmacological agents in controlled studies. In general, both compounds appear to be well-tolerated in clinical trials. However, our own clinical experience with both agents suggests that, in general, valproate is the better-tolerated drug.

LOADING DOSE STRATEGIES FOR LITHIUM AND VALPROATE

Loading dose strategies provide important treatment interventions for conditions in which rapid medicating is necessary to prevent significant morbidity or mortality. Thus, in mania, which can progress rapidly to severe impairment, agitation, and even delirium, the ability to load mood-stabilizing medication to rapidly achieve therapeutic serum levels could significantly reduce disability. Loading dose strategies have been reported for both lithium and valproate.

Attempts to load lithium to rapidly achieve therapeutic levels have been, in general, limited by concerns about the narrow therapeutic index of the drug, coupled with significant morbidity associated with lithium toxicity. Nonetheless, two groups of investigators have reported successful loading dose strategies with lithium. T. B. Cooper et al. (1973) developed a strategy to predict the necessary daily lithium dose needed to achieve a steady-state lithium serum trough level of 0.6–1.2 mEq/L. They gave patients a single dose of 600 mg of lithium, then obtained the 24-hour serum level. They then correlated the 24-hour level with the lithium dose needed to achieve the desired steady-state range and found a robust correlation ($r = 0.97$). They did not comment on patient tolerability of this technique. Subsequently, several studies used this method in patient samples and confirmed the accuracy, reliability, and tolerability of this method (T. B. Cooper and Simpson 1976; G. A. Fava et al. 1984; Gengo et al. 1980). Only one study by Naiman and colleagues (1981) reported that 31% of their 13 patients failed to achieve the defined steady-state range following this paradigm. Kook et al. (1985) reported the results of loading 30 mg/kg of slow-release lithium carbonate (Lithobid), which was predicted to give a steady-state trough level of 0.9–1.2 mEq/L. Thirty-eight patients (20 men, 18 women) participated in the study, and marked sex-differences were observed. Whereas the prediction error for men was -0.16 ± 0.09 mEq/L and no men had a level of > 1.1 and only one had a level of < 0.6, the prediction error for women was 0.28 ± 0.14 mEq/L, and four women developed potentially toxic levels of > 1.2 and one had a level of < 0.5. Nonetheless, the procedure was well-tolerated by all patients. Despite the relative success of these procedures, lithium loading is rarely used in clinical practice, probably because of clinician worries, valid or not, about exceeding the narrow therapeutic index. Moreover, whether these loading techniques actually decrease the time required to treat patients with mania is unknown.

In contrast, because of its wider therapeutic margin, valproate loading strategies have been used in neurological settings for many years (Keck et al. 1993) and recently have been applied to patients with mania. Keck et al. (1993) studied the efficacy of giving valproate 20 mg/kg in divided doses for 5 days in 19 patients with bipolar mania. Serum valproate concentrations were measured by a blinded rater after 1 and 4 days of treatment, and improvement was measured by a blinded rater using Young's Mania Rating Scale (MRS) (R. C. Young et al. 1978). Therapeutic serum valproate concentrations (>50 mg/L) were reached in all 15 patients who completed the study. Ten patients (53%) had a $> 50\%$ reduction in the MRS score during the 5 days of the study. No patient experienced significant side effects or toxicity. Similar results were obtained in an unblinded follow-up study, in which 10 of 13 patients with mania demonstrated a moderate or marked response to valproate using the loading strategy (McElroy et al. 1993). We have subsequently used this strategy as a routine part of our clinical treatment of patients on the Psychobiology Unit at the University of Cincinnati Hospital with continued effective results and few adverse events. Thus, valproate appears to be safe to initiate in this fashion, and manic symptoms improve rapidly with this technique in many patients.

SUMMARY AND CONCLUSION

From the above discussion, it appears that both lithium and valproate are equally effective pharmacological treatments for acute mania. Lithium is also established as an effective prophylactic agent, particularly for prevention of future manic episodes, whereas this has not yet been demonstrated for valproate in controlled clinical trials. Nonetheless, uncontrolled and anecdotal data suggest that valproate is likely to be an effective prophylactic agent as well. Lithium has also been shown to have some antidepressant efficacy in bipolar disorder, although this effect appears less robust than the antimanic effects. In contrast, to date, little evidence suggests that valproate is an effective antidepressant for acute bipolar depression. Lithium nonresponse is associated with mixed states, rapid cycling, and a history of lithium failure. In comparison and contrast, valproate acute nonresponse is associated with acute bipolar depression. It is important to note, however, that clinical predictors of lithium and valproate response have, in general, been determined retrospectively, using post hoc analyses of uncontrolled studies. More definitive, controlled studies directly comparing lithium and valproate are needed to clarify whether specific patient subgroups may be selectively responsive to one or the other pharmacological agent.

Advantages of lithium include its long history of use, its relatively low cost, and its established efficacy for prophylaxis and treatment of bipolar depression. Disadvantages include a narrow therapeutic index, a relatively slow treatment response time, and an often intolerable side-effect profile. Advantages of valproate include its potential utility in specific bipolar subgroups (e.g., rapid cyclers), its efficacy in lithium nonresponders, a relatively wide therapeutic margin, a more tolerable side-effect profile, and the ability to easily load the drug to potentially produce a more rapid antimanic response. Disadvantages include its cost and lack of established efficacy for prophylaxis and for treatment of acute depression. These considerations suggest that patients most likely to benefit immediately from lithium are those currently manic with "classic" manic symptoms (i.e., grandiosity, euphoria, activation, and minimal psychotic symptoms). Patients most likely to benefit prophylactically from lithium are those who do not exhibit rapid cycling and who do not abuse substances. Patients more likely to exhibit a valproate acute and prophylactic response are those with mixed affective states, a history of rapid cycling, and a history of lithium failure. Valproate may also be effective in patients with comorbid substance abuse. Moreover, the use of loading dose strategies with valproate, as well as its potential for a rapid treatment response, suggest that it may be the preferred mood stabilizer for hospitalized patients who are severely ill and require a rapid treatment effect. The limits to hospitalization imposed by managed care settings, in which the number of insured treatment days tends to be increasingly smaller, may therefore favor the use of valproate. Finally, it is likely that both agents are less effective in schizoaffective disorder than in bipolar disorder (Keck et al. 1994). It is hoped that future studies will clarify which patients might benefit most from which compound, and, perhaps, identify those who would respond best to the combination. Regardless, the addition of valproate to the armamentarium of treatment for bipolar disorder can only lead to improvement in the management of this condition.

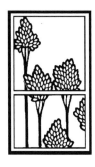

CHAPTER 9

Therapeutic Potential of Inositol Treatment in Depression, Panic, Dementia, and Lithium Side Effects

Joseph Levine, M.D.,
Yoram Barak, M.D.,
Jonathan Benjamin, M.D.,
Yuly Bersudsky, M.D.,
Ora Kofman, Ph.D., and
Robert H. Belmaker, M.D.

Inositol is a simple substance present normally in the diet at about 1 g/day and is an isomer of glucose. The phosphatidylinositol (PI) cycle is an important second messenger system for several brain neurotransmitters (Figure 9–1). Receptor (R) stimulation by an activator (A) leads to breakdown of membrane phosphatidylinositol 4,5-biphosphate (PIP_2) to

The animal work was supported by Grant I-245–098.02/92 from the German-Israel Foundation. The clinical studies were supported by a contract from the New Medications Development Program, National Institute of Mental Health, Bethesda, Maryland to R.H.B.

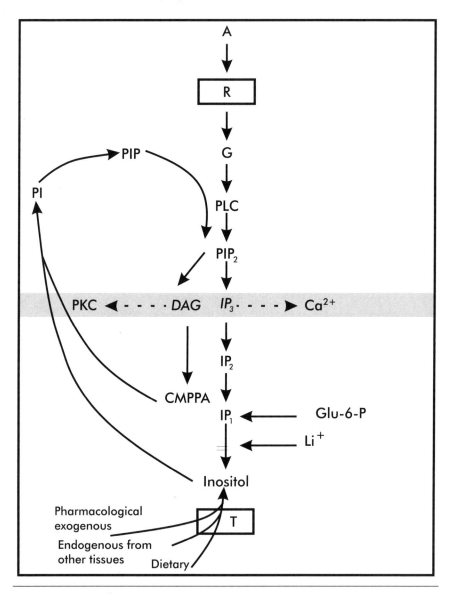

FIGURE 9–1.   Phosphatidylinositol cycle. A = activator; CMPPA = cytidine monophosphate phosphatidic acid; DAG = diacylglycerol; G = G protein; Glu-6-P, glucose 6-phosphate; IP_1 = inositol monophosphate; IP_2 = inositol biphosphate; IP_3 = 1,4,5-inositol triphosphate; PI = phosphatidylinositol; PIP = phosphatidylinositol phosphate; PIP_2 = phosphatidylinositol 4,5-biphosphate; PKC = protein kinase C; PLC = phospholipase C; R = receptor; T = transporter.

two second messengers, inositol 1,4,5-triphosphate (IP_3) and diacylglycerol (DAG), which induce intracellular effects: release of calcium (Ca^{2+}) and activation of protein kinase C (PKC). IP_3 is then sequentially dephosphorylated to inositol biphosphate (IP_2) and then to inositol monophosphate (IP_1). IP_1 is dephosphorylated to inositol via inositol monophosphatase. Inositol monophosphatase is inhibited by lithium (Li^+). Inositol, which is present in brain in very high concentrations, has several sources other than the PI cycle: 1) glucose 6-phosphate (Glu-6-P), which is converted to IP_1 to be dephosphorylated by inositol monophosphatase (inhibited by Li^+) to inositol; 2) exogenous dietary inositol; 3) endogenous inositol transported from other tissues; and 4) exogenous inositol given in pharmacological doses as a therapeutic drug.

The last three sources are transported into the cell via inositol transporter (T). Inositol combines with cytidine monophosphate phosphatidic acid (CMPPA) to be converted to PI, which is then phosphorylated to phosphatidylinositol phosphate (PIP) and to PIP_2 to be reused to form the PI cycle-derived second messengers IP_3 and DAG (Kofman and Belmaker 1993).

INOSITOL REVERSES LITHIUM EFFECTS ON ANIMAL BEHAVIOR

W. R. Sherman (1991) first reported that Li^+ reduces brain levels of inositol by inhibiting inositol monophosphatase. Berridge et al. (1982) noted the possible psychiatric implications of Li^+ inhibition of inositol monophosphatase and hypothesized that lowering of inositol might dampen the PI cycle. Based on Berridge's theory, several groups have used inositol reversal as a technique to study the role of Li^+ on the PI system. Li^+-induced suppression of rearing is a well-described behavioral effect of Li^+ in rats. Rats received LiCl or NaCl (5 mEq/kg, intraperitoneally), and then activity was measured 24 hours later after inositol or vehicle administration intracerebroventricularly. Rats that received an injection of Li^+ showed less rearing than did rats treated with saline. Administration of inositol intracerebroventricularly reversed the Li^+ effect. This was the first finding suggesting that inositol could reverse a behavioral effect of Li^+ (Kofman and Belmaker 1990).

Although exploratory rearing and its suppression has some face value as an animal model of mania and its treatment, this behavior has a large variance and is not always replicable. We sought a behavior that would give us a robust and consistent Li^+ effect, which could then be modified by administering inositol intracerebroventricularly. We examined the effect of inositol on limbic seizures induced by Li^+-pilocarpine (Kofman et al. 1993). We first used the standard doses of Li^+ pretreatment (3 mEq/kg) 24 hours before administering pilocarpine (20 mg/kg) in Sprague-Dawley rats. Inositol significantly increased the latency to exhibit clonus and lowered the seizure score. Fifty percent of rats treated with inositol did not have limbic seizures at all, whereas only 1 of the 14 vehicle-treated rats did not exhibit clonus. All the rats treated with chiro-inositol had limbic seizures. The ability of inositol to prevent seizures was highly significant (Kofman et al. 1993).

PHARMACODYNAMICS OF INOSITOL

The dramatic antagonism of limbic seizures by intracerebroventricularly administered inositol is a useful paradigm to study the time-course and dose response of behavioral effects of inositol. We injected rats with Li^+ and 10 mg of inositol intracerebroventricularly at different time intervals before the subcutaneous injection of pilocarpine. Inositol was effective at 1, 4, and 8 hours before pilocarpine administration. When injected immediately before or 24 hours before pilocarpine injection, inositol did not prevent seizures in any rat; when injected 12 hours before pilocarpine, 50% of rats had seizures. This time-course suggests that inositol must have time to distribute within the brain and to enter cells and that it is extruded from the brain or metabolized within 8–24 hours after injection. This time-course is long enough that therapeutic use of inositol seemed possible (Bersudsky et al. 1993b).

To obtain a dose-response curve for inositol effects, rats were injected intracerebroventricularly with either vehicle, 5 mg or 10 mg of inositol, 1 hour before pilocarpine injection. The prevention of seizures by giving 5 mg of inositol intracerebroventricularly was significantly less than the dramatic effect of 10 mg of inositol intracerebroventricularly. Brain concentrations of inositol are very high, about 10 mM, and apparently large doses of exogenous inositol are required to replenish inositol depletion induced by Li^+ (Bersudsky et al. 1993b). Thus, inositol might be similar to monoamine precursors such as L-dopa or tryptophan, of which doses of several grams per day are necessary for behavioral effects.

INOSITOL IS INEFFECTIVE IN LITHIUM TOXICITY

We attempted to prevent Li^+-overdose death with intracerebroventricularly administered inositol. Sprague-Dawley rats were implanted with guide cannulae in the lateral ventricle. Rats were injected intracerebroventricularly with either control, inositol, or chiro-inositol and 90 minutes later with LiCl at a median lethal dose. No difference was found among the treatment conditions in the number of rats dying. Thus, Li^+ lethality apparently has a different biochemical basis than the other behavioral and biochemical effects of Li^+ described above, and inositol is not likely to be useful as an antidote in clinical overdosage (Bersudsky et al. 1993a).

INOSITOL REVERSES LITHIUM-INDUCED POLYURIA

Polyuria is a common side effect of Li^+ treatment. To test whether inositol would mitigate Li^+-induced polydipsia-polyuria, rats were given either 2.5% mannitol or inositol in water. Half the rats in each group were injected intraperitoneally daily with either LiCl or NaCl. A fifth group was injected with LiCl daily but drank tap water. Li^+ induced marked polydipsia, and Li^+-treated rats that drank the inositol solution had significantly less polydipsia than Li^+-treated rats that drank tap water or mannitol in water (Bersudsky et al. 1992).

Berridge had emphasized that inositol enters brain very poorly (W. R. Sherman 1991). We therefore considered whether it might be possible to reverse Li^+ side effects in patients with low-dose inositol that would not reverse Li^+'s therapeutic effect in brain. To test whether inositol can alleviate polyuria-polydipsia in patients treated with Li^+, patients complaining of Li^+-induced polyuria-polydipsia were recruited for an open study with administration of 3 g of inositol daily for 5 days. The dose of inositol given was low, and the treatment period short because of the ethical consideration that inositol might reverse Li^+'s therapeutic benefit in these patients. Five of 11 patients reported a dramatic improvement in polyuria-polydipsia, whereas another four showed a mild improvement. Two patients also showed reversal of Li^+-induced skin lesions (Bersudsky et al. 1992).

HIGH-DOSE INOSITOL ENTERS BRAIN

Inositol enters the brain poorly. However, high doses of inositol may penetrate the blood-brain barrier sufficiently to influence behavior. Male rats were injected with LiCl intraperitoneally (3 mEq/kg), followed 18 hours later by inositol 12 g/kg intraperitoneally or an equal volume of glucose. Six hours after the peripheral inositol injection, rats were injected subcutaneously with pilocarpine and rated for limbic seizures. Peripheral high-dose inositol significantly reduced Li^+-pilocarpine seizures. Cortical inositol levels were measured in rats treated intraperitoneally with glucose or inositol. Inositol-treated rats had a 35% increase in cortical inositol (Agam et al. 1994; Belmaker et al. 1992). In a human study, 12 g/day of inositol was shown to raise inositol levels in the cerebrospinal fluid by 70% (Levine et al. 1993).

INOSITOL IS THERAPEUTIC IN DEPRESSION AND PANIC

Barkai et al. (1978) reported that cerebrospinal fluid levels of inositol were lower in patients with depression than in psychiatrically healthy subjects. We hypothesized that inositol may be deficient in some brain systems in depression. This does not contradict the concept that Li^+ reduces inositol levels and that Li^+ is an antidepressant, because the PI cycle serves as a second messenger for several balancing and mutually interactive neurotransmitters. Li^+ could alleviate depression by reducing inositol and a primary hyperactivity of one hypothetical brain system; low inositol levels in another system could cause second messenger dysfunction and thereby depression.

Therefore, we performed a double-blind controlled trial in which 12 g/day of inositol was administered for 4 weeks to 28 patients with depression (Levine et al. 1995a). Significant overall benefit from inositol compared with placebo was found at week 4 but not at week 2 as measured by the Hamilton Rating Scale for Depression (HRS-D; M. Hamilton 1960). Item analysis of the HRS-D found significant effects of inositol compared with placebo on mood, insomnia, anxiety, agitation, diurnal variation, and hopelessness. No changes were noted in hematology or kidney or liver function. One patient in the placebo group developed a mania after week 2, but none in the inositol group did so.

Because many antidepressant compounds are also effective in panic disorder, we performed a trial of inositol in panic (Benjamin et al. 1995). Twenty-one patients with panic disorder with or without agoraphobia completed a double-blind, random assignment crossover treatment trial of inositol 12 g/day versus placebo, with 4 weeks in each treatment phase. Frequency of panic attacks and severity of panic disorder and of agoraphobia declined significantly more on inositol than on placebo; the effect was comparable to that of imipramine in previous studies. Side effects were minimal.

SAFETY OF INOSITOL

A review of our safety data to date shows that 107 patients have been treated with inositol. Of these, 61 have had full chemistry and hematology before and after inositol. Only two patients, both in the depression study, showed any changes in blood chemistry. Both showed a mild increase in blood glucose that disappeared on repeat in one but continued in the other several weeks after discontinuation of inositol. Total side effects were flatus in four patients, nausea in one, sleepiness in two, and insomnia in two. These side effects were similar to those reported in the placebo group.

Inositol has been given in cases of diabetes for possible therapeutic effects on peripheral neuropathy at doses of 20 g/day with no side effects (Arendrup et al. 1989). Recently, newborns were treated with inositol 80 mg/kg with marked benefit in respiratory distress syndrome, and no side effects were reported (Hallman et al. 1992). In addition to the above, 10 psychiatrically healthy volunteers were given 12 g of inositol in a single dose, and no side effects or mood effects were reported (Levine et al. 1994); 15 patients were treated for 5 days each with 6 g of inositol daily for electroconvulsive therapy–induced confusion, with no clinical effects and no side effects (Levine et al. 1995b); and 4 patients with Li^+-induced electroencephalographic (EEG) abnormalities were treated for 7 days with 6 g daily of inositol (Barak et al. 1994) with minimal EEG effects and no side effects.

The most serious theoretical side effect of inositol treatment could be reversal of therapeutic effects of Li^+ or induction of mania in patients with bipolar disorder. So far, this has not been definitely seen in four patients with bipolar depression who were treated with full 12 g of inositol daily for depression (Levine et al. 1995a) or in 18 Li^+-treated patients with bipolar disorder who were treated with low-dose inositol for polyuria (Bersudsky et al. 1992) or EEG abnormalities (Barak et al. 1994). The pathophysiological relationship of inositol reversal of Li^+ side effects and inositol therapeutic efficacy in depression and panic is not clear.

SUMMARY

Inositol is a simple component of diet that is an important precursor in the PI cycle. Li^+ lowers tissue inositol levels. An open study of low-dose inositol in Li^+-induced polyuria-polydipsia showed marked attenuation of these side effects. A double-blind controlled trial of 12 g of inositol daily for 4 weeks in

28 patients with depression showed significant antidepressant effects of inositol with minimal side effects. A controlled, double-blind, crossover study of inositol versus placebo for 1 month each in panic disorder showed marked benefit for inositol.

CHAPTER 10

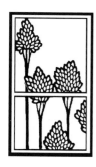

Electroconvulsive Therapy: Current Practice and Future Directions

Mitchell S. Nobler, M.D.,
Harold A. Sackeim, Ph.D., and
Davangere P. Devanand, M.D.

Electroconvulsive therapy (ECT) is one of the oldest so-matic treatments in psychiatry. The emergence of the field of psycho-pharmacology in the 1960s eclipsed advancement in ECT practice and research. To some extent, the pendulum has swung back in the past 15 years, as there has been intensive rediscovery of the basic science of ECT and an in-crease in its clinical use. Contemporary research has reexamined clinical is-sues, such as indications for treatment, response prediction, and relapse prevention, given the changing nature of psychiatric treatment and referral patterns. At the same time, more sophisticated approaches to treatment

Preparation of this chapter was supported in part by National Institute of Mental Health Grants MH35636 and MH47739 and by a Young Investigator Award from the National Alliance for Research on Schizophrenia and Depression.

technique, and advances in related areas of biological psychiatry, have led to a greater understanding of the strengths and limitations of ECT.

TECHNICAL ASPECTS OF TREATMENT

Following the introduction of ECT, much of the early research focused on basic properties of the electrical stimulus. This work was largely abandoned following the introduction of psychopharmacological treatments in psychiatry, and there was little technical progress in the administration of ECT. In the last 15 years, there has been renewed research interest in this area, which has in turn led to modifications in treatment technique.

Stimulus Characteristics

The physical properties of the ECT electrical stimulus have become a source of intensive investigation, given evidence that both cognitive side effects and clinical efficacy are partly determined by stimulus parameters (Sackeim et al. 1991, 1993). The basic electrical concepts important for an understanding of the physical properties of the ECT stimulus include voltage, current, and resistance. Discussion of these topics is beyond the scope of this chapter and can be found elsewhere (Sackeim et al. 1994). The stimulus wave form refers to the actual electrical stimulus that is produced by a given ECT device. Numerous devices have been in use, delivering a variety of wave forms. Broadly, the stimulus is either sinusoidal or pulse, and the current flow is unidirectional or bidirectional. Sinusoidal wave forms were the first to be used and involve a continuous flow of electrons in alternating positive and negative deflections at a frequency in the United States of 60 wave-pairs per second (60 Hz). The continuous electrical stimulation produced by sine wave stimuli has been associated with greater adverse cognitive effects (R. D. Weiner et al. 1986). Pulse stimuli are typically square-wave and are characterized by a rapid rise and fall of current. Pulse stimuli may be further subdivided into brief pulse (pulse width of 1–2 msec) and ultrabrief pulse (pulse width < 1 msec). Other parameters that can be manipulated by the practitioner include the amplitude (current) and frequency of the pulses and the duration of the pulse train. Astonishingly few systematic studies of how manipulation of specific stimulus parameters affect the safety and efficacy of ECT have been conducted.

Seizure Threshold

The term *seizure threshold* refers to the minimum amount of electrical energy necessary to produce a generalized seizure. Because the seizure threshold may show interindividual variability up to 40-fold (Sackeim et al. 1991), depending on how ECT is delivered, patients may be treated with grossly excessive amounts of electrical charge. Independent of seizure threshold, electrical wave forms differ in their efficiency in eliciting seizures. The slow onset to peak current and slow offset of sine wave stimuli result in inefficiency. For instance, R. D. Weiner (1980) compared the effects of stimulus wave form on seizure threshold and found that, on average, sine wave stimuli required nearly three times as much energy to elicit adequate seizures as brief pulse stimuli. Stimulus electrode placement also has a bearing on the seizure threshold. Several research groups have confirmed that the seizure threshold is higher with bilateral electrode placement than with unilateral placement (Beale et al. 1994; Coffey et al. 1995a; Enns and Karvelas 1995; McCall et al. 1993a; Sackeim et al. 1987b, 1993).

Several clinical variables also affect the seizure threshold. For example, gender was a fairly strong predictor of seizure threshold in our first study of constant current, brief pulse stimulation: men had a higher seizure threshold than did women, requiring approximately 70% more electrical dosage, as measured in charge, to elicit seizures (Sackeim et al. 1987b). Other groups have replicated this finding (Coffey et al. 1995a; Enns and Karvelas 1995; McCall et al. 1993a), although Beale et al. (1994) found no significant difference between men and women.

A moderate association between increasing age and elevated seizure threshold was documented by several early researchers (e.g., Shankel et al. 1960; Watterson 1945). R. D. Weiner (1980) also examined the relation of age to seizure threshold and found a significant positive correlation. Our work has shown a similar positive correlation, with older patients having a higher seizure threshold. However, this association is also somewhat sex-dependent, with men showing a stronger positive correlation than did women overall and a significant aging effect for both right unilateral and bilateral ECT, and women showing an aging effect for right unilateral but not bilateral ECT (Sackeim et al. 1991). Others have also found that increasing age predicts higher seizure thresholds (Beale et al. 1994; Coffey et al. 1995a; Enns and Karvelas 1995).

Little is known about possible relations between psychiatric diagnosis and seizure threshold. A few reports have suggested that patients with mania may have lower seizure thresholds than patients with depression (Mukherjee

1989; I. F. Small et al. 1986), and in our experience the same may hold true for some young patients with schizophrenia. However, confounding variables such as age and gender have not been addressed in these studies. In patients with major depressive disorder, we found no relation between seizure threshold and unipolar versus bipolar or psychotic versus nonpsychotic subtypes. Similarly, Coffey et al. (1995a) found no correlation between initial seizure threshold and severity of depressive illness or the unipolar-bipolar distinction. Finally, we found that history of ECT did not predict seizure threshold (Krueger et al. 1993).

Effects of Medication on the Electroconvulsive Therapy Seizure

The effect of medications on ECT seizure threshold and/or duration (i.e., proconvulsant or anticonvulsant effects) is a valuable yet still largely unexplored area of investigation (Nobler and Sackeim 1993). For instance, adenosine antagonists, such as theophylline, may lead to prolonged seizures. Indeed, there are reports of status epilepticus following ECT in patients at therapeutic plasma levels of theophylline (Devanand et al. 1988). This proconvulsant effect has been exploited in studies designed to use pharmacological strategies to lengthen seizures or to minimize stimulus dose during ECT (Coffey et al. 1990; Swartz and Lewis 1991).

Perhaps more immediately relevant to ECT are the effects of concurrent psychotropic medications. For example, benzodiazepines are known to possess anticonvulsant properties, and at high doses have been associated with decreased seizure duration (Krueger et al. 1993). Concerns are that benzodiazepines concurrent with ECT may result in diminished antidepressant efficacy (e.g., Pettinati et al. 1990), but this is a controversial issue, involving considerations of how best to manage extremely anxious or agitated patients during the ECT course (Nobler and Sackeim 1993). We generally recommend that an agent, such as lorazepam, with a shorter half-life be used, and then only on an as required basis, if possible. Neuroleptics have both proconvulsant and anticonvulsant effects, but appear generally safe when given concurrent with ECT. Of note, Coffey et al. (1995a) found that patients receiving neuroleptics had lower seizure thresholds. Tricyclic antidepressants most likely have minimal effects on seizures during ECT. However, despite some early uncontrolled studies to the contrary, tricyclic antidepressants have not been shown to augment antidepressant effects of treatment and are probably best to be avoided during the course of ECT (C. H. Kellner et al. 1991). Prolonged seizures and confusional states have been reported with concurrent lithium use, and the American Psychiatric Association Task Force on Electroconvulsive Therapy (1990) recommends that the drug either be discontinued or plasma levels be kept at a minimum during the ECT course.

Electrode Placement and Stimulus Dosing

In the past decade, studies in depression have focused on how electrode placement and electrical stimulus intensity affect both efficacy and side effects. Classic work by Ottosson (1960) indicated that 1) lidocaine (which possesses anticonvulsant properties) aborted the seizure discharge and interfered with clinical efficacy, and 2) increasing stimulus intensity to grossly suprathreshold levels offered no advantage for efficacy (but did worsen cognitive side effects). These findings suggested that the elicitation of an adequate generalized seizure was both necessary and sufficient for clinical efficacy, whereas a stimulus intensity administered well above threshold produces only greater adverse effects. Further, it had also long been recognized that unilateral ECT resulted in fewer cognitive side effects than bilateral ECT. Given that some studies had reported equal efficacy between unilateral and bilateral ECT, this led to the recommendation that unilateral treatment be the preferred method in almost all cases (American Psychiatric Association Task Force on Electroconvulsive Therapy 1978). A series of studies has challenged this fundamental perspective. Sackeim et al. (1987a) demonstrated that generalized seizures of adequate duration were elicited with low-dosage unilateral ECT (i.e., stimulus dose just barely above seizure threshold) that reliably lacked antidepressant properties. In contrast, low-dosage bilateral ECT was an effective antidepressant. This contradicted the notion that generalized seizures are both necessary and sufficient for the efficacy of ECT. This finding was replicated in a second study, in which unilateral and bilateral ECT was given either just above or 2.5 times the individual's seizure threshold (Sackeim et al. 1993). In this second study, the higher-dose unilateral ECT condition was more effective than low-dose unilateral ECT, but was still not as effective as low- or high-dose bilateral ECT. However, greater cognitive side effects appeared during the week following ECT in the patients who received bilateral ECT. In a third study, unilateral ECT given at a stimulus dose of 6 above seizure threshold achieved the same efficacy as high-dose bilateral ECT, while resulting in fewer cognitive side effects (H. A. Sackeim, J. Prudic, et al: "Effects of Electrode Placement and Stimulus Intensity on the Efficacy and Cognitive Effects of Electroconvulsive Therapy," manuscript submitted for publication). Thus, there appears to be a dose-response function for the antidepressant efficacy of unilateral ECT (Abrams et al. 1991; Sackeim et al.

1993). Moreover, the critical factor determining this dose-response curve is not the absolute electrical dose administered, but rather the relative dose, or the degree to which the absolute dose exceeds the individual's seizure threshold (Sackeim et al. 1987b, 1993).

Finally, traditional electrode placements have also been reexamined. Letemendia et al. (1993) compared the efficacy of unilateral ECT, standard bilateral ECT (i.e., bifrontotemporal electrode placement), and bilateral ECT using a bifrontal placement. Both forms of bilateral ECT had superior antidepressant efficacy compared with that of unilateral ECT, and the bifrontal condition was somewhat superior to the standard bilateral placement. This finding further challenges the idea that the elicitation of a generalized seizure in and of itself is both necessary and sufficient for the antidepressant effect of ECT. Rather, the site or sites of seizure initiation, and perhaps propagation, may be critical determinants of therapeutic efficacy.

Treatment Schedule

Traditionally, ECT is administered two to three times per week, with practitioners in the United States favoring the latter frequency. Investigation of how the treatment schedule has a bearing on efficacy or cognitive side effects has been limited. Lerer et al. (1995) randomly assigned patients with depression to ECT three times per week or to two real ECT and one sham ECT per week. Both groups received bilateral ECT, with electrical stimulus dose at 1.5 times the seizure threshold. Patients underwent blinded ratings of both clinical state and cognitive functioning. Three patients dropped out of the three-ECT-per-week group because of the development of an organic mental syndrome. Although patients showed the same overall antidepressant response at the end of the trial, clinical improvement was more rapid in the three ECT per week group. However, acute cognitive side effects were also more prominent in this group.

The results of Lerer et al. (1995) are consistent with clinical experience. When there is a need for rapid response with ECT (e.g., food refusal), treatment three times per week is indicated. On the other hand, if a patient appears to be at risk for cognitive side effects (e.g., frail elderly), reducing the frequency of treatment to two times per week is justified.

Pharmacological Augmentation of Electroconvulsive Therapy

From several standpoints, pharmacological agents can affect the safety and efficacy of ECT (Nobler and Sackeim 1993). On the one hand, the pharmacological effects may be mediated by the psychotropic properties of the medication acting additively or synergistically with the antidepressant, antimanic, or antipsychotic properties of ECT. For example, the combination of neuroleptics and ECT may be superior to neuroleptics alone in the treatment of schizophrenic spectrum illnesses (see Krueger and Sackeim 1995 for a review). Alternatively, as mentioned earlier, pharmacological agents may influence the outcome of ECT by their ability to alter major aspects of seizure physiology, such as the convulsive threshold or seizure propagation. For instance, both theophylline (Swartz and Lewis 1991) and the related compound, caffeine (Coffey et al. 1990), have been used to augment duration in situations where the ECT device cannot elicit an adequate seizure. With respect to caffeine, the mechanism appears to involve seizure prolongation, as it was found not to lower seizure threshold at ECT (McCall et al. 1993b). As yet, there is no conclusive evidence that caffeine enhances the efficacy or reduces the cognitive effects of ECT. However, preliminary data from an open, nonrandom assignment trial support this notion (Calev et al. 1993).

Based on the rationale that patients with depression may have abnormalities in the hypothalamic-pituitary-thyroid axis and that thyroid supplementation may augment antidepressant medications, R. A. Stern et al. (1991) compared augmentation with 50 μg of liothyronine with placebo in a double-blind study involving 20 male patients undergoing ECT. The medication was given nightly from before the first ECT until 7–10 days following the ECT course. The major finding of this preliminary report was that patients taking liothyronine required fewer ECT treatments than did patients on placebo. This finding merits independent replication, as there was also the suggestion of attenuation of certain cognitive side effects with liothyronine augmentation.

CLINICAL ASPECTS

Nearly 60 years of clinical experience with ECT have provided us with good information on the type of patients who respond to this treatment. However, some of the older conceptions of which patients are likely to respond to ECT may need revision as patterns of referral have changed. Although we are beginning to learn more about the patient characteristics associated with greater vulnerability to complications during the treatment course, we know little about the clinical features that predict relapse following ECT.

Diagnostic Indications

Major depression.   Although ECT was first developed for use in schizophrenia, the efficacy of ECT in depressive disorders was quickly established. In fact, some of the early work in defining which depressed patients were likely to respond to treatment led to the development of rating scales for depression, such as the Newcastle Index (Carney et al. 1965) and the Hamilton Rating Scale for Depression (J. M. Roberts 1959). The robust efficacy in depressive disorders has been verified in open clinical studies, in comparison with antidepressant medications and in comparisons between "real" ECT and "sham" ECT (i.e., the administration of general anesthesia without the passage of electrical current) (see Sackeim et al. 1995 for detailed review). The efficacy rate in clinical samples is traditionally quoted to be greater than 80% (Abrams 1992), which is superior to any somatic treatment in psychiatry. In carefully selected research samples employing rigorous response criteria, efficacy rates in major depression are 60%–80% (Sackeim et al. 1987a, 1993).

Mania.   In addition to being indicated as a treatment for major depression, ECT is clearly indicated as a treatment for manic episodes, and may even be a lifesaving measure in cases of manic delirium. This topic was extensively reviewed by Mukherjee et al. (1994), who found that, of 589 patients with mania receiving ECT described in the world literature, there was nearly an 80% response rate. (This is comparable, and even superior, to response rates for lithium, neuroleptics, and anticonvulsants.) Although most of these reports were based on case series or uncontrolled trials, they were corroborated by two prospective controlled studies in acute mania (Muhkerjee et al. 1988; J. G. Small et al. 1988). Overall, the literature supports the conclusion that ECT is an effective treatment of acute manic episodes and may possibly be of value in patients with mania who are medication-resistant. A study from India (Sikdar et al. 1994) compared patients with mania who were maintained on chlorpromazine and then randomly assigned to either eight bilateral ECT treatments or eight sham ECT treatments. Twelve of the 15 patients in the real ECT group showed clinical remission, compared with only 1 of the 15 patients with mania in the sham group.

Schizophrenia.   Although there is some controversy, schizophrenia is a recognized indication for ECT. This topic was recently reviewed in detail (Krueger and Sackeim 1995). The major points to be considered include the following: 1) although methodologically flawed resulting from lack of operationalized diagnostic criteria, early uncontrolled trials indicated that

ECT was generally inferior or equivalent to treatment with neuroleptics alone in terms of short-term outcome; 2) in contrast, long-term outcome in these early studies appeared to favor ECT over medications; 3) the combination of ECT and neuroleptic may be more effective than ECT or neuroleptic alone; and 4) although we lack controlled studies, several reports have indicated that ECT may be of benefit in neuroleptic-resistant patients with schizophrenia.

Other diagnostic indications.   A few less well-known diagnostic indications for ECT exist. The use of ECT in patients with Parkinson's disease is receiving greater interest. ECT is an effective treatment for depressions associated with this illness and may also be of benefit for the motor manifestations (see C. H. Kellner et al. 1994 for review). Other conditions in which the use of ECT may be appropriate include catatonia and the neuroleptic malignant syndrome (Sackeim et al. 1995).

Patterns of Usage

Despite overwhelming data supporting the efficacy of ECT treatment for major depression, marked variation in the extent and pattern of its usage continues. Use of ECT declined in the 1970s but then appeared to stabilize or increase in the 1980s (J. W. Thompson et al. 1994). ECT is used far more commonly in private hospitals than in public institutions and is more commonly administered to older patients and to women. Its more common administration to women may be the result of higher rates of depression in women (J. W. Thompson et al. 1994). Olfson et al. (1998) similarly reported that ECT is used more often in white persons, those with higher incomes, and the elderly.

A study by R. C. Hermann et al. (1995) examined factors that contribute to this wide variation in ECT use. These researchers analyzed responses to a survey of practitioners in 317 urban centers in the United States. No ECT use was reported in 115 (36%) of these metropolitan areas, whereas in the remaining 64% there was considerable variation in usage. ECT use was found to be strongly associated with the presence of an academic medical center. In a regression analysis, the strongest determinants of ECT use were 1) the number of psychiatrists per capita, 2) the number of primary care physicians per capita, and 3) the number of private hospital beds per capita. R. C. Hermann et al. (1995) also found that the stringency of state regulation was negatively associated with the use of ECT. Of interest, these investigators noted that among medical procedures ECT is among the highest in variability of utilization.

Prediction of Outcome

Much of the early research in predicting response to ECT stimulated interest in the subtyping of depressive disorders, especially the distinction between endogenous/melancholic and reactive/neurotic depression. For instance, Carney et al. (1965) noted that each of the phenomena that positively correlated with a diagnosis of endogenous depression also had a positive correlation with favorable outcome with ECT. Indeed, this study formed the basis of the Newcastle Scale, used to rate endogenous major depression. A major criticism of early research has been that the predictive rating scales were in essence singling out patients with severe (perhaps melancholic or delusional) depressions from those with more chronic low-grade or characterological depressive disorders. It is not surprising that the former group of patients would have a better outcome with ECT. Indeed, the ability to predict outcome based on symptom features alone may be greatly diminished once patient samples are more diagnostically homogeneous. Thus, Pande et al. (1988) and Andrade et al. (1988) found little utility for the older predictive scales within more diagnostically homogeneous, contemporary samples of patients with major depression.

Psychotic depression.   ECT is believed to be a particularly effective treatment for depressions with associated psychotic features. Stated differently, most clinicians believe that the presence of delusions among patients with major depression predicts good response to ECT. Overall, there is considerable empirical support for this contention. In the large British trials of real versus sham ECT, a consistent predictor of response to real ECT was the presence of delusions (Buchan et al. 1992; Clinical Research Centre, Division of Psychiatry 1984). In a retrospective study, C. G. Dunn and Quinlan (1978) also found that the presence of delusions predicted good ECT response. Further, in a sample of medication-resistant patients, Mandel et al. (1977) found that delusions predicted positive outcome. Others have also found that the presence of delusions predicts better outcome at discharge (Coryell and Zimmerman 1984; Pande et al. 1990). However, C. L. Rich et al. (1986) found that psychotic and nonpsychotic patients with depression showed equal benefit from ECT. It is worth noting that patients in this study were allowed to remain on concurrent medications, including antipsychotics. More recently, J. Smith et al. (1994) noted that the presence of psychotic symptoms was associated with rapid initial response, although not with longer-term outcome. One early study found that the absence of paranoid symptoms was related to better response to ECT (M. Hamilton and White 1960). On the whole, however, most studies found that the presence of psychotic symptoms is predictive of good outcome with ECT, or at least makes no measurable difference. The interpretation of this empirical observation remains open. At face value, it may be that psychotic depression is uniquely responsive to ECT and at a rate that exceeds that in nonpsychotic depression. This would indicate a double dissociation with pharmacotherapy, in that it is generally believed that patients with delusional depression have a lower rate of response to antidepressant medications (Spiker et al. 1985). An alternative explanation derives from the finding that patients with demonstrated medication resistance are less likely to respond to ECT than patients without such medication resistance (Prudic et al. 1990). Particularly because monotherapy with antidepressant medication is not an adequate treatment for delusional depression (Spiker et al. 1985), many patients with this illness are referred for ECT without adequate medication trials. It would be predicted that such patients would fare better with ECT than nonpsychotic patients who had failed adequate medication trials.

Duration of illness. In his classic study, R. F. Hobson (1953) indicated that a shorter duration of the index episode of depression (1-year cutoff) was a predictor of good ECT response. This finding was subsequently confirmed by several other groups (Coryell and Zimmerman 1984; C. G. Dunn and Quinlan 1978; Fraser and Glass 1980; M. Hamilton and White 1960; Kindler et al. 1991), although some studies found no relations or weaker relations between duration of index episode and clinical outcome (Andrade et al. 1988; Mendels 1967; Sackeim et al. 1987a). If anything, then, a shorter index episode of depression may be associated with an increased likelihood of favorable ECT response.

Severity of illness. J. M. Roberts (1959) originally reported that higher symptom scores at baseline predicted better ECT response. In contrast, Andrade et al. (1988) and Sackeim et al. (1987a) found no differences between responders and nonresponders in initial severity, while others reported that ECT nonresponders had greater initial severity of depression (Kindler et al. 1991; Pande et al. 1988). Thus, there is no consensus on how symptom severity, independent of the presence of psychosis or melancholia, is predictive of ECT response.

Patient age. An association between increased age and favorable response to ECT has been reported by many investigators (Carney et al. 1965; Coryell and Zimmerman 1984; Mendels 1967; Nystrom 1964; J. M. Roberts 1959; Sackeim et al. 1987b). In contrast, Ottosson (1960) and C. L. Rich et al. (1984) found increasing age to be associated with a slower rate of ECT response. Others have reported that age has no relation to outcome (Andrade et al. 1988; M. Hamilton and White 1960; R. F. Hobson 1953). Seizure threshold increases with age (Coffey et al. 1995a; Sackeim et al. 1991). Almost all of this research involved a fixed electrical stimulus dose independent of age. Because stimulus dose relative to threshold contributes to efficacy (Sackeim et al. 1993), relations between age and clinical outcome may have been underestimated. However, although statistically significant associations between age and clinical outcome may exist, these are not sufficiently robust to serve for clinical prediction.

Medication resistance.   As ECT has become a second- and third-line treatment for depression, response rates have been affected. Many years ago it was suggested that ECT outcome was poorer for medication-resistant patients compared with patients who had not failed an adequate antidepressant trial (M. Hamilton 1974; Medical Research Council 1965). More recently, Prudic et al. (1990) rated 53 patients as to the adequacy of pre-ECT medication trials during the index episode. There was only a 50% response rate to bilateral ECT in medication-resistant patients, compared with an 86% response rate among patients who were not known to be medication resistant. These findings stood in contrast to the long-held clinical impression that ECT has consistently good outcome, regardless of medication treatment history. This finding was subsequently replicated in a multicenter trial, involving a larger sample of patients drawn from diverse clinical settings (Prudic et al. 1996). It should be emphasized that response rates of approximately 50% are still impressive, especially among patients with established resistance to other somatic treatments. Still, the presence of medication resistance may predict poorer outcome with ECT relative to its absence. Furthermore, medication resistance may underlie the associations of ECT outcome with episode duration and the presence of delusions. Patients with longer depressive episodes often receive lengthier and more numerous medication trials before ECT and are more likely to qualify as medication resistant (Prudic et al. 1990). In contrast, patients with psychotic depression often receive inadequate pharmacological treatment (i.e., fail to receive adequate trials of combination antipsychotic-antidepressant medication) and are often referred for ECT earlier in their episode or as a first-line treatment.

Potential Biochemical Predictors of Outcome

A broad range of biochemical indices have been evaluated as possibly related to the therapeutic outcome of ECT (Sackeim et al. 1995). However, no good predictor has emerged from this list. Some recent studies have provided some new insights into this arena.

Neurophysins.   Neurophysins are carrier peptides for the posterior pituitary hormones oxytocin and vasopressin. The oxytocin-associated neurophysin is referred to as hNpII, which can be assayed in blood. Scott and colleagues (1989, 1991) reported that the acute surge in hNpII immediately following the first ECT predicted clinical response at the end of the treatment course. The same group demonstrated that the amount of oxytocin released following an ECT-induced seizure is greater with higher intensity simulation (W. J. R. Riddle et al. 1993). They speculated that the relation of the oxytocin (and consequently, hNpII) surge and clinical response is mediated by effects of stimulus intensity. Indeed, there is evidence that the degree to which stimulus intensity exceeds the patient's seizure threshold is a strong determinant of ECT response, at least for unilateral ECT (Sackeim et al. 1987a, 1993).

The work with oxytocin and hNpII had several methodological flaws, including the use of concurrent psychotropic medications during the ECT course, and separate analyses for response to bilateral and unilateral ECT. J. Smith et al. (1994) directly assayed plasma oxytocin levels and found that the surge immediately following ECT was greatest at the first treatment. These investigators were unable to replicate the finding that the acute oxytocin surge post-ECT predicted clinical response. As a whole, these data highlight the possibility that biological changes sensitive to stimulus intensity may be greater at initial ECT treatments relative to those later in the course.

Biopterin.   Abnormalities in biopterin metabolism have been reported in depression (Coppen et al. 1989). Tetrahydrobiopterin (BH_4) is a cofactor crucial to the biosynthetic pathways of the biogenic amines, including the conversion of phenylalanine (P) to tyrosine (T). The relative ratio of neopterins to biopterins (N:B) in the urine is an index of the synthesis of BH_4, with an elevated ratio implying a failure to produce BH_4. D. N. Anderson et al. (1992) measured the urinary N:B ratio in 23 patients with depression before and after a course of ECT and in 26 psychiatrically healthy control subjects. At baseline, patients with depression had a higher N:B ratio than did the control subjects. On further analysis, patients who went on to respond to ECT had higher ratios than did control subjects, whereas nonresponders did not differ from control subjects. D. N. Anderson et al. (1994) examined the effect of bilateral ECT on the biosynthesis of tyrosine in 26 patients with major depression by measuring the P:T ratio. Responders had significant reductions in the P:T ratio following the ECT course compared with nonresponders. This finding suggested an increased conversion of phenylalanine to tyrosine and that recovery with ECT is associated with increased BH_4 activity.

Prediction of Relapse

Perhaps the most pressing clinical issue facing the field of ECT is the high rate of relapse following treatment. There has been very limited study of clinical or biological predictors of relapse (Nobler and Sackeim 1996).

Medication resistance.   Sackeim et al. (1990) conducted a prospective, naturalistic study of relapse rates in 58 patients who were followed up to 1 year after ECT. The investigators used methods similar to those of Prudic et al. (1990): the patients were rated for their degree of medication resistance during the index episode before ECT. In most cases, continuation pharmacotherapy was at the discretion of the patient's private physician. Relapse following ECT was twice as common in patients who were medication resistant before ECT than in nonresistant patients (64% versus 32%). Furthermore, among medication-resistant patients, the adequacy of continuation pharmacotherapy had no effect on relapse rates. In a lithium continuation trial post-ECT, Shapira et al. (1995) also found that patients who were medication-resistant were more likely to relapse than were patients who were not known to be medication-resistant before ECT.

Biochemical measures.   Based both on reports of abnormal glucose metabolism in depression and on ECT's alteration of glucose metabolism, K. Williams et al. (1992) monitored plasma insulin and glucose during a course of ECT in 20 patients. Both insulin and glucose peaked immediately after ECT administration. The greatest insulin peak occurred following the first ECT. The nine patients who relapsed at 2 months had significantly lower insulin peaks at the fifth ECT, relative to patients who remained euthymic.

Scott et al. (1989) initially reported that baseline serum hNpII was lower in patients with sustained clinical improvement at 2 months following ECT. This finding was not replicated in their subsequent expanded sample (Scott et al. 1991). In contrast to their finding that maximum hNpII release after the first ECT predicted initial clinical improvement, they found no significant relation between maximal hNpII release and clinical outcome at 2 months (Scott et al. 1991).

Relapse Prevention

Traditionally, following clinical response to ECT, patients are placed on antidepressants and/or mood stabilizers as prophylaxis. Indeed, patients are often placed back on the medications that may have failed during the acute episode before ECT. The findings of Sackeim et al. (1990) called this practice into question. Indeed, for the medication-resistant patient who does respond to ECT, careful thought should be given to alternative psychopharmacological strategies, although we lack critical data in this regard. For many patients, continuation pharmacotherapy is not a viable option, either because these patients cannot tolerate side effects of medication or they have already relapsed on medication in prior episodes following successful ECT. For such patients, continuation ECT presents a useful treatment option. Indeed, the use of continuation ECT appears to be increasing, despite that there are no controlled, prospective studies and the evidence for its efficacy draws only from case series (Monroe 1991). Sackeim (1994b) provides a detailed discussion of the nature and difficulties in conducting a controlled, randomized trial of continuation ECT.

Prediction and Prevention of Cognitive Side Effects

Fairly characteristic cognitive side effects follow ECT. These include disorientation immediately following treatment, a transient inability to retain newly learned information (anterograde amnesia), and a more prolonged retrograde amnesia for events learned before the course of ECT, particularly for autobiographical information (Sackeim 1992). At the same time, some measures of cognitive performance, such as intelligence testing, may improve following ECT. The magnitude of these acute and short-term cognitive side effects are generally greater with bilateral electrode placement and with high stimulus intensity. However, there are wide individual differences among patients, and we lack reliable predictors of which patients will be most vulnerable. To examine this issue, Sobin et al. (1995) focused on the duration of acute disorientation following seizures and pretreatment global cognitive status (based on the Mini-Mental State Exam [Folstein et al. 1975]) as possible predictors of retrograde amnesia for autobiographical information following ECT. The results indicated that, regardless of electrode placement and stimulus intensity, patients who manifested global cognitive impairment at baseline and/or patients who had prolonged disorientation in the acute postictal period were the most vulnerable to persistent retrograde amnesia. This finding has important clinical implications. Prolonged disorientation after the first ECT should alert the clinician to the increased likelihood of severe cognitive impairment at the end of the ECT course. Appropriate modifications can be made at subsequent treatment, for example, decreasing stimulus intensity.

One of the central goals in current ECT research is to identify a form of treatment that will optimize clinical efficacy, while resulting in minimal cognitive side effects. At present, the use of high-dose, unilateral ECT or moderate-dose bilateral ECT are the best options. An alternative approach may be to employ pharmacological strategies designed to minimize the cognitive effects of ECT. Such studies are based both on animal models in which drugs are shown to decrease electroconvulsive shock–induced amnesia and on clinical studies of elderly patients with cognitive impairment (Krueger et al. 1992). One example of this type of investigation involves the opioid antagonist naloxone. Nasrallah et al. (1986) were unable to find any benefit of intravenously administered naloxone (0.1 mg/kg) on cognitive effects of ECT in their placebo-controlled study. This was disappointing, as there is good preclinical evidence that endorphins have naloxone-reversible amnestic effects and that naloxone may reverse electroconvulsive shock–induced amnesia (Krueger et al. 1992). Two possible explanations for the null findings were that the dose used was too small and that naloxone was given 3–5 days after the course of ECT, as opposed to administration at each treatment. Accordingly, our group recently found evidence that naloxone, when given at much higher doses and immediately before individual ECT treatments, improved measures of verbal fluency, attention, and anterograde amnesia relative to placebo (Prudic et al., in press).

Prediction of Cardiac Side Effects

In general terms, ECT is considered to be a very safe procedure, with low rates of morbidity and an extremely low mortality rate (as low as that for general anesthesia alone) (Abrams 1992; American Psychiatric Association Task Force on Electroconvulsive Therapy 1990). Among the most serious immediate side effects are myocardial ischemic events and ventricular tachyarrhythmias. Yet, as conditions that were once considered contraindications for ECT are shown to be successfully treated (e.g., vascular aneurysms), ECT practitioners have become more comfortable treating more medically ill patients. This has led to larger numbers of patients with fairly severe cardiac disease being treated with ECT. Indeed, such patients are often not even considered candidates for treatment with antidepressants. The question arises as to whether these patients are indeed more likely to experience adverse cardiac effects with ECT. Rice et al. (1994) compared a series of patients with a clinical history of cardiac disease with a matched sample with no cardiac illness. These authors reported that major complications were rare and were no more likely in the high-risk group. Minor complications, however, were more common in this group.

Zielinski et al. (1993) assessed cardiac side effects in 40 patients undergoing ECT who had preexisting cardiac disease documented by low ejection fraction, conduction disease on electrocardiogram, or frequent ventricular ectopy on 24-hour electrocardiogram. Twenty-two of the patients had at least one cardiac complication: 14 were minor and 8 were major. In a comparison group without cardiac disease, only three patients had cardiac complications (all minor). In the cardiac group, all the ischemic events occurred in patients with known history of ischemic heart disease, while the presence of baseline ventricular arrhythmia was strongly associated with the development of ventricular arrhythmia following ECT. Therefore, the particular nature of preexisting cardiac disease predicted the type of cardiac side effect during ECT.

The patients in the Zielinski et al. (1993) study developed more severe cardiac complications than did those of Rice et al. (1994). This discrepancy may result from the former study requiring rigorous evaluation of cardiac illness, with strict inclusion criteria, and thus may have involved relatively sicker patients. Nonetheless, even in the Zielinski et al. (1993) study, 38 of 40 cardiac patients completed a course of ECT. Indeed, with proper monitoring and management, patients with cardiac disease can be safely treated with ECT (American Psychiatric Association Task Force on Electroconvulsive Therapy 1990).

NEUROBIOLOGICAL MARKERS OF EFFECTIVE ELECTROCONVULSIVE THERAPY

Electroconvulsive therapy produces an extraordinary number of physiological and biochemical changes. A central challenge in uncovering mechanisms of therapeutic action is the separation of relevant effects from those that are epiphenomena of generalized seizure activity. This topic was reviewed in detail (Sackeim 1994a). From a practical standpoint, efforts are under way to identify markers of when an optimally therapeutic form of ECT has been administered.

Alterations in the Seizure Threshold

ECT itself has long been recognized to possess anticonvulsant properties, which have been hypothesized to underlie its antidepressant and antimanic effects (Mukherjee 1989; Post et al. 1986c; Sackeim et al. 1983). This anticonvulsant effect is demonstrated in the phenomenon that seizure threshold often becomes elevated during the course of ECT, whereas the duration of individual seizures decreases. There is empirical evidence that this increase in threshold varies with electrode placement and cumulative number of treatments. In a study of low-dosage treatment, Sackeim et al. (1987b) found that the total sample averaged a 64.6% increase in seizure threshold from the beginning of the course to the final treatment. Both the absolute and the proportional increase in seizure threshold were greater with bilateral than with right unilateral ECT, despite that bilateral ECT had a higher initial threshold. On average, seizure threshold increased by 87.1% during the course of treatment with bilateral ECT, as compared with only a 40.3% increase in threshold with unilateral ECT. This pattern was replicated in a second study (Sackeim et al. 1993).

Coffey et al. (1995b) assessed seizure threshold at the first and sixth treatments in 62 patients (50 patients received unilateral and 12 patients received bilateral ECT). Across the sample, seizure threshold increased by 47%. Only 56% of the patients demonstrated an increase in threshold, and electrode placement had no bearing on change in threshold. However, a fundamental limitation in this study was that the majority of patients had seizures at the first stimulation in the titration schedule. This overestimation of initial seizure threshold led to an underestimation of subsequent rise in threshold.

The extent of the rise in seizure threshold during a course of ECT is a potential marker of the potency and/or adequacy of treatment. In a study comparing the efficacy of bilateral and right unilateral ECT, given at stimulus doses just above the seizure threshold, we found that greater increase in seizure threshold over a course of ECT was significantly associated with greater symptom reduction (Sackeim et al. 1987c). In the same study, no increase or minimal increase in seizure threshold during the ECT course predicted poor clinical response. Others have also reported that the absence of a significant rise in seizure threshold during a course of ECT is associated with poor outcome (Roemer et al. 1990; Yatham et al. 1989). In contrast, Coffey et al. (1995b) found no relation between response status or change in depression rating scale scores and change in seizure threshold, despite an overall increase in seizure threshold across a sample of 62 patients. Those authors concluded that the anticonvulsant effect of ECT, as evidenced in increased seizure threshold may be a necessary, but not sufficient, condition for therapeutic effects. However, some methodological problems in this study limit interpretation of the results.

Biochemical Studies

Prolactin.   Prolactin is one of several hormones released following seizures. The magnitude of prolactin release has been shown to be greater with bilateral ECT than with unilateral ECT (Lisanby et al. 1998; Swartz and Abrams 1984) and with higher-intensity stimulation than with low-intensity stimulation (Lisanby et al. 1998; Robin et al. 1985; Zis et al. 1993). Despite these clear associations, the prolactin rise with ECT has not proven to be a marker of clinical improvement (Lisanby et al. 1998), although C. P. Clark et al. (1995) reported a trend association between percentage of prolactin increase following the first ECT and lower depression scores at the end of the ECT course.

γ-Aminobutyric acid.   Based partly on the hypothesis that increased γ-aminobutyric acid (GABA)-ergic transmission mediates the anticonvulsant mechanisms of ECT and that low levels of plasma and cerebrospinal fluid GABA have been reported in patients with depression, Devanand et al. (1995) investigated the effects of ECT on plasma GABA. In contrast to expectations, plasma GABA was found to be reduced immediately following a seizure, and this decrease did not appear associated with electrode placement or stimulus intensity. Of note, patients with higher plasma GABA levels at baseline were more likely to respond to ECT.

Electroencephalogram Correlates

Research has highlighted the potential usefulness of the electroencephalogram (EEG) in determining the adequacy of seizures elicited at ECT. For instance, Sackeim et al. (1996) found that the induction of slow-wave activity in prefrontal cortex in the interictal EEG is linked to the efficacy of ECT. Nobler et al. (1993) demonstrated that forms of ECT that differ in therapeutic efficacy also had characteristic EEG patterns. Low-dose unilateral ECT, the weakest form of treatment, resulted in seizures that had the longest latency to reach full slow-wave activity and had the least amount of immediate postictal bioelectric suppression. In contrast, high-dose bilateral ECT, the form of ECT associated with marked and rapid clinical response, resulted in seizures with the greatest peak slow-wave EEG amplitude. Across all forms of ECT, immediate postictal suppression was significantly associated with positive clinical outcome (Nobler et al. 1993).

Krystal and colleagues (1993, 1995) have similarly demonstrated differences in the EEG according to electrode placement and stimulus intensity, using both intraindividual and interindividual study designs. This group has developed an EEG model that was able to differentiate low-dose and high-dose unilateral ECT with sensitivity and specificity greater than 80% (Krystal et al. 1995). Thus the ictal EEG holds promise as a marker of ECT treatment adequacy and as an "on line" tool for the clinician to help guide the selection of stimulus dose.

Cerebral Blood Flow

Neuroimaging techniques assessing cerebral blood flow (CBF) and cerebral metabolic rate provide powerful windows onto the effects of ECT. Nobler et al. (1994) assessed cortical CBF using the planar xenon-133 inhalation technique in 54 patients. The patients were studied just before and 50 minutes after the sixth ECT treatment. At this acute time point, unilateral ECT led to postictal reductions of CBF in the stimulated hemisphere, whereas bilateral ECT led to symmetric anterior frontal CBF reductions. Regardless of electrode placement and stimulus intensity, patients who went on to respond to a course of ECT manifested anterior frontal CBF reductions in this acute postictal period, whereas nonresponders failed to show CBF reductions. Such frontal CBF reductions may reflect functional neural inhibition and may index anticonvulsant properties of ECT. A predictive discriminant function analysis revealed that the CBF changes were sufficiently robust to correctly classify both responders (68% accuracy) and nonresponders (85% accuracy). More powerful measures of CBF and/or cerebral metabolic rate, as can be obtained with positron-emission tomography, may provide even more sensitive markers of optimal ECT administration.

CONCLUSION

Our understanding of many of the basic principles underlying ECT has advanced in the past several years. The field has moved away from simplistic notions regarding the primacy of the generalized seizure toward elucidation of the subtleties of seizure threshold and dose-response functions. From a clinical standpoint, although the efficacy of ECT in the treatment of patients with severe depressive disorders is well-established, patterns of usage for these patients vary widely. The usefulness of ECT as treatment for mania is less well known, unfortunately resulting in underutilization. More recently, the role of ECT in the treatment of schizophrenia and Parkinson's disease has also received increased attention. The major clinical problem we now face is how to better predict and prevent relapse following a successful course of ECT.

ECT is unique in creating numerous biochemical and physiological changes in the brain. At the theoretical level, research into mechanisms of action has received new impetus from advances in fields such as neuroimaging. At the practical level, the use of techniques such as the EEG is leading to the ability to separate effective forms of ECT from those that lack antidepressant efficacy.

Despite these advances, ECT remains controversial in the public eye. Indeed, the high variability in its utilization reflects the fact that a wide range in attitudes toward ECT still exist, even among mental health practitioners. Part of this lack of consensus no doubt stems from lack of information. For instance, many are unaware that ECT can now be routinely delivered in a manner in which cognitive side effects can be minimized. Further, even the most medically compromised patients can safely undergo ECT.

From a research perspective, ECT is certainly a powerful treatment, which can provide new windows into the pathophysiology of mood disorders. More important, with further research, ECT can be provided to appropriate diagnostic groups and administered in a rational fashion, minimizing side effects while maximizing efficacy.

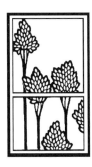

CHAPTER 11

Antidepressant and Mood Stabilization Potential of Transcranial Magnetic Stimulation

Amos Fleischmann, Ph.D.,
Daniel Silverberg, M.D., and
Robert H. Belmaker, M.D.

Electroconvulsive therapy (ECT) is an established and effective treatment of depression and some forms of schizophrenia. ECT is the treatment of choice in several types of depression (W. Z. Potter and Rudorfer 1993), especially severe depression (American Psychiatric Association Task Force on Electroconvulsive Therapy 1990; W. Z. Potter et al. 1991). The mechanism by which ECT exerts its antidepressant effect is still unknown. Studies of pharmacologically as well as of electrically induced convulsions suggest that the convulsion is a necessary condition for ECT's therapeutic effects (Cerletti and Bini 1938; Lerer 1987; Lerer et al. 1984). However, there is no satisfactory explanation for the clinical efficacy of convulsions.

This work was supported by a National Association for Research in Schizophrenia and Affective Disorder Senior Investigator Grant to R.H.B.

We propose that the therapeutic efficacy of ECT may be related to activation of specific brain areas and the whole brain need not convulse for an antidepressant effect. It is possible that neural discharge in specific brain regions (Bolwig 1984), and not the convulsion, is the key factor for ECT's antidepressive effects. External electrical stimulation as used for ECT may depolarize deep brain regions only by induction of convulsion. Local electrical brain stimulation in humans is not possible, of course; ECT initiates massive discharge in the central nervous system (Lerer et al. 1984), and activation of no specific brain area has been proven to be the cause for ECT's therapeutic action. Local electrical stimulation of various brain regions for examination of antidepressive effect in animal models of depression would be a tedious and complicated task.

A new method has been developed for stimulation of the brain: transcranial magnetic stimulation (TMS). Magnetic stimulation of the brain may offer a means to examine the importance of the convulsion for ECT effects. TMS is a novel noninvasive method for the stimulation of neurons (for review, see Barker 1991). High electrical current flow in a spiral of wire induces a magnetic field. The magnetic field produces an electric field that initiates ion flow and consequent membrane depolarization directly in brain tissues. Therefore, magnetic stimulation of deep structures may be achieved with relatively little induced current in the skin or skull and without convulsions (Barker 1991).

> The magnetically induced electric field falls off much less rapidly with distance than the fields from the surface electrodes, thus enabling structures at greater depths to be stimulated without the high fields at the surface that stimulate pain fibers. For example, relative to the surface field, the magnetically induced electric field at a depth of 40 mm will be approximately 10 times greater than that produced by the large electrode pair. (Barker 1991)

TMS is widely known in neurology and is routine in clinical electromyography today (Barker 1991). Clinical experience suggests that many brain structures may be stimulated by this procedure. Thus, for example, a magnetic stimulation above the left motor cortex may simultaneously stimulate the right hand as well as the left hand and the facial muscles. Several investigators have examined TMS effects on cognitive and motor performance as well as TMS effects on various cardiovascular and biochemical parameters. The data obtained from the studies of TMS safety as well as the data obtained from numerous stimulators in clinical use do not indicate hazards or cognitive deficits for patients who underwent TMS (Barker 1991; Hallett and Cohen 1989).

Preliminary clinical studies in patients with depression in Germany (Hoflich et al. 1993; Kolbinger et al. 1995), Israel (Grisaru et al. 1994), and the United States (M. S. George et al. 1995) suggest antidepressant efficacy for TMS in humans. Thus for example, relatively weak (0.3-tesla) and slow (0.25- to 0.5-Hz) TMS (250 stimuli per session for 5 consecutive days) improved the clinical status of patients ($N = 10$) with major depression (Kolbinger et al. 1995). The cumulative score in the Hamilton Rating Scale for Depression (M. Hamilton 1960) in these patients with depression was improved significantly. A recent study reported better antidepressive effects for rapid TMS. Daily repeated rapid TMS was able to improve dramatically two patients with depression (M. S. George et al. 1995) in a semicontrolled study.

Animal behavioral models can be used to evaluate the effect of antidepressants on depression (Thiebot et al. 1992). If TMS and ECT exert antidepressant effects by a similar mechanism, animal models for depression that are sensitive to electroconvulsive shock (ECS) should also be sensitive to TMS. ECS has effects on known animal models for depression. These effects may be displayed after recovery from the immediate effects of the convulsions (Thiebot et al. 1992). We evaluated the effects of TMS on the forced swimming test and on apomorphine-induced stereotypy, a sensitive behavioral measure for the effects of repeated ECS.

FORCED SWIMMING TEST

The forced swimming test model of depression is based on the hypothesis that the animal has lost the ability to escape an aversive situation (Thiebot et al. 1992). Rats swim in a restricted area and after unsuccessful attempts to escape become gradually immobile (Porsolt et al. 1979). The swimming-induced immobility is attenuated by most antidepressants (Thiebot et al. 1992), including ECS (Borsini and Meli 1988; Czyrak 1993; Kawashima et al. 1987).

APOMORPHINE-STIMULATED BEHAVIOR

Repeated ECS enhances apomorphine and other dopamine agonist–induced hyperactivity and stereotypy (Grahame-Smith et al. 1978; A. R. Green 1984; Modigh 1989). Although apomorphine-stimulated behavior is not a face valid model for depression, ECS sensitizes apomorphine-stimulated behavior very reliably, and this may give clues to the therapeutic efficacy of ECT. There is no consistent change after ECS in ligand-binding measures of dopamine receptors. Thus ECS may affect components other than the dopaminergic receptor itself.

INHIBITION OF SEIZURE

Postseizure anticonvulsive effect has been shown both in animals (Essig and Flanary 1966; Tortella and Cowan 1982) and in humans (Holmberg 1954; Kalinowsky and Kennedy 1943). In animals, postictal inhibition has been demonstrated after bilateral ECS through ear-clip electrodes as well as after electrical stimulation in localized regions (for review, see Krauss and Fisher 1993). It seems reasonable to suggest that TMS might have anticonvulsive effects if it stimulates brain areas that are responsible for seizure inhibition.

INHIBITION OF NEURAL ACTIVITY

Only few direct electrophysiological reports of TMS effects on neural activity exist. Effects of TMS on both inhibition and stimulation of neurons are based on indirect electromyographic studies (Ferbert et al. 1992; Pascual-Leone et al. 1994; Valls-Sole et al. 1992; Valzania et al. 1994). For better comprehension of the neural basis of TMS effects on rat behavior, it is useful to study the effects of the magnetic stimulation on activity of neurons. In this chapter, we report that rapid TMS affects rat behavioral models for ECT. We used rat brain slices for comparison of the behavioral effects with direct effects of rapid TMS on neurons. Some of the above behavioral studies (Fleischmann et al. 1994, 1995) have been reported elsewhere in partial form.

Is convulsion necessary for ECT therapeutic effects? Traditionally, it was agreed that generalized convulsion is both sufficient and necessary for ECT therapeutic effects (Bolwig 1984; Cerletti and Bini 1938; Lerer 1987; Lerer et al. 1984; for review, Sackeim et al. 1991). It was shown that current intensity has importance for ECT therapeutic effects (Sackeim et al. 1991, 1993). Sackeim et al. (1991) have shown that low-intensity right unilateral ECT may induce a general convulsion that lacks therapeutic effects. Convulsion might be a disadvantageous inevitable outcome of surface electrodes that are used for ECT (Zyss 1994) because such surface electrodes can activate deep brain regions only if a convulsion is induced. Magnetic fields are not affected by tissue impedance such as electrical fields (Barker 1991). Therefore, TMS may activate deep brain areas without the need for intense depolarization at the skull (Barker 1991). Consequently, TMS could conceivably exert antidepressive effects without convulsion (Zyss 1994). This speculation remains to be proven.

Transcranial Magnetic Stimulation Effect on Apomorphine-Induced Stereotypy

Our data indicate that rapid TMS and ECS have similar effects on several aspects of rat behavior. Our study confirms former studies of potentiation induced by repeated ECS on apomorphine and other dopamine agonists' stimulation of behavior (Grahame-Smith et al. 1978; A. R. Green 1984; Modigh 1989). Rapid-rate TMS augments apomorphine stereotypy at both apomorphine doses. ECS has effects of similar magnitude to TMS, but of greater statistical significance. Slow magnetic stimulation shows no effect at 0.25 mg of apomorphine/kg and a small effect, if any, with 0.5 mg of apomorphine/kg. Rapid-rate TMS may be more potent as high-rate stimuli lead to expansion of cortical excitability (Pascual-Leone et al. 1993, 1994). The increased efficacy of TMS at high-rate magnetic stimulation may be the result of potentiation of the synaptic response during the stimulus (Pascual-Leone et al. 1994).

Transcranial Magnetic Stimulation Effect on the Porsolt Swim Test

TMS reduced mouse immobility in the swim test. It has been shown that most antidepressants, including ECT, reverse immobility in the swim test (Thiebot et al. 1992). The Porsolt swim test in mice is well established and is sensitive for antidepressants regardless of mechanism of action (Thiebot et al. 1992). Although there are many false-positive values for this test, the Porsolt swim test is considered to be a reliable test for depression. Thus, the TMS effect in the Porsolt swim test suggests that TMS might have antidepressive potential in humans. Indeed, pilot studies revealed that slow TMS might have moderate antidepressant effects (Grisaru et al. 1994; Hoflich et al. 1993; Kolbinger et al. 1995). A recent study suggests better antidepressive effects for rapid TMS. Daily rapid low-intensity TMS was applied to the left frontal cortex of six patients with depression that did not respond to medications. The mood of two patients improved dramatically, the mood of two others improved moderately, and two patients did not respond at all to TMS. These last two patients did not respond also to ECT (M. S. George et al. 1995).

Transcranial Magnetic Stimulation Inhibition of Convulsion

Our study verifies former reports in which postseizure anticonvulsive effects have been displayed in animals (Essig and Flanary 1966; Herberg and Watkins 1966; Herberg et al. 1969; Meglio et al. 1976; Mucha and Pineal 1968; Prince and Wilder 1967; Stock et al. 1980; Tortella and Cowan 1982). Similar results have been reported for humans (Efron 1961; Gowers 1881/1964; Holmberg 1954; Kalinowsky and Kennedy 1943). It was suggested that postictal inhibition of seizures is not an outcome of neuronal fatigue (Caspers and Speckmann 1972; Plum et al. 1968). The postictal refractoriness seems to be an active mechanism (Caspers and Speckmann 1972; Engel et al. 1981; Moshe and Albala 1983). Indeed, postictal refractoriness appears to be a result of equilibrium between excitatory and inhibitory processes in the central nervous system (Moshe and Albala 1983). It seems that ECT enhances the inhibitory mechanisms in the central nervous system (Sackeim et al. 1991). Activation of γ-aminobutyric acid (GABA)-ergic (A. R. Green et al. 1982; Sackeim et al. 1986) or opiate (Tortella and Cowan 1982) neurotransmission might be responsible for these inhibitory mechanisms.

Our data indicate that ECT and TMS decreased the duration as well as threshold of a subsequent seizure. Decrease in seizure duration may serve on some occasions as an indication for antiseizure effects. For example, human subjects with high threshold for convulsion have shorter convulsions. Similarly, treatments that decrease seizure threshold are considered to be anticonvulsant agents (Sackeim et al. 1991). Patients that receive high doses of anesthetics with anticonvulsive effects have shorter convulsions (Sackeim et al. 1991). A course of ECT reduces seizure duration at subsequent treatments. However, in humans, short seizure duration is not necessarily an outcome of inhibited seizure. In humans, the relations between current intensity and seizure duration are complex. Approximately at the threshold for convulsion, intensification of the electrical dosage will elongate seizure duration. However, the opposite is true for substantially suprathreshold stimulus dose (Sackeim et al. 1991). More intense stimulus dose will then decrease seizure duration. Nevertheless, our data in rats indicates that ECS and TMS decrease seizure percent as well as seizure duration. ECS inhibition of subsequent convulsion duration continued after ECS failed to decrease seizure percent. Hence, inhibition of seizure duration might serve as a sensitive tool for detection of postictal inhibitory effects in rats. Increasing the rate of TMS and TMS duration augmented the inhibition of seizure duration. Thus it appears that stronger magnetic stimulation is correlated with stronger seizure inhibition.

Postictal inhibition has been demonstrated after bilateral ECS through ear-clip electrodes as well as after direct electrical stimulation of specific brain areas (for review, see Krauss and Fisher 1993). TMS might exert anticonvulsive effects by stimulation of brain areas that are responsible for seizure inhibition. Alternatively, TMS might inhibit by direct inhibition of neural excitability in brain regions that are responsible for seizure initiation and spreading. Indeed, the TMS-induced decrease in postsynaptic action potentials hints that TMS might generate direct inhibitory mechanisms on neural excitability.

Transcranial Magnetic Stimulation Inhibitory Effects on Neural Mechanisms

TMS of the motor cortex in humans induces short-latency, motor-evoked potentials in contralateral muscles. This activation is followed by cortical inhibition of the contralateral muscles. Such inhibitory mechanisms induced by TMS may be revealed by studying effects of paired TMS or a train of TMS on motor-evoked potentials (Ferbert et al. 1992; Pascual-Leone et al. 1994; Valls-Sole et al. 1992; Valzania et al. 1994). Indeed, transcranial cortical stimulation generates an inhibition of voluntary activity, called the silent period. The silent period can persist up to several hundred milliseconds (Cantello et al. 1992; Inghilleri et al. 1993; Triggs et al. 1993; Uncini et al. 1993; Wassermann et al. 1993). Thus, for example, TMS of the motor cortex induced an electromyographic silent period in abductor pollicis brevis and flexor carpi radialis muscles. TMS-induced, motor-evoked potentials were also inhibited during this poststimulation silent period. Consequently, it appears that TMS inhibits some cortical elements (Triggs et al. 1993; Wassermann et al. 1993). Similarly, it seems that TMS inhibits brain stem motor neuron excitability and cortical control of brain stem reflexes in psychiatrically healthy subjects (Leis et al. 1993).

Repeated stimulation of a variety of brain structures can lead to long-term potentiation (LTP) or long-term depression (LTD) of synaptic transmission (Malgaroli 1994). A cascade of events, including presynaptic and postsynaptic mechanisms such as depolarization of neurons, release of glutamate, activation of excitatory amino acid receptors, increase in cellular calcium, which is followed by more second messenger mechanisms, were suggested to induce both LTP and LTD (B. R. Christie et al. 1994; Malenka et al. 1989; Malgaroli 1994; D. Muller et al. 1991). This cascade of events might also be evoked by repeated TMS stimulation. The relationship between the repeated magnetic stimulation to LTP and LTD is still unknown.

The above project represents a novel approach and a possible new treatment for psychiatric disorder. The possibility that neuronal discharge short of total brain convulsion may have psychiatric effects would be a major advance in understanding the action of ECT. Moreover, a possible substitute treatment for ECT would be a major clinical breakthrough. TMS might allow us to stimulate deep brain regions without convulsions, pain, or known hazards. Before one widens the use of TMS in humans, further evaluation of the effectiveness of TMS in animal models for depression is necessary. Our hypothesis is that ECT exerts its therapeutic effects by stimulation of specific brain regions. We suggest that TMS may exert therapeutic effects without need for total brain convulsion.

SUMMARY

Recently, a method for TMS of the brain has been developed. By using TMS it is possible to noninvasively depolarize neurons located deep in the brain without induction of seizures or pain. Thus, it may be possible to compare behavioral effects of TMS and known effects of repeated ECS and other antidepressants in rats. ECS reverses behavioral despair in the swim test and enhances apomorphine hyperactivity and stereotypy. TMS appears to have similar effects to ECS on reversal of the despair in the swim test. Rapid (25-Hz) TMS but not slow (0.2-Hz) TMS potentiated apomorphine stereotypy. ECS is followed by a postictal inhibitory period for further seizures. In this study, TMS as well as ECS increased the seizure threshold for subsequent stimulation and decreased the duration of subsequent seizure. Rapid (25-Hz) TMS but not slow (5- or 1-Hz) TMS decreases the duration of seizure induced by electrical current.

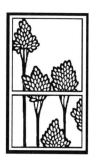

SECTION III

Antidepressants

Alan F. Schatzberg, M.D., Section Editor

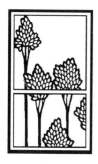

CHAPTER 12

Changing Targets of Antidepressant Therapy: Serotonin and Beyond

Stuart A. Montgomery, M.D.

Over the past 10–15 years, much of the discussion of new antidepressant action has centered on serotonin (5-hydroxytryptamine [5-HT]). For a time, this caused other possible mechanisms to be neglected to some extent. It is appropriate to review the limitations of the serotonergic approach and examine what might lie beyond serotonin for the treatment of depression.

CURRENT SEROTONIN REUPTAKE INHIBITORS

The selective serotonin reuptake inhibitors (SSRIs) are established and accepted antidepressants. Their easy tolerability and simplicity of use have led to their widespread use: it has been estimated that at least 50 million people who would not otherwise have received treatment for their depression have received these drugs. It appears that the proportion of patients treated with tricyclic antidepressants (TCAs) has remained relatively stable and the contribution of the SSRIs has been to increase substantially the size of the patient pool receiving treatment for depression. It is fair to say that the advent of the SSRIs has facilitated more ready discussion of depression and has reduced to some extent the stigma of mental illness. The development of the SSRIs has made it more acceptable for patients to come forward for treatment, although recent epidemiological studies suggest that there is still a long way to go because effective treatment for depression is provided only to a small proportion of those who have this debilitating disorder (Keller et al. 1986; Lepine et al. 1997).

Strengths of Selective Serotonin Reuptake Inhibitors

A major advantage with the SSRIs is that they have been thoroughly investigated in the course of their clinical development. More is known about their efficacy in short-term and long-term treatment, their side effects, and possible drug interactions before they have reached clinical use than was ever the case with the older TCAs. Fixed-dose studies have identified for us the optimum therapeutic dose and enabled us to estimate the range within which an adequate therapeutic dose lies (S. A. Montgomery et al. 1994a). This information is generally not available for the older TCAs. In some cases, the studies have identified a subtherapeutic dose by which efficacy is demonstrated, but the level can be judged insufficient for clinical use. In the case of paroxetine, for example, the 10-mg dose was found to be significantly less effective than the 20-mg dose, and no extra efficacy was seen on raising the dose above 20 mg in conventional major depression (Dunner and Dunbar 1992). In the studies of fluoxetine, although the 5-mg dose was superior to placebo, the quality of the response seen was not as good as the response seen with 20 mg. Nor was any extra efficacy seen with this drug if the dose was raised above 20 mg in conventional major depression (Wernicke et al. 1987, 1988).

Establishing a minimum effective dose is a difficult task. Lower doses of antidepressants have some effect, and a judgment has therefore customarily been made to establish the dose at which a minimum therapeutically relevant response is seen. In cases in which the TCAs are poorly tolerated, clinicians have tended to use low doses in an attempt to alleviate some of the side effects; these doses are often subtherapeutic. Surveys of prescriptions given in primary care in the United Kingdom indicate that as few as 25% of those treated with older TCAs received an adequate therapeutic dose, accepting a fairly modest dosage as being adequate, compared with 100% treated with SSRIs (Donoghue and Tylee 1996).

The light-side-effects burden of the SSRIs, particularly when compared with the older TCAs, has important consequences for improving treatment. Several meta-analyses of published studies have reported a significant advantage in terms of tolerability and safety for the SSRIs. Significantly lower rates of withdrawal from treatment due to side effects are consistently found with

SSRIs compared with those of TCAs (I. M. Anderson and Tomenson 1995; S. A. Montgomery and Kasper 1995; S. A. Montgomery et al. 1994b). This is the more remarkable because many of the studies used low doses of TCAs, which would be expected to be relatively well tolerated. A criticism has been made of these meta-analyses that only the published literature was examined and the exclusion of unpublished data might introduce a bias. However, analysis of the complete database of all studies, published and unpublished, found concordant results (Jenner 1992; Pande and Sayler 1993). This advantage in terms of tolerability and consequent improved compliance with treatment has been interpreted by pharmacoeconomists as leading to a lower pharmacoeconomic burden from relapses, admissions to hospital, further interventions, and so on (Jonsson and Bebbington 1994; S. A. Montgomery et al. 1996). Many experts claim that the cost savings of a better tolerated drug more than compensate for the extra tablet cost of the SSRIs.

The SSRIs are associated with low cardiotoxicity, particularly when compared with the TCAs, and this feature of their pharmacological profile gives them a low potential for lethality in overdose. It has been estimated from coroners' reports in the United Kingdom that the SSRIs are associated with deaths in only 1–2 overdoses per million prescriptions compared with 35 per million prescriptions for the TCAs (Henry et al. 1995).

Whether there is a close link between the suicidal ideation associated with depression and suicide attempts remains unclear. Nevertheless, it is of interest that the SSRIs appear to have some beneficial effects on suicidal thoughts. Comparisons between the improvement in suicidal thoughts during treatment with SSRIs compared with that during treatment with TCAs show that with at least some of these compounds a faster and more complete reduction in suicidal thoughts is achieved (S. A. Montgomery et al. 1981, 1995; Wakelin 1988). It has been observed that, during treatment of depression, symptoms may fluctuate and suicidal thoughts may emerge. High levels of apparently new suicidal thoughts have been observed during treatment with placebo. It appears that SSRIs may have some protective effect against the appearance of suicidal ideation in those with fluctuating symptoms (S. A. Montgomery et al. 1995).

The rates of provocation of mania reported with SSRIs appear to be lower than rates with the TCAs and may therefore be a more appropriate therapeutic option in the treatment of depression in patients with bipolar disorder. It is of course difficult to distinguish the beneficial effect of a drug in relation to rare events, but the meta-analysis of the database of one of the SSRIs reported a switch rate of between 2% and 3%, which compares favorably with 11% reported with TCAs (S. A. Montgomery 1995d).

Weaknesses of Selective
Serotonin Reuptake Inhibitors

The side effects seen with the SSRIs, although fewer and generally less troublesome than side effects of the TCAs, are still of some concern. Nausea, nervousness, and sexual side effects are the most bothersome. The nausea appears to be dose related, and, when a full dose is used immediately, it may not be tolerated in some individuals. The nausea tends to reduce and cease to be a problem with further treatment so that in sensitive patients lower initial doses may be the best approach followed by raising the dose later (Jenner 1992). The mechanism by which the nausea is produced relates to the direct effects of the SSRIs on 5-HT$_3$ receptors. The 5-HT$_3$ antagonist ondansetron is primarily used to control nausea associated with cancer treatments, and some reports indicate that 5-HT$_3$ antagonists are helpful in reducing the nausea associated with SSRIs. Mirtazapine, which has 5-HT$_3$ antagonist properties, is believed to induce less nausea than the SSRIs induce and indeed has been used as adjunctive treatment in controlling the nausea of the SSRIs (S. A. Montgomery 1995d).

Nervousness and agitation in some patients early in treatment are characteristic side effects of the SSRIs. These too have been reported to be dose related. In the fluoxetine database, these side effects were more common with the 60-mg dose than with the 20-mg dose and were associated with some insomnia (G. L. Cooper 1988). Although in general the various SSRIs differ little one from the other, there appear to be some differences in their propensity for producing nausea and nervousness.

Sexual dysfunction is commonly associated with depressive illness, with approximately 83% of men and 53% of women reporting loss of libido (Cassidy et al. 1957). It appears that sexual dysfunction also often develops during treatment with psychotropic drugs, and the true prevalence may have been underestimated (Baldwin 1996). The sexual side effects were not adequately reported in the early studies with SSRIs, and it was thought that they were uncommon. However, an increasing number of studies report failure to ejaculate in men and anorgasmia in women during treatment for depression with SSRIs. Estimates vary from study to study, but one review suggested that as many as 34% of patients taking fluoxetine report some sexual dysfunction when asked specifically about the symptoms (Jacobsen 1992). The sexual dysfunction may be related to 5-HT$_2$ receptors, and some evidence indicates that nefazodone, which is an SSRI, plus 5-HT$_2$ antagonist activity is associated with less sexual dysfunction than, for example, the SSRI sertraline. Levels of sexual dysfunction with mirtazapine, which has 5-HT$_2$

antagonist properties, are reported to be the same as those of placebo (S. A. Montgomery 1995c).

Some questions have been raised about the relative efficacy of the SSRIs, particularly in severe depression. The pooled analyses of the data from blinded, controlled trials have tended to find similar levels of efficacy between the SSRIs and the comparator TCA, imipramine. Paroxetine and fluvoxamine were both found in subanalyses of patients with severe depression included in large placebo- and imipramine-controlled studies to be more effective than imipramine in severe depression (S. A. Montgomery 1992a; Ottevanger 1991; Tignol et al. 1992; Wakelin 1988). However, imipramine may not be the TCA that is most effective in severe depression or may not have been used in the trials at an adequate dose.

A significant advantage compared with the SSRI fluoxetine has been reported with the newer double-action antidepressants venlafaxine (Clerc et al. 1994), milnacipran (López-Ibor et al. 1996), and mirtazapine (S. A. Montgomery 1996), which have all been found to be significantly more effective than fluoxetine. These studies were conducted for the most part in inpatients with depression with a greater severity than is normally included in studies. A series of studies comparing clomipramine with citalopram (Danish University Antidepressant Group 1986) and paroxetine (Danish University Antidepressant Group 1990) reported that clomipramine was more effective in inpatients. The methodology of these studies is open to criticism because not all of these patients were severely depressed and imprecise diagnostic criteria were used. Nevertheless, these studies have given rise to some concern on the part of clinicians that, in some with severe depression, SSRIs may not be the optimum treatment (Martensson and Aberg-Wistedt 1996).

Selective Specificity

Much evidence suggests that drugs with a potent effect on the reuptake of serotonin have a different therapeutic profile than do drugs without this pharmacological action or with only a small effect. The SSRIs and clomipramine have, for example, been found to have therapeutic efficacy in obsessive-compulsive disorder (OCD) (S. A. Montgomery 1994), whereas less potent inhibitors of serotonin reuptake do not appear to possess this antiobsessional activity (W. K. Goodman et al. 1990b). OCD appears at present to be the psychiatric illness most specifically related to the serotonergic system in that the only drugs with established efficacy are either the SSRIs fluvoxamine (Greist et al. 1995c; S. A. Montgomery and Mancaux 1992), paroxetine

(Wheadon et al. 1993), fluoxetine (S. A. Montgomery et al. 1993b; Tollefson et al. 1994), and sertraline (Greist et al. 1995a, 1995b) or clomipramine (S. A. Montgomery 1994), which is unique among the TCAs in having potent effects on the reuptake of serotonin.

Some evidence indicates that other drugs with action on the serotonergic system may be associated with efficacy in OCD. Tryptophan, a precursor of serotonin, was shown in a small placebo-controlled study to have an effect size similar to that of the SSRIs (S. A. Montgomery et al. 1992). Mianserin, which has $5-HT_{1D}$ and $5-HT_{2C}$ receptor affinities, has also been reported in a small placebo-controlled study to be more effective than placebo. This last result raises the possibility that $5-HT_{1D}$ or $5-HT_{2C}$ may be the more specific receptors for OCD. The provocation of obsessional symptoms by m-chloro-phenylpiperazine (mCPP), which also has affinities for $5-HT_{1D}$ and $5-HT_{2C}$, reinforces this concept (Zohar et al. 1988a).

SSRIs have been reported to have a beneficial effect on the anxiety associated with depression which is greater than that conferred by treatment with TCAs (Dunbar and Fuell 1992; S. A. Montgomery et al. 1981; Wakelin 1988). This finding suggested that the SSRIs may be effective in the anxiety disorders per se. Good evidence now exists indicating that SSRIs are effective in treating panic disorder with or without concomitant major depression. Paroxetine has been licensed additionally for the treatment of panic disorder in many countries, based on evidence of efficacy from placebo-controlled short-term and long-term studies. The distinction between depression with panic attacks and panic disorder with major depression has not been clearly drawn. In those studies that have investigated pure panic disorder without major depression, some evidence shows that a selective beneficial effect may be found for the SSRIs compared with that for the TCAs (Den Boer and Westenberg 1988). On the other hand, depression with secondary panic attacks appears to respond to a variety of antidepressants with different mechanisms of action. It is possible that pure panic disorder is more specifically related to serotonin, but further studies are needed to clarify this issue.

Some evidence indicates that social phobia responds to SSRIs, and case reports and studies with fluoxetine (B. Black et al. 1992; Van Ameringen et al. 1993), fluvoxamine (Mendels et al. 1995), paroxetine (Pitts et al. 1996; Ringold 1994), and sertraline (Katzelnick et al. 1995) have reported positive results. Although the full details of these studies have not been published, it seems that SSRIs might well prove, in due course, to be effective treatments for social phobia. At the moment, the only treatment licensed for social phobia is moclobemide, which is a reversible inhibitor of monoamine oxidase-A (Nutt and Montgomery 1996; Versiani et al. 1992), and it is possible that it exerts its therapeutic effect via an action on serotonin. TCAs are thought to be ineffective in this condition, and this may encourage investigations to determine whether social phobia might have a direct therapeutic relationship with serotonergic drugs.

As other indications are sought for the SSRIs, it is clear that their action extends beyond depression, dysthymia, and the anxiety disorders, and the broad spectrum of therapeutic action of these antidepressants becomes apparent. For example, based on the evidence from placebo-controlled studies (A. Wood 1993), fluoxetine has been licensed in Europe for the treatment of bulimia, and several SSRIs are reported to be effective in the treatment of premenstrual syndrome.

Nefazodone

Nefazodone is an SSRI with 5-HT_2 antagonist properties. Nefazodone is licensed as an antidepressant in many countries, and the evidence for efficacy from placebo-controlled and reference-controlled studies does not suggest that this drug is associated with superior efficacy (Dillier 1982; R. Fontaine et al. 1994; Mendels et al. 1995; Rickels et al. 1994). The 5-HT_2 antagonism does not appear to confer extra efficacy, which appears to be similar to that of SSRIs. However, a beneficial effect on sleep and on anxiety symptoms of depression is reported. This may be attributable to 5-HT_2 blockade, but some studies have demonstrated nefazodone's superior efficacy to SSRIs. One attribute of nefazodone that may be related to 5-HT_2 blockade is that it is associated with rather little in the way of sexual side effects. A direct comparison between nefazodone and sertraline reported significantly fewer sexual side effects with nefazodone (Baldwin 1996).

PINDOLOL PLUS

To answer questions about the relative lack of efficacy of the SSRIs in certain groups of patients, it should be possible to test whether additional receptor effects could enhance response. Various adjunctive treatments have been considered as augmentation strategies. Currently the most interesting of these approaches is the investigation of the use of pindolol to augment treatment with SSRIs. It has been suggested that the 5-HT_{1A} autoreceptor antagonist might accelerate the response to SSRIs by blocking the 1A receptor on the cell body, which would have the effect of stopping the initial reduction in activity found at the beginning of SSRI treatment (Artigas et al. 1994; Blier and Bergeron 1995). Pindolol appears to be specific in that it blocks the presynaptic autoreceptor but not the postsynaptic 1A receptors.

The initial reports from open studies (Artigas et al. 1994; Blier and Bergeron 1995) suggest that the combination is associated with improved efficacy with probable faster onset of action. This rapid response was reported with augmentation of fluoxetine and paroxetine, and more recently with nefazodone (Bakish et al. 1997), but interestingly not with sertraline or low doses of fluvoxamine. These results needed to be confirmed in placebo-controlled studies, and the reports from large studies do indeed find an acceleration of response measured as time to response and possible superiority of action with some antidepressants at the end of treatment (Perez et al. 1997; Tome de la Granja et al. 1997).

It is important for this type of study to be of adequate size because to demonstrate differences between two active treatments requires larger numbers than a difference between an active antidepressant and placebo. Caution is needed in accepting the negative results from underpowered small studies.

The phenomena of early onset of response and of final improved response at the end of treatment are probably closely related. Stassen and colleagues (1993, 1994), who carried out a large pooled analysis of two placebo- and reference-controlled development programs for different antidepressants, reported that response to both placebo and conventional antidepressants follow the same time-course. In those with an earlier onset of improvement, there should also be a later improved overall response at the end of treatment. A higher proportion of early improvers should be reflected in a higher proportion of later responders (S. A. Montgomery 1995a).

An intriguing finding is that this rapid onset of action appears to be concentrated in those patients who were expected to have a good response to treatment (Tome de la Granja et al. 1997). Little response is seen in the more chronic or resistant patients. This finding is in contrast to the results of Blier and Bergeron (1995), who reported some effect in those with resistant depression. Berman and colleagues (1997) have reported that pindolol augmentation of fluoxetine was not effective in a small group of 50 patients treated with either fluoxetine or fluoxetine plus pindolol under controlled conditions. The patients included in this study largely had resistant depression, and half of them were reported to have a duration of illness that suggested they had chronic depression. The acceleration of response may be achieved only in those in whom response is expected but not in those who would not respond to an SSRI at all. The diagnostic issues need to be examined far more closely before any conclusions can be drawn.

These interesting results suggest that there are ways of improving the response to SSRIs by rapidly increasing the serotonergic activity. However, pindolol is not simply a 5-HT$_{1A}$ autoreceptor antagonist. It is also a β-adrenergic antagonist, and this activity may also add some extra therapeutic effect.

NORADRENALINE PLUS

The addition of a nonselective noradrenaline reuptake inhibitor, desipramine, to an SSRI, fluoxetine, has been reported to be associated with a more rapid downregulation of β-adrenoceptors in rats than seen with either treatment on its own (B. M. Baron et al. 1988). This observation suggests that the addition of desipramine to fluoxetine might be associated with more rapid response and therefore possibly improved response.

The only current evidence to support this view is the finding that the addition of desipramine to fluoxetine was better than desipramine alone in the treatment of patients with depression (J. C. Nelson et al. 1991). Desipramine alone resulted in the expected improvement of approximately 20% at week 1 and 40% at 2 weeks in 52 patients. In patients treated with the combination of fluoxetine and desipramine, the response was greatly accelerated, and a response of 42% was seen at the first week of treatment. At the end of 4 weeks of treatment, 71% of the 14 patients on combined treatment were in complete remission compared with only 14% of those receiving desipramine alone. This study provides some evidence of the better efficacy seen with a double action on both noradrenaline and serotonin, but firm conclusions cannot be drawn because of the open nature of the investigation.

An interesting series of studies has used tryptophan depletion to test the functional integrity of the serotonin system and α-methyl-*p*-tyrosine (AMPT) to investigate the integrity of the catecholamine system (Delgado et al. 1990b; H. L. Miller et al. 1996a, 1996b). In these studies, 80% of the patients with depression who had been successfully treated with monoamine oxidase inhibitors or fluvoxamine were found to relapse rapidly once plasma tryptophan levels were reduced. In those who responded to desipramine, only 18% relapsed. This implies that the SSRI was producing a response in those patients with a compromised serotonin system. Similarly, AMPT caused a relapse in those successfully treated with desipramine, but not in those successfully treated with SSRIs.

These elegant studies indicate that the response with SSRIs depends on depression related to a compromised serotonergic system, whereas the response to a noradrenaline reuptake inhibitor depends on a depression related to a compromised noradrenergic system. Although the proportion of responders may be similar in any group of patients treated with a noradrenergic reuptake inhibitor or SSRI, these studies suggest that the biological dysfunction producing the depression may be different in the two groups. The addition of a noradrenaline reuptake inhibitor to an SSRI should produce an increase in the number of patients responding in a particular sample.

DOUBLE ACTION OF SEROTONIN AND NORADRENALINE INHIBITION

Venlafaxine and milnacipran are two members of a new class of antidepressants that have selective effects on the reuptake of both serotonin and noradrenaline—serotonin noradrenaline reuptake inhibitors (SNRIs). In theory, based on the findings of B. M. Baron and colleagues (1988) and of J. C. Nelson and colleagues (1991), the combination of these two pharmacological actions should be associated with superior efficacy either in terms of rapid onset of action or extra efficacy at the end of treatment.

Venlafaxine

Venlafaxine appears to produce a rapid desensitization of the β-adrenergic receptors, and this may be important for the time course of antidepressant response. In an early study, venlafaxine was found to be associated with a significant difference from placebo at 4 days measured on the Montgomery and Asberg Depression Rating Scale (MADRS) (S. A. Montgomery and Asberg 1979) and a clinically relevant 4-point difference from placebo from 1 week onward (Guelfi et al. 1995; S. A. Montgomery 1995b). This response, which was seen far earlier than would normally be expected, suggested that venlafaxine is a drug associated with rapid onset of action and response. The comparison of different doses of venlafaxine with placebo showed that the rapid response appeared to be associated with the medium (150–225 mg/day) and high doses (300–375 mg/day) of the drug rather than with the more conventional dose of 75 mg.

The advantage of venlafaxine in terms of more rapid onset of action is apparently only seen when the drug is escalated rapidly to the high dose. In a recent study comparing venlafaxine with imipramine in inpatients with severe depression, a significant difference was observed between the two active treatments by the second week (Benkert et al. 1996).

Studies need to be designed specifically to test early onset of action, and these would require frequent observations, at least twice a week. These studies on venlafaxine were not specifically designed to test early onset of action, and they were generally underpowered for a comparison between two active drugs. The demonstration of significant differences between treatments is therefore of considerable interest. The labeling of the early onset of action of venlafaxine is now recognized in many European countries.

Several studies have indicated that venlafaxine is associated with superior efficacy. In particular, venlafaxine has been found to have a significant advantage compared with that of fluoxetine given in a dose of 40 mg in the treatment of inpatients with severe depression (Clerc et al. 1994). There are several indications that venlafaxine in appropriate dosing is associated with superior efficacy both in the short term and in the long term. However, specific studies, adequately powered to find differences between two active treatments, have not been carried out. The early onset of antidepressant response and the suggestions of superior efficacy at the end of treatment should be viewed together as a related phenomenon, and the evidence that venlafaxine in medium to high doses is a different kind of antidepressant to low-dose venlafaxine or the SSRIs should be taken seriously.

Milnacipran

Milnacipran is a rather newer SNRI licensed as an antidepressant in France. It is associated with clear-cut efficacy judged on the placebo-controlled studies (Lecrubier et al. 1996; Macher et al. 1989). Milnacipran inhibits the reuptake of both noradrenaline and serotonin (Moret et al. 1985). It has a relatively short half-life and is given optimally in a dose of 50 mg twice daily. The proportion of reuptake inhibition between serotonin and noradrenaline is approximately equal with this antidepressant, and so one would expect that milnacipran would be more effective than SSRIs, assuming the theory is correct that two actions are better than one.

Two studies have compared milnacipran, in the recommended dose of 50 mg twice daily, with SSRIs in patients with severe depression, reviewed recently by López-Ibor and colleagues (1996). Both studies reported a significant advantage for milnacipran, measured on the MADRS, compared with fluoxetine given in a dose of 20 mg/day or fluvoxamine given in a dose of 100 mg twice a day. The size of the effect was substantial: in the combined studies, the advantage for milnacipran compared with that for the SSRIs was more than 4 points.

The dual action of milnacipran would also make it an appropriate candidate for testing whether this type of compound could bring about more rapid onset of response. However, studies requiring more frequent assessments have not yet been carried out.

Mirtazapine

Mirtazapine is also designed to have effects on both serotonin and noradrenaline simultaneously. The mechanism of action is rather more complicated in that it preferentially blocks the noradrenergic α_2 autoreceptors, which seem to be responsible for controlling noradrenaline release. Mirtazapine increases serotonergic firing but, because it blocks 5-HT$_2$ and 5-HT$_3$, only the 5-HT$_1$ transmission is enhanced. The effect is therefore to produce increased 5-HT$_1$ and noradrenergic transmission. Animal studies show that acute administration of mirtazapine produces a rapid increase in both noradrenaline and serotonin transmission (Haddjeri et al. 1995). Because mirtazapine blocks 5-HT$_2$ and 5-HT$_2$ receptors, the nausea and sexual side effects (the typical side effects of serotonergic antidepressants) are likely to be avoided (S. A. Montgomery 1996).

On the basis of the large placebo-controlled studies, mirtazapine has undoubted antidepressant action and is licensed in both Europe and the United States (Claghorn and Lesem 1995; Sitsen et al. 1995). The evidence for superior efficacy is again limited by the failure to set up studies that were large enough to provide an adequate test of two active antidepressants. Nevertheless, mirtazapine has been shown to be more effective than trazodone in hospitalized patients with major depression (van Moffaert et al. 1995); and in a more recent study, mirtazapine was more effective than fluoxetine given in a dose of 20 mg (S. A. Montgomery 1996).

Mirtazapine has been investigated in long-term treatment, and interestingly, although both amitriptyline, the comparator, and mirtazapine were effective, mirtazapine was associated with fewer relapses than was amitriptyline (S. A. Montgomery 1996).

Mirtazapine has a benevolent side-effect profile, and in particular the claims of lower levels of nausea and sexual difficulties appear to be supported by the results of the clinical trials (S. A. Montgomery 1995c).

NORADRENALINE REUPTAKE INHIBITORS

Reboxetine

Reboxetine is a pure noradrenaline reuptake inhibitor that is licensed as an antidepressant in the United Kingdom. Reboxetine has established efficacy based on placebo-controlled studies both in the short and the long term. Previous noradrenaline reuptake inhibitors, such as desipramine, nortriptyline, and maprotiline, have been relatively selective for noradrenaline compared with serotonin but have not avoided affinities with α_1, muscarinic, and histaminergic receptors. The lack of selectivity of these drugs has the consequence that the levels of cardiotoxicity are those expected with TCAs. Reboxetine is the first pure noradrenaline reuptake inhibitor, and therefore it may also provide a more appropriate agent to consider for the investigation of possible adjunctive treatments with SSRIs.

Dopamine

The role of dopamine is discussed more thoroughly in Pinder, Chapter 14, in this volume. Several antidepressants are thought to have enhanced antidepressant action attributed to extra effects on the dopamine system. Bupropion, which is available as an antidepressant in the United States only, has an indirect effect on dopamine. An appropriate minimum effective dose was not established in the early clinical trial development program, and the rather high doses used in clinical practice may have contributed to the number of reports of convulsions. The rate, which is acceptable at lower doses of 450 mg/day, rises to unacceptable levels at higher doses (J. A. Johnston et al. 1991).

Amineptine, which is available as an antidepressant in some countries in Europe, is a selective dopamine reuptake inhibitor. Amineptine is an old drug and was not subjected to the rigorous trial methodology applied to more recent antidepressants. There are suggestions that amineptine may be associated with early onset of antidepressant action, but this has not been thoroughly studied (Garattini 1997). Some concerns have been expressed that amineptine may be associated with abuse potential, and theoretically these two phenomena may be linked through the dopamine system because of an amphetamine-like effect.

Other compounds with a predominant effect on the dopamine system have been investigated as antidepressants, but the results have not been particularly promising. A poorer response was seen with high doses of minaprine compared with lower doses, which compromised the use of this drug (S. A. Montgomery et al. 1991), and similar results were reported with GBR12909, a purer dopamine reuptake inhibitor (Danion 1991).

CONCLUSION

Over the past 30 years, considerable improvements have been made in the treatment of depression. Much effort has been devoted in the past 15 years to the development and use of newer drugs devoid of unnecessary, counter-therapeutic side effects. Drugs such as the SSRIs, because of their significantly greater tolerability compared with that of the TCAs, have made an important impact on drawing more people with depression to seek treatment.

It is recognized that conventional antidepressants including the SSRIs have limitations in terms of efficacy. There are a large number of non-responders and the response is slow. Current development of antidepressants is focusing on increased efficacy both in increasing the response rate and in accelerating the response. These developments have largely centered on the additive benefits of action on both the noradrenaline and the serotonin systems. We look forward to the more imaginative development of novel compounds designed on the basis of their receptor interactions to achieve more effective treatments.

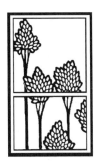

CHAPTER 13

New Emerging Serotonergic Antidepressants

Jogin H. Thakore, Ph.D., M.R.C.Psych.,
Carlo Berti, M.B., M.F.P.M., and
Timothy G. Dinan, M.D., Ph.D.,
F.R.C.P.I., F.R.C.Psych.

SPECIFIC SEROTONERGIC AGENTS IN THE TREATMENT OF DEPRESSION

In this chapter, we review the pharmacology of several selective serotonin reuptake inhibitors (SSRIs) and other drugs that act on the serotonergic system. That these developments have enhanced safety and tolerability is now beyond dispute, but it is also clear that these agents are no more effective than the old-style tricyclic antidepressants (TCAs). (For a comprehensive discussion of serotonergic medication, see Montgomery, Chapter 12, in this volume.) Here, several compounds are discussed in detail.

Citalopram

Basic pharmacology. Claims that citalopram is the "most selective" SSRI are based on two types of in vitro evidence (Hyttel 1994): IC_{50} (concentration required to inhibit uptake by 50%) ratios between noradrenaline (NA) and serotonin (5-HT) and its binding profile for a variety of receptor sub-types. The $IC_{50}NA/IC_{50}$5-HT ratio for citalopram is 3,400, and citalopram binds to the serotonin reuptake sites, with an order of magnitude 200 times greater than that for the dopaminergic type-2 receptor, $5\text{-}HT_{1A}$ receptor, $5\text{-}HT_2$ receptor, cholinergic receptors, histaminergic type-1 receptors, β-adrenergic receptors, NA reuptake sites, and dopaminergic reuptake sites (Hyttel 1982). Demethylcitalopram and didemethylcitalopram, metabolites of citalopram, are less potent and selective than the parent compound (Hyttel and Larsen 1985).

Clinical pharmacology.   A bicyclic isobenzofurane derivative, citalopram is nearly completely absorbed after oral administration, with 80% available after first-pass metabolism. Eighty-three percent of that absorbed is protein bound, and peak plasma concentrations are reached in 3 hours (range 1–6 hours) (Milne and Goa 1991). Even though citalopram's half-life is 33–35 hours, steady-state levels are achieved only after 1–2 weeks, reflecting the longer half-life of its metabolites demethylcitalopram (half-life = 49 hours) and didemethylcitalopram (half-life = 102 hours) (P. Baumann 1992). Mainly eliminated by hepatic metabolism, citalopram's biotransformation is not fully understood as the parent compound, and its two metabolites account for only 45%–50% of the dose in urine (Van Harten 1993).

Dose ranges of 20–60 mg/day have been recommended based on a series of studies with patients with differing severities of depression (S. A. Montgomery et al. 1994a). Dosing studies have revealed that elderly patients achieve four times greater plasma concentrations for an equivalent dose given to a younger subject (Fredericson Overo et al. 1985).

Efficacy.   Citalopram is licensed in the United Kingdom and several other countries for the acute treatment of depression and for 6 months thereafter to prevent relapse. Evidence for citalopram's effectiveness in the long-term prophylaxis of depression comes from a single double-blind, placebo-controlled study, in which 20–40 mg of citalopram was found to be superior to placebo in terms of efficacy and time to relapse (S. A. Montgomery et al. 1993a). Citalopram was found to have similar efficacy in comparison with amitriptyline, imipramine, and various other TCAs (Bech 1989; Bouchard et al. 1987; Gravem et al. 1987; Rosenberg et al. 1994; D. M. Shaw et al. 1986). In contrast, the Danish University Antidepressant Group (1986) found that clomipramine was more effective than citalopram in major depressive disorder.

Adverse effects. More than 500,000 people have been treated with citalopram; the tolerability of the compound has been evaluated in 2,420 patients and volunteers in phase II and III clinical trials, with more than 6,700 patients having been recruited into phase IV trials. Adverse effects of citalopram that occurred by ≥5% over placebo were nausea, dry mouth, and somnolence. Elderly patients appear to tolerate citalopram well, and their adverse-effect profile is similar to that of younger patients (Gottfries and Nyth 1991). The 6-month relapse prevention study has shown that citalopram and placebo do not differ in side-effect frequency at weeks 12 and 24 (S. A. Montgomery et al. 1993a). Withdrawal phenomena have not been reported to occur on abrupt termination of this compound. Three fatal events have been reported involving citalopram, although these deaths, possibly as a result of the serotonin syndrome, have been attributed to citalopram use in combination with another agent, moclobemide (Neuvonen et al. 1993).

Fluvoxamine

Basic pharmacology. Fluvoxamine is an effective serotonin reuptake inhibitor with an IC_{50} value of 0.3 μmol/L; comparable IC_{50} values for desipramine and fluoxetine are 0.8 μmol/L and 1.3 μmol/L, respectively (Bradford 1984). The IC_{50} values for NA and dopamine were 100 times higher than those for serotonin (Bradford 1984). In vitro data indicate that fluvoxamine has little or no affinity for α_1, α_2, β_1, β_2, D_2, 5-HT_2, muscarinic, or histaminergic receptors (Benfield and Ward 1986). Fluvoxamine has a total of 11 metabolites, and the 2 principal ones have little or no pharmacological activity (Claassen 1983).

Clinical pharmacology. Peak plasma concentrations are reached within 2–8 hours (DeBree et al. 1983), and steady-state concentrations are achieved at about 10 days, reflecting a half-life of 19–22 hours (DeVries et al. 1992). Fluvoxamine is 77% bound to plasma proteins and is extensively metabolized by the liver (Claassen 1983). Optimal dosing regimens for fluvoxamine range from 100 mg/day to 200 mg/day, with the maximum recommended dose being 300 mg/day. Lower doses should be used in those with significant hepatic impairment.

Efficacy. To date, more than 15 clinical trials have been conducted comparing fluvoxamine with other active agents and placebo. Imipramine was the most common comparator drug used, and studies have indicated that fluvoxamine was effective as the reference drug, although significantly superior to placebo (Amore et al. 1989; Fabre et al. 1992; Gonella et al. 1990; Lapierre et al. 1987; March et al. 1990; Ottevanger 1991). In comparison with other TCAs, fluvoxamine is as effective as amitriptyline, dothiepin, and clomipramine (Coleman and Block 1982; P. Dick and Ferrero 1983; Harris et al. 1991; Mullin et al. 1988; Rahman et al. 1991). Clinical trials involving other non-TCAs have shown fluvoxamine to be an effective antidepressant (for review, see Wilde et al. 1993).

Adverse effects.   Postmarketing surveillance, in which more than 34,000 patients were studied, revealed that fluvoxamine is generally well tolerated if initial dose titration is employed (Wilde et al. 1993). By far the most common side effect reported was nausea (15.7%); other adverse effects included somnolence (6.4%), asthenia (5.1%), headache (4.8%), and dry mouth (4.8%); these events had an incidence of ≥1%. On reviewing the manufacturer's database, Henry (1991) found that 310 cases of overdose with fluvoxamine had been reported worldwide. The overwhelming majority recovered with no sequelae; the 13 fatalities were associated with multiple substance ingestion, making the contribution of any single substance difficult to assess.

Nefazodone

Basic pharmacology.   A phenylpiperazine, nefazodone has been shown to inhibit serotonin uptake and inhibit 5-HT$_2$ receptor binding in a dose-dependent manner. Its IC$_{50}$ for serotonin uptake sites is 181 nM and for 5-HT$_2$ receptors is 32 nM. Nefazodone has no affinity for dopaminergic or α_2-adrenergic sites, has weak cholinergic antagonistic and histaminergic activity, and shows reduced α_1-adrenergic activity relative to TCAs (D. P. Taylor et al. 1986). Hydroxynefazodone and to a lesser extent m-chlorophenyl-piperazine are the principal metabolites of nefazodone and may exhibit clinically significant effects.

Clinical pharmacology.   Following absorption, peak plasma concentrations occur 1–3 hours after oral administration (Franc et al. 1991). Following extensive hepatic metabolism, the bioavailability of nefazodone is between 15% and 23%, after which it is 99% protein bound. Nefazodone reaches steady-state plasma levels in 3 days and is eliminated from the body within 24 hours, reflecting its half-life of 2–4 hours (Franc et al. 1991). Therapeutic doses in young adults have been found to range from 100 to 300 mg twice daily (E. Fontaine 1994). Lower doses are recommended in patients with concomitant liver disease and the elderly, as plasma concentrations can be double those seen in younger patients.

Efficacy. Several double-blind clinical trials comparing nefazodone to other antidepressants and placebo are in print (Feighner et al. 1989a, 1989b; R. Fontaine et al. 1994; Mendels et al. 1991; Rickels et al. 1994; van Moffaert et al. 1994). Nefazodone was superior to placebo, although equally efficacious in comparison with imipramine in these studies. To date, no study has been published comparing nefazodone with SSRIs. Studies in psychiatrically healthy volunteers and patients with major depression have indicated that nefazodone is capable of normalizing disrupted sleep patterns (Armitage et al. 1994; Sharpley and Cowen 1995). Yet, this property may not be unique to nefazodone, as no comparison trials have been performed with other active agents. Long-term efficacy is indicated by a single study, an amalgamation of several 6- to 8-week trials that were extended for up to 240 days (S. F. Anton et al. 1994).

Adverse effects. Side effects that occurred with nefazodone to a greater degree than with placebo and that were dose related included somnolence, dry mouth, nausea, and dizziness. Furthermore, there is no need to taper the dose if discontinuation is being considered (L. Friedman et al. 1992; L. H. Gold and Balster 1991). More than 2,256 patients have been studied in clinical trials, and, to date, only two cases of overdose (>3,600 mg ingested) have been reported; both patients recovered with no sequelae.

Tianeptine

Basic pharmacology. Although sharing a structure similar to TCAs, tianeptine has the unusual property of increasing the uptake of serotonin. This has been demonstrated ex vivo in rat brain (Mennini et al. 1987), rat platelets (Kato and Weitsch 1988), and human platelets (Chamba et al. 1991). Further evidence of this presynaptic effect of tianeptine has come from a variety of sources, the most convincing evidence being presented by Whitton et al. (1991). The increased serotonin uptake is the result of an increase in rate of uptake and not the result of an increased affinity for the uptake site (Mennini et al. 1987). Tianeptine has little affinity for D_2, adrenergic, γ-aminobutyric acid, benzodiazepine, muscarinic, or histamine sites (Kato and Weitsch 1988; Mennini et al. 1987). Neither does it bind to either presynaptic serotonin sites or postsynaptic 5-HT$_1$ and 5-HT$_2$ sites (Hamon et al. 1988). The two principal metabolites of tianeptine, MC_5 and MC_3, appear to have biological activity.

Clinical pharmacology. Peak plasma levels are reached within 1 hour of ingestion, and tianeptine does not appear to undergo any first-pass hepatic metabolism. Though tianeptine has a short half-life (1.4–3.6 hours), its principal metabolite, MC5, has a half-life of 7.2 hours, and so, steady-state levels are reached within 1 week. Tianeptine undergoes extensive hepatic metabolism, with the resulting compounds having shortened side chains. The recommended daily dose for tianeptine is 12.5 mg in three divided doses. Doses should be reduced in the elderly and those with chronic renal failure.

Efficacy.   Five double-blind trials comparing tianeptine with imipramine, nomifensine, and amitriptyline have found that tianeptine has a therapeutic efficacy similar to that of the reference drug (Guelfi et al. 1989; Loo et al. 1988). Even though Mennini et al. (1987) and Mocaer et al. (1988) suggested that tianeptine is unique in increasing serotonin reuptake, others have found this to occur with other TCAs and certain SSRIs, following chronic dosing (Manias and Taylor 1983).

Adverse effects.   Common side effects on taking tianeptine include drowsiness, irritability, and gastrointestinal upset. Long-term safety data on tianeptine indicate that it is well tolerated in overdose, with drowsiness being the major problem (Loo et al. 1988).

CONCLUSION

In most Western countries, SSRIs are gradually becoming the first-line treatment of choice for major depressive illness. There is also an increasing tendency to use these drugs in the management of obsessive-compulsive disorder, panic disorder, premenstrual syndrome, and bulimia nervosa (see Montgomery, Chapter 12, in this volume). This increasing use, although undoubtedly partly driven by the effective marketing by multinational pharmaceutical companies, is nonetheless significantly the result of the SSRIs being such a well-tolerated group of compounds.

That SSRIs are more acceptable from the patient's perspective than traditional TCAs is largely accepted by clinicians but has recently been questioned in an article by F. Song et al. (1993). These researchers conducted a meta-analysis of 63 randomized controlled trials comparing the efficacy and acceptability of SSRIs with those of tricyclic and related antidepressants. The article has been cited widely, especially in the United Kingdom. The authors suggest that the dropout rate in patients receiving SSRIs is similar to that of patients receiving TCAs in controlled studies. They concluded that the routine use of SSRIs as the first-line treatment of depressive illness was not cost-effective. The article is obviously based on the false assumption that dropout rates in clinical trials are a true reflection of drug tolerability in normal clinical practice. This, as most clinicians will agree, is not the case. Patients withdraw from clinical trials for a myriad of reasons: on some occasions, because of adverse side effects; on other occasions, because they have responded to treatment. The conclusions that one can draw from this paper are also not helped by the fact that a variety of drugs are consistently miscategorized throughout the text. That SSRIs are more expensive than traditional TCAs is beyond doubt, although the differences are decreasing at a rapid rate. Nonetheless, it seems likely that, with improved patient awareness, patients will themselves choose the newer line of treatment.

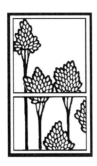

CHAPTER 14

Dopamine Receptors and Antidepressant Development

Roger M. Pinder, Ph.D., D.Sc.

In an era preoccupied with serotonin (5-HT) research in depression and the emergence of the selective serotonin reuptake inhibitors (SSRIs) as antidepressants, other neurotransmitters such as noradrenaline (NA) and dopamine (DA) have been neglected (Blier and de Montigny 1994). DA was not part of the original biogenic amine hypotheses for depression, and its involvement was first proposed by Randrup et al. (1975), who subsequently showed that many of the then-newer antidepressants exhibited rather potent inhibition of DA reuptake (Randrup and Braestrup 1977). Led by nomifensine, an effective antidepressant that was withdrawn in 1986 because of its association with hemolytic anemia, a series of antidepressants was developed having a primary effect on central dopaminergic mechanisms, principally on reuptake. These included the still available products aminep-tine, bupropion, and minaprine, as well as two drugs whose clinical develop-ment was discontinued, the most potent known inhibitors of DA reuptake, diclofensine and GBR 12909 (Pinder and Wieringa 1993). Substantial evi-dence suggests that DA precursors and agonists have antidepressant efficacy, whereas standard antidepressant treatments and electroconvulsive therapy enhance DA function. Results from studies of depression and Parkinson's disease, as well as of animal models of depression, favor a deficiency of DA in depressive disorders (A. S. Brown and Gershon 1993; Diehl and Gershon 1992; Kapur and Mann 1992).

Nevertheless, despite the wealth of evidence supporting a role for DA in depression, dopaminergic mechanisms no longer seem to be fashionable targets for the design of new antidepressants (D. Leysen and Pinder 1994; Pinder and Wieringa 1993). Paradoxically, the potential for obtaining more selective agents is better than ever with the recent identification of multiple subtypes of DA receptors (P. Seeman and Van Tol 1994) and the complete molecular characterization of the DA uptake transporter (Giros and Caron 1993). Application of this new knowledge, particularly that on DA receptors, is largely channeled into antipsychotic research, but it is also an appropriate time to reassess the role of the dopaminergic system in depression. In this chapter, we therefore explore new information that suggests that dopaminergic mechanisms may be fertile ground for the design and development of novel antidepressant treatments.

DOPAMINE IN THE BRAIN

Most DA-containing neurons in the brain belong to the nigrostriatal pathway, which arises from cells in the midbrain areas A8 and A9 and ascends to the striatum, and are involved in modulating motor behavior. DA-containing neurons involved in cognition and the modulation of motivation and reward ascend from area A10 and project to limbic and cortical areas, the so-called mesolimbic and mesocortical pathways, respectively. Hypothalamic DA cell bodies, which project to the median eminence and the neurohypophysis, mediate neuroendocrine regulation of prolactin secretion. The mesolimbic and mesocortical pathways are those that are most likely to be involved in the pathophysiology of affective disorders (Willner and Scheel-Krüger 1991).

The effects of DA in the brain are mediated by DA receptors, of which five types have been identified, cloned, and characterized in humans (Sibley and Monsma 1992). All are members of the large group of 7-transmembranal G protein–coupled receptors, and they fall broadly into two families: D_1-like receptors, which activate the adenylate cyclase system, and D_2-like receptors, which inhibit it (Table 14–1). D_1 and D_5 receptors are coded by genes on chromosomes 5 and 4, respectively, but the D_5 receptor has two related pseudogenes on chromosomes 1 and 2 that result in heavily truncated versions of the normal receptor. D_3 and D_4 receptors belong to the D_2 family, all of which have many variants (P. Seeman and Van Tol 1994). Most antipsychotic drugs block D_2 receptors in direct correlation to clinical potency except for clozapine, which prefers D_4 receptors. D_1 and D_2 receptors can enhance each other's actions, possibly through subunits of the G pro-

TABLE 14-1. Properties of cloned human dopamine receptors

	D_1	D_5	D_2	D_3	D_4
Number of amino acids	446	477	443	400	387
Number of variants	1	3	5[a]	5	12[b]
Human chromosome	5	4	11	3	11
Introns in gene	No	No	Yes	Yes	Yes
Effector pathways	↑ cAMP	↑ cAMP	↓ cAMP	↓ cAMP	↓ cAMP

Note. cAMP = cyclic adenosine monophosphate.
[a]Three of these variants are rare in humans; the most common are D_{2L} with 443 and D_{2S} with 414 amino acids.
[b]Three of these variants have not yet been found in humans.

teins. Although both families exist postsynaptically, only D_2 and D_3 receptors seem to be involved in presynaptic autoreceptor control of DA release (Tang et al. 1994), with D_2 autoreceptors having been identified in human cortex (Fedele et al. 1993). Presynaptic D_1 receptors may facilitate the release of other neurotransmitters, particularly γ-aminobutyric acid, in the midbrain (D. L. Cameron and Williams 1993). Both main families of DA receptors tend to be localized in midbrain and limbic areas, but the D_2 family predominates in cortical regions (Sibley and Monsma 1992).

Optimal dopaminergic neurotransmission in the human brain is maintained by two principal presynaptic mechanisms, autoregulation by D_2 (and perhaps D_3) receptors and reuptake via the DA transporter (Giros and Caron 1993). Deficiencies in transmission can be rectified in principle by three mechanisms: reuptake inhibition, thereby making more DA available to its receptors; stimulation of postsynaptic DA receptors with DA agonists; or increase of the release of DA from its terminals by blocking DA autoreceptors. If depression is indeed associated with a deficiency of DA, then antidepressant treatment could theoretically be effected with DA reuptake inhibitors, D_1 or D_2 postsynaptic agonists, or D_2 autoreceptor antagonists.

DOPAMINE AND DEPRESSION: CLINICAL STUDIES

The most consistent finding in clinical studies has been decreased turnover of DA in patients with depressive disorders, as measured by cerebrospinal fluid (CSF) levels and urinary output of its principal metabolite homovanillic acid (HVA) (A. S. Brown and Gershon 1993; Kapur and Mann 1992). Patients with depression who attempt suicide as well as those who succeed seem to have the lowest turnover of DA (Bowden et al. 1994a; A. Roy et al. 1992). Depression is common in patients with Parkinson's disease (Cummings 1992), and, although this may be more associated with lower CSF levels of the principal serotonin metabolite 5-hydroxyindole-3-acetic acid (5-HIAA), a distinct pattern of neuropsychological deficits associated with low HVA has been noted across diagnostic categories, including major depression and Parkinson's disease (Wolfe et al. 1990). The association may not extend to seasonal affective disorder, which is characterized by normal turnover of DA (Rudorfer et al. 1993) and unresponsiveness to the DA precursor levodopa (Oren et al. 1994), despite previous circumstantial evidence implicating abnormal dopaminergic regulation in seasonal affective disorder (Depue et al. 1989).

The sensitivity of DA receptors may be changed in depressive disorders. A significantly greater growth hormone response to the D_2 agonist apomorphine was observed in women with affective psychosis after childbirth, indicating enhanced D_2 receptor sensitivity in the hypothalamus and possibly elsewhere in the brain during depression (Wieck et al. 1991). More direct investigations in vivo using positron-emission tomography (PET) or single photon emission computed tomography (SPECT) have largely confirmed such changes, although one earlier PET study failed to differentiate between D_2 receptors in psychiatrically healthy control subjects or patients with bipolar disorder (D. F. Wong et al. 1985). Thus, SPECT studies have demonstrated that uptake of high-affinity ligands for D_2 receptors into the basal ganglia is higher in patients with depression than in psychiatrically healthy control subjects, indicating increased D_2 receptor density in depression (D'haenen and Bossuyt 1994), whereas responders to total sleep deprivation showed a significant decrease of basal ganglia D_2 receptor occupancy compared with that of nonresponders (Ebert et al. 1994). SPECT studies of brain perfusion implicate the basal ganglia and cingulate cortex in recovery from major depressive episodes and suggest that state changes in depressive illness are confined largely to inferior limbic and subcortical regions (G. M. Goodwin et al. 1993). D_1 receptor binding seems to be decreased in the frontal cortex of patients with depression as compared with control subjects, independently of their thymic state (Suhara et al. 1992).

Although considerable evidence suggests significant genetic transmission of both bipolar disorders and recurrent depressive illness, linkage analyses of DA receptor genes in affected families have failed to establish a role for D_1, D_2, or D_3 receptor genes (S. Jensen et al. 1992; Mitchell et al. 1992, 1993). Because DA receptor genes, particularly the D_3 type, are expressed largely in the limbic system, which is the brain area responsible for control of emotions, it had been anticipated that such linkages might be found especially in bipolar disorders.

DOPAMINE AND DEPRESSION: ANIMAL STUDIES

Several animal models of depression appear to involve dopaminergic mechanisms, and accumulating evidence suggests that some antidepressant treatments can increase the functional output of the mesolimbic DA system (Kapur and Mann 1992; Willner 1991). For example, exposure of rats to long-term mild stress induces a state of anhedonia characterized primarily by a desensitization of postsynaptic D_2 receptors in the nucleus accumbens (Willner et al. 1992), which is associated with a prolonged and persistent increase in mesolimbic DA release (Imperato et al. 1993). Postsynaptic D_2 agonists such as bromocriptine and quinpirole, given intermittently, can reverse the effects of long-term stress, a reversal that is blocked by D_2 antagonists (Muscat et al. 1992). Tricyclic antidepressants can also reverse the effects of chronic stress when administered long term and, as with DA agonists, their actions are blocked by D_2, but also by D_1, receptor antagonists (Sampson et al. 1991). In this model of depression, the effects of long-term treatment with antidepressants are additive with intermittent treatment with quinpirole (Papp et al. 1992). It has been proposed, on the basis that the effects of antidepressants of diverse pharmacology are reversed by D_2 antagonists in this model, that sensitization of postsynaptic D_2 receptors in the nucleus accumbens is a final common pathway for antidepressant action (Willner et al. 1992).

Similar results have been observed in other animal models involving stress (Willner et al. 1992). Electric footshock–induced aggression in rats was abolished by long-term antidepressant treatment only in animals not pretreated with the DA receptor antagonists haloperidol and sulpiride (Zebrowska-Lupina et al. 1992). Exposure of rats to forced swimming in the behavioral despair test resulted in a long-lasting depletion of mesolimbic DA, which was partially prevented by long-term pretreatment with imipramine (Rossetti et al. 1993). That mesolimbic DA is involved is confirmed by findings that the antidepressant-like effect of clonidine in reversing behavioral despair was antagonized by intraperitoneal or intra-accumbens injections of the D_2 antagonist sulpiride, but not intracerebroventricular injection of 5,7-dihydroxytryptamine, which destroys serotonin neurons (Cervo et al. 1992). Although earlier reports had suggested that D_2 but not D_1 receptor agonists were effective in reducing behavioral despair in both rats (Borsini et al. 1988) and mice (Duterte-Boucher et al. 1988), more recent studies have indicated that selective D_1 agonists are effective and their action is blocked by D_1 antagonists (D'Aquila et al. 1994).

Two mechanisms have been proposed to account for antidepressant-induced increases in the functional activity of the mesolimbic DA system: desensitization of presynaptic inhibitory autoreceptors or sensitization of postsynaptic receptors. Because reductions in mesolimbic DA autoreceptor sensitivity have also been observed in rats exposed to long-term stress without antidepressant treatment (Muscat et al. 1988), it is highly likely that the postsynaptic mechanism is responsible (Willner et al. 1992). Thus, antidepressants of diverse types, when given repeatedly, increased the locomotor hyperactivity induced in rats by the D_2 agonist quinpirole, a postsynaptic effect that was blocked by the D_2 antagonist sulpiride (J. Maj et al. 1989). Hypermotility induced in rats by intra-accumbens injection of high doses of the D_2 agonist apomorphine, an effect mediated by postsynaptic receptors, was consistently facilitated by long-term antidepressant treatments, whereas the hypomotility induced by low-dose apomorphine acting at presynaptic autoreceptors was differentially affected by individual antidepressants (Durlach-Misteli and Van Ree 1992). Long-term administration of desipramine had no effect on interstitial DA levels in the nucleus accumbens of rats and did not attenuate the autoreceptor-mediated decrease in interstitial DA induced by low-dose apomorphine (Nomikos et al. 1991). Changes in behavioral responses to DA agonists such as apomorphine observed after long-term antidepressant treatment were also not associated with presynaptic changes in DA uptake sites (K. Allison et al. 1993).

Single doses of antidepressants of diverse pharmacology (Tanda et al. 1994), as well as single application of electroshock (McGarvey et al. 1993), shared the ability to raise extracellular levels of DA in the rat prefrontal cortex and striatum, respectively. DA release was dependent on the dose of antidepressant and was enhanced by coadministration of an antagonist of N-methyl-D-aspartate (NMDA) receptors (Wedzony and Gofembiowska 1993), or it was dependent on the duration and voltage of electroshock administered. Long-term treatment of rats with imipramine or repeated electroshock produced a decrease in D_1 receptor density in limbic brain areas and a reduced potency of DA to stimulate adenylate cyclase activity as well as increased sensitivity to D_2 agonists (G. M. De Montis et al. 1990), effects that were prevented by blockade of NMDA receptors (D'Aquila et al. 1992;

M. G. De Montis et al. 1993). D_1 receptor density in rat striatum was also reduced by long-term administration of desipramine or monoamine oxidase inhibitors (Paetsch and Greenshaw 1992). Despite the apparent lack of effect of long-term desipramine treatment on either D_1 receptor density or D_2 receptor function in the nucleus accumbens of rats (Reyneke et al. 1989) and of long-term imipramine treatment on striatal D_2 receptor density (Nowak and Zak 1991), a consistent finding has been that repeated administration of antidepressants or electroshock reduces D_2 receptor density and enhances affinity for D_2 agonists in the limbic system (Klimek and Maj 1989; Nowak and Zak 1991). Sensitization of the D_2 receptor has also been observed in hippocampus taken from rats treated with repeated doses of different antidepressants, although this increase in quinpirole-induced neuronal firing in vitro (Bijak 1993) was not matched by an enhancement in vivo of the effects of intrahippocampal injection of quinpirole (Przegalinski and Jurkowska 1990).

DOPAMINERGIC AGENTS AS ANTIDEPRESSANTS

Precursor Therapy

Precursor therapy as a means of increasing dopaminergic transmissions is limited to L-tyrosine and L-dopa. Although under basal conditions the exogenous administration of tyrosine leads to specific enhancement of noradrenergic transmission, it can enhance dopaminergic transmission in conditions of DA deficiency (Kapur and Mann 1992). Only one adequately controlled clinical trial has been reported, in which 65 patients with major depression were randomly selected to treatment for 4 weeks with oral L-tyrosine 100 mg/kg/day, imipramine 2.5 mg/kg/day, or placebo (Gelenberg et al. 1990). Tyrosine increased and imipramine decreased excretion of the main metabolite of NA, but no evidence was found that tyrosine had antidepressant activity in contrast with imipramine.

Evidence on the potential antidepressant efficacy of L-dopa is more voluminous, but also discouraging (Kapur and Mann 1992; Oren et al. 1994). Despite the definite effects of L-dopa on mood, its antidepressant efficacy, given with or without a peripheral decarboxylase inhibitor, is not established even in the subset of patients with psychomotor retardation and low pretreatment CSF HVA who are supposed to be particularly sensitive to its effects. Standard antidepressants or electroconvulsive therapy are the methods of choice in treating depression in patients with Parkinson's disease, in whom L-dopa appears to have limited or no antidepressant efficacy and has been suspected of producing depression (Cummings 1992). Furthermore, prospective and retrospective studies suggest that the frequency of depression reported in patients with Parkinson's disease who are being treated with L-dopa is within the range of that observed in patients with Parkinson's disease before the introduction of L-dopa therapy (Cummings 1992). Nevertheless, selegiline (L-deprenyl), a monoamine oxidase-B (MAO-B) inhibitor thought to slow progression of Parkinson's disease by limiting generation of neurotoxic free radicals specifically in dopaminergic neurons, may have mild antidepressant properties when combined with L-dopa. Thus, the prevalence of depression in patients with Parkinson's disease who are treated with L-dopa and selegiline is lower than that in those receiving the DA precursor alone (Cummings 1992). Even so, the evidence for selegiline itself being an antidepressant is equivocal, with most of the positive controlled trials being conducted at high, and not MAO-B–selective, doses, whereas lower and selective doses have resulted in mostly negative results (A. S. Brown and Gershon 1993; Kapur and Mann 1992; Pinder and Wieringa 1993). Thus, selegiline's antidepressant properties may have less to do with specific effects on brain DA than with a nonselective inhibition of MAO-B.

Dopamine Agonists

DA agonists such as the central nervous system (CNS) stimulants piribedil, bromocriptine, and pergolide have been disappointing as antidepressants, displaying limited efficacy and producing psychiatric side effects (Bouckoms and Mangini 1993; A. S. Brown and Gershon 1993; Kapur and Mann 1992). CNS stimulants such as amphetamine, methylphenidate, and pemoline, which act in part as indirect DA agonists by promoting release of DA, produce transient improvement of mood accompanied by dysphoria. These agents may be useful in augmentation therapy, and recent open-label studies have demonstrated that pemoline improved response to fluoxetine (Metz and Shader 1991), whereas methylphenidate shortened the latency of response to classic tricyclic antidepressants (Gwirtsman et al. 1994). The ability of CNS stimulants to enhance DA release in rat brain is more related to their mobilization of the inert storage pools of DA to releasable sites than to any blockade of D_2 presynaptic autoreceptors (Butcher et al. 1991; Hafizi et al. 1992). Another indirect DA agonist is the phenylpyridazine derivative minaprine, which shares with the CNS stimulants their ability to release DA in limbic areas of rat brain, but after moderate-term and not short-term treatment (Imperato et al. 1994). However, minaprine does not mobilize DA pools, and the precise mechanism of its DA-releasing effect is unknown. Furthermore, minaprine also facilitates serotonergic and cholinergic transmission, and its undoubted antidepressant efficacy in several placebo- and active-controlled clinical trials cannot be attributed solely to effects on DA (Amsterdam et al. 1989b; Del Zompo et al. 1991).

Piribedil is a more direct DA agonist than is minaprine or CNS stimulants, lacking the effects of the former on the serotonergic and of the latter on the noradrenergic system. Like apomorphine, piribedil can stimulate presynaptic DA autoreceptors at low doses, but acts as a postsynaptic DA agonist at higher doses. Unlike apomorphine, which has pronounced emetic properties and has not been studied in depression, piribedil appeared to have modest antidepressant effects in patients with low pretreatment CSF levels of HVA and 5-HIAA and may be especially effective in those with particular poly-somnographic features (Kapur and Mann 1992).

More substantial information is available on the antidepressant potential of the direct DA agonists bromocriptine (Sitland-Marken et al. 1990) and pergolide (Bouckoms and Mangini 1993), which are more familiar in the treatment of Parkinson's disease as adjuvants to L-dopa or for the therapy of hyperprolactinemia. Both are ergolines derived from lysergic acid, but in contrast to bromocriptine, which is a potent D_2 agonist with additional D_1 antagonism, pergolide stimulates D_2, and to a lesser extent, D_1, receptors. Controlled trials with bromocriptine have been reported only in patients who do not respond to tricyclic antidepressant treatment, and these trials demonstrate comparable efficacy to tricyclic antidepressants. Response to bromocriptine resembled that to DA precursors and CNS stimulants in being rapid but associated with a higher incidence of psychomotor activation and precipitation of mania. The more potent D_2 agonist pergolide produced rapid improvement in patients with depression who did not respond to treatment with tricyclic antidepressants and monoamine oxidase inhibitors, but pergolide has not been studied as monotherapy. No information is yet available on the antidepressant potential of those agonists highly selective for the D_2-like receptor family, such as quinpirole or quinelorane, which retain a partial ergoline structure (Foreman et al. 1995), or on selective D_1 receptor agonists such as the isochroman derivative A-68930 (DeNinno et al. 1991), although the D_2 agonists were more potent than bromocriptine in the behavioral despair model of depression in rats.

Paradoxically, perhaps, DA antagonists have antidepressant properties (Robertson and Trimble 1982). Controlled trials have established that some neuroleptics have antidepressant effects characterized by an early onset of action and relative lack of side effects. Furthermore, two drugs that are chemically related to the established neuroleptics loxapine and flupentixol and that retain substantial DA antagonism are marketed in various countries as antidepressants (viz. amoxapine and flupentixol). The best-studied example is the neuroleptic sulpiride, a selective D_2 antagonist, which has been evaluated in double-blind, placebo-controlled trials and in comparative studies against standard antidepressants (Benkert et al. 1992; Kapur and Mann 1992; Robertson and Trimble 1982). The lower doses of sulpiride used in the treatment of depression may reflect antagonism at presynaptic D_2 autoreceptors, thereby promoting DA release and activating dopaminergic transmission in a manner akin to that of antidepressants of the α_2-adrenoceptor antagonist type such as mianserin and mirtazapine for the noradrenergic system (Serra et al. 1990a). Alternatively, or additionally, sulpiride may preferentially block mesocortical DA transmission at the level of the frontal cortex (Kaneno et al. 1991).

Although postsynaptic DA agonists and presynaptic D_2 autoreceptor antagonists share a common property of enhancing DA transmission, D_2 autoreceptor agonists have been developed specifically to block DA transmission as an alternative approach to antipsychotic therapy (Benkert et al. 1992). A variety of such compounds are available (Seyfried and Boettcher 1990), four of which—talipexole, pramipexole, roxindole, and OPC-4392 —have been evaluated as antipsychotics in schizophrenic patients (Benkert et al. 1992). Only roxindole has been tested in depression, and then only in two uncontrolled pilot studies over 4 weeks of treatment (Benkert et al. 1992; M. Kellner et al. 1994). Response rates similar to those of imipramine were observed, with a fast onset of action in some patients. Roxindole's antidepressant action may lie in its ability to selectively stimulate supersensitive postsynaptic D_2 receptors, and thereby enhance DA function, or in its additional properties as an inhibitor of serotonin reuptake and as a 5-HT_{1A} receptor agonist (Benkert et al. 1992; Seyfried et al. 1989).

Dopamine Reuptake Inhibitors

Proven antidepressant activity among agents affecting dopaminergic mechanisms is restricted to those that, among other things, inhibit DA reuptake, including nomifensine, bupropion, and amineptine. The two most potent inhibitors of DA reuptake, diclofensine and GBR 12909, the latter of which might have provided the acid test for the concept in that it is highly selective for DA reuptake (Table 14–2), were insufficiently evaluated in clinical trials before their discontinuation (Pinder and Wieringa 1993). Inhibition of DA reuptake is a minor feature of the neurochemical profile of many more antidepressants (Randrup and Braestrup 1977) and prompted the inclusion of DA, with the original NA and serotonin, as an important biogenic amine in the

TABLE 14–2. Potency and selectivity of some dopamine reuptake inhibitors in vitro

Compound	IC$_{50}$ (nM), rat brain synaptosomes[a]			K$_i$ (nM), cloned human DA transporter[b]
	DA (striatum)	NA (cortex)	5-HT (whole brain)	
Mazindol	29.4	8	NT	11
GBR 12909	1	440	170	17
Diclofensine	16.8	15.7	51	NT
Nomifensine	134	11.2	1,820	17
Bupropion	648	940	>10,000	330

Note. DA = dopamine; 5-HT = serotonin; IC$_{50}$ = concentration that inhibits 50%; NA = noradrenaline; NT = not tested.
[a]Andersen 1989.
[b]Giros and Caron 1993.

etiology of depression (Randrup et al. 1975). Nevertheless, newly developed antidepressant drugs largely lack effects on DA reuptake (Bolden-Watson and Richelson 1993), and the mechanism is no longer a target in the search for novel antidepressants (D. Leysen and Pinder 1994; Pinder and Wieringa 1993).

Nomifensine is a tetrahydroisoquinoline derivative whose undoubted antidepressant efficacy was associated with a specific activating effect on psychomotor retardation (Kapur and Mann 1992). Nomifensine inhibits the reuptake of both DA and NA, the latter more so (Table 14–2), although a PET study in primates and humans using ^{11}C-nomifensine demonstrated its high affinity and selectivity for the DA reuptake sites (Aquilonius et al. 1987). Furthermore, nomifensine shows higher-than-expected affinity for the human DA transporter (Table 14–2). Nomifensine and its major human metabolites also appear to enhance DA release in rat brain, probably via a mobilizing effect on the storage pool of DA and not via blockade of D$_2$ autoreceptors, in which respect it resembles classic CNS stimulants such as methylphenidate (Butcher et al. 1991; Hafizi et al. 1992). Nomifensine is no longer available because of its association with hemolytic anemia, an effect that is probably unrelated to its dopaminergic action. Diclofensine is a close structural relative of nomifensine that showed potent inhibition of DA reuptake with significant effects also on the reuptake of other monoamines such as NA and serotonin (Table 14–2). Its in vivo pharmacological profile was quite different from that of nomifensine, lacking stimulant character, probably because of a lesser propensity than nomifensine for releasing DA and its biotransformation to non-catechol-like metabolites with reduced potency as DA reuptake inhibitors. Antidepressant efficacy had been demonstrated in controlled trials before development was discontinued in 1986 at the time that nomifensine was itself withdrawn from the market (Pinder and Wieringa 1993). The anorectic drug mazindol has a neurochemical profile rather similar to that of nomifensine, being selective for NA over DA reuptake, but with a higher than expected affinity for the human DA transporter (Table 14–2). The potential antidepressant properties of mazindol have not been properly explored in controlled clinical trials, although a close structural relative ciclazindol, which is more selective for NA reuptake, was probably antidepressant (Pinder and Wieringa 1993).

The propiophenone derivative bupropion is structurally related to the sympathomimetic agents diethylpropion and amphetamine, both of which have pronounced dopaminergic effects. However, bupropion is a relatively weak inhibitor of DA and NA reuptake and has low affinity for the human DA transporter (Table 14–2). Nevertheless, long-term, but not short-term, administration of bupropion elevates interstitial concentrations of DA specifically in the nucleus accumbens and not in the striatum, whereas short-term doses raised DA levels in both brain areas of freely moving rats (Nomikos et al. 1992). These changes were associated with an enhancement by bupropion of locomotor stimulation and were not accompanied by alterations in regional NA concentrations. Like other activators of dopaminergic transmission, bupropion acutely increased D_2 receptor binding in vivo in rats, an effect that was time- and dose-dependent, greatest in the striatum, and paralleled by behavioral stimulation (Vassout et al. 1993). Because bupropion was inactive in vitro and ex vivo, the authors have proposed that it modifies D_2 binding through the intervention of a dynamic regulation of the receptors by the neurotransmitter itself, which is consistent with an in vivo enhancing effect on DA levels. Bupropion is now an accepted standard antidepressant with proven efficacy and mild stimulating properties. Its association with seizures has hindered its more widespread introduction and use, and its availability is confined to the United States.

The development of GBR 12909, which had shown preliminary evidence of antidepressant efficacy (Fensbo et al. 1990), was discontinued because of lack of efficacy in a subsequent placebo-controlled trial. GBR 12909 is the most potent and selective inhibitor of DA reuptake to be tested in humans (Søgaard et al. 1990), and its affinity for the human DA transporter is similar to that of nomifensine (Table 14–2). It appears to block DA reuptake by binding to the DA binding site on the transporter protein, thereby blocking the carrier function (Andersen 1989). In contrast to GBR 12909, the efficacy of amineptine is established in large-scale double-blind trials (Kapur and Mann 1992), and, like most dopaminergic agents, it seems to be preferentially effective in patients with psychomotor retardation (Rampello et al. 1991). Amineptine is only about 10 times less effective in inhibiting NA than DA reuptake in vitro and is also markedly less potent at DA sites than is GBR 12909 (Garattini and Mennini 1989). Mesolimbic D_2 autoreceptor sensitivity in mice was reduced by long-term administration of amineptine (Chagraoui et al. 1990), an effect common to many antidepressants (Willner et al. 1992). Amineptine after short-term administration to rats raised extracellular levels of DA in the nucleus accumbens and striatum, similarly to some other inhibitors of DA reuptake such as bupropion, but additionally increased cortical DA and NA levels probably as a result of its inhibition of NA uptake (R. Invernizzi et al. 1992b). This suggests that amineptine may not be as selective in vivo as in vitro and begs the question whether a selective increase of mesolimbic DA via DA reuptake is sufficient to cause antidepressant effects. Furthermore, the amineptine analogue tianeptine, also an effective antidepressant but lacking inhibitory effects on catecholamine reuptake and indeed specifically increasing uptake of serotonin, increases both cortical (Louilot et al. 1990) and nucleus accumbens levels of DA (R. Invernizzi et al. 1992a) in rats by a serotonin-independent mechanism. Proper evaluation of a highly selective agent such as GBR 12909 is needed to answer such doubts. Amineptine has recently been withdrawn from some markets because of potential for abuse.

FUTURE TRENDS

The DA transporter is known to be a glycoprotein of 620 amino acids having 12 hydrophobic membrane-spanning regions with the amino-terminal and the carboxyl-terminal ends of the polypeptide located intracellularly (Giros and Caron 1993; Kuhar 1994). Although there is evidence for only a single gene for the DA transporter, it is clear that heterogeneity exists, resulting principally from differential glycosylation. Thus, the molecular weight of the DA transporter increases significantly with human age, whereas that in the nucleus accumbens differs from the striatal transporter. If such differences represent real physiologically distinct subtypes of transporter, it may well be possible to design more regioselective inhibitors of DA reuptake than have presently been evaluated in treating depression. Certainly the construction of chimeric DA-NA transporters has demonstrated that the binding domains for tricyclic antidepressants and neurotransmitter substrates are discretely located in different regions (Giros et al. 1994). At the very least, the use of the cloned human transporters for different monoamines will allow the issue to be readdressed of which neurotransmitter system is actually activated when antidepressant drugs of dopaminergic action are used.

The existing DA receptors have been fully characterized as 7-trans-membranal G protein–coupled receptors in their five subtypes and multiple variants (Table 14–1). The availability of cloned human receptors will permit the discovery of more selective drugs for the purposes already partially achieved in depression by the relatively nonselective agonists and antagonists described earlier. New D_2 postsynaptic agonists and autoreceptor-selective D_2 antagonists may offer the best prospects. It is entirely likely that further subtypes and variants will be added to the present list (P. Seeman and Van Tol 1994; Sibley and Monsma 1992).

The interaction between brain DA and other neurotransmitters may also become important factors in new antidepressant development. 5-HT_{1A} receptor agonists and 5-HT_{2A} receptor antagonists are able to enhance the functioning of mesencephalic and mesocortical DA systems in rat brain by, respectively, increasing the electrical activity of DA neurons and elevating DA efflux (Arborelius et al. 1993; C. J. Schmidt and Fadayel 1995). 5-HT_{1A} agonists are anxiolytic and are being touted as putative antidepressant agents (D. Leysen and Pinder 1994; Pinder and Wieringa 1993), whereas 5-HT_{2A} antagonists may be appropriate for treating the negative symptoms of schizophrenia including lack of affect and anhedonia. Although NMDA antagonists prevent imipramine-induced supersensitivity to the D_2 agonist quinpirole (D'Aquila et al. 1992; M. G. De Montis et al. 1993), coadministration of antidepressants and NMDA antagonists enhances extracellular concentrations of DA in rat prefrontal cortex (Wedzony and Gofembiowska 1993) and potentiates antidepressant-like effects in animal models of depression (J. Maj et al. 1992). Finally, long-term administration of the angiotensin II-1 receptor antagonist losartan increased dopaminergic transmission in rat striatum via a compensatory response resulting from its antagonism at striatal angiotensin II-1 receptors (Dwoskin et al. 1992). Undoubtedly more links remain to be identified between dopaminergic and other systems in the brain than these examples, but these examples demonstrate that DA function can be enhanced by means other than those purely dopaminergic in nature.

CONCLUSION

Substantial evidence suggests a deficiency of DA in depressive disorders and the involvement of mesolimbic dopaminergic mechanisms in antidepressant action. The lack of antidepressants of sufficiently selective action on DA receptors or reuptake has limited our ability to confirm unequivocally the role of DA. New techniques for studying DA receptors in the human brain in vivo, as well as the full molecular characterization of DA receptors and the DA transporter, will provide the means for greater insight. It is entirely possible, although not currently fashionable, that new antidepressant treatments could be developed on the basis of this new knowledge. Given the beneficial effects of dopaminergic antidepressants on psychomotor retardation and the general acceptance in the past of nomifensine as a particularly advantageous drug for the treatment of selected patient groups, including the elderly, such antidepressants would be welcomed.

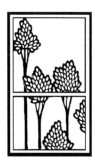

CHAPTER 15

Noradrenergic and Other New Antidepressants

William Z. Potter, M.D., Ph.D., and
Mark E. Schmidt, M.D.

The catecholamine and indolamine hypotheses of mood disorders have proven to be enduring attempts at defining the pathophysiology of mood disorders (Bunney and Davis 1965; Schildkraut 1965). Originally the hypotheses evolved from astute clinical observations of precipitation of mania by the monoamine oxidase–inhibiting antitubercular drug iproniazid and of depression by the storage vesicle–depleting drug reserpine. For 30 years, these hypotheses have served as heuristic organizing principles for many clinicians and researchers confronted with the growing maze of knowledge of human neurochemistry. Although there remains intuitive appeal in the original parallel between depletion or excess of a neurotransmitter and the psychic "depletion" of depression or frantic "excess" of mania, there are few data to directly support the catecholamine hypotheses as accurate models of mood disorders and their treatment and much data to argue against them. Nonetheless, compounds targeted to increasing availability or function of the amine neurotransmitters norepinephrine and serotonin, those most commonly associated with the hypotheses, are viewed as likely antidepressants. Two other chapters focus in detail on drugs targeted to serotonin and on those targeted to dopamine. Here, we focus on norepinephrine and start with a brief review of efforts to understand its function in depression so as to put the biochemical effects of putatively noradrenergic antidepressants into perspective.

As the principal neurotransmitter for the sympathetic nervous system, norepinephrine and its major metabolites are present in blood and urine at concentrations that can be reliably measured. Under proper experimental conditions, the relative amounts and changes in the concentrations of the neurotransmitter and its metabolites can be related to the activity of the sympathetic nervous system. The brain noradrenergic system, however, is distinct in distribution and function from the peripheral sympathetic nervous system. The activity of the noradrenergic system in the brain cannot readily be deduced from the measured concentrations of norepinephrine and its metabolites in any of the peripheral fluids, including cerebrospinal fluid (CSF). Indeed, most of the variability of 3-methoxy-4-hydroxyphenylglycol (MHPG) in CSF (MHPG being the principal metabolite of norepinephrine) can be accounted for by the concentration in blood resulting from the ready diffusion of MHPG from plasma into CSF. Nonetheless, there are similarities between the central and peripheral noradrenergic system in the regulation of norepinephrine synthesis, release, and turnover. As a consequence, drug effects on the peripheral system (e.g., inhibition of monoamine oxidase) can be used as reliable "surrogate" indicators of effects on brain norepinephrine, especially when considered in conjunction with preclinical data. Moreover, with adequate controls, the relationship between the activity of the two systems is strong enough that, using plasma and urine measures, estimates of norepinephrine turnover can cautiously be used as an index of some aspects of central norepinephrine activity. These data can then be used in studies of treatment effect and/or pathophysiology of depression.

What then, is the current evidence to support a role of norepinephrine in depression, such that manipulation of noradrenergic activity bears particular relevance to the successful treatment of mood disorders? Interpretation of studies depends on the continually evolving conceptualizations of the roles of brain noradrenergic systems. A potentially useful way of thinking about the function of the norepinephrine in the brain can be derived from examining the neuroanatomy of the noradrenergic system. A summary of findings (primarily from rodents and primates) is as follows.

Norepinephrine is widely distributed throughout brain in a nonuniform pattern, discrete from that of other amine systems such as dopamine and serotonin, although overlapping in several areas. The majority of noradrenergic axons and nerve endings found in the brain originate from the locus coeruleus, a small, well-delineated cluster of cell bodies located in the pontine brain stem, just below the floor of the fourth ventricle. Given the wide distribution of norepinephrine in the brain (widely documented in the psychiatric literature), remarkably few neurons, estimated as 12,000 neurons on each side of the human brain, are in this nucleus. These neurons then project along five distinct tracts, of which three are directed to either the midbrain (particularly hypothalamus), the limbic system (notably the hippocampus), or the cerebral cortex (J. R. Cooper et al. 1991).

The noradrenergic neurons innervating the primate cerebral cortex project to the frontal cortex and then run in a parallel fashion to the occipital cortex. As they course through deep cortical layers, frequent branching occurs, directed out toward the cortical surface. These branches, in turn, form characteristic T-shaped branches that parallel the superficial (molecular) lamina of the cortex. Multiple varicosities appear along these branches, forming presynaptic neurotransmitter release sites. The density of varicosities on the terminal branches in the molecular layer is high, estimated at $300,000/mm^3$ of cortex. Only a small number of these release sites form synapses with other neurons. Rather than releasing norepinephrine to a specific postsynaptic neuron, they appear instead to allow for release of neurotransmitter on any population of nearby neurons.

These characteristics of diffuse distribution throughout the brain, and wide dissemination of neurotransmitter initiated from a single brain-stem nucleus, readily suggest the hypothesized function of the noradrenergic system as modulating neuronal activity in many areas of the brain, following stimuli that activate or inhibit the locus coeruleus. The noradrenergic system then has the potential of generally influencing multiple central nervous system areas that by themselves are involved in various discrete functions that use other neurotransmitters in their primary functions. One hypothesis is that norepinephrine can increase the "signal-to-noise" ratio of a specific incoming stimulus (e.g., pain, visual perception, noise) by suppressing random tonic activity or "noise" (Foote et al. 1975). Thus, noradrenergic activation, although widely present, is functionally relevant only in terms of some more specifically activated pathway.

Additionally, the noradrenergic system can achieve some regional specificity in its effects by regional differences in the density of noradrenergic fibers. For example, in many species studied to date, the primary somatosensory cortex has a high density of noradrenergic fibers relative to other cortical areas. Moreover, the response in the noradrenergic projection fields will be influenced by the highly regional distribution of noradrenergic receptor subtypes in the brain. To illustrate the importance of this fact, it is through this system that the same neurotransmitter can produce both vasoconstriction (through α_1 and α_2 receptors on peripheral vessels) and vasodilation (through β receptors on coronary vessels).

Each of the principal adrenergic receptors, α_1, α_2, β_1, and β_2, has been identified and mapped in the human brain using autoradiography of labeled receptor-specific ligands in postmortem brain slices, and each of these receptor types has a unique, highly regional distribution (De Vos et al. 1992; Gross et al. 1989; Pascual et al. 1992; Reznikoff et al. 1986). This raises the possibility of targeting particular receptor populations to enhance therapeutic effects or reduce side effects of antidepressants. Such a strategy is explicitly being pursued in the development of new medications for the negative symptoms of schizophrenia (Litman et al. 1993) as well as in the attempt to use α_2 antagonism as a primary and/or adjunctive principle in antidepressant development (see below); β receptors have particular relevance to any discussion of antidepressants. In preclinical models, decreased number and activity or "downregulation" of receptors occur following long-term exposure to many compounds with proven antidepressant effects. Consequently, β-receptor downregulation was regarded for many years as a sine qua non phenomenon in screening for potential new antidepressants. It has subsequently been demonstrated that some antidepressants do not result in β-receptor downregulation, including citalopram, a selective serotonin reuptake inhibitor (SSRI), and mianserin, currently classified as a mixed α_2-adrenergic and serotonergic 5-HT$_2$ antagonist (Nalepa and Vetulani 1993, 1994).

It is a considerable conceptual leap to go from the modulation of noradrenergic receptors or even electrophysiological measures of a signal-to-noise ratio in animals to the pathophysiology of mood disorders and their treatment in humans. One may draw a rough parallel between the actions and the neuroanatomical distribution of the noradrenergic system and the symptoms of depression. Symptoms potentially generated in brain regions with known noradrenergic input include sleep and appetite patterns mediated in the midbrain, mood symptoms mediated by the limbic system, and the cognitive response to environmental stimuli by the neocortex. Until more can be learned about the function of norepinephrine in humans, the connection between the noradrenergic system and mood relies on the pharmacological bridge, created by comparing the effect of different drugs on mood with what we know of their effects on aspects of noradrenergic activity.

ANTIDEPRESSANTS WITH EFFECTS ON THE NORADRENERGIC SYSTEM

Nearly all antidepressants, including many not thought of as noradrenergic compounds, have downstream, if not primary, short-term effects on the noradrenergic system in humans. Following long-term treatment with zimeldine, an SSRI, significant reductions were seen in CSF MHPG (W. Z. Potter et al. 1985). Treatment with the aminoketone bupropion, commonly thought of as a dopaminergic compound, was found to result in a reduction in "whole body" turnover of norepinephrine (Golden 1988). The magnitude of change in norepinephrine parameters following either drug was not related to clinical outcome, suggesting that the effect on norepinephrine was related to the drug treatment and was not a consequence of a change in clinical state. The simple cation lithium has been found to increase resting plasma norepinephrine concentrations as well as adenylate cyclase activity in lymphocytes in psychiatrically healthy volunteers (Manji et al. 1991a; Risby et al. 1991). Conversely, in one of the same long-term treatment studies cited above, desmethylimipramine, the most selective norepinephrine reuptake inhibitor among the tricyclics, had as profound an effect on the serotonin metabolite 5-hydroxyindoleacetic acid (5-HIAA) as did zimeldine and other more recent SSRIs. Pharmacologically, the apparent lack of specificity of these antidepressant treatments appears to reflect actions that go beyond those identified by in vitro affinities for receptors or uptake sites, including possible long-term adaptive changes to interactions between, for instance, norepinephrine and serotonin.

Physiologically, there are mechanisms, examples of which are described below, for reciprocal regulation between the monoamine systems in the central nervous system at a receptor level. Additionally, when postsynaptic receptors for two or more of the monoamine systems are present on a neuron, these systems can have integrated effects by postreceptor mechanisms, through "cross-talk" between the second-messenger pathways associated with the different receptors. Therefore, discussion of noradrenergic mechanisms has limitations when studying living systems, and the definition of noradrenergic antidepressants could be quite broad. For the sake of clarity, the antidepressants that are discussed include only those with potent effects on the synaptic elements of noradrenergic neurons in vitro or demonstrable short-term effects on norepinephrine in vivo in animals.

One can simply classify a drug as noradrenergic on the basis of interaction with the transporter or specific receptor subtypes. But this does not really address the functional consequences, such as the extent to which, for instance, a drug affects the intrasynaptic concentration of norepinephrine. The latter requires some knowledge of the pathway followed by norepinephrine from synthesis, storage, release, and clearance. This pathway is depicted in Figure 15–1.

As can be seen in the figure, a number of sites are not only for pharmaco-

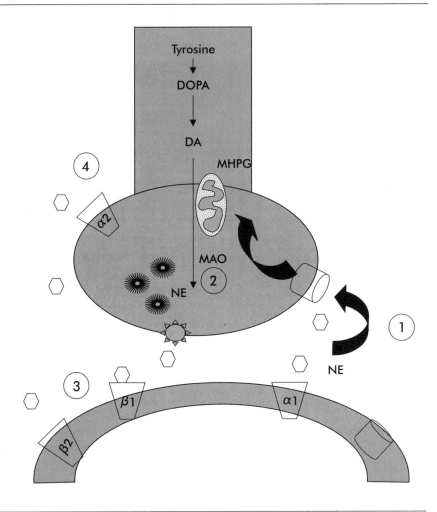

FIGURE 15–1.   Pathway followed by norepinephrine (NE) from synthesis, storage, release, and clearance: 1) inhibition of norepinephrine reuptake; 2) inhibition of deamination by monoamine oxidase (MAO); 3) direct agonism/antagonism of postsynaptic receptors; 4) antagonism of autoinhibitory presynaptic receptors. DA = dopamine; DOPA = dihydroxyphenylalanine; MHPG = 3-methoxy-4-hydroxyphenylglycol.

logical intervention but also for autoregulating processes responding to norepinephrine. The only specifically noradrenergic site that is generally implicated in the action of any class of marketed antidepressants is the presynaptic norepinephrine transporter. This is hypothesized to be the initial site of action of the so-called norepinephrine uptake inhibitors (Table 15–1A).

TABLE 15–1A. Drugs marketed in the United States as tricyclic antidepressants (and one tetracyclic, maprotiline) that inhibit norepinephrine (NE) uptake through either parent drug or a major metabolite

Mixed NE/serotonin uptake inhibitors
  Imipramine
  Amitriptyline
  Clomipramine
  Doxepin
Preferential NE uptake inhibitors
  Desipramine
  Nortriptyline
  Protriptyline
  Maprotiline
Tricyclics with additional actions
  Trimipramine
  Amoxapine

Although many of the drugs in Table 15–1A that inhibit norepinephrine uptake also inhibit that of serotonin, we include these as noradrenergic compounds because all available evidence indicates that they do have substantial effects on at least some components of noradrenergic function in humans. The ways in which the short- and long-term effects of these compounds, all of which except maprotiline are classified as tricyclic antidepressants (TCAs), have been studied at the preclinical and clinical levels have recently been reviewed elsewhere (W. Z. Potter et al. 1990, 1995). Our interpretation is that the downregulation of β- and α_2-adrenergic receptors observed in various regions of rat brain, the decreased "turnover" (total synthesis and metabolism of norepinephrine) measurable in rats and humans, and the increased extracellular norepinephrine detectable in rat brain via microdialysis and in human CSF and plasma are consistent with the supposition that norepinephrine uptake inhibitors produce sustained increases of intrasynaptic norepinephrine. By rather different mechanisms, that is, inhibition of intraneuronal degradation so that more norepinephrine is stored and released per vesicle, monoamine oxidase inhibitors (MAOIs) are also thought to increase intrasynaptic norepinephrine (as well as serotonin and dopamine).

Thus, it can be argued that the two oldest classes of antidepressants, TCAs and MAOIs, can include sustained increases of intrasynaptic norepinephrine among their actions. In recent years, drugs that affect norepinephrine through the same mechanisms, but with a much more limited range of effects on sites associated with side effects, have become available either on the market or for clinical trials. These drugs are shown in Table 15–1B and include venlafaxine and duloxetine, mixed norepinephrine/serotonin uptake inhibitors, and moclobemide, a reversible inhibitor of MAO type A. Recently, a far more selective series of compounds has emerged from the same molecular platform that gave rise to fluoxetine. These include nisoxetine (D. T. Wong and Bymaster 1976), tomoxetine (Fuller and Hemrick-Luecke 1983), and reboxetine, which has been recently marketed as an antidepressant (Dostert et al. 1997; Melloni et al. 1984). Unlike the tricyclics, reboxetine has no significant affinity for muscarinic, cholinergic, or α-adrenergic receptors (Riva et al. 1989), so that side effects attributable to such pharmacology should be substantially reduced.

Two major classes of action on norepinephrine truly distinct from those produced by the classic TCAs and MAOIs are provided by drugs that selectively inhibit α_2 (and certain subtypes of serotonin) receptors and drugs that are agonists at β receptors (Table 15–2). There is also at least one putatively selective indirect agonist, modafinil, but the basis for its apparent action via α_1 receptors is unknown. Finally, long-term, but not short-term, studies implicate changes of norepinephrine function in the mode of action of bupropion, although the short-term action that leads to the longer term changes remains to be elucidated (Golden et al. 1988).

The clinical efficacy of classic TCAs and MAOIs in major affective disorder is not in question. Controlled studies also support the efficacy of bupropion, although dose-response relationships have not been established.

TABLE 15–1B. Compounds marketed since 1990 or under development as selective or combination norepinephrine/serotonin uptake inhibitors or selective monoamine oxidase inhibitors (MAOIs)

Selective norepinephrine uptake inhibitors
  Reboxetine
  Tomoxetine
Mixed norepinephrine/serotonin uptake inhibitors
  Duloxetine
  Venlafaxine
Selective reversible MAOI type A
  Moclobemide

TABLE 15–2. Drugs acting on the noradrenergic system not involving an action at uptake sites or on monoamine oxidase

Adrenergic compounds			
Agonists		Antagonists	Indirect noradrenergic
β_1/β_2	α_1	α_2	(unknown mechanism)
Albuterol	Adrafanil	Fluparoxan	Bupropion
Salbutamol	Modafinil	Idazoxan	
Clenbuterol		?Mirtazapine (also 5-HT$_2$)	
Fenoterol		Yohimbine	
		Clozapine	

Note. 5-HT$_2$ = serotonin type 2 receptor.

This lack of information may well relate to bupropion's complex metabolism, whereby biologically active metabolites predominate several-fold over the parent compound; these metabolites may ultimately prove to be the basis for therapeutic effects (Golden et al. 1988). Furthermore, because the full spectrum of action of the metabolites has not been explored, it is difficult to confidently characterize the "primary" biochemical action of bupropion as noradrenergic. One must therefore be cautious in interpreting any distinct aspects of bupropion's clinical actions as reflecting some noradrenergic mechanisms. And to our knowledge, bupropion is unique in that no other compound available for use in humans has a similar overall profile of preclinical and clinical biochemical effects.

Interestingly, other drugs, such as agonists (Table 15–2), that have a much more clearly demonstrable noradrenergic action show, at best, transient therapeutic effects. We were not able to find any recent controlled or open clinical trials using more contemporary β agonists (albuterol [salbutamol], clenbuterol, fenoterol) in depression. The conclusions of an earlier review of studies from the 1980s (W. Z. Potter et al. 1990) would therefore seem to stand, that is, that available agonists are unlikely to prove to be antidepressants. Moreover, given the profile of major peripheral effects associated with the theoretically more relevant α_1 agonists, it is unlikely that drugs of this class will be developed as psychopharmacological agents.

As for β antagonists, it is clear that they are sometimes useful in psychopharmacological practice, but not as antidepressants. Fears that β antagonists would be depressogenic have not been realized, although some evidence did suggest that propranolol could precipitate depression in susceptible individuals. The main role of β antagonists in practice is for so-called performance anxiety (Brantigan et al. 1982; Siitonen et al, 1977) and as an adjunct to lithium or valproic acid to reduce tremor. Nonselective blockers, such as propranolol, may be the most effective. Nonetheless, low doses of the β_2 selective antagonists (atenolol or metoprolol) can be tried for tremor and are clearly effective for protecting against TCA-induced tachycardia, especially that associated with use of the secondary amines, nortriptyline and desipramine.

Other specific noradrenergic sites at which drugs can act (Figure 15–1) are provided by α_1 and α_2 adrenoreceptors. Direct α_1 agonists (e.g., phenylephrine) are vasoconstrictors and have no known role in psychopharmacology. An antagonist of α_1 (and α_2) adrenoreceptors, phentolamine, used to be the first-line treatment for "cheese" or drug-related hypertensive reactions in individuals on MAOIs; now the calcium channel antagonists of the nifedipine type, which rapidly reduce peripheral resistance, are being recommended by some (Clary and Schweizer 1987; Gifford 1991). In fact, α_1 antagonism is usually viewed as producing undesirable side effects if included in the action of psychopharmacological agents and is implicated in the orthostatic hypotensive effects, especially of tertiary amine TCAs. In contrast, a long-standing theoretical argument supports α_2 adrenoreceptor antagonism as a basis for antidepressant action or potentiating the rate of onset of antidepressant effects (see below). This class of compounds is discussed in greater detail.

α_2 Antagonists

Currently recognized as a subfamily of at least three different molecular subtypes in humans (Bylund 1992), the α_2 adrenoreceptors most generally considered to be of interest to psychopharmacology are those located on presynaptic nerve endings, either of noradrenergic neurons (autoreceptors) or serotonin neurons (heteroreceptors) (S. Z. Langer 1974; Raiteri et al. 1990). In the former instance, the autoreceptors provide feedback inhibition of norepinephrine release. Accordingly, short-term treatment with α_2 antagonists can enhance release of norepinephrine in both peripheral (Grossman et al. 1991; van Veldhuizen et al. 1993) and central compartments, actions that can be linked to at least transient augmentation of norepinephrine-mediated processes.

In the brain, however, many and possibly most α_2 receptors are located postsynaptically or extrasynaptically to noradrenergic neurons. To date, α_2 receptors have been associated with not only serotonergic nerve endings, as noted above, but also cholinergic, dopaminergic, and GABA-ergic neurons, where, when activated, they can inhibit release of the neurotransmitter (Beani et al. 1986; V. A. Russell et al. 1993). Because α_2 antagonists may thereby alter the release of a number of neurotransmitters besides norepinephrine, caution is necessary in interpreting their effects as being mediated primarily through the noradrenergic system. Nonetheless, whatever the ultimate cascade of biochemical events, the initial effect of these agents remains α_2 antagonism.

Several available medications show sufficient α_2 antagonism, at least in preclinical systems, to suggest that this action might be relevant to their effects in humans. These include mianserin, mirtazapine, and, most obviously, yohimbine, for which there is clinical pharmacological evidence of α_2 antagonism (Table 15–2). Clozapine has also been found to antagonize α_2 receptors (Richelson and Nelson 1984). Following long-term treatment with clozapine, both norepinephrine and its metabolites are increased, consistent with producing central and/or peripheral α_2 blockade (Pickar et al. 1992). These findings are particularly notable in that other neuroleptics studied, to date, *reduce* indices of norepinephrine output and in that clozapine offers advantages for the negative (depressed?) symptoms of schizophrenia and perhaps for mixed states (combined symptoms of depression and mania) in bipolar disorder (McElroy et al. 1991a; Suppes et al. 1992).

Yohimbine is an alkaloid derived from plants of the *Rauwolfia* genus, which is available in health food stores and marketed as a legitimate pharmaceutical for certain forms of impotency. At least one case report suggests that yohimbine can augment the antidepressant response to bupropion (Pollack and Hammerness 1993) and be used as an adjunct to tricyclics to treat orthostatic hypotension symptoms and/or treat anorgasmia/impotency associated with SSRI use (S. J. Jacobson 1992). Of particular interest would be a test of the theoretical formulation that the acceleration and increase of β-receptor downregulation produced in rodent models by combining yohimbine and norepinephrine uptake inhibitors will translate into increased speed or degree of response with the combination in humans. Because the rate of β-receptor downregulation measured in animal models was hypothesized to be related to the time of onset of antidepressant effects in humans (Sulser et al. 1978), it made sense to look for agents that would produce more rapid downregulation. And, as predicted from the current model of a noradrenergic synapse, when both α_2 adrenoceptors and norepinephrine uptake sites are inhibited (by combining tricyclics and α_2 antagonists), receptor downregulation is both more rapid and more extensive (Crews et al. 1981; R. W. Johnson et al. 1980).

To date, however, no direct test of this possibility in humans has been conducted, presumably because of fears that the combination of acute α_2 adrenoceptor and norepinephrine uptake blockage might produce unacceptable increases in blood pressure. Two studies do test the *addition* of yohimbine to treatment of patients who had not responded to a full trial of a tricyclic—in both instances, however, without therapeutic success (Charney et al. 1986; Schmauss et al. 1988). The failure of yohimbine addition to convert tricyclic nonresponders to responders does not, of course, address the question of whether yohimbine (or a more selective α_2 antagonist) added to a tricyclic at the outset would significantly accelerate or improve response in patients who typically show response at 4–6 weeks. An adequate test may have to wait for the availability of more selective α_2 antagonists than yohimbine or even those described in what follows.

Mianserin and Mirtazapine

As has been reviewed in detail elsewhere (Vinar et al. 1991), mianserin, which in some systems can be shown to antagonize both α_2 adrenoceptors and 5-HT$_2$ serotonergic receptors, enjoys a wide market outside of the United States and shows similar antidepressant efficacy to other nontricyclic antidepressants developed in the last two decades. It is not completely clear why no attempt was made to introduce it in this country, although reports of agranulocytosis and aplastic anemia (Coulter and Edwards 1990; Mashford 1984) probably discouraged potential sponsors. Controversy remains concerning the extent to which therapeutic doses of mianserin carry a significant risk of blood dyscrasias (reviewed in Rudorfer et al. 1994). The European manufacturer (Organon, Oss, The Netherlands) of this compound has developed an analogue, mirtazapine, which is reported to show equivalent efficacy to tricyclics and superiority over placebo (Claghorn and Lesem 1995; Zivkov and De Jongh 1995). Preclinically, mirtazapine has been shown to inhibit α_2 adrenoceptors as well as 5-HT$_2$ and 5-HT$_3$ receptors, a combination of effects argued to facilitate postsynaptic 5-HT$_{1A}$ throughput (de Boer and Ruigt 1995). The model on which this interpretation is based depends on arguments about the net changes produced by direct and indirect effects of α_2 antagonism at serotonin nerve endings and cell bodies coupled with antagonism of 5-HT$_2$ and 5-HT$_3$ receptors.

We are not aware, however, of any studies, to date, that show that either mianserin or mirtazapine produces sustained α_2 adrenoceptor or 5-HT$_2$ receptor blockade in humans. Indeed, in animals, mianserin has been reported *not* to block α_2 adrenoceptors following long-term administration (Sugrue 1980). Elsewhere it has been argued that the 5-HT$_2$ antagonism might be important in the action of mianserin because the more selective α_2 antagonists tested, to date, do not, by themselves, appear to be clearly effective antidepressants in unipolar depression (D. L. Murphy et al. 1995) (also see below). It should also be noted that, at least in vitro, mianserin can inhibit norepinephrine uptake (de Boer et al. 1988; Goodlet et al. 1977), although preclinical ex vivo studies have been interpreted to rule this out as a relevant action (Pinder and Fink 1982). There are, however, no biochemical studies in humans that adequately test whether or not norepinephrine uptake inhibition occurs at therapeutic doses. The analogue, mirtazapine, does not have norepinephrine uptake blocking activity, even in vitro (de Boer et al. 1988).

Idazoxan

Idazoxan is an imidazoline compound developed to be a potent and highly selective α_2-adrenoceptor antagonist with little interaction at α_1 and β adrenoceptor or other major neurotransmitter receptors. However, like many of the imidazolines that show high affinity for adrenoceptors, idazoxan has equal or higher affinities for the recently identified imidazoline receptors. Imidazoline receptors have been shown to be present in many tissues, including human brain (De Vos et al. 1994), and have been hypothesized to be involved with the regulation of blood pressure and possibly norepinephrine release (Ernsberger et al. 1990).

The oral form of idazoxan is readily absorbed and has a mean bioavailability of only 34% in humans, indicative of a high first-pass metabolism associated with a plasma half-life of only 5.6 hours. The drug lacks any affinity for muscarinic or histaminergic receptors and does not have any cholinergic or sedative side effects. Side effects that have been reported are consistent with idazoxan-enhancing sympathoneural activity, namely, exertional tachycardia.

Preclinical studies provide strong biochemical and functional evidence that short-term idazoxan administration selectively antagonizes α_2 adrenoceptors. Following long-term administration using implanted minipumps, α_2 antagonism persists. In humans, short-term effects such as increased plasma norepinephrine (and blood pressure) are consistent with α_2 antagonism (Elliott et al. 1984), whereas effects following long-term oral administration are more equivocal (no sustained increase of plasma norepinephrine) (Glue et al. 1991). Whether these discrepancies reflect compensatory mechanisms or too low doses of idazoxan given its short half-life is unknown.

Studies in outpatients with depression who are administered idazoxan are therefore difficult to interpret as adequate tests of the ability of sustained α_2 antagonism to produce antidepressant effects. Although initial open trials were suggestive of antidepressant efficacy, unpublished controlled trials undertaken by the manufacturer must be assumed to have been negative. We found no evidence of efficacy (at doses of 120 mg) in a small group of inpatients with unipolar depression who were referred for failure to respond to standard agents, but, surprisingly, we did observe responses in patients with bipolar depression (most of whom were receiving maintenance lithium) (Osman et al. 1989). Interestingly, another compound developed as an α_2 antagonist, fluparoxan (Table 15–2), is also said to have failed to show sufficiently robust effects in outpatients with depression to motivate further development (Corn 1994). We are aware of no data to demonstrate that sustained α_2 antagonism was produced by the doses of fluparoxan used in these patients.

Perhaps the clearest evidence that long-term administration of an α_2 antagonist produces sustained beneficial clinical changes emerged from a study in which idazoxan was added to fluphenazine in patients with schizophrenia. Both positive and negative symptoms improved to the same degree seen with clozapine (Litman et al. 1996). This is of particular interest because in humans, as noted above, clozapine has been shown to produce long-term biochemical changes consistent with preclinical demonstrations that it can block α_2-adrenergic as well as dopaminergic, serotonergic, and cholinergic receptors. As in the case of idazoxan showing positive effects in bipolar depression, combination treatment was involved, or in the case of clozapine, de facto combination therapy, because this compound has interactions with many neurotransmitter receptors. It may be that, by itself, even sustained α_2 antagonism is sufficiently compensated for so that no functional changes are produced. Available cardiovascular data, however, do suggest that some degree of the blood pressure elevation seen following short-term administration of α_2 antagonism persists with long-term treatment.

Finally, while on the subject of possible clinical effects of α_2 antagonism, it should be noted that many of the 5-HT$_{1A}$ agonists (e.g., buspirone, gepirone, and ipsapirone) that were developed or tested for antianxiety and antidepressant effects are extensively metabolized to 1-(2-pyrimidyl)-piperazine, itself an active α_2-adrenoceptor antagonist (G. Bianchi et al. 1988). Whether this is relevant in vivo in humans remains to be seen.

POSSIBLE CLINICAL DISTINCTIONS OF MORE NORADRENERGIC ANTIDEPRESSANTS

In the preceding discussion, the focus is mainly on whether an initial action at some noradrenergic site is likely to be involved in the therapeutic action of various antidepressants. Here, we directly address the question of whether specifically noradrenergic action appears related to special clinical features. Three questions of major clinical importance are suggested by the literature. First, does the combination of norepinephrine- *and* serotonin-uptake inhibition yield a broader spectrum antidepressant with overall greater efficacy in patients with more serious depression? Second, can the addition of an α_2-adrenoceptor antagonist accelerate response to classic tricyclics (and possibly other antidepressants)? Third, are certain subclasses of noradrenergic antidepressants better or uniquely useful for bipolar as opposed to unipolar depression?

Does the combination of norepinephrine- and serotonin-uptake inhibition yield a broader spectrum antidepressant with overall greater efficacy in patients with more serious depression? In terms of presumed core biochemical effects, TCAs are best distinguished from SSRIs by their universal ability to potently inhibit norepinephrine uptake and more variably inhibit serotonin uptake. Thus, TCAs are more "broad spectrum" in their effects on neurotransmitter systems than are SSRIs and hence may ultimately prove to have a different spectrum of clinical effects. In keeping with this suggestion, a series of Danish studies concluded that SSRIs may not be as effective in inpatients with severe depression as is clomipramine, although the latter clearly has more severe side effects (Danish University Antidepressant Group 1986, 1990). The apparent ability of a combination of a non-MAOI with fluoxetine to convert nonresponders or partial responders to a single treatment to full responders indirectly supports this notion (Weilburg et al. 1989). It has also been reported that venlafaxine is more effective than is fluoxetine or placebo for hospitalized patients with depression (Clerc et al. 1994).

Can the addition of an α_2-adrenoceptor antagonist accelerate response to classic tricyclics (and possibly other antidepressants)? An accelerated antidepressant response has been reported following initiating treatment with a combination of desipramine and fluoxetine (J. C. Nelson et al. 1991) in keeping with the prediction from preclinical studies showing that the combination produced more rapid downregulation of β receptors than did desipramine alone (B. M. Baron et al. 1988). Moreover, the mixed norepinephrine/serotonin uptake inhibitor, venlafaxine, has been reported at various meetings to produce more rapid response when high doses (250 mg or more) are attained early in treatment (Rudolph et al. 1991).

As already noted, initiating treatment with the combination of an α_2 antagonist with a norepinephrine uptake inhibitor (or serotonin uptake inhibitor for that matter) is yet to be tested. Although there are limitations to all of the available α_2 antagonists as definitive "concept testing" compounds, such a trial, say with idazoxan and imipramine, coupled with appropriate measures of norepinephrine and its metabolites to indicate that α_2 antagonism was achieved, would be of great interest.

Are certain subclasses of noradrenergic antidepressants better or uniquely useful for bipolar as opposed to unipolar depression? As suggested by the success of adding the α_2 antagonist idazoxan to fluphenazine in a subgroup of patients with schizophrenia (Litman et al. 1996), noradrenergic effects may prove particularly useful for selected patients. Interesting data in this regard continue to emerge from our earlier observation of antidepressant responses to idazoxan in two previously treated patients with bipolar disorder who were nonresponsive to treatment (Osman et al. 1989). Subsequently, we have treated nine inpatients with unipolar depression and nine inpatients with bipolar disorder with 80–120 mg of idazoxan alone or idazoxan added to a stable dose of lithium in the majority of the patients with bipolar disorder using a double-blinded protocol design. Among the patients with bipolar disorder, seven of nine responded; among those with unipolar depression, one of nine responded ($\chi^2 < 0.05$). This supports previous impressions that monotherapy with α_2 antagonists is not particularly useful for unipolar depression; whether in combination with lithium it would have been more effective is unknown. Nonetheless, the favorable response in the bipolar group is striking, particularly because this group had a history of poor antidepressant response to agents other than MAOIs. It should be of interest to see if our experience can be replicated or if other α_2 antagonists prove selectively effective for bipolar depression, as monotherapy in patients with bipolar II and added to lithium in those with bipolar I illness.

CONCLUSION

There is no question that certain drugs marketed as antidepressants as well as other compounds targeted to noradrenergic sites produce short- and long-term biochemical changes that differentiate them from the SSRIs trazodone and nefazodone. These "noradrenergic" agents cannot be differentiated in terms of clinical efficacy in the outpatient populations with depression that are typically available for studies. Patients with far more severe depression, however, especially those who are hospitalized, including treatment with a noradrenergic component, may produce superior antidepressant efficacy.

More targeted studies may answer the question of whether enhancing short-term noradrenergic effects will yield more rapidly acting antidepressants or ones that have special efficacy in subgroups such as bipolar depression.

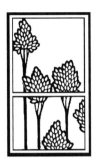

CHAPTER 16

Sleep in Depression and the Effects of Antidepressants on Sleep

Constantin R. Soldatos, M.D., and
Joanne D. Bergiannaki, M.D.

Sleep disturbance has been long recognized as one of the main symptoms of depression. Actually, the diagnoses of insomnia and hypersomnia "associated with mood disorders," such as major depression, were included in various official classification systems (DSM-III-R and DSM-IV [American Psychiatric Association 1987, 1994]; ICSD [American Sleep Disorders Association 1990]; ICD-10 [World Health Organization 1992]). Moreover, the close relationship between disturbed sleep and depression has been documented repeatedly in many epidemiological studies establishing a high prevalence of depression among patients with insomnia (Bixler et al. 1979; Ford and Kamerow 1985; Frisoni et al. 1992; Liljenberg et al. 1989; Mellinger et al. 1985; Soldatos 1994) and a high prevalence of insomnia among patients with depression (Brabbins et al. 1993; Dryman and Eaton 1991; Livingston et al. 1990; Quera-Salva et al. 1991; Soldatos 1994).

With the advent of a standardized sleep laboratory recording technique and scoring system (Rechtschaffen and Kales 1968) and the development of the computerized sleep electroencephalogram (EEG) analysis method (Borbely et al. 1984; Feinberg et al. 1980; Ktonas 1987; Kupfer et al. 1984; Mendelson et al. 1987a; J. E. Shipley et al. 1988; Soldatos 1979), the study of sleep in depression became one of the major areas of sleep research. The sleep recordings of depressed patients were shown to be distinctly different from those of nondepressed control subjects (Benca et al. 1992; C. Chen 1979; Gillin et al. 1984; Kupfer 1984; Mendlewicz and Kerkhofs 1991; C. F. Reynolds and Kupfer 1987; Sakkas et al. 1990; Soldatos et al. 1987). Early hopes, however, that certain sleep EEG aberrations are unique to major depression (Kupfer 1976) were not proven valid because similarly aberrant sleep EEG patterns were observed in various subtypes of depression and many other psychiatric disorders (Akiskal et al. 1982; Benca et al. 1992; Bergiannaki et al. 1987; Gierz et al. 1987; Insel et al. 1982b; J. L. Katz et al. 1984; Riemann et al. 1991; Tandon et al. 1988; Thase et al. 1984; Uhde et al. 1984; Wehr 1990; Zarcone et al. 1987).

Sleep researchers also were involved in assessing the effects of antidepressant drugs on sleep (C. Chen 1979; Montero and Berger 1995; Sandor and Shapiro 1994; Sharpley and Cowen 1995; Soldatos et al. 1990; van Bemmel 1993; G. W. Vogel et al. 1990). Their interest related basically to the assessment of the sedative or stimulant side effects of a given antidepressant. Moreover, they were hoping that the drug-induced sleep EEG changes would enable them to gain better insight into the mechanism of action of antidepressants (G. W. Vogel et al. 1990). Unfortunately, this rather ambitious aim does not seem to have been fulfilled as yet (Montero and Berger 1995; Sandor and Shapiro 1994; Sharpley and Cowen 1995; Soldatos et al. 1990; van Bemmel 1993).

The purpose of this chapter is to provide an update of research on 1) the sleep laboratory and computerized sleep EEG findings in depression and 2) the effects of antidepressants on sleep efficiency and sleep stages as well as on computerized sleep EEG patterns. Documentation was based on a MEDLINE library search and on references provided in extensive reviews, such as those by C. F. Reynolds and Kupfer (1987), G. W. Vogel et al. (1990), Benca et al. (1992), van Bemmel (1993), M. Berger and Riemann (1993), Armitage (1995), Montero and Berger (1995).

SLEEP IN DEPRESSION

Sleep Efficiency Characteristics

When sleep patterns are recorded in the laboratory, depressed patients as a group show significantly less total sleep time than do noninsomniac control subjects; more specifically, although both groups spend the same amount of time in bed, the depressed patients have a longer sleep-onset latency, more wakefulness during the night, and an earlier awakening in the morning (Benca et al. 1992; Kupfer 1984; Mendlewicz and Kerkhofs 1991; C. F. Reynolds and

Kupfer 1987; Soldatos et al. 1987). However, despite these intergroup differences, a subgroup of depressed patients may actually sleep more than the control subjects (Garvey et al. 1984; Kupfer 1984; Michaelis and Hofmann 1973); this subgroup includes mainly patients with seasonal affective disorder (Rosenthal et al. 1984) and those with anergic depression of the bipolar type (Detre et al. 1972; Kupfer et al. 1972).

Comparisons of sleep laboratory findings in depressed patients with those in patients with other psychiatric disorders, such as schizophrenia, dementia, anorexia, and anxiety disorders, showed that a reduction in sleep efficiency is not only seen in depression (Benca et al. 1992; Ganguli et al. 1987; Hiatt et al. 1985; Insel et al. 1982b; Levy et al. 1988; Loewenstein et al. 1982; T. A. Mellman and Uhde 1989; Neil et al. 1980; Papadimitriou et al. 1988; Prinz et al. 1982; C. F. Reynolds et al. 1983; Stern et al. 1969; Walsh et al. 1985). Nonetheless, with the exception of schizophrenic patients, depressed patients have the most severely affected indices of sleep induction and maintenance (Benca et al. 1992).

Sleep Stages in Depression

Based on standardized scoring procedures (Rechtschaffen and Kales 1968), the entire sleep period is internally characterized as either rapid eye movement (REM) sleep or non-REM sleep, the latter including stages 1, 2, 3, and 4. Furthermore, stages 3 and 4 form the so-called slow-wave sleep (SWS). In this section, we describe the sleep stage characteristics of depression.

In non-REM sleep patterns in depression, stage 1 sleep increases and SWS decreases (Benca et al. 1992; Gillin 1983a; Kupfer and Foster 1978; W. B. Mendelson et al. 1977). These findings, in conjunction with the numerous shifts from one stage to another observed in depressed patients, indicate that sleep in depression usually is not only reduced in quantity but also quite unstable and shallow (Soldatos et al. 1987). The non-REM sleep characteristics of depression also have been seen in many other psychiatric and medical conditions (Benca et al. 1992; Soldatos et al. 1987). Thus, they do not distinguish depression from other disorders.

REM sleep time is preserved in depression (Benca et al. 1992; Mendlewicz and Kerkhofs 1991). Yet, REM sleep percentage is slightly increased, and the density of rapid eye movements is enhanced (Benca et al. 1992; Gillin et al. 1981; Mendlewicz and Kerkhofs 1991). Most notable of all REM sleep characteristics in depression is a short latency to the onset of REM sleep (C. F. Reynolds and Kupfer 1987). These REM sleep patterns were considered to be unique to depression; in particular, the short REM latency was originally claimed to be a marker for primary depression (Kupfer 1976, 1984). Unfortunately, this did not prove to be the case. Short REM latency with other REM sleep alterations have been seen not only in primary depression but also in almost every subtype of depression and in mania, schizophrenia, obsessive-compulsive disorder, borderline personality disorder, eating disorders, and other disorders (Akiskal et al. 1982; Benca et al. 1992; Bergiannaki et al. 1987; Gierz et al. 1987; Insel et al. 1982b; J. L. Katz et al. 1984; Riemann et al. 1991; Tandon et al. 1988; Thase et al. 1984; Uhde et al. 1984; Wehr 1990; Zarcone et al. 1987). Thus, REM sleep characteristics cannot differentiate depression from other psychiatric disorders (Benca et al. 1992) nor can they distinguish among the various subtypes of depression itself (M. Berger and Riemann 1993).

Depressed patients, when compared with nondepressed control subjects, have been shown repeatedly to have an earlier occurrence of REM sleep onset induced by intravenous administration of cholinomimetics (M. Berger and Riemann 1993; Gillin et al. 1991; Riemann et al. 1994; Sitaram et al. 1980). This well-established supersensitive response to cholinomimetics, however, also has been observed in schizophrenic patients (M. Berger and Riemann 1993; Riemann et al. 1991). Yet, an increase in the density of rapid eye movements through cholinergic stimulation appears to be specific to depression (Riemann et al. 1994).

When using sleep research methods to elucidate the nature of depression, an important consideration is whether REM patterns themselves and REM alterations through pharmacological manipulations of the cholinergic system are state or trait characteristics of depression. The findings are inconsistent across studies regarding the persistence of REM sleep abnormalities following remission from depression (Cartwright 1983; Knowles et al. 1986; Rush et al. 1986; Steiger et al. 1989). However, these findings suggest that the abnormalities of REM sleep likely denote the presence of a vulnerability toward relapses of depression (M. Berger and Riemann 1993). Evidence for vulnerability toward relapses also stems from the results of family studies of depressed patients in the sleep laboratory (D. E. Giles et al. 1987, 1988; Schreiber et al. 1992; Sitaram et al. 1987). In any case, a supersensitive response to the cholinergic REM induction test has been repeatedly shown to be not only a state but also a trait characteristic of depression (M. Berger and Riemann 1993; Gillin et al. 1991; Riemann et al. 1994).

Computerized Sleep EEG Findings

Computer-assisted techniques for the analysis of sleep EEG have been used to investigate the intensity and distribution of various frequency bands throughout the night (Armitage 1995; Armitage et al. 1992a; Borbely et al. 1984; Feinberg et al. 1980; Ktonas 1987; Kupfer et al. 1984, 1986, 1989a, 1989b; W. B. Mendelson et al. 1987a; Soldatos 1979). Most studies suggested that depressed patients compared with nondepressed control subjects have a significantly reduced overall power in the delta frequency band (Kupfer et al. 1989a, 1989b), but some did not (Armitage 1995). Furthermore, contrary to what happens in nondepressed individuals, depressed patients show a lower level of delta wave intensity during the first non-REM period than in the second non-REM period (Kupfer et al. 1990). According to subsequent findings, however, the ratio of delta activity in the first two non-REM periods does not seem to differentiate depressed patients from nondepressed control subjects (Armitage et al. 1992b).

Regarding EEG frequencies outside the delta band, several microarchitectural sleep EEG characteristics of depression have been sought in both the remitted and the symptomatic state (Armitage 1995). Based on preliminary data, certain computerized sleep EEG patterns appear to be relatively specific to depression (e.g., an elevated fast frequency activity on the right hemisphere and a reduced beta and theta interhemispheric coherence) (Armitage et al. 1991, 1992c, 1993). The consistency of all these findings, however, has not yet been established.

Clinical Significance and Theoretical Implications

The usefulness of the sleep laboratory patterns as a diagnostic tool for depression has not been demonstrated (Benca et al. 1992). Moreover, no special clinical significance has been attributed to any sleep stage or computerized EEG changes in depression. A drug-free period of 2–4 weeks is required before obtaining "uncontaminated" sleep laboratory data, which is practically impossible for obvious ethical reasons (Soldatos et al. 1990). For research purposes, however, sleep laboratory recordings, especially when they are combined with computerized EEG analysis, can become of appreciable value. They may eventually prove to be quite helpful in elucidating the pathophysiology of sleep in depression. Furthermore, studying sleep more thoroughly may clarify certain aspects of the multifaceted pathophysiology of depression itself. It could, eventually, provide important information about the biological and genetic heterogeneity of affective disorders with potential taxonomic, prognostic, and therapeutic implications (Soldatos and Paparrigopoulos 1995).

Of all the sleep alterations in depression, those pertaining to REM sleep have been given special consideration (M. Berger and Riemann 1993; C. F.

Reynolds and Kupfer 1987; van Bemmel 1993). Actually, several hypotheses have been raised to explain their occurrence. One hypothesis suggests that an increased pressure of REM sleep is responsible (Snyder 1969; G. W. Vogel et al. 1975, 1977, 1980). Another hypothesis suggests that a weakness of the non-REM sleep, as explained by the two-process model of sleep regulation, may be underlying (Borbely 1982, 1987; Borbely and Wirz-Justice 1982; Daan et al. 1984). A third hypothesis, however—that of the cholinergic versus aminergic imbalance (Gillin and Shiromani 1990; Janowsky et al. 1972; Sitaram et al. 1982)—appears to have the most merit (M. Berger and Riemann 1993). This hypothesis explains the occurrence of a short REM latency in conjunction with a supersensitive response to the cholinergic REM induction test. It is based on experimental evidence that the activity of the cholinergic system is priming the REM-on process, whereas the activity of the aminergic systems promotes the REM-off process (J. A. Hobson et al. 1975, 1986; McCarley 1982; McCarley and Hobson 1975).

An imbalance in the cholinergic/aminergic interactions may result from the deficient activity of a certain aminergic system or the hyperactivity of the cholinergic system or any quantitative combination of the two, which could very well be responsible for the pathophysiology of depression (M. Berger and Riemann 1993; Soldatos and Paparrigopoulos 1995).

Because a short REM latency (Benca et al. 1992) and a supersensitive response to the cholinergic REM induction test (M. Berger and Riemann 1993) also can be observed in schizophrenia and other disorders, an imbalance of the cholinergic/aminergic interactions may underlie not only the pathogenesis of depression but also the symptom formation of schizophrenia or other psychiatric disorders (Soldatos and Paparrigopoulos 1995). Specific research information about the exact link between psychiatric disorders and associated sleep alterations is currently lacking. Several disorders may share common fundamental features in their pathophysiology, or, alternatively, certain psychiatric disorders each have unique biological mechanisms that lead to common final pathways affecting complex behaviors, including sleep (Benca et al. 1992).

ANTIDEPRESSANTS AND SLEEP

Effects on Sleep Efficiency

The study of antidepressants in the sleep laboratory has shown that some of them disturb sleep, whereas others either do not affect it considerably or actually increase total sleep time (van Bemmel 1993). These differential effects on sleep appear to be independent of the specific category of each antidepressant. Thus, drugs disturbing sleep include the tricyclic antidepressants (TCAs) clomipramine (E. Klein et al. 1984b; Riemann and Berger 1990) and imipramine (Kupfer et al. 1979; Ware et al. 1989); the monoamine oxidase inhibitors (MAOIs) clorgiline (R. M. Cohen et al. 1982) and tranylcypromine (Nolen et al. 1993); the selective serotonin reuptake inhibitors (SSRIs) fluoxetine (Kerkhofs et al. 1990; Nicholson and Pascoe 1988), fluvoxamine (Kupfer et al. 1991), indalpine (Nicholson and Pascoe 1986), and paroxetine (Oswald and Adam 1986; Saletu et al. 1991); and other antidepressants, such as nomifensin (Nicholson and Pascoe 1986). However, some drugs in these same categories either do not considerably affect sleep or may actually increase its amount; these antidepressants include the TCAs amitriptyline (Gillin et al. 1978; Hartmann and Cravens 1973; Kupfer et al. 1978; Mendlewicz et al. 1991; Riemann et al. 1990), desipramine (Kupfer et al. 1991; J. E. Shipley et al. 1985), doxepine (Dunleavy et al. 1972; Roth et al. 1982), and trimipramine (Feuillade et al. 1992; Wiegand et al. 1986); the MAOIs moclobemide (Monti et al. 1990) and pargyline (R. M. Cohen et al. 1982); the SSRI citalopram (van Bemmel et al. 1993a); and other antidepressants, such as amineptine (Di Perri et al. 1987), maprotiline (C. Chen et al. 1977; Jovanovic 1977), mianserin (Maeda et al. 1990; Mendlewicz et al. 1985), nefazodone (Sharpley et al. 1992), S 3344 (Soldatos et al. 1988), and trazodone (Mouret et al. 1988; van Bemmel et al. 1992a; Ware 1990). Consequently, based on their effects on sleep efficiency, antidepressants can be differentiated into energizing and nonenergizing (Table 16–1).

Effects on Non-REM Sleep

The energizing antidepressants either increase stage 1 sleep or do not affect it (R. M. Cohen et al. 1982; Kerkhofs et al. 1990; E. Klein et al. 1984b; Kupfer et al. 1979, 1991; Nicholson and Pascoe 1986, 1988; Nolen et al. 1993; Oswald and Adam 1986; Riemann and Berger 1990; Saletu et al. 1991; Ware et al. 1989). Most of the nonenergizing antidepressants do not significantly affect stage 1 sleep (R. M. Cohen et al. 1982; Di Perri et al. 1987; Dunleavy et al. 1972; Mendlewicz et al. 1985; Monti et al. 1990; Sharpley et al. 1992; Soldatos et al. 1988; van Bemmel et al. 1993a); some of them, however, have somewhat inconsistent effects on stage 1 sleep (Feuillade et al. 1992; Gillin et al. 1978; Kupfer et al. 1978, 1991; Mendlewicz et al. 1991; Mouret et al. 1988; J. E. Shipley et al. 1985; van Bemmel et al. 1992a; Ware 1990; Wiegand et al. 1986). Many antidepressants increase stage 2 sleep indepen-

TABLE 16–1. Grouping antidepressants based on their effects on sleep efficiency

	Energizing	Nonenergizing
Tricyclic antidepressants	Clomipramine	Amitriptyline
	Imipramine	Desipramine
		Doxepin
		Trimipramine
Monoamine oxidase inhibitors	Clorgiline	Moclobemide
	Tranylcypromine	Pargyline
Selective serotonin reuptake inhibitors	Fluoxetine	Citalopram
	Fluvoxamine	
	Indalpine	
	Paroxetine	
Other	Nomifensin	Amineptine
		Maprotiline
		Mianserin
		Nefazodone
		S 3344
		Trazodone

dent of their energizing or nonenergizing effects (Blois and Gaillard 1990; R. M. Cohen et al. 1982; Dunleavy et al. 1972; Feuillade et al. 1992; Gillin et al. 1978; Hartmann and Cravens 1973; Kupfer et al. 1978, 1979, 1991; Mendlewicz et al. 1985; Monti et al. 1990; Mouret et al. 1988; Nicholson et al. 1989a; Passouant et al. 1975; Riemann et al. 1990; Saletu et al. 1991; J. E. Shipley et al. 1985; van Bemmel et al. 1993a). Obviously, the increase in stage 2 sleep with the energizing drugs does not parallel an increase in total sleep time. Rather, it should be considered as compensatory to drug-induced suppression of SWS and/or REM sleep. Furthermore, although certain drugs did not alter stage 2 sleep (Bramanti et al. 1985; Di Perri et al. 1987; Kerkhofs et al. 1990; E. Klein et al. 1984b; Mendlewicz et al. 1991; Nicholson and Pascoe 1988; Nolen et al. 1993; Oswald and Adam 1986; Riemann et al. 1990; Saletu et al. 1991; Sharpley et al. 1992; Soldatos et al. 1988; Ware 1990; Ware et al. 1989; Wiegand et al. 1986), none decreased it.

Most antidepressants did not considerably change SWS. Nonetheless, evidence indicates that doxepine (Roth et al. 1982), imipramine (Kupfer et al. 1979), and fluoxetine (Kerkhofs et al. 1990) suppress SWS, whereas paroxetine (Oswald and Adam 1986) and trazodone (I. Montgomery et al. 1983; Mouret et al. 1988) may enhance it.

Effects on REM Sleep

Initially, antidepressants were consistently found to exert a powerful REM suppressant effect, followed by REM rebound on discontinuation (R. M. Cohen et al. 1982; Dunleavy et al. 1972; Gaillard et al. 1983; Gillin et al. 1976, 1978; Hartmann and Cravens 1973; Kupfer and Bowers 1972; Kupfer et al. 1982b; Monti et al. 1990; Nicholson et al. 1989b; Steiger et al. 1988; G. W. Vogel 1975; Wyatt et al. 1971). This type of REM suppression was considered to be analogous to REM deprivation induced through arousals, which had been shown to have clear-cut therapeutic efficacy for depression (G. W. Vogel et al. 1975, 1980). Actually, the efficacy of antidepressants was somehow ascribed to their REM suppressant effects (G. W. Vogel et al. 1980). As research data were accumulated from studies of more antidepressants, however, this assumption did not prove to be as valid as originally thought (Di Perri et al. 1987; Feuillade et al. 1992; Jovanovic 1977; Mendlewicz et al. 1985; Mouret et al. 1988; Sharpley et al. 1992; Soldatos et al. 1988; Wiegand et al. 1986).

As Table 16–2 shows, most antidepressants studied in the sleep laboratory have been found to suppress REM sleep. The TCAs amitriptyline (Gillin et al. 1978; Hartmann and Cravens 1973; Kerkhofs et al. 1990; Kupfer et al. 1978; Mendlewicz et al. 1991; J. E. Shipley et al. 1985), clomipramine (Dunleavy et al. 1972; E. Klein et al. 1984b; Kupfer et al. 1989a; Passouant et al. 1975; Riemann and Berger 1990), desipramine (Dunleavy et al. 1972; Gaillard et al. 1983; Kupfer et al. 1991; J. E. Shipley et al. 1985; Zung 1969), doxepin (Dunleavy et al. 1972; Roth et al. 1982), and imipramine (Dunleavy et al. 1972; Kupfer et al. 1979; Ware et al. 1989); the MAOIs clorgyline (R. M. Cohen et al. 1982; Gillin et al. 1976), pargyline (R. M. Cohen et al. 1982; Gillin et al. 1976), phenelzine (Akindele et al. 1970; Dunleavy and Oswald 1973; Kupfer and Bowers 1972; Wyatt et al. 1971), and tranylcypromine (Nolen et al. 1993); the SSRIs citalopram (van Bemmel et al. 1993a, 1993b), fluoxetine (Bardeleben et al. 1989; Kerkhofs et al. 1990; Nicholson and Pascoe 1988), fluvoxamine (M. Berger et al. 1986; Kupfer et al. 1991), indalpine (Oswald and Adam 1986), and paroxetine (Nicholson and Pascoe 1986); and some other antidepressants, such as maprotiline (Nicholson and Pascoe 1986), mianserin (Maeda et al. 1990; Morgan et al. 1980; Nicholson et al. 1986), and nomifensin (Nicholson and Pascoe 1986) are indeed REM suppressors. Actually, for about half of these

TABLE 16–2. Grouping antidepressants based on their effects on rapid eye movement sleep

	Suppressors	Nonsuppressors
Tricyclic antidepressants	Amitriptyline	Trimipramine
	Clomipramine	
	Desipramine	
	Doxepin	
	Imipramine	
Monoamine oxidase inhibitors	Clorgiline	Moclobemide
	Pargyline	Iprindole
	Phenelzine	
	Tranylcypromine	
Selective serotonin reuptake inhibitors	Citalopram	
	Fluoxetine	
	Fluvoxamine	
	Indalpine	
	Paroxetine	
Other	Maprotiline	Amineptine
	Mianserin	Nefazodone
	Nomifensin	S 3344
		Trazodone

antidepressants, the respective sleep laboratory studies included a withdrawal period, and, in most cases, they found a REM rebound following discontinuation of the medication that was similar to the effect following termination of the arousal-induced REM deprivation (Blois and Gaillard 1990; R. M. Cohen et al. 1982; Dunleavy et al. 1972; Feuillade et al. 1992; Gaillard et al. 1983; Gillin et al. 1976, 1978; Hartmann and Cravens 1973; Kupfer and Bowers 1972; Monti et al. 1990; Steiger et al. 1988; Wyatt et al. 1971). Yet, several antidepressants belonging to various categories either did not change REM sleep, such as iprindole (Dunleavy et al. 1972) and trazodone (Mouret et al. 1988; van Bemmel et al. 1992a, 1992b; Ware 1990), or enhanced REM sleep, such as trimipramine (Wiegand et al. 1986), moclobemide (Monti 1989), amineptine (Bramanti et al. 1985; Di Perri et al. 1987), nefazodone (Sharpley et al. 1992), and S 3344 (Soldatos et al. 1988).

A frequent concomitant of REM suppression is a lengthening of REM latency. Thus, one would expect to see prolonged REM latency with the antidepressants that suppress REM sleep and shortened REM latency with those that enhance REM sleep. This is indeed the case for the REM suppressants without exception (Akindele et al. 1970; Bardeleben et al. 1989; M. Berger et al. 1986; R. M. Cohen et al. 1982; Dunleavy and Oswald 1973; Gillin et al. 1976, 1978; Kerkhofs et al. 1990; Kupfer and Bowers 1972; Kupfer et al. 1978, 1979, 1989a; Maeda et al. 1990; Mendlewicz et al. 1985, 1991; Morgan et al. 1980; Nicholson et al. 1986; Nolen et al. 1993; Oswald and Adam 1986; Riemann and Berger 1990; Roth et al. 1982; Saletu et al. 1991; J. E. Shipley et al. 1985; van Bemmel et al. 1993a, 1993b; Ware et al. 1989; Wyatt et al. 1971). However, among the REM-enhancing drugs, only amineptine administration was associated with a shortening of REM latency (Bramanti et al. 1985; Di Perri et al. 1987); REM latency was unchanged with S 3344 and nefazodone (Sharpley et al. 1992; Soldatos et al. 1988) and was actually lengthened with trimipramine, trazodone, and moclobemide (Feuillade et al. 1992; Monti et al. 1990; Mouret et al. 1988; Steiger et al. 1988; van Bemmel et al. 1992a; Ware 1990; Wiegand et al. 1986).

Effects on Computerized Sleep EEG

Only seven published studies exist regarding the effects of a small number of antidepressants on computerized sleep EEG patterns (Jarrett et al. 1988; Kupfer et al. 1991, 1994; Minot et al. 1993). In these studies, only 118 total patients were included, and no confirmatory study was done for any of the drugs. Moreover, the length of the drug administration period varied from 1 day (Jarrett et al. 1988) to 3 years (Kupfer et al. 1994), and the method of computerized analysis was not uniform: some studies used period analysis (Jarrett et al. 1988; Kupfer et al. 1991), others used fast Fourier transform (Minot et al. 1993; van Bemmel et al. 1992b, 1993b), and some others used both period analysis and fast Fourier transform (Kupfer et al. 1994).

Taking into account the aforementioned limitations, it is not surprising that the results of the existing computerized sleep EEG studies of antidepressants are rather disparate (Table 16–3). Thus, after acute administration of 50 mg of imipramine, delta counts increased in the first non-REM period (Jarrett et al. 1988), whereas after chronic administration of 150–300 mg of imipramine, delta counts and delta and theta power decreased, coupled with an increase in fast beta power in every non-REM period (Kupfer et al. 1994). Clomipramine, 150–200 mg given over a 2-week period, increased delta counts and delta power for the first part of the night (Kupfer et al. 1989a), whereas desipramine, 100–250 mg, and fluvoxamine, 200–300 mg, did not significantly change delta counts throughout the night over a 4-week period (Kupfer et al. 1991). Trazodone, 300 mg, increased slow delta power and de-

TABLE 16–3.   Computerized sleep electroencephalogram (CSEEG) effects of antidepressants

Antidepressant/Time of tests	CSEEG effects	Clinical correlates
Imipramine, 50 mg, acute[a]	↑δ counts in first NREM period	Independent of GH change
Imipramine, 150–300 mg, chronic[b]	↓δ counts ↓δ and θ power ↑β power	
Clomipramine, 150–200 mg, acute, fifth day, second week[c]	↑δ counts ↑δ power in early night	Relation to treatment outcome
Desipramine, 150–250 mg, acute, first week, third week[d]	No change in δ counts	
Fluvoxamine, 200–300 mg, acute, first week, third week[d]	No change in δ counts	
Trazodone, 300 mg, acute, fourth week, withdrawal[e]	↑ slow δ power ↓ slow β power On withdrawal, return to baseline	No relation to treatment outcome
Citalopram, 40 mg, acute, fourth week, withdrawal[f]	↓ slow α power ↓ α, maintained on withdrawal	No relation to treatment outcome
Moclobemide, 450 mg, acute, first week, fourth week, withdrawal[g]	↑δ power ↓β power in REM	

Note.   GH = growth hormone; NREM = non rapid eye movement; REM = rapid eye movement.
[a]Jarrett et al. 1988. [b]Kupfer et al. 1994. [c]Kupfer et al. 1989a. [d]Kupfer et al. 1991. [e]van Bemmel et al. 1992a. [f]van Bemmel et al. 1993a. [g]Minot et al. 1993.

creased slow beta power over 1 month of drug administration (van Bemmel et al. 1992a), whereas citalopram, 40 mg, decreased slow alpha power at the end of the 1-month administration period (van Bemmel et al. 1993a). Trazodone and citalopram also differed in terms of their withdrawal effects: drug-induced power spectra changes were maintained during the 1-week period of withdrawal from citalopram (van Bemmel et al. 1993a), whereas computerized sleep EEG spectra returned to predrug levels after trazodone withdrawal (van Bemmel et al. 1992a). Finally, moclobemide, 450 mg administered for 4 weeks, increased delta power and decreased beta power during REM sleep (Minot et al. 1993).

Clinical Significance and Theoretical Implications

Ample evidence indicates that manipulations of sleep, such as total sleep deprivation (Christodoulou et al. 1978; Gillin 1983b; Papadimitriou et al. 1993; Pflug and Tolle 1971; van den Burg and van den Hoofdakker 1975; Wehr et al. 1985) and selective REM sleep deprivation (G. W. Vogel et al. 1975, 1980), exert a beneficial effect in some depressed patients. This suggests that the remarkable influence of most antidepressants on sleep may not be merely an epiphenomenon of depression and the changes during its clinical course (van Bemmel 1993). Nonetheless, despite the large amount of data regarding the effects of antidepressants on sleep, the empirical foundation of the prevailing model of physiological mechanisms involved in sleep-wake regulation during the treatment of depression is still lacking.

Based on their effects on sleep efficiency, antidepressants can be differentiated into energizing and nonenergizing (Table 16–1). This distinction is of obvious practical usefulness for the prescription of antidepressants. It has been suggested that drugs inhibiting noradrenergic reuptake are more likely to induce sedation, whereas the serotonin reuptake inhibitors promote alertness during the day and often cause sleep continuity problems at night (Nicholson and Pascoe 1986, 1991). According to our review of the literature, this theory does not appear to hold true entirely. Improvement in sleep continuity should not be merely considered as a matter of sedation; rather, the complex interactions among the various pharmacological effects of a given antidepressant may be involved (Sharpley and Cowen 1995). It should be also noted that different antidepressants have been studied for different periods of drug administration (van Bemmel 1993). Moreover, certain drugs, such as amitryptiline and desipramine, have been thoroughly studied in large samples of both depressed and healthy individuals (Dunleavy et al. 1972; Gaillard et al. 1983; Gillin et al. 1978; Hartmann and Cravens 1973; Kerkhofs et al. 1990; Kupfer et al. 1978, 1991; Mendlewicz et al. 1991; Riemann et al. 1990; J. E. Shipley et al. 1985; Zung 1969), whereas others, such as indalpine and nefazodone, have been studied in just a few healthy subjects (Nicholson et al. 1986; Sharpley et al. 1992). Thus, the confidence of drawing conclusions about drug-induced sleep alterations across antidepressants varies accordingly.

After four decades of sleep research, the clinical significance of sleep stages has not yet been determined. Nonetheless, as already mentioned in the previous "Sleep Stages in Depression" section of this chapter, considerable progress has been made in terms of raising plausible hypotheses pertaining to the neurophysiological mechanisms underlying the regulation of sleep stages in nondepressed individuals (Borbely 1982; Daan et al. 1984; Gillin and Shiromani 1990; Hobson et al. 1986; McCarley and Hobson 1975). Thus, studies of drug-induced sleep stage alterations may eventually contribute to the elucidation of the mechanism of action of antidepressants. The effects of these drugs on non-REM sleep stages are either compensatory and therefore without any particular significance, as is the case with stage 2, or rather inconsistent and difficult to interpret, as is the case with SWS. The effects on REM sleep, however, deserve special consideration.

Although there are some exceptions, antidepressants generally tend to suppress REM sleep (Table 16–2). The question is whether seven antidepressants are indeed REM nonsuppressors or whether they actually may be suppressors but, for some reason, were not detected as such. It appears certain that at least iprindole, trazodone, and trimipramine are actually REM nonsuppressors because more than one study found a lack of REM suppression with their administration (Baxter and Gluckman 1969; Dunleavy et al. 1972; Feuillade et al. 1992; Mouret et al. 1988; Steiger et al. 1988; van Bemmel et al. 1992a, 1992b; Ware 1990; Wiegand et al. 1986). Yet, even with trazodone and trimipramine, REM latency lengthened instead of shortening, as expected (Feuillade et al. 1992; Mouret et al. 1988; van Bemmel et al. 1992a, 1992b; Ware 1990; Wiegand et al. 1986). Thus, the REM suppressant effect of antidepressants, whenever present, is quite robust (G. W. Vogel et al. 1990), whereas its absence with some antidepressants does not always seem to be very convincing. However, certain methodological problems, such as dose equivalence and time of drug administration (Montero and Berger 1995), may have contributed to divergent results across studies of the REM suppressant effects of antidepressants.

Many psychotropic drugs from various classes other than antidepressants have been shown over the years also to suppress REM sleep, but they do not have any antidepressant efficacy (Kales 1995). A review, however, indicated that, compared with other REM suppressant drugs, antidepressants produce a suppression of REM sleep that is larger, more persistent, and followed more frequently by REM rebound on drug discontinuation (G. W. Vogel et al. 1990). Thus, differences across drug classes indeed make antidepressants unique, with their REM suppressant effect paralleling only that of the arousal-induced REM sleep deprivation.

It has been assumed that the REM suppressing properties are a prerequisite for the antidepressant efficacy of a drug (G. W. Vogel 1975, 1983). It is now clear that this position was an oversimplification (Montero and Berger 1995). Actually, G. W. Vogel et al. (1990) admitted that only a correlation exists between antidepressant efficacy and drug effect on REM sleep, and, of course, causality cannot be inferred from correlation alone.

Several hypotheses have been elaborated to explain the REM suppressant effects of antidepressants (van Bemmel 1993). Among these hypotheses, the one using the acetylcholine-monoaminergic imbalance model seemed to have had the highest merit (M. Berger and Riemann 1993) because it was based on a presumed common pathophysiological mechanism underlying both REM sleep disturbance in depression and drug-induced REM sleep alterations. This hypothesis could not be tested clinically because the acetylcholine-monoaminergic balance cannot be measured directly in relevant brain structures of depressed individuals with or without antidepressant drug treatment (van Bemmel 1993). Nonetheless, the ability of many antidepressants to decrease REM sleep was attributed to their facilitation of noradrenergic and/or serotonergic uptake blockade (Sharpley and Cowen 1995). Thus, it can be inferred that the acetylcholine-monoaminergic imbalance may be involved in the mechanism of the REM sleep alterations induced by most antidepressants.

The computerized analysis of the sleep EEG appeared to be a promising method for the detection of drug-induced sleep changes. Beersma and van den Hoofdakker (1992) hypothesized that the efficacy of antidepressants might be the result of the suppression of the non-REM sleep power rather than the suppression of REM sleep. Furthermore, these investigators argued that even nonpharmacological sleep manipulations with antidepressant effects, such as total or partial sleep deprivation, all share the non-REM sleep suppressing element (Beersma and van den Hoofdakker 1992). They predicted that antidepressant effects must be expected from suppression of non-REM sleep intensity. Our review of the relatively limited literature on the computerized sleep EEG changes during administration of antidepressants showed that these drugs have rather inconsistent effects on delta counts and/or power. Thus, the results of the studies reviewed in this chapter do not seem to favor the hypothesis of Beersma and van den Hoofdakker.

Albeit limited, research on the computerized sleep EEG effects of antidepressants has provided some results suggesting certain clinical correlates of these effects. Thus, one study showed that the increase in delta counts in the first non-REM period after acute administration of imipramine was independent of the changes in growth hormone secretion (Jarrett et al. 1988). This finding confirms previous observations that growth hormone secretion and SWS are not necessarily related (Bixler et al. 1976; Rubin et al. 1973). Another study documented a correlation between the increase in delta power in the early part of the night with clomipramine administration and the treatment outcome with this drug (Kupfer et al. 1989a). However, no correlation was found between drug-induced computerized sleep EEG changes and treatment outcome with trazodone or citalopram (van Bemmel et al. 1992a, 1992b, 1993a, 1993b). Therefore, the clinical significance of computerized sleep EEG changes caused by antidepressants has not yet been firmly established.

FUTURE DIRECTIONS

Despite the striking similarity among various psychiatric conditions in the direction of alterations of sleep patterns, these alterations are more profound and widespread in depression than in other psychiatric disorders (Benca et al. 1992). It is also noteworthy that manipulations of sleep wakefulness in depression are frequently associated with significant mood changes (i.e., improvement with sleep deprivation and worsening with subsequent napping) (M. Berger and Riemann 1993), suggesting a close relationship between sleep and depression. Yet, no single sleep characteristic reliably distinguishes depression from other psychiatric conditions (Soldatos and Paparrigopoulos 1995). Even a short REM latency, which was originally considered a biological marker for depression, proved to be rather a quantitative index of the severity of any psychiatric condition (Benca et al. 1992).

Multivariate analysis could eventually be helpful in differentiating among various diagnostic groups of psychiatric disorders based on their sleep characteristics (Benca et al. 1992). In this type of analysis, several confounding factors should be considered, including age, psychoticism, anxiety, level of stress, inpatient versus outpatient status, physical exercise, ambient and body temperature, concurrent medical illnesses and drugs used, and psychiatric family history. Other methodological issues that must be taken into account in future research include standardized and accurate psychiatric diagnoses, sharp distinction among diagnostic categories and subtypes, and precise definitions of sleep variables (Soldatos and Paparrigopoulos 1995).

The distinction between energizing and nonenergizing antidepressants and between REM suppressors and REM nonsuppressors that is being made in this chapter is based on sleep laboratory studies, whose data may not be comparable across drugs because of a number of methodological reasons. Therefore, further studies are needed to obtain definitive results. Although difficult to conduct, large-scale studies simultaneously comparing equivalent doses of various antidepressants should be done. The timing of drug intake should be given special consideration to ensure that the peak plasma level of each drug studied occurs during sleep (Montero and Berger 1995). Also, the drug administration periods should be long enough to provide sufficient information interfacing sleep changes with antidepressant efficacy (Soldatos et al. 1990).

Studies in healthy individuals are useful to assess the effects of drugs on sleep patterns free of the aberrations due to depression itself (Soldatos et al. 1990). However, before drawing any conclusions on a given drug's effects on sleep, studies in depressed patients are also necessary because the antidepressants are intended for these patients. Studies in depressed patients may eventually provide indispensable data relevant to the mechanisms of drug action as well as to the pathophysiology of depression (Soldatos et al. 1990). It should also be noted that the action of most newer antidepressants is targeted toward specified receptors, thus allowing for the application of true pharmacological probes in the elucidation of the pathogenesis of depression.

To date, studies of the effects of antidepressants on computerized sleep EEG are sparse and have provided rather inconsistent results. The recommendations outlined for future studies of drug-induced changes of conventionally recorded sleep patterns also should be observed in the studies of computerized sleep EEG effects of antidepressants. In addition, special attention should be given to the application of standardized computerized sleep EEG analysis methods as well as to sampling rates, band pass filters, frequency characteristics, and so forth. Various rating scales, psychological inventories, and neuropsychological tests also should be used, preferably in a computerized form, to determine how the computerized sleep EEG changes interface with mood changes and other relevant psychometric data. In this context, issues related to bioavailability and bioequivalence should be considered when assessing the significance of pharmacodynamic measurements (Itil and Itil 1986). Clearly, comprehensive studies combining a variety of scientific methodologies will produce results that need to be approached in an integrative multidisciplinary fashion.

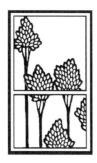

CHAPTER 17

Hormonal Interventions as Antidepressants or Adjunct Therapy: Treatment Implications

Uriel Halbreich, M.D.

The notion that mood and behavior are influenced by peripheral body fluids or by other events outside the brain has been accepted since antiquity. Even some current terminology is derived from this concept, for example, melancholia and dysthymia—just to mention the depressions. It has also been observed that changes in affect, behavior, and cognition are an integral part of the core symptoms of many hormonal disorders. Hypothyroidism, hyperthyroidism, Cushing's and Addison's diseases (hyperadrenaline and hypoadrenaline function), hypoparathyroidism, hyperprolactinemia, diabetes, and abnormalities of the hypothalamic-pituitary-gonadal system are only a partial list of these disorders.

The concept of peripheral-hormonal influence on mood was pivotal to psychoendocrinology until the mid-20th century. In the early 1960s, with the development of hormones as "windows into the brain," the emphasis shifted to understanding the influence of the brain on the periphery. How-

Preparation of this chapter was supported by National Institute of Mental Health Grant RO1-MH-46901.

ever, during the last two decades, our knowledge of the influence and effect of peripheral hormones on mood and behavior has been accumulating at an exponential pace. That effect of hormones is on multiple levels including cerebral blood flow, receptors, enzymes, cell membrane, signal transduction, and other processes in the central nervous system (CNS) that are putatively involved in regulation of mood and behavior. Several steroid and neuropeptide hormones bind directly to specific receptors in specific brain regions that are hypothesized to be key locations for the processes influenced by these hormones. The discovery of the neurosteroids, which are secreted in the brain itself, add another important dimension to the field. From the other side, there is an increasing pool of data on hormonal abnormalities associated with several mental disorders; some of the hormonal abnormalities are state-related and others might be traits. The best known of these findings, widely documented, mostly in patients with depression, is the non-suppression of cortisol in response to administration of dexamethasone.

The cause-and-effect relations of some of the hormonal abnormalities are unclear. It is plausible that at least in some cases the hormonal abnormalities are not "biological markers" for the mental disorder or for a symptomatic state; rather they might be the causative factor. Therefore, hormonal interventions might be applied as psychotropic vehicles or as psychotropic medications.

Most attempts of using hormones as psychotropic medications were conducted with gonadal or with thyroid hormones, mainly because of the apparent mood changes associated with physiological or disorder-associated changes in levels or activity of these hormones. However, as shown in Table 17–1, current applications are broader and involve several hormones and systems. It is anticipated that, with acquired knowledge on mood effects of several other hormones, that list will continue to expand. Here, I focus on psychotropic effects of gonadal and thyroid hormones. Cortisol and melatonin are only briefly discussed.

ESTROGEN

The "use of folliculin in involutional stress" was proposed already in the early 1930s (Sevringhaus 1933). Since then, there were several early attempts to use estrogen for treatment of postmenopausal depression (Wiesbader and Kurzrok 1938).

The effect of estrogen on the CNS and its processes might substantiate the notion that estrogen can be applied as an antidepressant (e.g., McEwen 1991). Estrogen generally increases the activity of monoamines—

TABLE 17-1. Hormones and hormonal interventions with psychotropic activity

Some hormones with demonstrated psychotropic activity
  Gonadal hormones
    Estrogens
    Progestins
    Androgens
  Neurosteroids
  Thyroid hormones
  Melatonin
  Vasopressin
  Oxytocin
Hormonal interventions with psychotropic activity
  Cortisol antagonists
  Cholecystokinin antagonists
  Ovulation suppressors
  Antiestrogens?
  Prolactin inhibitors

norepinephrine, dopamine, and serotonin—by a combined influence on synthesis, receptor sensitivity, and metabolism. It even possesses some of the adverse effects of common antidepressants by its effects on the cholinergic system.

However, actual clinical reports of the efficacy of estrogen as an antidepressant were almost consistently negative. To my knowledge, only one published observation indicated that the administration of high doses of estrogen had a positive effect on women with major depressive disorder (MDD) (Klaiber et al. 1979). Other attempts for application of estrogen as an antidepressant were not successful (Coope 1981; Coope et al. 1975; Oppenheim 1986; Schneider et al. 1977; Shapira et al. 1985). One study was even aborted because of several intolerable cholinergic side effects (Prange 1972). These disappointing results might be of general heuristic interest for the understanding of the mechanism of action of antidepressant medications, suggesting that some other mechanisms that are not influenced by estrogen might be responsible for the antidepressant main effect. This issue is of special interest because there are clinical observations that estrogen is an effective adjunct or an augmentation agent for postmenopausal women who are treatment-resistant to tricyclic antidepressants (TCAs) or to selective serotonin reuptake inhibitors (SSRIs). Estrogen might complement the SSRI activity by its inhibitory effect on monoamine oxidase, its postsynaptic effect on serotonergic receptors, its enhancement of catecholamine activity, as well as its effect on intracellular signal transduction. The combination SSRI-estrogen might be clinically more effective than TCA-estrogen because of the reported (Prange 1972) amplification of cholinergic TCA side effects by estrogen. However, despite the accumulation of anecdotal clinical reports, the efficacy of estrogen augmentation has not been satisfactorily demonstrated in a double-blind, placebo-controlled study. Such a firm confirmation of clinical experience is certainly needed.

The clinical similarities between the effect of estrogen on postmenopausal women who are otherwise nonresponsive to treatment and the effects of thyroid on the same group are of interest. It has been previously shown that estrogen and thyroid receptors belong to the same superfamily. Recent studies on the postreceptor-intracellular cascade of signal transduction (Pfaff 1996) are destined to shed light on the involvement of estrogen and thyroid hormones in regulation of mood and behavior and also, it is hoped, on the mechanism of their action as adjunct treatments.

The role of estrogen as a psychotropic medication is of further interest because of numerous reports that psychiatrically healthy postmenopausal women who receive estrogen replacement therapy (ERT) for prevention of osteoporosis or cardiovascular diseases also show improvement of mood and general well-being as well as improved libido and increased energy (Aylward 1976; Daly et al. 1993; Limouzin-Lamothe et al. 1994; Michael et al. 1970). The underlying mechanisms of action of increased general well-being might be related to the ability of estrogen to augment antidepressant response and its inability to serve as an antidepressant in its own right. Indeed, further studies comparing these two situations are needed.

Although the role of estrogen as an antidepressant is not clear yet, its role as a cognitive enhancer is recently becoming more apparent. Simultaneously, the complexities of estrogen's influence on cognition are unveiled. The diversity of the cognitive effects of estrogen and its dependence on the cognitive construct studied were suggested already in the early 1950s (Caldwell and Watson 1952). Therefore, it is interesting that generalizations still prevail. The selective influence of estrogen on cognitive tasks can be demonstrated from two studies of Sherwin's group. These studies (Phillips and Sherwin 1992) have shown that women who had improved immediate recall and association learning in response to estradiol did not show improvement of delayed recall, visual reproduction, or digit span. Similar selectivity was shown in another study (Kampen and Sherwin 1994) in which selective reminding tests and paragraph recall tests (verbal memory) were improved, whereas spatial ability and attention span were not. Similarly, I (Halbreich 1997) showed estrogen-induced improvement in complex integrative cognitive tasks that require integration of several cognitive constructs, such as recognition, interpretation, decision making, eye-hand coordination and reaction, as well as tests of short-term memory, but not some other cognitive functions. The mechanism of action of improvement of cognitive tests in psychiatrically healthy women might be related also to recent reports (e.g., Honjo et al. 1989; Ohkura et al. 1994) of improved or delayed dementia in women with Alzheimer's disease who were treated with estrogens.

At present, several key issues that are related to ERT, mood, and cognition are still far from being clear. ERT might be a measure to prevent deterioration of cognition and a general feeling of well-being in postmenopausal women, in a similar way to its preventive effects on bone and cardiovascular impairments. This notion, however, still requires confirmation by longitudinal follow-up studies. If women are more vulnerable to depression during their premenopausal or early menopausal years (e.g., Weissman 1996), then it is still unclear if estrogen might decrease this vulnerability and also serve as a preventive measure for mood disorders or dysphorias. It is unknown yet if all estrogens are alike as far as their effect on mood and cognition. Our own preliminary results (Halbreich 1997) suggest that at least estradiol transdermal patches and conjugated estrogens might differ from each other. It is known though that the addition of progesterone to estrogen as part of hormonal replacement therapy might counteract the positive effect of estrogen (Ohkura et al. 1994), especially if it is applied in sequential fashion (Hammarback and Backstrom 1988). It is suggested, but not yet confirmed, that women who develop dysphoric symptoms in response to sequential administration of progestins are those who had dysphoric premenstrual syndrome (PMS) during their reproductive life and who are also vulnerable to other dysphoric states.

The accumulation of data on the psychotropic effects of estrogen as well as the cumulative knowledge on estrogen's effects in animals and in vitro studies promise that estrogen itself or similar synthetic derivatives would eventually have an important role as antidepressants and/or cognition enhancers.

PROGESTINS AND ANTIPROGESTINS

Dysphoric adverse effects, mostly depression and anxiety, of progesterone are well-documented and might be responsible for some side effects of combined oral contraceptives as well as hormonal replacement therapy. Progesterone receptors in selected mood and cognitive related areas of the brain have been demonstrated already more than 20 years ago (Luine et al. 1975). However, an interesting development during the last decade is the recognition that various progesterone metabolites or various progestins might have opposing effects on mood and behavior, and the metabolic pathway of progesterone might determine the overall effect. Anxiolytic, anesthetic, and antiepileptic effects of pregnenolone and allopregnanolone as well as some other progestins have been reported (Gee 1988; Majewska 1992; Majewska and Schwartz 1987; Majewska et al. 1986; Norberg et al. 1987).

These effects are probably related to a potent agonist effect on the brain γ-aminobutyric acid type A receptor (S. M. Paul and Purdy 1992) and complementing effects of benzodiazepine action. The interaction among γ-aminobutyric acid, benzodiazepines, and progesterone led also to a speculation that progesterone might be beneficial to attenuate withdrawal symptoms of patients who are benzodiazepine-dependent (Schweizer et al. 1995), but this has not been confirmed. Nonetheless, the development of progestins as anxiolytics and antiepilepsy medications is promising and should be followed closely in the near future.

If progesterone is anxiogenic and dysphoric, then it might be of interest to explore the possibility of progesterone antagonists, for example, RU 486 (mifepristone), as a psychotropic medication. Such application for dysphoric PMS has been suggested (Halbreich 1990). However, administration of RU 486 to a small group of women with dysphoric PMS did not alleviate their symptoms, probably because it was administered in the mid luteal phase, when progesterone was already at its peak, and not during the early luteal phase before it starts its increase. The psychotropic activity of RU 486 and other progesterone antagonists might be the result of more general antisteroid action, which is not necessarily limited to progesterone, especially when higher dosages are administered. In such a case, corticosteroids and glucosteroids are also suppressed, an effect that by itself might improve mood and cognition.

CORTISOL ANTAGONISTS AND LIMBIC-HYPOTHALAMIC-PITUITARY-ADRENAL SYSTEM STABILIZERS

Hyperactivity and dysregulation of the limbic-hypothalamic-pituitary-adrenal (LHPA) system in patients with affective disorders, is well documented (e.g.,

Halbreich et al. 1985a, 1985b). The most apparent manifestation of that hyperactivity is hypercortisolemia, which with the dexamethasone suppression test (which is an indication of abnormality of feedback mechanisms in the LHPA) has been widely used as a biological marker for MDD. However, it has been shown that cortisol and other corticosteroids also affect mood, behavior, and cognition through genomic and nongenomic mechanisms (e.g., McEwen et al. 1992). It is also well documented that psychotropic and iatrogenic disorders, which are associated with high levels of corticosteroids (e.g., Cushing's syndrome), are also associated with dysphoric mood (Starkman et al. 1981), which is alleviated when cortisol levels are lowered. Interpretation of these facts is complicated because patients who have Addison's disease, in which cortisol levels are low, also have dysphoric mood, which is alleviated with corticosteroid administration.

It has been demonstrated that many antidepressants increase levels of corticosteroid receptors and increase patient sensitivity to corticosteroid feedback inhibition (Barden et al. 1995). Therefore, stimulation of corticosteroid receptor expression and enhanced negative feedback and lowered levels of corticotropin-releasing hormone (CRH) and cortisol have been suggested as an important common mechanism of action of antidepressants. If correct, this intriguing possibility might lead (Wolkowitz 1996) to the development of hormones or other synthetic compounds that directly increase corticosteroid sensitivity and would be applied as antidepressants. Indeed, this effect, though a common denominator of many current antidepressants, might be an epiphenomenon, and not necessarily the main therapeutic mechanism, as is the case with several other prevalent suggested common mechanisms. Another and more feasible possibility is compatible with the notion that MDD is a cluster of symptoms or syndromes that might be the end result of several biological pathways. One of them might be dysregulation of the LHPA system. In this subgroup of patients, such LHPA stabilizers might be effective antidepressants. Future studies and future compounds will prove or disconfirm this hypothesis.

The same issue of validity of current sensitivity and specificity data on biological processes in MDD is also pertinent to the nearly 20 studies that have reported antidepressant and cognitive-enhancing effects of cortisol-lowering pharmacological, radiological, or surgical interventions (B. E. P. Murphy and Wolkowitz 1993). The antidepressant effects of ketoconazole, metyrapone, and aminoglutethimide are probably more significant in patients who have high baseline levels of cortisol and in whom the anticorticosteroids administered decrease these levels (Wolkowitz et al. 1996a).

In the early 1980s, when the dexamethasone suppression test was in vogue, sporadic reports of a transient improvement of mood in response to cortisol suppression with that test appeared. Recent studies (Arana et al. 1995) demonstrated that administration of high dosages of dexamethasone do have an antidepressant effect. This effect might be limited to only a subgroup of patients with depression, as has been suggested by another recent study (Wolkowitz et al. 1996b).

In this context, it is worthwhile to mention the possible psychotropic effect of the corticosteroid dehydroepiandrosterone (DHEA). Its exogenous administration is associated with antiglucosteroid effect. DHEA has been shown (Wolkowitz et al. 1997) to have antidepressant and cognitive-enhancement effects in patients with MDD and also to enhance general well-being in psychiatrically healthy people. However, DHEA is also a pro-androgen, and its mood-enhancing effect might also be through increased androgenic effects, especially in elderly men. Larger-scale current studies may shed more light on this issue and establish the psychotropic role of DHEA.

Although recently the focus of LHPA system interventions is on the more remote steps in the system—mainly those that involve the adrenal cortex or related feedback mechanisms—there are already signs that at least some attention might shift to the initial steps, those involving the CRH (or corticotropin-releasing factor [CRF]) functions. CRH putatively plays a major role in the stress response as well as in the translation of acute and chronic stress to depression (Nemeroff 1992). A CRH antagonist has been recently studied in animals. This compound, α-helical CRF_{9-41}, which acts on the CRF receptor, has been shown (Heinrichs et al. 1994) to reduce stress behavior in animals. Two other CRF analogues also were reported to antagonize CRF-mediated stress-induced behavioral changes in rats (Menzaghi et al. 1994). The picture here is complex because CRF might be involved in the pathobiology of some depressions as well as anxiety disorders, and its influence might or might not be derived by driving lower steps in the LHPA cascade. This complexity is also demonstrated by elucidation of the role of the pituitary hormone adrenocorticotropic hormone (ACTH). An analogue to $ACTH_{4-9}$, ORG 2766 was developed with the assumption that it will be an anxiolytic, but this has not been the case (Den Boer et al. 1992). On the other hand, several components of the pro-opiomelanocortin molecule, including $ACTH_{4-9}$, might have cognitive effects, and not necessarily mood effects (DeWied and Jolles 1992).

It remains unclear whether interventions in different levels of the LHPA system would induce different mood and behavior results, because each of the LHPA system components probably has an independent direct psychotropic effect as well as indirect effects that result from its influence on other steps in the system. It is premature to attempt to distinguish among these effects, but the interest and thrust in this area are promising.

THYROID HORMONES

The thyroid hormone tetraiodothyronine (thyroxine; T_4) and its active metabolite 3,5,5-triiodothyronine (T_3) are the peripheral products of the hypothalamic-pituitary-thyroid (HPT) system. Normally, these hormones are in a homeostatically balanced state with the hypothalamic hormone thyrotropin-releasing hormone, which regulates the secretion of the pituitary thyroid–stimulating hormone. The three main steps in this axis influence one another by a series of feedback loops. Abnormalities of the HPT system have been shown to be associated with dysphoria. Hypothyroidism has been reported (e.g., Asher 1949) to be associated with retarded depression; and hyperthyroidism, with anxiety, irritation, and increased energy. The similarities between disorders of the HPT axis and affective disorders have been well-noted (e.g., M. S. Gold et al. 1981; Prange et al. 1969), and the value of treatment trials with thyroid hormones and of thyroid hormones as adjuncts to TCAs was noted already in the early 1960s (Prange 1963). Some of the rationale for such treatment has been the notion that some depressed patients, especially women, have relative hypothyroidism, or subclinical hypothyroidism (Haggerty et al. 1993; Wenzel et al. 1974), which might be a trait of this subgroup and make them more vulnerable to depression.

Much of the existing data on the use of thyroid hormones as antidepressants were accumulated by Prange and his colleagues (Prange, in press) and later by Whybrow and colleagues (Whybrow 1996).

T_3 by itself probably is not beneficial as an antidepressant and causes intolerable thyrotoxicity (Prange et al. 1976). We are unaware of early studies with T_4 alone, but in a single study (Gjessing and Jenner 1976), T_4 was used to treat "periodic catatonia" with moderate success. This issue is not clear yet. To my knowledge, at least one ongoing current study addresses the possibility of stand-alone T_4 as treatment for depression.

A body of literature indicates that thyroid hormones are effective as adjuncts to antidepressants and that they enhance antidepressant activity, accelerate rate of response, and decrease treatment resistance. The accumulated literature is convincing that 25–50 mg of T_3 is very effective as an adjunct to TCA when added to TCA nonresponders (Aronson et al. 1996). Of special interest is the short period, 1 week, that is necessary for the T_3

added effect. T_3 also accelerates time to response to TCA of patients with depression who are not necessarily nonresponders, especially women (Prange et al. 1976, 1984). Data on the effects of T_4 are more scarce, as are data on the use of T_4 or T_3 as adjuncts to monoamine oxidase inhibitors or to SSRIs.

It is worthwhile noting that the combined treatment of T_4 and lithium for patients with rapid-cycling bipolar disorder is reported to be more effective than lithium alone (Whybrow 1994), whereas T_4 by itself is not effective and in high dosages may even cause hypomania or manic states.

The mechanisms by which thyroid hormones enhance antidepressant activity are still unknown. It is of interest that thyroid hormone increases net activity of several neurotransmitters that are putatively involved in the pathophysiology of depression in a way that is descriptively similar to that of estrogens. Receptors for the two hormones belong to the same superfamily. As was previously mentioned (Pfaff 1996), these issues are currently being explored, and clarifications are expected shortly.

MELATONIN

Melatonin is synthesized from serotonin in the pineal gland. Melatonin's main synthesizing and production-limiting enzyme is N-acetyltransferase, which is under regulation of norepinephrine and is substantially influenced by darkness. Light decreases its production (for review, R. J. Reiter, in press a, in press b). Melatonin crosses the blood-brain barrier, and melatonin-specific membrane (Reppert et al. 1995) and nucleus (Carlberg and Wiesenberg 1995) receptors have been demonstrated in the brain. Direct free radical scavenging action of the hormone has also been reported (R. J. Reiter et al. 1995).

The finding that the influence of light on melatonin production is conveyed through the retinohypothalamus tract to the suprachiasmatic nuclei (which play an important role as endogenous circadian pacemakers, which, in their turn, influence rhythm in the paraventricular nuclei and, through sympathetic neurons, stimulate N-acetyltransferase in the pineal gland) was important to the understanding of that hormone. The involvement of the above pacemakers in the regulation of melatonin and its light-dark association naturally led to its study in situations where the light-dark rhythm or length is altered, such as seasonal affective disorder or the hormone involvement in the light therapy of this situation (for review, Lewy et al., in press). Later the hormone was studied as treatment for another situation, jet lag, that involves a substantial change in circadian rhythm and for which it has been the subject of much media publicity. Another related situation is adaptation to work shift (Sack et al. 1995). In both cases, melatonin is probably effective, but this has yet to be confirmed. If confirmed, effective dosages have to be adequately studied.

Because melatonin is sold over the counter and its production is not the subject of strict regulation as is that of prescribed medications, it is in wide use, but insufficient scientifically controlled information is available. Another consequence of the popularity and availability of the hormone is its use in a wide array of situations in which its efficacy has not been proven yet; for instance, as treatment for neurodegenerative diseases or as a sleep-inducing medication. It also has been tried as an antidepressant, but that effect is still unclear. The administration of melatonin to patients with bipolar depression, especially to rapid cyclers, is of interest, especially if its use is associated with the presumed decrease in nocturnal hormonal levels and increase in sensitivity to light (Lewy et al. 1985). The possibility that melatonin also serves as a stabilizer of rhythm in these patients is in accord with the homeostatic effect of several other hormones that have been previously discussed here.

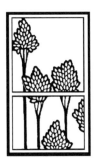

CHAPTER 18

Mechanisms and Management of Treatment-Resistant Depression

John P. O'Reardon, M.D., and
Jay D. Amsterdam, M.D.

As the selective serotonin reuptake inhibitors (SSRIs) have become widely prescribed in primary care settings, the clinical efforts of psychiatrists are increasingly being focused more on patients with treatment-resistant depression (TRD). Viewed in a broader framework (i.e., failure to achieve complete remission of depressive symptoms), TRD characterizes most patients treated in the primary care setting, as well as by psychiatrists. Treatment resistance may be defined at a simple, but practical, level as a failure of the patient to respond sufficiently to a treatment known to be effective for depression. When taken in this context, some level of treatment resistance is the norm rather than the exception. Only approximately 30% of patients will have a full response, that is, will be "cured" of their depressive episode; approximately 30%–50% will experience only a partial response; and approximately 20% will have no response at all (Fawcett 1994; Roose et al. 1986). Many patients who have heretofore been considered as having successful outcomes in the framework of clinical trials (i.e., those with a reduction in baseline values in the Hamilton Rating Scale for Depression [M. Hamilton 1960] of 50% or more) may still have substantial residual symptoms. Thus, the comforting statistic of a 60%–70% response rate to this or that antidepressant has lulled physicians into a false sense of security. In this regard, morbidity and potential mortality rates remain substantial, even in patients with more mild symptoms of depression. In addition, when one takes into account the high relapse rates during maintenance treatment, it is clear that most patients with either unipolar or bipolar depression display at some point in the course of their illness some degree of treatment resistance. Thus, the study of TRD must be of critical importance to all clinicians.

TRD can best be conceptualized as occurring along a continuum rather than as an all or none phenomenon. Some patients have a relatively low level of therapy resistance, which can be easily handled in practice by straightforward clinical procedures; other patients will follow a much more malignant course. From longitudinal studies (Keller et al. 1992), it is now clear that as many as 15% of patients with depression follow a long-term course and eventually become treatment resistant to almost all antidepressants.

DEFINITION OF TREATMENT-RESISTANT DEPRESSION

Research in this field has been significantly hampered by the lack of consensus on a clear definition of TRD, resulting in studies of patients with widely varying levels of prior treatment resistance, making the studies not readily comparable. In addition, the goalposts have been shifting over the years, and what was considered adequate treatment 20 years ago is considered inadequate today. In 1974, the World Psychiatric Association in its symposium on TRD proposed that the definition of TRD be divided into terms of *absolute* and *relative* treatment resistance. *Absolute* TRD was defined as failure of one adequate antidepressant trial, defined as 4 weeks of imipramine therapy at 150 mg/day or its equivalent. In contrast, *relative* TRD was applied to patients failing an inadequate antidepressant trial (Heimann 1974). This latter definition is clearly illogical, as a condition can hardly be conceived of as resistant to treatment when no adequate treatment has been administered. These patients can better be construed as having a "pseudo" TRD and not relative resistance. Table 18–1 outlines a putative schema for classifying TRD, as proposed by Thase and Rush (1997), from a genuine but relatively mild level of TRD, stage I, in which a patient has failed a single adequate antidepressant

TABLE 18-1. A simple system for staging antidepressant resistance

Stage I	Failure of at least one adequate trial of one major class of antidepressants
Stage II	Failure of at least two adequate trials of at least two distinctly different classes of antidepressant
Stage III	Stage II resistance plus failure of an adequate trial of a TCA
Stage IV	Stage III resistance plus failure of an adequate trial of an MAOI
Stage V	Stage IV resistance plus a course of bilateral ECT

Note. ECT = electroconvulsive therapy; MAOI = monoamine oxidase inhibitor; TCA = tricyclic antidepressant.
Source. Adapted from Thase and Rush 1997.

trial, to much more severe levels of TRD, stages IV and V, in which patients are resistant to multiple drug trials and even electroconvulsive therapy (ECT). It is therefore helpful to "stage" the degree of TRD to better understand its relative severity and to determine appropriate future treatment algorithms.

WHAT IS AN ADEQUATE ANTIDEPRESSANT TRIAL?

The criteria for defining adequacy of treatment have become more stringent since 1974. Factors to be considered include dose, duration of treatment, and pharmacokinetic and pharmacodynamic issues. Initially it was felt that a 4-week trial at sufficient dose was adequate duration. Schatzberg et al. (1983) suggested that an adequate treatment would last a minimum of 3 weeks at two-thirds of the maximum recommended dose. In contrast, Quitkin et al. (1984) found that a substantial number of patients were late responders, that is, they responded between weeks 4 and 6, and that the proportion of responders increased from 33% at week 4 to 53% by week 6. Thus, an unimproved patient at week 4 still had a 40% chance of improving by week 6 (compared with a 12% chance on placebo). These investigators suggested that a minimum dose equivalent of imipramine at 300 mg/day or phenelzine at 90 mg/day be given for at least 6 weeks before concluding the presence of TRD (Quitkin 1985). Although this finding has been questioned on the basis that the upward titration of medication dose had been slow in these studies, nevertheless these findings have been influential. At this point, 6 weeks is taken as the minimal duration necessary to judge response in the majority of clinical trials (M. Fava and Davidson 1996). Some have argued for even longer duration to ensure adequacy. For instance, Greenhouse et al. (1987) found a 50% response in patients with major depression after 10 weeks of treatment with imipramine at 150–300 mg/day; patient response then increased to 75% after 17 weeks of medication. Applying this research to clinical reality, it may be difficult for the clinician, when faced with a nonresponding patient, to persist beyond 4 weeks at full dosage in the complete absence of any response; and, for patients who respond partially, the clinician may well elect to extend the trial rather than switch medications.

Over the past two decades, a consensus has emerged that aggressive dosing is necessary. Now there seems to be general agreement that 300 mg/day equivalent of imipramine or 90 mg/day equivalent of phenelzine constitutes an adequate trial (Ravaris et al. 1976; G. M. Simpson et al. 1976). However, because of compliance differences and individual pharmacokinetic differences, dosing ranges need to be bolstered by blood levels wherever therapeutic ranges have been established. Although plasma level ranges for some tricyclic antidepressants (TCAs) (nortriptyline, amitriptyline, desipramine) have been established (Hollister 1979), and for monoamine oxidase inhibitors (MAOIs) a level of platelet MAO inhibition of at least 80% has been suggested (D. S. Robinson et al. 1978), as yet, little consensus exists on the value of SSRI plasma levels (Amsterdam et al. 1997).

For the SSRIs, it remains unclear as to the best approach to dosing and treatment duration. Schweizer et al. (1990) showed that there was no significant difference in response rates if nonresponders to fluoxetine at 20 mg at 3 weeks were randomly selected to fluoxetine at either 20 or 60 mg/day for a further 5 weeks (response rates of 49% versus 50%, respectively), illustrating that at least for the first 8 weeks the "tincture of time" may be more important than dosage increase. Whether the dose-response curve remains flat for patients beyond that time is unclear. M. Fava (1992) did find that more than 80% of patients resistant at 8 weeks to fluoxetine 20 mg/day did respond when the dose was raised to 40 mg/day. These two findings may be reconciled by taking the view that time is more important than increasing the dose for the early nonresponders, but for persistent nonresponders there appears to be an advantage in pushing the dose to 40 mg/day. As yet, no analogous data exist to guide the clinician with respect to treating TRD with paroxetine and sertraline.

In summary then, the first stage of valid treatment resistance can be defined as when the patient fails to respond to a trial of an antidepressant for at least 6 weeks, meeting the dosing requirements as outlined above. Beyond this, little consensus exists on how to define further stages of TRD and/or treatment adequacy. Some researchers have leaned on the number of prior failed treatment trials, including those with antidepressants from different classes (Amsterdam and Berwish 1987, 1989; Fawcett and Kravitz 1985; Schatzberg et al. 1986), usually defining resistance as failure of at least two antidepressant trials. Malizia and Bridges (1992) classified treatment resistance based on depressive subtype: major depression without psychosis, major depression with psychosis, and bipolar depression. Feighner et al. (1985) included duration (at least 2 years) of the depressive episode as well, whereas others would not consider a patient as treatment resistant without a trial of ECT (M. Fink 1987, 1991).

Nierenberg et al. (1994b), in their study with venlafaxine, used rigorous criteria to define what could be considered an advanced stage of TRD. Patients had to have failed at least three adequate drug trials with antidepressants from two different classes, at least one of which had to be a tricyclic, plus an augmentation trial. A course of ECT counted toward a single trial. Table 18–2, adapted from Nierenberg et al. (1994b), outlines criteria for adequacy of antidepressant treatment, with a duration of 4–6 weeks accepted as "probably" adequate and 6 weeks required for a "definitely" adequate trial of a therapy. Finally, a series of consensus meetings to define TRD have been held in Europe to bring standardization to the field. Ultimately, a clear advantage of agreement of the clinical staging of TRD will be the more precise identification of homogeneous patient populations with TRD at discrete levels of severity to whom systematic treatment algorithms can then be applied.

MECHANISMS OF TREATMENT RESISTANCE

The many factors that may result in treatment resistance may be considered under adequacy of treatment issues, diagnostic issues in subtyping of depression, psychiatric comorbidity, medical mimics of depression, medical factors contributing to depression, and possibly iatrogenic factors, namely, decreasing response over time to each new treatment (Amsterdam et al. 1994b). Finally, evidence is emerging that in the future some biological markers may be indices and predictors of treatment resistance.

ADEQUACY OF TREATMENT CONSIDERATIONS OR PSEUDORESISTANCE TO TREATMENT

As indicated in the above discussion, many patients initially labeled as treatment resistant have not received adequate treatment. Schatzberg et al.

TABLE 18–2.   Criteria for adequacy of antidepressant trials

Treatment	Daily dose	
	Definite adequacy (duration > 6 weeks)	Probable adequacy (duration between 4 and 6 weeks)
Tricyclics		
IMI, DMI	> 250 mg (or plasma levels > 125 ng/mL) DMI > 200 ng/mL IMI	200–249 mg
Nortriptyline	> 100 mg (or plasma levels in 50–150 ng/mL range)	75–99 mg
AMI, doxepin	> 250 mg	200–249 mg
Protriptyline	> 60 mg	40–59 mg
MAOIs		
Phenelzine	> 60 mg	45–59 mg
Tranylcypromine	> 40 mg	30–39 mg
Fluoxetine	> 20 mg	5–19 mg
Bupropion	> 400 mg	300–399 mg
Trazodone	> 300 mg	200–299 mg
Lithium	(Plasma level 0.7–1.1 mEq/L)	(Level 0.4–0.69 mEq/L)
ECT	(> 12 total, at least 6 bilateral)	(> 9–11 unilateral)
Augmenting agents		
Lithium	(Plasma level 0.7–1.1 mEq/L)	D-Amphetamine 10 mg
T_4	0.1 mg	Methylphenidate 15 mg
T_3	25 µg	L-Tryptophan 2.0 g

Note.   AMI = amitriptyline; DMI = desipramine; ECT = electroconvulsive therapy; IMI = imipramine; MAOI = monoamine oxidase inhibitor; T_3 = triiodothyronine; T_4 = thyroxine.
Source.   Adapted from Nirenberg et al. 1994b.

(1983) studied the records of 110 patients with depression referred because of treatment resistance. Only 39% of the 170 antidepressant trials were judged to be adequate (two-thirds of maximum recommended dose for 4 weeks). Community-based studies reveal that less than 50% receive adequate dosing or treatment duration (Nelsen and Dunner 1993). Moreover, many family practitioners and general psychiatrists rarely prescribe MAOIs (Clary et al. 1990), even though research supports their use preferentially in atypical depression. These and other considerations result in many patients being prematurely labeled as treatment resistant. Until the patient has had at least one adequate medication trial, his or her depressive episode cannot be classed as TRD or, restating the obvious, a patient is only resistant to treatment after some adequate treatment has been given.

Moreover, what is adequate treatment for one patient may not be adequate for another because of diagnostic, pharmacokinetic, and pharmacodynamic considerations. Often what has been called a treatment failure turns out to be treatment intolerance, as the patient failed to tolerate an adequate dose for sufficient duration to receive any benefit. It has been estimated that approximately 20% of cases called treatment resistant are instead treatment intolerant (Schatzberg at al. 1983). The vast majority of intolerant drug trials are, as one would expect, inadequate trials—92% in the study by Schatzberg et al. (1983). So the first task of the clinician is to distinguish what is resistance from what was inadequate treatment for whatever reason. In this way, the group that is pseudoresistant to treatment can be identified and managed appropriately.

DIAGNOSTIC CONSIDERATIONS

Depressive Subtype

Major depression represents a syndrome of different etiologies. Thus, various depressive subtypes may respond differently to different treatments. Unfortunately, to date, no litmus test for matching the depressive subtype to the appropriate treatment has been identified. Therefore, what we now call stage I TRD may often be more accurately construed as treatment mismatching.

Atypical depression. DSM-IV (American Psychiatric Association 1994) defines atypical depression as characterized by mood reactivity and at least two of the following features: significant weight gain or increase in appetite, hypersomnia, leaden paralysis (i.e., a heavy leaden feeling in the arms or legs), and a long-standing pattern of interpersonal rejection sensitivity. In the study by Liebowitz et al. (1984) of 119 patients meeting criteria for atypical depression, phenelzine was compared with imipramine and placebo over 6 weeks. The best response was observed with phenelzine (71%) versus imipramine (50%) and placebo (28%). A subsequent study by McGrath et al. (1987) compared imipramine (200–300 mg/day) with phenelzine (60–90 mg/day) in a double-blind crossover design. Nonresponders to imipramine were almost twice as likely to respond to a subsequent 6-week trial of phenelzine (65%) versus continued treatment with imipramine (29%), supporting the earlier observation that patients with atypical depression may respond preferentially to MAOIs. Yet how many clinicians would use an MAOI as a first-line treatment for their patients with atypical depression?

Bipolar depression. Few controlled data exist to guide the specifics of treatment with bipolar depression. Several studies suggest that MAOIs may be more effective than TCAs (F. K. Goodwin and Roy-Byrne 1987; Nierenberg and Amsterdam 1990). Also, a substantial literature suggests that, for bipolar depression, lithium may be an effective antidepressant. J. C. Nelson and Mazure (1986) examined 30 delusional patients with depression (21 unipolar, 9 bipolar) who did not respond to 3 or more weeks of treatment with desipramine plus an antipsychotic. Twenty-one of the 30 patients had a 1- to 2-week trial of lithium augmentation, with 8 of 9 (89%) patients with bipolar depression responding versus only 3 of 12 (25%) patients with unipolar depression responding. Although the trial of desipramine and an antipsychotic drug can be considered to be too brief, the substantial response in the group with bipolar depression suggests that lithium was preferentially effective for patients with bipolar depression. Moreover, Himmelhoch et al. (1991) observed a superior treatment outcome with tranylcypromine (versus imipramine) in patients with bipolar I and II depression. Although clinicians are not likely to use MAOIs as a first-line drug for bipolar depression, Amsterdam et al. (1998) recently observed similar efficacy for fluoxetine monotherapy in 89 patients with bipolar II depression (versus 89 matched patients with unipolar depression) with a hypomanic switch rate of only 3.8%.

Major depression with psychotic features. Clear evidence exists that TCAs by themselves may be less effective in depression with psychotic features. A double-blind randomized study by Spiker at al. (1985) showed clear superiority for the combination of a amitriptyline plus perphenazine (78%) compared with perphenazine alone (41%). A review by Chan et al. (1987) revealed an overall response rate to TCAs of 67% in nondelusional patients with depression compared with only a 33% response rate in patients with depression and psychotic features. Although some analyses suggest that SSRIs may be effective in the treatment of psychotic depression (Nierenberg 1994), these data need to be confirmed in prospective studies. Given the low response rate to antidepressant monotherapy, some clinicians have suggested initiating ECT as a first-line therapy for TRD with psychosis rather than holding it in reserve as the final arbiter. It has been known since the 1960s that the presence of delusions is a positive predictor of response to ECT (Carney et al. 1965), with about an 80% response rate in this condition (Kroessler 1985).

PSYCHIATRIC COMORBIDITY CONSIDERATIONS

Many studies have reported the association between the presence of comorbid psychiatric conditions and TRD (Akiskal et al. 1982; D. W. Black et al. 1988a; Coryell et al. 1988; Fawcett and Kravitz 1988; Pfohl et al. 1984). It is often unclear clinically which came first. Nevertheless, the implications for treatment are to address both conditions simultaneously, regardless of the linkage, to avoid consolidating a TRD condition.

Comorbid anxiety and depressive features are common in clinical practice, and DSM-IV has included mixed anxiety-depression in its appendix of conditions needing nosological refinement. The presence of comorbid anxiety has prognostic implications. For example, prospective studies of patients with depression have found that the co-occurrence of panic attacks was correlated with a poor outcome (Coryell et al. 1988; van Valkenburg et al. 1984). Some evidence suggests that such patients do better with MAOIs. Likewise, patients with depression and obsessive-compulsive disorder may be more resistant to treatment, even with SSRIs (Hollander et al. 1991)

Similarly, covert substance abuse is also common in depression (Akiskal 1982; MacEwan and Remick 1988) and a leading cause of TRD. In a survey of 6,355 patients with substance abuse, M. S. Gold et al. (1994) found that 43.7% had a lifetime prevalence of major depression. Not only does comorbid substance abuse lead to TRD, but the presence of resulting hepatic disease alters antidepressant pharmacokinetics, making these patients more difficult to treat (Ciraulo and Jaffe 1981; Ciraulo et al. 1988; Mason and Kocsis 1991). In this regard, SSRIs may offer some advantages over other antidepressants. One recent study of alcoholic patients with depression found a modest advantage for an SSRI over a TCA (G. Invernizzi et al. 1994).

Comorbid personality disorders have long been associated with TRD and a poor response to antidepressant treatment. For example, Pfohl et al. (1984) observed only a 16% response rate in inpatients with comorbid depression and personality disorder compared with a 50% response rate in patients with pure depression. Similar results were reported from a study by D. W. Black et al. (1987), in which, with the use of ECT in addition to a TCA, the response rate among those with a comorbid Axis II disorder was lower, 42% compared with a 60% recovery in those without Axis II pathology. The best approach for these patients may be a combination of psychotherapy and medication. This approach was recently borne out by the Treatment of Depression Collaborative Research Project (Shea et al. 1990), which found that cognitive-behavioral therapy yielded a better response than either impramine or interpersonal therapy. Finally, other disorders such as comorbid sleep apnea (James et al. 1991) have sometimes been associated with chronic TRD.

MEDICAL COMORBIDITY CONSIDERATIONS

Unrecognized Medical Problems

Organic factors may cause or contribute to affective illness in up to 50% of patients (Hall et al. 1981). In a patient with TRD, it is critical to rule out the presence of underlying medical disorders (Akiskal 1982; MacEwan and Remick 1988). Moreover, iatrogenic depression may result from the coadministration of medications for acute and chronic medical illnesses (Metzger and Friedman 1994). A partial list of organic causes of TRD with references is presented in Table 18–3.

Among medical causes of depression, the most frequent appear to be endocrine, particularly thyroid (M. S. Gold et al. 1981; Prange et al. 1990). Grade I, or clinically overt, hypothyroidism will manifest depression in up to 40% of cases (Jain 1972), but even subtler subclinical grades of hypothyroidism may also contribute. These are grade II, in which only thyroid-stimulating hormone (TSH) is elevated (with normal thyroxine [T_4] and triiodothyronine [T_3]), and grade III, in which T_4, T_3, and TSH are all normal, and the only abnormality is a TSH rise above normal in response to a thyrotropin-releasing hormone (TRH) stimulation test (Gorman and Hatterer 1994; Joffe and Levitt 1992; Targum et al. 1984). Hyperthyroidism is a less common cause of depression (Gadde and Krishnan 1994). Overall, uncontrolled studies suggest a high frequency of thyroid dysfunction in patients with refractory depression compared with unselected populations with depression (Howland 1993). Hypothalamic-pituitary-adrenocortical (HPA) axis dysfunction with elevated cortisol is also frequently reported in depression followed by normalization of the axis after remission of depression (Amsterdam et al. 1989a, 1989b, 1994a, 1994b; P. W. Gold et al. 1986, 1988a, 1988b). Moreover, Reus and Berlant (1986) estimated that 40%–90% of patients with Cushing's syndrome will manifest affective disturbances—in particular, depression. Neurological disorders, both cortical and subcortical, have been associated with depression. An important cortical cause is poststroke depression, in which vulnerability to depression seems to correlate with proximity of the lesion to the anterior part of the left hemisphere (Cummings 1994). In some clinical situations, the onset of depression may

TABLE 18-3. Medical illnesses associated with treatment-resistant depression

Illness	References
Endocrine diseases	
Hypothyroidism and hyperthyroidism	Gadde and Krishnan 1994; Jain 1972; Joffe and Levitt 1992; Reus 1993; Targum et al. 1984
Hypoadrenalism and hyperadrenalism	Amsterdam et al. 1987a, 1987b; P. W. Gold et al. 1986, 1988a, 1988b; Hornig-Rohan et al. 1994; Reus and Berlant 1986
Neurological disorders	
Strokes	Cummings 1994
Parkinson's disease	Cummings 1992; Hantz et al. 1994
Huntington's disease	Lishman 1987b
Seizure disorders	Himmelhoch 1984
Dementias, brain tumors, multiple sclerosis	Caplan and Ahmed 1992; Skuster et al. 1992
Neoplasms	
Pancreatic carcinoma	A. I. Green and Austin 1993
Lymphoma, bronchogenic carcinoma	Lishman 1998
Infectious diseases	
AIDS	G. R. Brown and Rundell 1993
Influenza, Epstein-Barr virus	Lishman 1987a
Lyme disease	J. F. Jones 1993

be a harbinger of a malignant process, as with pancreatic cancer, in which up to two-thirds of patients experience psychiatric symptoms before local symptoms of the tumor (A. I. Green and Austin 1993).

THERAPEUTIC DECREMENT

A *therapeutic decrement* may be inherent in the repeated application of antidepressant treatments. In this context, patients who are repeatedly treated with antidepressants appear to become increasingly more resistant to subsequent treatment strategies, including ECT (Amsterdam et al. 1994b). A number of clinical and biochemical factors, including progressive virulence of recurrent depressive episodes, reduced plasticity of neuronal receptor regulatory mechanisms, and the development of secondary (and even tertiary depressive syndromes) in individuals with chronic depression, may contribute to this condition. Several clinical conditions appear to characterize the syndrome of therapeutic decrement (Table 18–4).

Clinical observations have shown that patients with inadequate response to multiple treatments appear to become increasingly resistant to successive antidepressant trials (Amsterdam et al. 1994b; Nierenberg et al. 1994b; Thase and Rush 1997). In a review of sequential treatment strategies, Thase and Rush (1997) point out that patients who have failed to respond to an initial SSRI will have only a 48% response to a subsequent trial with another SSRI. Similarly, in a prospective trial of venlafaxine in patients with stages IV and V TRD, Nierenberg et al. (1994b) observed a 42% response rate in stage IV patients and only a 15% response rate in stage V patients who did not respond to ECT.

The likelihood of producing progressive treatment resistance has recently been further supported in a study of 149 patients with depression who received fixed-dose fluoxetine 20 mg daily for at least 6 weeks, 84 (56%) of whom had received prior antidepressant therapy (Amsterdam and Maislin 1994). A multivariate logistic regression analysis was undertaken to identify clinical predictors of fluoxetine response. Odds ratios were generated to estimate the likelihood of a clinical factor to predict a good outcome to fluoxetine therapy. Although none predicted a good outcome to fluoxetine therapy, the variable "number of prior treatments" predicted a negative outcome to treatment (parameter estimate = -0.22, odds ratio = 0.80, $P < .03$). Thus, with each prior treatment received, the likelihood of responding to the next antidepressant diminished by about 20%. These disturbing data support the 30% decrement suggested by Thase and Rush (1997) in their review. Given that a pattern of progressive treatment resistance may be established early in therapy, these observations indicate that adequate and aggressive therapy be rendered in the initial stages of antidepressant therapy and that treatment be continued indefinitely in patients with multiple prior drug trials.

TABLE 18–4.   Syndromes characterized by therapeutic decrement

Progressive treatment resistance to successive antidepressant drug trials

Progressive drug intolerance to successive antidepressant drug trials

Antidepressant tachyphylaxis ("poop out") or partial relapse during maintenance therapy

Loss of efficacy on switching antidepressants caused by adverse events

BIOLOGICAL PREDICTORS OF TREATMENT RESPONSE

Dexamethasone Suppression Test

Early reports suggested that an abnormal overnight 1-mg dexamethasone suppression test (DST) result might be associated with "biochemical" depression (Carroll et al. 1968; Stokes et al. 1975). Although more recent studies have attempted to use the DST as a predictor of antidepressant response (Amsterdam et al. 1983; Arana et al. 1985; Georgotas et al. 1986), a meta-analysis of 28 predictive DST studies found no relationship (Ribeiro et al. 1993). However, other tests of HPA axis function, such as the corticotropin-releasing hormone and the adrenocorticotropic hormone (ACTH) stimulation tests (Amsterdam et al. 1987a, 1987c), tomographic and magnetic resonance imaging volume estimates of the adrenal glands (Amsterdam et al. 1987b; Nemeroff et al. 1992) and pituitary glands (Axelson et al. 1992), may in the future provide biological markers for TRD and/or antidepressant response.

Thyrotropin-Releasing Hormone Stimulation Test

Similarly, TRH stimulation test abnormalities have been demonstrated in 25%–40% of patients in studies of thyrotropin (TSH) response to TRH stimulation (Kirkegaard 1981; Winokur et al. 1983). Krog-Meyer et al. (1985) and Winokur et al. (1989) suggested that change in TSH after repeat TRH stimulation tests predicts difference in long-term treatment outcome. G. Langer et al. (1986) also observed a relationship between pretreatment TSH value and clinical outcome, with a 36% 1-year relapse rate in patients with a persistently blunted TSH response. More recently, however, we (Amsterdam et al. 1995b) found no association between response to fluoxetine and change in TRH test results in outcome in response to long-term fluoxetine treatment.

Brain Imaging

Finally, brain imaging techniques may be useful in characterizing TRD. For example, the technique of single photon emission computed tomography (SPECT) or positron-emission tomography with various radioligands has been used to investigate TRD. In one study, [123I]iodoamphetamine SPECT demonstrated asymmetry in the temporal lobe area. Increased [123I]iodoamphetamine activity in the right anterior temporal lobe was found in 63% of patients with depression (12/19) compared with 8% of medical comparison subjects (1/12) ($P < .005$) (Amsterdam and Mozley 1992). The ^{123}I asymmetry seemed to be more evident in patients with TRD. A "normalization" of temporal lobe [^{123}I]iodoamphetamine asymmetry was noted to occur after clinical improvement in TRD patients (Amsterdam et al. 1995/1996). A more recent controlled SPECT study with ^{99m}Tc-hexamethylpropyleneamine oxime (^{99m}Tc-HMPAO), a putative cerebral blood flow marker, in patients with and without TRD indicated bilateral increases in the hippocampus and amygdala in patients with TRD (Hornig et al. 1997). Thus, various sites in the limbic circuitry, including the entire temporal lobe, the hippocampus and amygdala, may mediate treatment refractoriness in certain patients with TRD.

TREATMENT ALGORITHMS

There are as many approaches to treating TRD as there are antidepressants available. More than 300 potential treatment options are available. However, given the possibility of a substantial therapeutic decrement, it is imperative to apply adequate aggressive treatments early in therapy.

We recommend the application of systematic treatment algorithms, which represent a method of clinical decision making driven by a logical, stepped-care approach. Algorithms are intended to limit or attenuate therapeutic decrement in the absence of specific predictors of treatment response. Until recently, most algorithms for treating TRD started with TCAs as first-line drugs (Amsterdam and Hornig-Rohan 1996; Nierenberg and Amsterdam 1990).

OPTIMIZATION

Optimization strategies refer to maximizing the dose and/or treatment duration of the current medication. Unfortunately, little consensus on these parameters exists. Table 18–1 presents suggested criteria for determination of trial adequacy.

Optimization of Treatment Duration

Inadequate treatment duration is a rarely considered cause of TRD (Keller et al. 1982a, 1982b, 1982c). In the context of TRD, a 4- to 6-week trial is inadequate to determine potential treatment efficacy. Most outcome studies have found only a 25%–30% remission rate by week 6 of treatment. Georgotas et al. (1989) observed a mean time to clinical response with nortriptyline to be 6 weeks, with patients with severe depression taking longer. These investigators attributed the delay in response to the presence of low doses (and plasma levels) in the early weeks of treatment. Moreover, Greenhouse et al. (1987) observed increasing remission rates during progressively longer treatment duration in patients taking adequate doses (and plasma levels) of imipramine beyond 4 weeks. Thus, remission rates rose from 25% after 4 weeks to 50% by 3 months and 89% by 6 months of therapy. Therefore, it appears that a longer duration of treatment (at adequate dosage) is associated with a greater response rate.

Optimization of Dosage and Plasma Concentrations

Many patients with TRD receive inadequate doses of antidepressant medication. Dosage optimization must be achieved (along with therapeutic plasma levels, where available) in patients with TRD. For some TCAs, therapeutic plasma level ranges have been identified whereby antidepressant efficacy can be maximized (Amsterdam at al. 1980). Steady-state plasma levels are, however, partially dependent on the metabolic half-life of each medication, taking approximately 5–6 half-lives to reach steady-state plasma concentrations. Given that there is a 30-fold range of steady-state plasma levels among individuals taking antidepressants (Amsterdam et al. 1980; Åsberg 1976), it would be likely that some patients may have TRD as a result of less than optimal plasma concentrations.

AUGMENTATION

Lithium

The addition of lithium to a failed antidepressant trial is rapidly becoming a standard operational procedure, with studies supporting its efficacy in TRD (de Montigny 1994). Although it is hypothesized that lithium augmentation enhances serotonergic neurotransmission, its mechanism of action is unknown, and lithium appears to be equally effective when added to noradrenergic agents (L. H. Price et al. 1986). Latency of response to lithium augmentation may range from several days to as much as 6 weeks (de Montigny 1994). Attempts to identify predictors of response to lithium augmentation have been unsuccessful, with the exception of the report by J. C. Nelson and Mazure (1986) that delusional patients with bipolar depression may be more responsive to lithium augmentation than patients with unipolar depression may be. However, in spite of these shortcomings, lithium augmentation is rapidly becoming the standard first-line strategy for TRD.

Thyroid Hormones

The addition of thyroid hormone to a failed antidepressant trial has also received much attention. T_3 augmentation has been employed more often than T_4. After obtaining baseline thyroid function laboratory tests, T_3 is typically initiated at 25 µg/day and then increased to 50 µg/day, depending on the clinical response. T_3 augmentation has been successfully used with a variety of antidepressants (Gorman and Hatterer 1994; Joffe and Levitt 1993). Although the literature suggests that T_3 may be superior to T_4 in TRD, comparative efficacy has received limited attention. One randomized, double-blind comparison of T_3 and T_4 augmentation in patients unresponsive to TCA showed superior efficacy with T_3 versus T_4 (Joffe and Singer 1990). In contrast, high-dose T_4 augmentation and T_4 monotherapy at hypermetabolic levels have been shown to diminish rapid-cycling bipolar episodes (Gorman and Hatterer 1994; Joffe and Levitt 1993).

Selective Serotonin Reuptake Inhibitor Augmenting Agents

Several open trials have investigated agents, including buspirone (a partial serotonin type 1A agonist) and pindolol (a β-blocker and antagonist of presynaptic serotonin type 1A autoreceptors), that are thought to enhance serotonin neurotransmission. Joffe and Schuller (1993) examined buspirone efficacy in TRD patients taking either fluvoxamine or fluoxetine for more than 5 weeks. Buspirone (20–50 mg/day) was added for an additional 3 weeks. A marked or complete response was observed in 17 of 25 patients with TRD (Joffe and Schuller 1993). Similarly, in a retrospective analysis, 6 of 14 (43%) patients with TRD (12 of whom had failed to respond to ECT) showed a "rapid and significant improvement" when buspirone was added to their SSRI (Bouwer and Stein 1997). Other reports have supported these observations (Bakish 1991; Jacobsen 1991).

Pindolol augmentation has also been used successfully with either SSRIs or MAOIs. Artigas et al. (1994) noted a 100% response in 12 patients given pindolol 2.5 mg three times a day along with an SSRI or an MAOI. Blier and Bergeron (1995) found that 7 of 9 patients without TRD who were given pindolol plus paroxetine responded and that 10 of 19 patients with TRD who were given pindolol and a SSRI or MAOI responded. To date, only one double-blind study with pindolol versus placebo has been performed (Perez et al.

1997). After 6 weeks of treatment, 41 of 55 (75%) patients given fluoxetine plus pindolol versus 33 of 56 (59%) patients given fluoxetine plus placebo responded ($P = .04$). Interestingly, no difference was found in the speed of onset of response. Although not limited to patients with TRD, these data do suggest a putative efficacy for patients who are nonresponsive to SSRIs.

Combinations

The combination of two antidepressants with different modes of action has long been suggested for the management of TRD. The combination of a TCA with an SSRI and the addition of an MAOI to a failed TCA trial have emerged as two common strategies for treating TRD. Yet there are few controlled studies directly assessing the efficacy of drug combinations in TRD (M. Fava et al. 1994; Pande et al. 1991). In this regard, the efficacy of MAOI/TCA combinations in TRD has not been well established in controlled studies. Yet a substantial proportion of TCA nonresponders will benefit from the cautious addition of an MAOI. Moreover, the tolerability of the MAOI/TCA combination, although less frequently used, has been found to be similar to that of the MAOI and TCA alone (Pande et al. 1991; Razani et al. 1983). However, the combination of clomipramine and an MAOI is fraught with the risk of serotonin syndrome and should generally be avoided (Amsterdam et al. 1995a). More commonly, drug combinations are applied to a failed SSRI monotherapy trial. Most studies suggest that the addition of a TCA or lithium to an SSRI may enhance efficacy (M. Fava et al. 1994). However, a recent double-blind study compared the addition of desipramine (50 mg/day) or lithium (600 mg/day) to fluoxetine (20 mg/day) versus increasing the fluoxetine to 60 mg/day (M. Fava et al. 1994). The best outcome was seen in the patients with TRD whose fluoxetine dose was increased.

High-Dose Antidepressant Therapy

Therapeutic plasma level ranges have been established for several TCAs. Thus, it is now relatively easy to achieve adequate TCA dosing based on plasma level determination. However, because of the potentially serious cardiotoxicity for exceeding established therapeutic ranges, little justification exists for pursuing high-dose TCA therapy beyond established ranges. This paradigm does not necessarily follow for other antidepressant agents. For example, 16 of 22 patients with TRD responded when trazodone was administered at doses higher than 600 mg daily (Wheatley 1980). Similarly, tranylcypromine may also be effective in TRD. In one open study, Amsterdam

(1991) administered up to 180 mg/day in 14 patients with severe TRD. These investigators observed substantial response in 50% of patients. Moreover, no hypertensive events were observed, and the most common adverse event to be seen was hypotension (which usually attenuated at the higher dosage range, >90 mg/day).

More recently, an open label study with venlafaxine in patients with TRD, who were nonresponsive to an average of five prior adequate treatments including various augmentation strategies and ECT, demonstrated almost a 40% response at a dose of 300–450 mg/day (Nierenberg et al. 1994b).

NOVEL TREATMENT STRATEGIES FOR TREATMENT-RESISTANT DEPRESSION

As our knowledge expands regarding potential etiologies of TRD, additional treatment approaches have been developed. One recent strategy involves reducing cortisol production by manipulating HPA axis function in TRD (Amsterdam et al. 1994a). Hypercortisolemia may play a pathophysiological role in major depression, particularly in TRD. Attempts have been made to lower cortisol levels in TRD by inhibiting its synthesis in the adrenal gland. Ghadirian et al. (1995) administered either ketoconazole or aminoglutethimide (in combination with metyrapone) to 20 patients with TRD and observed a 65% response rate. Similar results were reported by Thakore and Dinan (1995) in 8 patients treated with ketoconazole for 4 weeks, and these observations have been confirmed by others (B. E. P. Murphy et al. 1991; Wolkowitz et al. 1993). Recently, however, Amsterdam et al. (1994a) stratified patients with TRD into those with and without hypercortisolemia and found only modest response during ketoconazole augmentation in 2 of the 10 patients with hypercortisolemia.

Anticonvulsants and Partial Anticonvulsants

Well known for their clinical role as antimanic agents, anticonvulsants such as carbamazepine and valproate have also been used in both bipolar and unipolar TRD (Post et al. 1994a, 1994b). In one series, Post et al. (1994a) found a greater response in patients with bipolar (15/40) versus those with unipolar (2/17) TRD. Open studies of valproate also suggest limited antidepressant efficacy, but only a paucity of data with anticonvulsants on TRD exists. More recently, in open trials, lamotrigine (a partial anticonvulsant that inhibits glutamate release) has been shown to have efficacy in bipolar TRD (Weisler et al. 1994), although other agents (such as the benzodiazepines) with anticonvulsant properties have not been carefully studied in TRD (Rickels et al. 1985). Finally, a variety of other agents have been used in TRD with variable success. These include *S*-adenosylmethionine (Janicak et al. 1989), reserpine, amphetamine, amino acids, and anxiolytics.

NONPHARMACOLOGICAL TREATMENTS

A range of nonpharmacological therapies for TRD have included ECT (M. Fink 1987, 1991), narcotherapy (Karazman et al. 1991), and psychosurgery (Ballantine et al. 1987). Of these, ECT has been consistently found effective in TRD. In fact, some investigators have suggested that patients do not have TRD unless they have failed a course of bilateral ECT (M. Fink 1987, 1991). However, there appears to be a lower response to ECT among patients with TRD compared with those with non-TRD, about 50% (Prudic et al. 1990), as well as the concern of rapid relapse in patients with TRD after successful ECT. Finally, there has been a revival of interest in the use of psychosurgical techniques in TRD (Ballantine et al. 1987). Selective stereotactic procedures have enabled neurosurgeons to undertake these surgical procedures with minimal postoperative morbidity. Although several patient series have suggested surgical approaches may be helpful in TRD (Ballantine et al. 1987; Bouckoms 1991), a careful analysis of Ballantine et al.'s (1987) large patient sample suggests that outcome in TRD with psychosurgical techniques is not superior to aggressive pharmacological intervention. Thus, although few controlled studies have been performed using nonpharmacological interventions for TRD, future controlled studies may clarify the role of these interventions in TRD. Lastly, treatment of the patient who is severely ill and resistant to treatment may sometimes, though rarely, include psychosurgical techniques. In one large prospective series, stereotactic bilateral cingulotomy was associated with low mortality, low morbidity, and substantial improvement in 65% of surgically treated patients with affective disorder (Ballantine et al. 1987).

Thus, although few controlled studies have been performed in well-characterized treatment-resistant populations, further studies using these techniques would prove useful in determining the role of these interventions in the treatment of refractory major depressive disorder.

CONCLUSION

This chapter represents a highly selective description of the most common clinical and biological factors contributing to TRD and has attempted to review some of the general strategies for managing TRD. Our ability to avoid or limit the occurrence of TRD has been expanding along with the application of new systematic treatment algorithms and a better understanding of the clinical and biological factors that contribute to TRD. The absence of specific biological markers that can reliably identify those patients who will go on to develop TRD and the failure of clinical variables to reliably predict the type of antidepressant to which particular patients will respond suggest that much work remains to be done. The developments of systematic diagnostic and treatment algorithms for TRD, critically tested in well-controlled prospective trials, will likely assist in eliminating much of the present confusion and therapeutic nihilism that currently characterize the field.

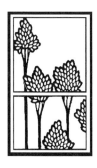

CHAPTER 19

Treatment of Psychotic Depression

Charles DeBattista, D.M.H., M.D.,
Joseph K. Belanoff, M.D., and
Alan F. Schatzberg, M.D.

Substantial evidence supports the theory that psychotic depression represents a distinct type of major depression (Schatzberg and Rothschild 1992). Statistically significant differences between psychotic and nonpsychotic major depression have been noted along many axes, including presenting features (Coryell et al. 1984; Frances et al. 1981; Glassman and Roose 1981; Lykouras et al. 1986; J. C. Nelson and Bowers 1978), biology (Carroll et al. 1976a; Coryell et al. 1982; Rihmer et al. 1984; Rudorfer et al. 1982), familial transmission (Leckman et al. 1984; W. H. Nelson et al. 1984), course of illness (D. G. Robinson and Spiker 1985), and response to treatment (Chan et al. 1987; Glassman and Roose 1981; Kantor and Glassman 1977; J. C. Nelson and Bowers 1978; Rothschild 1985).

Many centers have reported specific abnormalities on measures of hypothalamic-pituitary-adrenal axis activity in patients with psychotic depression. Patients with psychotic major depression (PMD) are among those with the highest rates of nonsuppression on the dexamethasone suppression test, and many of them have markedly elevated posttest levels (Carroll et al. 1976c, 1980; Coryell et al. 1982). Significant differences have been observed in 24-hour measures of urinary free cortisol between patients with psychotic and those with nonpsychotic major depression (NPMD) (R. F. Anton 1987).

Evidence has also accumulated that patients with PMD have higher dopaminergic activity than do patients with NPMD (Wolkowitz et al. 1989). It also appears that patients with PMD differ from patients with NPMD in measures of serotonin function (Healy et al. 1986), sleep architecture (Kupfer et al. 1980), and perhaps even anatomically. For example, some computed tomography studies have indicated that patients with PMD may have a larger ventricle-to-brain ratio than do patients with NPMD (Targum et al. 1983). In the single functional imaging study done to date, patients with PMD demonstrated hypofunction in the prefrontal cortex and hyperfunction in the limbic areas (M. P. Austin et al. 1992).

With the many physiological and anatomical variables that appear to distinguish PMD from NPMD, it is not surprising that significant differences in treatment response between the two groups exist (R. F. Anton and Burch 1990, 1993; Glassman and Roose 1981; Kantor and Glassman 1977; J. C. Nelson and Bowers 1978). Among the more substantial differences is the relatively poor response of PMD to antidepressants alone.

ANTIDEPRESSANT MONOTHERAPY

Since the advent of tricyclic antidepressants (TCAs) in the late 1950s, it has been noted that PMD responds less robustly to TCAs alone than does NPMD. Angst (1961) noted that the presence of hypochondriacal delusions in 200 patients with depression that he studied predicted poor response to open-label treatment to 200 mg/day of imipramine in divided intramuscular injections. Similarly, Hordern and colleagues (1963), in a study of 137 patients with depression, found that approximately 79% of patients with NPMD responded to either amitriptyline or imipramine, whereas only 14% of patients with NPMD responded robustly to either of these TCAs. Furthermore, in an open-label study of 13 delusional and 21 nondelusional patients with depression treated with 3.5 mg/kg/day of imipramine for 28 days, Glassman et al. (1975) found that 67% of patients with PMD responded, whereas only 24% of patients with NPMD responded. Finally, in one of the largest prospective studies completed, Avery and Lubrano (1979) compared 265 delusional inpatients with depression with 256 nondelusional inpatients with depression. Using doses averaging more than 200 mg/day of imipramine, approximately 60% of patients with NPMD responded, whereas only 40% of patients with PMD did equally well.

Although these studies suggest that PMD predicts a relatively poor response to TCA treatment, there are a number of methodological problems in these studies. Among the problems is that the criteria for diagnosing PMD and NPMD were not standardized. Except in the Glassman et al. (1975)

study, plasma levels of TCAs were not measured. Furthermore, placebo-control groups, a double-blind design, and adequate randomization were rarely employed. Finally, the criteria for treatment response were often not discussed or standardized.

Two later studies attempted to amend some of these deficiencies. One study by W. H. Nelson and colleagues (1984) used a double-blind randomized design to evaluate response in 13 patients with PMD and 12 patients with NPMD who received 150 mg of either imipramine or amitriptyline over a 4-week period. At the end of this trial, 2 of 13 patients with PMD had a Hamilton Rating Scale for Depression (M. Hamilton 1960) score of less than 8 (complete remission of symptoms), whereas 7 of 12 patients with NPMD had achieved remission.

In a similar, but larger, double-blind study, 107 patients with unipolar and bipolar depression and 25 patients with PMD were randomly selected to either amitriptyline or imipramine after a 2-week placebo washout (Kocsis et al. 1990). Doses of both drugs averaged >200 mg/day for 4 weeks. Approximately 67% of the moderately depressed patients with NPMD responded to pharmacotherapy, whereas only 32% of the patients with PMD experienced significant improvement with either drug. However, when severely depressed patients with NPMD (with Hamilton Rating Scale for Depression scores of >27) were compared with the patients with PMD, no difference in response rate was noted.

Some investigators have also suggested that the poor response of PMD to TCAs is the result of the severity of the illness rather than the presence of psychotic symptoms per se. Glassman et al. (1977) and Avery and Lubrano (1979) both found that severity of depression predicted poorer response to TCAs. In contrast, Chan et al. (1987) found that the severity of depression did not predict poor response, but found that the presence of delusions predicted a less robust response rate.

Virtually all studies on the monotherapy of PMD have employed TCAs. At this time, no data exist on the utility of the selective serotonin reuptake blockers (SSRIs), serotonin type 2 antagonists (trazodone or nefazodone), or other newer agents such as venlafaxine in the monotherapy of PMD.

To date, only one antidepressant, amoxapine, has proven effective in the treatment of PMD as the sole therapy. Amoxapine is a chemical congener of the antipsychotic drug loxapine, so it possesses both dopamine-blocking and monoamine-enhancing properties. One double-blind study has confirmed that amoxapine appears to be as effective as the combination of a TCA and an antipsychotic. R. F. Anton and Burch (1990) randomly selected 46 inpatients with psychotic depression to either amoxapine (to 400 mg/day) or amitriptyline (to 200 mg/day) and perphenazine (to 32 mg/day). The investigators found no significant difference between the groups, with 85% of the amitriptyline/perphenazine group responding and 82% of the amoxapine group responding.

The TCAs do not appear to be effective single agents in the treatment of PMD as they are in NPMD. This discrepancy may be as much a function of PMD tending to be more severe than the depression in the NPMD population. Antidepressants other than the TCAs have not been extensively tested in the monotherapy of PMD. Amoxapine is the single antidepressant that does appear effective as a sole therapy for PMD.

ANTIDEPRESSANT/ANTIPSYCHOTIC COMBINATION TREATMENT

Although the data are fairly convincing that TCAs alone are not as efficacious in PMD as they are in NPMD, the data are equally convincing that combination therapy of a TCA with an antipsychotic is an effective strategy for PMD.

Several small, open-label studies have supported TCA/antipsychotic combinations in the treatment of PMD. Minter and Mandel (1979) studied 54 inpatients with PMD who were treated openly with either TCAs alone, TCAs and antipsychotic combination, antipsychotics alone, or electroconvulsive therapy (ECT) in treatment failures. Although only 3 of 11 patients treated with TCAs alone responded, 16 of 16 patients treated with the combination of a TCA and an antipsychotic responded. Interestingly, 14 of 15 patients treated with antipsychotic drugs alone also responded, which is contrary to findings in other studies (Spiker et al. 1985). Several other open-label studies have confirmed the utility of the combination treatment for PMD (Charney and Nelson 1981; Frances et al. 1981), but few controlled studies have been completed.

One of the more methodologically rigorous studies on the utility of TCA/antipsychotic combinations in treating PMD was completed by Spiker et al. (1985). In this study, 54 patients who met criteria for depression with psychotic features on the Schedule for Affective Disorders and Schizophrenia (Endicott and Spitzer 1978) and by Research Diagnostic Criteria (Spitzer et al. 1985) were randomly selected to treatment with amitriptyline alone, perphenazine alone, or the combination of two drugs. After a 7-day placebo washout, patients were treated for 35 days with doses averaging approximately 50 mg/day of perphenazine and approximately 200 mg/day of amitriptyline. The authors found that 78% of patients treated with the combination of drugs responded. However, only 41% of the patients treated with amitriptyline alone and only 19% of those treated with perphenazine alone responded.

To date, only one study has been completed with an antidepressant other than a TCA combined with an antipsychotic in the treatment of PMD. Rothschild and colleagues (1993) investigated the efficacy of fluoxetine and perphenazine in the treatment of PMD and found that approximately 73% of 30 patients who met DSM-III-R (American Psychiatric Association 1987) criteria for major depression with psychotic features had at least a 50% reduction on their Hamilton Rating Scale for Depression scores over 5 weeks. Furthermore, the combination of fluoxetine and perphenazine appeared to be better tolerated than the combination of TCAs with antipsychotics. Although there is no evidence that monotherapy with an antidepressant other than amoxapine is efficacious, the combination therapy with many antidepressants other than the TCAs may prove useful.

ELECTROCONVULSIVE THERAPY

ECT has been known to be an effective treatment for PMD since the 1940s. (This treatment modality is described in detail in Nobler et al., Chapter 10, in this volume.)

Given the generally favorable response of PMD to ECT, an important question is whether PMD responds to ECT preferentially over nonpsychotic subtypes of major depression. M. Greenblatt et al. (1964) found that psychotic depression did not show a significantly different response rate to ECT from bipolar depression or even psychoneurotic depression. In contrast, more recent studies (R. P. Brown et al. 1982; C. L. Rich et al. 1984) have found that patients with psychotic depression did not respond preferentially to ECT over other subtypes of depression. However, Charney and Nelson (1981) found that the presence of delusions predicted a more favorable response to ECT in 49 inpatients with depression. The question of whether PMD responds preferentially to ECT over other subtypes remains unanswered.

OTHER STRATEGIES

Over the past few years, several case reports suggested that other pharmacological strategies may have a role in the treatment of PMD. Dassa et al.

(1993) found that a 40-year-old woman with PMD who failed various antidepressant regimens in combination with neuroleptics responded to the atypical antipsychotic clozapine, alone. In addition, Parsa et al. (1991) found that clozapine was effective and well-tolerated in a case of PMD associated with Parkinson's disease. Anecdotal reports, but no published data, suggest that one of the other currently available atypical antipsychotics, risperidone, may also be effective monotherapy in the treatment of psychotic depression. Interestingly, at least one report describes a refractory psychotic depression in an elderly patient responding to the calcium channel blocker verapamil (Dassa et al. 1993).

An intriguing hypothesis first proposed by Schatzberg and colleagues (1985) is that the development of delusions in patients with depression is secondary to the effects of hypercortisolism on dopaminergic systems.

Glucocorticoids appear to increase the levels of dopamine in the brain, and this may lead to psychosis in some patients. Some new strategies for the treatment of PMD have therefore focused on medications, including aminoglutethimide (Ghadirian et al. 1995), ketoconazole (Thigore and Dinan 1995), metyrapone (B. E. P. Murphy et al. 1991), and mitotane (Starkman et al. 1985), that inhibit steroid biosynthesis. Similarly, drugs that are glucocorticoid receptor antagonists may prove effective in reducing psychotic symptoms in PMD (A. F. Schatzberg et al., unpublished data).

Further study of the efficacy of alternative strategies, including clozapine, steroid antagonists, and verapamil, for the treatment of PMD appears worthwhile.

CLINICAL RECOMMENDATIONS

Several conclusions can be drawn from the current literature on the treatment of psychotic depression:

- PMD responds less well to a TCA alone than does NPMD. It is unknown, but unlikely, whether other antidepressants alone would fare any better.
- The combination of an antidepressant and an antipsychotic appears effective in most cases of PMD. Preliminary data suggest no differences in the combination of an SSRI and an antipsychotic versus a TCA and an antipsychotic. However, the vast majority of studies have employed TCA and antipsychotic combinations.
- The tetracyclic agent amoxapine appears as efficacious in the treatment of PMD as the combination of a TCA and an antipsychotic.

- ECT is an effective option even in patients with PMD who do not respond to antidepressants alone, an antipsychotic alone, or the combination of an antidepressant with an antipsychotic. However, unilateral ECT treatments may be ineffective.

Given the available data, it is extremely important that clinicians evaluate patients with major depression for features of psychosis, because the failure to do so may result in inadequate treatment for the patient. A practical problem encountered by clinicians, however, is the subtlety of delusions. For example, it is not unusual in geriatric depression for patients to present with a somatic preoccupation that borders on delusional. These so-called near delusions may put the patient into the arena of psychotic depression. Some evidence exists that patients with depression with near delusions may respond more favorably to combinations of antidepressants and antipsychotics or ECT. Once the presence of both major depression and psychosis is determined, other psychotic disorders including bipolar disorder and schizophrenic spectrum illness must also be ruled out because this may influence long-term treatment decisions.

After the diagnosis of psychotic unipolar depression is established, the next decision may be whether to pursue ECT as a first line of treatment. According to the American Psychiatric Association Guidelines for the Treatment of Depression (American Psychiatric Association 1993), ECT is an acceptable first-line treatment in PMD. Given the consistent efficacy of ECT in multiple studies of PMD (even in cases in which other treatments failed), ECT appears to be reasonable first option for many patients. Those patients with a life-threatening PMD, particularly those at risk for suicide or who become cachectic secondary to PMD, as well as patients who have had a good past response to ECT, would seem particularly good candidates for immediate use of ECT. If ECT is pursued, the limited available data suggest that bilateral treatments may be more effective than unilateral treatments. It is unclear what roles prophylactic pharmacotherapy or maintenance ECT have in preventing recurrences after the successful treatment of PMD with psychotic depression because maintenance treatments have not been studied thus far.

Some patients will decline ECT, and the available data suggest that combination antidepressant/antipsychotic treatment or amoxapine may be equally effective. Given the preponderance of data supporting TCA/antipsychotic combinations in the treatment of PMD, it may be reasonable to consider TCA combinations before other antidepressant combinations. Currently, the literature shows debates as to whether the SSRIs are as efficacious as the

TCAs in more serious forms of depression such as melancholic or psychotic depression. Some studies have suggested that the SSRIs do not work as well as the TCAs in melancholic depression (Roose et al. 1994). Likewise, one study has suggested that venlafaxine, a drug with a mechanism of action similar to that of the TCAs, was superior to fluoxetine in the treatment of inpatients with melancholic depression (Clerc et al. 1994). Still, other meta-analyses have failed to find a difference in the efficacy of SSRIs versus TCAs in serious forms of depression (Nierenberg 1994). Nonetheless, given that most studies have employed TCAs, and some debate exists about the utility of SSRIs in severe subtypes, it may be prudent to start with a TCA in most patients until the debate is further resolved. For patients who present a significant suicide risk or who have not been able to tolerate TCAs, the SSRIs in combination with a standard antipsychotic appears an effective option.

Some clinicians adhere to the maxim *never use two drugs when one will suffice* and will prefer amoxapine. This is a reasonable strategy. However, amoxapine may be difficult for many patients to tolerate, and using a combination of two drugs may afford the clinician a finer ability to determine the amount of antipsychotic to the doses of the antidepressant and the antipsychotic for maximum efficacy and minimum toxicity.

The available data indicate that patients with PMD will often respond to combination drug therapy or amoxapine at adequate doses (>200 mg/day for amoxapine or TCAs) for at least 4 weeks. However, the course of psychotic depression is often prolonged, and it may take several months of treatment before a remission is secured.

The choice of an antipsychotic is largely up to the clinician. No evidence exists at this time that any antipsychotic is more effective than any other in the treatment of PMD. In combination therapy, using TCAs with higher potency agents might be better tolerated in many patients because they add less anticholinergic load than lower potency agents. Risperidone, with its potent serotonin type 2 antagonism, may prove to be a useful alternative to standard antipsychotics in the combination treatment of PMD.

Patients who do not respond to combination trials or amoxapine should be considered for ECT if this treatment has not already been pursued. Unfortunately, some patients will not respond to any standard strategies including ECT. These patients represent a significant treatment challenge. Such patients may benefit from other strategies such as treatment with clozapine. Because of the potential toxicity of clozapine and the need for close monitoring, clozapine represents a second- or third-line treatment for refractory cases.

Clearly, the clinician has a number of viable treatment options for the patient with PMD. More study is needed on the role of newer antidepressants, atypical antipsychotics, and other strategies such as calcium channel blockers in the treatment of psychotic depression.

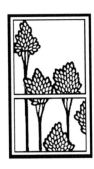

CHAPTER 20

Antidepressant Maintenance Medications

John F. Greden, M.D.

RECURRENT NATURE OF MAJOR DEPRESSIVE DISORDER

Depression for most people is an episodic recurrent disorder. Longitudinal assessments indicate that 50%–95% of patients with major depressive disorder (MDD) will have multiple episodes (75% is perhaps the most reasonable estimate) (Angst et al. 1973; Frank et al. 1990; F. K. Goodwin and Jamison 1990a; Greden 1993; P. Grof et al. 1973; Kraepelin 1921; S. A. Montgomery et al. 1988; NIMH/NIH Consensus Development Panel 1985; Thase 1990). If untreated, most patients not only will experience recurrences but also predictably will have many episodes over a lifetime, with an estimated median of five for those with unipolar depression and eight for those with manic-depressive disorder (F. K. Goodwin and Jamison 1990a; P. Grof et al. 1973; NIMH/NIH Consensus Development Panel 1985). For most patients, with each new episode, the severity tends to worsen, the duration tends to lengthen, the well interval between episodes tends to shorten, and treatment responsivity may lessen (P. Grof et al. 1973; Keller 1985; Keller et al. 1982a, 1982b; Kraepelin 1921; Post 1992, 1994; Post et al. 1986a; Roy-Byrne et al. 1985; Zis and Goodwin 1979). Using graphic techniques (Post et al. 1988; Squillace et al. 1984), the longitudinal courses of three representative patients are illustrated in Figure 20–1, revealing the pattern of cycle accelera-tion that is found in perhaps the majority of patients (Roy-Byrne et al. 1985).

STRATEGIES FOR PREVENTION OF RELAPSE OF MAJOR DEPRESSIVE DISORDER

Several treatment approaches, including maintenance medications, psy-chotherapies, a combination of medications and psychotherapies, and mainte-nance electroconvulsive therapy, for preventing recurrences of MDD have been considered by clinicians (American Psychiatric Association Task Force on Electroconvulsive Therapy 1990; Beck et al. 1979; Covi et al. 1974; Doogan and Caillard 1992; Elkin et al. 1989; Frank et al. 1993; N. S. Jacobson et al. 1991; Katon et al. 1992; Klerman et al. 1984; Kupfer 1991; Kupfer et al. 1992; S. A. Montgomery et al. 1988; Prien et al. 1984; Rehm 1979; Rush et al. 1977; Thase 1990). In this chapter, we focus on maintenance antidepres-sant medications. It is the only modality for which the database is reasonably extensive.

Antidepressant maintenance medications are effective in preventing re-lapses in the majority of patients with MDD (Doogan and Caillard 1992; Greden 1993; Katon et al. 1992; Kupfer 1991; S. A. Montgomery et al. 1988; Prien et al. 1984; Thase 1990). Indeed, maintenance antidepressants

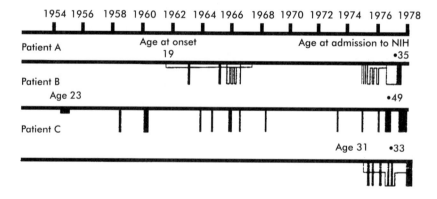

FIGURE 20–1.   Life course of illness in unipolar depression. NIH = National Institutes of Health.

Source.   Adapted from Greden JR: *Recurrent Depression: A Lifetime Disorder.* In-dianapolis, IN, Dista Products Division, Eli Lilly and Company, 1992 (video-tape/monograph). Used with permission.

represent the only intervention currently known to prevent relapses in the majority of patients. Over a long-term course, interpersonal psychotherapy has been shown to be superior to placebo treatment for patients with recurrent MDD, but not as effective as maintenance imipramine or combined imipramine plus interpersonal psychotherapy (Frank et al. 1990).

HISTORICAL NEGLECT OF LONG-TERM MAINTENANCE STUDIES

The study of antidepressant maintenance medications for patients with unipolar MDD has been historically neglected. Such neglect is puzzling. Considering that multiple recurrences may well be the sine qua non for unmedicated patients with manic depression (Coryell and Winokur 1982; NIMH/NIH Consensus Development Panel 1985; Prien et al. 1984; Suppes et al. 1991; Zis and Goodwin 1979; Zis et al. 1980) and that unipolar illness is pathophysiologically similar to bipolar disorder in many important respects, recurrences could have been presumed to be innate.

A number of reasons explain why recurrences were not prioritized until recently as an essential feature of unipolar disease:

1. Many initial episodes of depression tend to be mild enough so that they go unrecognized as a legitimate "episode" by the patient, family, or doctor. When a full-fledged episode of MDD does occur, these early episodes have often been forgotten or denied, and the developing, worsening pattern of recurrences remains undetected until late in the course.
2. Prevailing theories about the etiology of mood disorders traditionally emphasized the importance of precipitating events (stressors or traumatic life events). Although there is robust evidence that stressful life events play a role (G. W. Brown et al. 1977; Kendler et al. 1993; Paykel et al. 1969; Post 1994), many clinicians believed that, if the stressor had been addressed and the depressive symptoms resolved, the patient could be considered to have returned to "normal." The concept that "asymptomatic" patients in remission might have a persistent underlying pathophysiology was not widely held.
3. DSM-III, DSM-III-R, and DSM-IV (American Psychiatric Association 1980, 1987, 1994) specified arbitrary time criteria (e.g., 2 weeks' duration) before a person qualified for a diagnosis of MDD. Such arbitrariness meant that brief recurrences (e.g., 7–10 days) sometimes were not "officially" diagnosed as depression, and the relapsing pattern went undetected.

4. Even when medications were required for clinical resolution, treating clinicians often encouraged medication discontinuation as soon as stability was achieved, believing that medications interfered with the important clinical gains achieved during psychotherapy.

5. Long-term treatment by the same clinician has not been the norm for most patients. That meant fewer opportunities for consistent observation by the same psychiatrist, and recurrences were less likely to be detected.

6. Long-term studies are expensive, difficult to launch, methodologically complicated (Greenhouse et al. 1991), time-consuming, plagued by dropouts, and not especially conducive to academic promotion, because data sets take so long to develop. Long-term studies have received considerably less attention than short-term investigations.

7. Traditional cross-sectional treatment trials infrequently exceeded 4–6 weeks in length. Although trials have grown longer during the past decade and many now often approximate 8–12 weeks, even this length does not provide an adequate time frame for assessment of relapses (months and years are required).

8. Modest results from early maintenance studies dampened enthusiasm among a later generation of investigators or clinicians. The prevailing clinical practice of prior decades was that if a patient's acute episode was successfully treated with antidepressants and if some continuation treatment was prescribed, doses were characteristically reduced to approximately one-half of the short-term treatment dose (e.g., a 200 mg/day acute treatment dose would be reduced to a 100 mg/day maintenance dose). During the 1970s, maintenance imipramine and lithium were assessed systematically in a series of seminal studies (Prien and Kocsis 1995; Prien et al. 1984), and, although resulting data indicated that such treatments were clearly better than placebo, the maintenance of euthymia was only modestly successful, preventing relapse in approximately 37%–50% of patients over several years. It was documented only later that the relatively high rate of relapse almost certainly was influenced by the pattern of dosage reductions when patients entered their "maintenance" phase (Frank et al. 1990, 1993). The relapsing consequences of dosage reduction are still not well known among many clinicians.

MECHANISM OF RECURRENCES

No consensus exists about which pathophysiological mechanisms might explain recurrent episodes (F. K. Goodwin 1989; Kendler et al. 1993; Post

1992, 1994). Relevant hypotheses need to incorporate cycle acceleration (well intervals becoming shorter with each new episode), increasing severity, the suggestion that traumatic life events are more important during the early phases of the life cycle, and greater duration with additional episodes.

One hypothesis that has drawn considerable attention focuses on brain sensitization, or kindling (Post 1992, 1994; Post and Weiss 1995). To illustrate, assume that a patient with a genetic liability for unipolar depression experiences a severe early loss, such as the death of a parent. This event may sensitize key neurobiological networks, possibly altering expression of immediate early gene systems, the corticotropin-releasing hormone network (P. W. Gold et al. 1988a, 1988b), or some other neural network, and possibly, but not necessarily, being associated with depressive symptoms. Additional sensitizing stressors may occur in subsequent months or years, and at some point in time a stressful event such as a divorce or death may precipitate a depressive episode that meets DSM-IV criteria for MDD. The neurobiological changes associated with each new stressful event or the depressions themselves, the sustained alterations of stress mechanisms in the hypothalamic-pituitary-adrenal axis or elsewhere, or combinations of all are postulated to progressively produce an apparent brain "sensitization," with relatively sustained biochemical and/ or structural changes. Once the pattern is under way, medical illnesses, medications, substance abuse, chronobiological time-zone shifts (e.g., transmeridian jet travel), sleep disruptions, or other new traumatic life events (even those of lesser intensity) may set off subsequent episodes of depression. Similar to the pattern of electrophysiological or neuro-pharmacological kindling, depressive episodes eventually may seem to develop in response to seemingly innocuous occurrences or even in response to nothing at all.

Clinical documentation of sensitization, or kindling, patterns in humans is difficult to compile, but Post and colleagues have noted that traumatic life events become less evident with incremental episodes. Sixty percent of the patients who have symptoms that meet criteria for their first episode of MDD have identifiable precipitating events, as contrasted with 36% of those with two or more episodes (Post 1994).

Well-designed prospective investigations will be required to elucidate the pathophysiology of recurrent episodes of MDD. While waiting for data from such investigations, clinicians should recognize that effective interventions are available in the form of maintenance antidepressant medications.

PREVENTION OF RECURRENCES WITH ANTIDEPRESSANT MAINTENANCE MEDICATIONS: SUMMARY OF DATA

To qualify for valid interpretation, long-term studies should, at a minimum, incorporate the following methodologies: 1) a placebo control; 2) a treatment duration of at least 18–24 months, preferably longer; 3) adequate dosage during the maintenance phase; 4) monitoring of compliance; and 5) control for concomitant treatments. Few studies have incorporated all, but those that have the essential components strongly support the hypothesis that maintenance antidepressants prevent recurrences in most patients with MDD (Bjork 1983; Coppen et al. 1971, 1978; Doogan and Caillard 1992; Eric 1991; Frank et al. 1990; Georgotas et al. 1989; Glen et al. 1984; Jakovljevic and Mewett 1991; Kane et al. 1982; S. A. Montgomery et al. 1988, 1991; Old Age Depression Interest Group 1993; Prien et al. 1978, 1984; D. S. Robinson et al. 1991; Rouillon et al. 1991; Schou 1979; Souza et al. 1990). Data are summarized in Table 20–1. In none of the studies with placebo-control subjects did placebos do better than active medications, whereas in almost all studies, antidepressant maintenance medications performed significantly better. Considering that most of the early studies incorporated "maintenance" dosage reductions, even the most conservative interpretation is that the recurrence rate is approximately twice as great for those who were crossed over to placebo treatment as for those maintained on active antidepressant medications. With optimal clinical practice, results are likely to be considerably better. The clinical, fiscal, and social consequences of such differences are profound.

Perhaps the best controlled maintenance assessment was the one conducted by Frank and colleagues (1990). They prescribed full-dosage imipramine treatment and interpersonal therapy to achieve euthymia in 128 patients with recurrent depression. Once patients were no longer depressed, they were entered into a long-term treatment design and enrolled in one of five cells. Two of the five cells included active imipramine medication, with and without interpersonal therapy; two of the cells emphasized IPT, with and without placebo; and one involved placebo. All patients participated in a medication clinic. The four key findings were 1) those treated with active imipramine at mean dosages of approximately 200 mg/day (patients usually received the same dose that got them better) did significantly better than those who did not receive active antidepressant maintenance, and relapse rates were considerably greater in those transferred to the placebo cell; 2) the maintenance of euthymia was generally sustained over the 3-year fol-

TABLE 20–1. Efficacy of antidepressant maintenance versus placebo in prevention of unipolar depression

| Reference | Medication | % Relapse | | Significance |
		Placebo	Rx	
Prien et al. 1978	Imipramine	85	29	.01
Prien et al. 1978	Lithium	85	41	.05
Prien et al. 1978	Lithium	71	57	.05
Coppen et al. 1978	Amitriptyline	31	0	.01
Schou 1979	Lithium	84	29	.001
Kane et al. 1982	Lithium	100	29	.001
Kane et al. 1982	Imipramine	100	67	NS
Bjork 1983	Zimeldine	84	32	.001
Glen et al. 1984	Amitriptyline	88	43	.05
Glen et al. 1984	Lithium	88	42	.05
Prien et al. 1984	Imipramine	71	44	.05
S. A. Montgomery et al. 1988	Fluoxetine	57	26	.001
Georgotas et al. 1989	Phenelzine	65	13	.05
Rouillon et al. 1991	Maprotiline	32	16	.01
Frank et al. 1990	Imipramine	78	21	.001
S. A. Montgomery and Dunbar 1993	Paroxetine	39	15	.01
Jakovljevic and Mewett 1991	Paroxetine	23	14	NS
Jakovljevic and Mewett 1991	Imipramine	23	12	.05
D. S. Robinson et al. 1991	Phenelzine	75	10	.001
Doogan and Caillard 1992	Sertraline	46	13	.001

Note. NS = not significant; Rx = drug administered.

low-up; 3) interpersonal psychotherapy with or without placebo was better than placebo treatment alone but was meaningfully less effective than medication maintenance; interpersonal psychotherapy without medication failed to maintain euthymia in the majority of patients; and 4) relapses tended to occur early when active treatment was discontinued, with more than three-quarters of those who were switched to placebo relapsing within 1 year. In summary, discontinuation of full-dose maintenance imipramine treatment led to prompt relapse in the vast majority of patients with recurrent MDD.

As stated previously, maintenance assessments from the 1970s (Prien and Kocsis 1995) almost certainly would have been more impressive if they had employed full dosages of antidepressant medications during the maintenance phase (Frank et al. 1993). When effective dosages were maintained in the study by Frank et al. (1990, 1993), even when patients were followed for a longer time period (3 years versus 1 or 2 years in most earlier studies), the relapse rate was only 22%. Until dosage reductions are demonstrated to be comparably effective to full-dose treatment using well-controlled designs, it should be assumed that they are risky. The influence of dosage is illustrated in Table 20–2.

The decades-old question (Prien and Kupfer 1986; Quitkin et al. 1984) of how long maintenance treatment remains effective cannot yet be answered because the length of most studies has been limited. The longest controlled maintenance assessments were the ones conducted in Pittsburgh (Frank et al. 1990, Kupfer 1991). Most of those maintained at full treatment dose remained euthymic for 5 years. Longer studies clearly are needed.

SELECTION OF MEDICATIONS FOR MAINTENANCE ANTIDEPRESSANT TREATMENT

When selecting an antidepressant for resolution of an acute episode of MDD, clinicians traditionally have prioritized 1) efficacy (percentage of responders and degree of improvement); 2) time interval until euthymia (speed of on-

TABLE 20–2.   Comparisons of imipramine versus placebo for prevention of recurrences of major depressive disorder: effects of maintenance dosage

Reference	Length of study (year)	Approximate maintenance of IMI (mg)	Recurrence rate (%)	
			IMI	Placebo
Prien et al. 1978	2	< 135	48	92
Kane et al. 1982	2	< 135	83	100
Prien et al. 1984	2	< 135	46	71
Frank et al. 1990	3	≥ 200	22	78

Note. IMI = imipramine.

set); and 3) a constellation of factors, such as side effects, risk-benefit ratio, drug-drug interactions, pharmacokinetic or pharmacodynamic effects, cost, and subjective preferences (of the patient, family, doctor, and reimbursing agencies), known to influence compliance. These factors, clearly important when planning short-term treatment, are arguably more crucial for extended treatment and should be clearly linked with maintenance strategies. They warrant elaboration.

Efficacy: Percentage of Responders and Degree of Improvement

Because maintenance of euthymia first requires attainment of euthymia, initial efficacy is the logical starting point, but it is only the starting point. A deluge of studies have compared numerous antidepressants with placebo, and with each other, to determine if one might be better than another in ability to end the acute episode of depression. Most studies (Elkin et al. 1989) conclude that available antidepressants are approximately equal in their capacity to resolve acute episodes of "typical" MDD.

In contrast, a less extensive but still convincing database has identified important clinical differences in efficacy for antidepressants used to treat patients with "atypical" or comorbid depression. Individuals with "atypical" depression (distinct quality of mood, hyperphagia, hypersomnia, psychomotor retardation, rejection sensitivity, and such unusual atypical features as chocolate craving) have superior responses to monoamine oxidase inhibitors (MAOIs), selective serotonin reuptake inhibitors (SSRIs), and perhaps venlafaxine, and most do not respond well to tricyclic antidepressants (TCAs) (Davidson et al. 1982; Liebowitz et al. 1988; Quitkin et al. 1988, 1991). Despite these data, TCAs unfortunately have been the first choice for most atypical patients until SSRIs were introduced.

Similar differences in efficacy appear to exist for those with comorbid syndromes, when depression is accompanied by anorexia, bulimia, or obsessive-compulsive manifestations. For each of these comorbid conditions, TCAs again appear less efficacious than clomipramine, SSRIs, venlafaxine, and perhaps MAOIs, possibly because the comorbid syndrome may be linked to serotonin dysregulation, and these latter medications are more potent in altering serotonergic function (Grunhaus 1988; Herzog et al. 1988; Hudson et al. 1983; Schatzberg and Ballenger 1991). In summary, acute efficacy is required before considering maintenance efficacy, but three important "efficacy" or "effectiveness" questions emerge when selecting a medication for maintenance.

Is any single antidepressant more effective than another in sustaining euthymia? Few studies have compared one antidepressant to another for long-term maintenance (Prien et al. 1973a). Comparisons with placebos or "no treatment" provide the majority of the database. Thus, no one agent can be convincingly stated to be more effective than any other agent in sustaining maintenance.

Should a switch be made from the medication that induced euthymia to a different medication when seeking to sustain euthymia? No studies show that once a medication produces euthymia a "switch" can be made to a different maintenance medication without increasing the risk of relapse. In contrast, available data show that discontinuation of any antidepressant—often done as part of a switch—leads to a greater risk of relapse. Until systematic studies reveal differently, it is prudent to assume that the antidepressant that induces short-term remission will be best in sustaining long-term remission over the long term and to avoid decisions that require subsequent switches. Thus, it is crucial for clinicians who are prescribing antidepressants to think "long-term" or "maintenance" from the first moment onward, choosing an agent that resolves the acute episode and is effective and well-tolerated for indefinite, extended maintenance.

Will medications known to sustain maintenance over several years continue to do so indefinitely? Few studies have monitored antidepressant maintenance efficacy for periods exceeding several years (Prien and Kocsis 1995). Lacking data, the clinician can only hope that efficacy over several years will translate into sustained effectiveness over many years, decades, or indefinitely. This remains to be demonstrated. For imipramine, maintenance of euthymia has been systematically demonstrated in a small number of patients for at least 5 years (Kupfer 1992). Anecdotes suggest that SSRIs may lose some of their efficacy over time, but few convincing data support this to date. Considering the widespread use of SSRIs, research is sorely needed to address this question.

Time Interval Until Euthymia: Speed of Onset

No data link speed of onset during the acute episode with effectiveness in sustaining long-term maintenance, probably because most antidepressants are approximately equivalent in their speed of onset.

Factors That Affect Compliance: Side Effects, Risk-Benefit Ratio, Drug-Drug Interactions, Pharmacokinetic or Pharmacodynamic Effects, Cost, and Preferences

Maintenance antidepressants must be given in adequate dosages to sustain euthymia, and discontinuations may increase risk of relapse. Thus, compliance is essential if maintenance antidepressants are to work. Too few studies have paid adequate attention to reasons for noncompliance or lack of adherence (Axelrod and Wetzler 1989; Kelly et al. 1990; Meichenbaum and Turk 1987; L. S. Morris and Schulz 1992), but it appears to be most influenced by side effects, although for some patients, cost is a significant variable. In seeking to enhance adherence, clinicians must select a medication at the beginning of treatment that patients will find acceptable for years or decades to come.

Pharmacokinetics, pharmacodynamics, mechanisms of action, clearance, binding, and molecular actions differ considerably among antidepressants (Preskorn 1993). In general, the more mechanisms of action a medication possesses, the less tolerable it tends to be. Most studies agree that compliance rates differ considerably for different antidepressants (Eraker et al. 1984; E. D. Myers and Calvert 1984), and presumably these differences are based mostly on different side-effect profiles. Although all antidepressants have side effects when taken at effective doses, those for traditional TCAs and MAOIs are generally more annoying, severe, dangerous, or disabling. Although some tolerance often develops, side effects that occur during treatment of the acute episode generally continue to some degree. As a result, the patient requests to discontinue one medication and switch to another occur far more often with TCAs than with SSRIs (Katon et al. 1992).

Newer antidepressants (such as the SSRIs, bupropion, and venlafaxine) probably achieved their impressive popularity primarily because their side-effect profiles were more favorable. Because dry mouth, blurry vision, tachycardia, lethargy, constipation, urinary hesitancy, and arrhythmias are deeply distressing to many, paucity of anticholinergic side effects from SSRIs was especially noteworthy. Convenience and simplicity of use are also favorable qualities for some newer agents. However, the decreased libido, anorgasmia, and erectile problems caused by SSRIs are of note and should be taken into consideration for long-term therapy.

Lithium has been effective for maintenance treatment of manic-depressive disorder (Suppes et al. 1991), and some patients find the side-effect profile preferable. Lithium is an option for those with unipolar disease (Prien et al. 1973a). A consensus conference published in 1985 (NIMH/NIH

Consensus Development Panel 1985) confirmed that lithium salts were efficacious and should especially be considered for those considered "unipolar" but with a family history of bipolar disorder, because perhaps as many as 15% of patients with unipolar depression do subsequently experience hypomania or mania. Lithium may be the ideal maintenance agent for such "uncertain" patients for whom there is concern that administration of antidepressants may precipitate "highs" or increase the frequency of cycling and for those who dislike side effects of some antidepressant groups.

In summary, although it is difficult to recommend a specific agent for long-term maintenance, because of compliance, convenience, and safety reasons, the newer antidepressants (e.g., SSRIs, venlafaxine) appear to be agents of first choice. Because the long-term database for these agents is less extensive than that for TCAs, further studies are indicated.

SELECTION OF PATIENTS FOR MAINTENANCE ANTIDEPRESSANT TREATMENT

Indefinite treatment with antidepressant medications has been recommended for individuals with three or more documented episodes (Greden 1993). This is based on the high probability of relapse within 12–24 months for a high percentage of such patients. However, numeric "formulas" for number of prior episodes serve only as a rough guideline. The clinician should consider other variables as well. Patients with a strong family history of mood disorders, a history of severe episodes with suicidal behavior or psychosis, prior documented relapse following treatment discontinuation, demonstrated treatment refractoriness, coexisting medical problems, or complications of aging that would make another episode hazardous are candidates for extended treatment, even if they have had fewer than three episodes. Some data suggest that if the "first episode" occurred when the patient was older (Zis and Goodwin 1979), the risk of relapse is higher without maintenance treatment. It is probable that these observations are confounded by prior episodes, whether forgotten, ignored, overlooked, denied, or misdiagnosed. Because elderly patients are often more difficult to treat, however, older age at apparent onset of a first episode of serious MDD or melancholia can be considered an indicator for indefinite treatment (Greden 1993). Clinical indications that support consideration of indefinite antidepressant medications are summarized in Table 20–3.

TABLE 20-3. Clinical indications supporting indefinite antidepressant maintenance medications

Three or more episodes

One or two prior severe episodes with
   Suicidal behavior
   Treatment refractoriness
   Psychosis

Chronic dysthymia followed by major depressive disorder ("double depression")

Prompt relapse following prior treatment discontinuation

Strong "positive" family history of recurrent mood disorders

Coexisting medical problems or complication of aging that would make a future episode hazardous

Initial episode occurring after age 50

Personal or occupational circumstances that make any recurrence "unacceptable"

RISK-BENEFIT RATIO

Risks and benefits, important for any treatment, are especially relevant when considering extended treatment. When considering the risk-benefit ratio associated with long-term administration of medications, the database is less impressive than desired (Boyer and Blumhardt 1992; Doogan 1991; Henry 1992; Nora et al. 1974; Roose et al. 1986; Vorhees et al. 1979; Wernicke 1985), but appears extremely favorable, although infrequent complications must be acknowledged (e.g., long-term lithium treatment is known to induce distal renal tubular fibrosis in a very small percentage of users, bupropion is suggested to have an increased risk of seizures in selected patients [Davidson 1989], and usage of all medications during pregnancy must be approached with caution). Generally, available TCAs, SSRIs, or other antidepressants are not believed to cause long-term medical complications different from their short-term side effects. As experience grows, clinicians must continue to observe for long-term deleterious consequences. When doing so, they should recall that the risks of long-term maintenance treatment need not be identical to those for short-term treatment.

In contrast to minimal risks for long-term antidepressant administration, the risks of treatment discontinuation are profound, attributable to the greatly increased risk of recurrence. With each new episode, the patient is likely to have increased risk of occupational dysfunction, job loss, social impairment, problems with interpersonal relationships, marital discord, separation, divorce, eradication of the lifetime maximum insurance benefit for mental health coverage with subsequent financial strain, increased medical illnesses, greater utilization of health services, possible immune impairment with greater risk of cancer and other serious illnesses, increased risk of accidents, more suicide attempts, greater chance of a successful suicide, and further risk of brain sensitization, cycle acceleration, increasing severity, and the promise of even further deterioration (Greenberg et al. 1993a, 1993b; Katon and Sullivan 1990; Klerman and Weissman 1992; Wells et al. 1989, 1992). Summary recommendations are listed in Table 20–4.

DISCONTINUATION STRATEGIES

Although discontinuation of antidepressants *significantly* increases the risk of recurrence of depression for many patients and should not be considered a safe option, even when risks of relapse are conveyed, many patients still request that medications be stopped once they feel improved. Should it be impossible to dissuade the patient who is at risk for relapse, some clinically based guidelines for discontinuation are available (Greden 1993). First, the taper should be as slow as possible, perhaps as long as 6–12 months, because rapid discontinuation may increase the overall risk or the promptness of the recurrence, an extended time period provides ample time for brain receptors to undergo gradual regulatory readaptation, and it allows for the patient and clinician to have optimal opportunity to recognize and respond to any return of symptoms before a fully developed relapse occurs.

TABLE 20–4. Clinical recommendations for antidepressant maintenance medications

---

Indefinite (extended, lifetime) treatment for appropriate candidates (Table 20–3)

"Full-dose" treatment

Selection of agents with favorable side-effect profile

Active educational interventions and monitoring to promote compliance

No "drug holidays"

Dosage adjustment or augmentation if symptoms reemerge after sustained euthymia (avoid prescription "switch" to a different agent)

Regular, periodic use of clinical rating scales

Patient graphs, diaries, and life charts to monitor monthly, seasonal, and chronobiological changes

Special precautions during high-risk times (e.g., severe traumatic life events, sustained stress, transmeridian travel, seasonal changes, premenstrual period)

LIMITATIONS OF DATA

Many major questions about maintenance treatment remain unanswered. Few studies have assessed whether long-term maintenance is necessary or effective for patients with atypical depression; whether gender or age differences significantly alter risk of recurrence; whether antidepressants—especially the newer agents that have been studied for shorter periods—might lose effectiveness after years or decades of treatment; whether concomitant medical illnesses or treatment might interfere with maintenance or require changes in strategy; whether natural neurobiological milestones (such as menopause) dictate alterations in strategy (e.g., the addition of estrogen); whether sensitization, or kindling, might diminish or disappear after years of euthymia; whether extended antidepressant maintenance treatment might induce neurobiological changes that actually increase the likelihood of relapse if the medications are discontinued; whether other types of interventions such as phototherapy could play a role in maintenance treatment; whether laboratory correlates might help identify those most vulnerable to relapse; and most importantly, whether maintenance treatment can *ever* be safely discontinued.

As new projects are launched, it will be important to use operationalized definitions of remission, recurrence, and relapses (Frank et al. 1991); to consider and record chronobiological milestones, especially puberty, menstruation, menopause, and season; to employ life charting by the patient so that brief recurrences can be identified; to emphasize severity rather than dichotomous DSM-IV criteria; and to consider well-known confounds such as mood subtype, age, comorbid conditions, and associated medication or substance use.

Future clinical investigations designed to test sensitization hypotheses should consider the role of precipitating events in early mild episodes that heretofore have often been overlooked. Other confounds include 1) recent observations that many patients respond to "threats" (versus "losses"), with onset of anxiety or panic symptoms and only later drift toward depressive symptoms; 2) reports that patients who develop migraine headaches during adolescence or young adulthood may be at higher risk for anxiety and anxiety/depression during later years; 3) the contributions of comorbid conditions, especially obsessive-compulsive disorder, eating disorders, and substance abuse; and 4) the confounding effects of naturalistic antidepressant treatments.

CONCLUSION

Continuation of adequate-dose antidepressant medications prevents new episodes in most patients. Discontinuation leads to a significantly greater risk of recurrence for most patients. Maintenance treatment appears to be safe and cost-effective for most patients. These are strong conclusions. Important research questions remain unanswered, but, while striving to address them, it is reassuring to know that we have powerful tools and strategies (Table 20–4) to sustain relative euthymia and effective functioning. Successful treatment of an acute episode of depression is a commendable accomplishment; maintenance of euthymia is far more important.

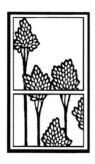

SECTION IV

Anxiolytics

Stephen M. Stahl, M.D., Ph.D.,
Section Editor

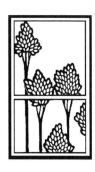

CHAPTER 21

Overview of New Anxiolytics

Stephen M. Stahl, M.D., Ph.D.,
Lewis L. Judd, M.D., and
Jelena L. Kunovac, M.D.

Although the benzodiazepines have been the treatment of choice for anxiety disorders for many years, unfavorable aspects to their side-effect profile have initiated efforts to develop new-generation antianxiety agents. Over the past decade, scientists have been searching for compounds that retain the robust anxiolytic efficacy of benzodiazepines, but lack a number of unwanted properties, including sedation, cognitive impairments such as memory disturbance, and drug dependence. Two major strategies for developing new anxiolytic agents have been used. The first is based on development of compounds that act as partial agonists at benzodiazepine receptors. The second is leading psychopharmacologists to focus on developing agents active at various other neurotransmitter receptors, including those for serotonin (5-hydroxytryptamine [5-HT]), cholecystokinin (CCK),

This work was supported in part by National Institute of Mental Health Research Grant 5 R01 MH45787-02 and by a Veterans Administration Merit Review Award to S.M.S. This work was also supported in part by Mental Health Clinical Research Center Grant MH30914 and General Clinical Research Center Grant M01-RR00827 to the University of California, San Diego.

333

neuropeptide Y, corticotropin-releasing factor (CRF), and glutamate. Because these various neurotransmitters are involved in the neurobiology of anxiety, compounds acting on these systems may be effective anxiolytics. Recent preclinical and clinical data, in fact, support the idea that selective ligands for 5-HT_{1A}, 5-HT_{2A}, 5-HT_{2C}, 5-HT_3, CCK-B, and N-methyl-D-aspartate (NMDA) subtype of glutamate receptors are of potential interest for the development of novel anxiolytics. In this chapter, we discuss research strategies based on both approaches and propose future directions for the development of new anxiolytics.

NOVEL ANXIOLYTICS ACTING AT BENZODIAZEPINE RECEPTORS

The anxiolytic, sedative, hypnotic, and muscle relaxant properties of benzodiazepines result from benzodiazepine interaction with central nervous system benzodiazepine receptors. Receptors for benzodiazepines in the central nervous system are part of a supramolecular complex that also includes binding sites for γ-aminobutyric acid (GABA), barbiturates, picrotoxin, β-carbolines, and an associated chloride ionophore that may be conceptualized as the effector of this receptor complex (Drugan and Philip 1991). All of the binding sites within this supramolecular complex are allosterically interrelated in that binding at any one of these positions alters the binding kinetics at other subunits of this complex (Drugan and Philip 1991). At least five benzodiazepine receptor subtypes have been identified. Diversity among various subtypes lies in the differences of their apparent sensitivity to GABA and in the structural and functional heterogeneity of the allosteric centers modulating the primary transmitter recognition site located on the supramolecular receptor complex (Slobodyansky et al. 1990). Benzodiazepine 1, or omega 1, receptor subtype seems to mediate anxiolytic action of benzodiazepines.

The novel imidazopyridazines alpidem and zolpidem have high selectivity for benzodiazepine 1 sites yet seem to be less deleterious than classic benzodiazepines acting at benzodiazepine 1 and 2 sites, with regard to memory and learning capacity (Zivkovic et al. 1990). Alpidem is registered in Europe as an anxiolytic and is proven to be effective in the treatment of generalized anxiety disorder, stress-induced anxiety, and adjustment disorder with anxious mood (Morselli 1990). Alpidem has a good safety profile, is well tolerated, and displays very low potential to induce dependence or to develop tolerance (Zivkovic et al. 1991). Zolpidem has been registered in the United States and Europe as a hypnotic agent and produces sedation without tolerance, dependence, or the withdrawal liability of sedative-hypnotic benzodiazepines (S. Z. Langer et al. 1990).

Abecarnil, a β-carboline-3-carboxylic-ester, has a selective pharmacological profile in animal studies and is under development for the treatment of generalized anxiety disorder. It has anxiolytic and anticonvulsant activity, with a low abuse liability and low dependence potential (Stephens et al. 1993). Although the initial results of phase II clinical trials were promising (Ballenger et al. 1991), they have not been yet confirmed in phase III clinical trials.

The promising anxiolytic-antipanic preclinical profile of bretazenil, an imidazobenzodiazepine congener of the benzodiazepine antagonist flumazenil (Katschnig et al. 1991), also has not been confirmed in large-scale clinical testing.

NEUROSTEROIDS

Neurosteroids are natural or synthetic steroids that rapidly alter the excitability of neurons by interacting at benzodiazepine receptors (S. M. Paul and Purdy 1992). Neurosteroid anxiolytics are still early in their development for application as possible anxiolytic agents. For example, allotetrahydrodeoxycorticosterone shows anxiolytic activity in animal models of anxiety (Crawley et al. 1986). This finding led to the suggestion that neurosteroids may represent an important class of new anxiolytic drugs with rapid onset of action (S. M. Paul and Purdy 1992). The 3α–hydroxy ring A-reduced metabolites of progesterone, such as alfaxalone, allopregnanolone, and allotetrahydrodeoxycorticosterone, augment inhibitory neurotransmission through interaction with the $GABA_A$-benzodiazepine-chloride channel receptor complex in the central nervous system and possess sedative-hypnotic action (S. M. Paul and Purdy 1992).

DRUGS ACTING ON SEROTONIN RECEPTORS

Evidence from numerous preclinical and clinical studies suggests that dysfunction of serotonin neurons plays a role in the pathophysiology of anxiety. Since the early 1980s, the classic hypothesis of serotonin function in anxiety has suggested that the serotonin system promotes anxiety, whereas suppression of this system diminishes it. The discovery of numerous serotonin receptor subtypes has extended our understanding of the role of the serotonin system in anxiety and is extending the simple classic hypothesis of serotonin function into a far more complex story involving multiple specific subtypes of serotonin receptors. For example, current knowledge suggests that even increased serotonin activity can reduce anxious behavior under certain circumstances and at certain serotonin receptor subtypes (Handley and McBlane 1993).

Researchers are currently attempting to develop new potential anxiolytic drugs by targeting various serotonin receptors selectively. Among 18 or more identified serotonin receptors subtypes, it seems that 5-HT_{1A}, 5-HT_{2A}, 5-HT_{2C}, and 5-HT_3 receptors may be especially involved in the serotonin system's response in anxiety. Most interest has focused around 5-HT_{1A} drugs (buspirone, ipsapirone, gepirone, tandospirone, flesinoxan, and others). Some preclinical data indicate that antagonists at 5-HT_{2A}, 5-HT_{2C}, and 5-HT_3 receptors may also exert anxiolytic activity, but so far these findings have not been consistently confirmed in clinical trials.

Drugs Acting on 5-HT_{1A} Receptors

Buspirone, a 5-HT_{1A} partial agonist, is the first drug acting on serotonin receptors to be approved in the United States for the treatment of anxiety. Its clinical efficacy is equivalent to that of benzodiazepines in patients with generalized anxiety disorder, with evidently lower incidence of adverse reactions (D. L. Murphy 1990). Moreover, buspirone produces no withdrawal symptoms or low-dose dependence (Keppel Hesselink 1992). However, the onset of anxiolytic effects is delayed compared with that of benzodiazepines (D. L. Murphy 1990), and some clinicians doubt that buspirone has efficacy comparable to that of benzodiazepines. A possibility of buspirone augmentation of benzodiazepines' activity has been suggested. Currently, several new compounds, such as ipsapirone and flesinoxan, acting on the 5-HT_{1A} receptor, are under evaluation in phase II and III clinical testing.

Drugs Acting on 5-HT_{2A} and 5-HT_{2C} Receptors

m-Chlorophenylpiperazine (mCPP) induces anxiety in human volunteers and laboratory animals. This effect can be blocked by the nonselective $5\text{-HT}_{2A}/5\text{-HT}_{2C}$ receptor antagonists (Kennett et al. 1994). In addition, several nonselective $5\text{-HT}_{2A}/5\text{-HT}_{2C}$ antagonists have been observed to possess anxiolytic profiles in animal models of anxiety, whereas selective 5-HT_{2A} receptor antagonists were found to have no effect (Kennett et al. 1994). These findings led to the hypothesis that selective 5-HT_{2C} antagonists might be useful in the treatment of anxiety. However, no such compound is yet available.

Drugs Acting on 5-HT_3 Receptors

The 5-HT_3 receptor is the only receptor among monoamine receptors coupled directly to a cation channel; therefore, the drug actions at this receptor subtype may be more rapid than drug actions at other serotonin receptor subtypes. Recently, many selective 5-HT_3 receptor antagonists including ondansetron, zacopride, tropisetron, granisetron, zatosetron, and nazasetron have been developed. The 5-HT_3 antagonists exhibit anxiolytic effects in animal models of anxiety (Fozard 1992). Preclinical data also indicate that 5-HT_3 antagonists are not sedative, do not have addictive liability, generate no problems withdrawing from chronic treatment, and can be used following benzodiazepine withdrawal (Costall and Naylor 1992a). Ondansetron, a 5-HT_3 antagonist, is under investigation as a potential treatment for generalized anxiety disorder, panic disorder, and social phobia (Lader 1991).

DRUGS ACTING ON NEUROPEPTIDE RECEPTORS

In the past decade, several major advances have been made with regard to understanding the functional role of peptides in anxiety, but without major breakthroughs in terms of showing a causal relation between a peptide and anxiety or the therapeutic utility of peptide drugs for the treatment of anxiety. The major achievement in recent years has been the development of second-generation peptide antagonists, which are small molecules of nonpeptide nature that pass the blood-brain barrier. Several neuropeptides have been implicated in the neurobiology of anxiety, including CCK, CRF, and neuropeptide Y, which are reviewed here.

Cholecystokinin

A gastrinlike neuropeptide, CCK exists in the central nervous system both as an octapeptide (CCK-8) and as a tetrapeptide (CCK-4) (Rex et al. 1994b). The octapeptide CCK-8 occurs predominantly in sulfated form and is one of the most abundant neuropeptides in the central nervous system (Rex et al. 1994b). Two major subtypes of CCK receptors, labeled as CCK-A and CCK-B receptors, have been identified (Hill et al. 1993). At this point, the most promising neuropeptide receptor to target for the treatment of anxiety may be the CCK-B receptor. This receptor is widely distributed throughout the brain, with particular distribution in limbic structures and cortical areas (Derrien et al. 1994). Agonists acting at CCK-B receptors have anxiogenic-like effects in various animal tests, whereas human studies have demonstrated panicogenic effects of the CCK-B agonist CCK-4 (Bradwejn et al. 1992a, 1992b, 1992c; de Montigny 1989). Recently developed CCK-B receptor antagonists, such as RB-211, CI-988, and L-365,260, have shown anxiolytic-like actions (Bradwejn et al. 1993; Rex et al. 1994a), probably mediated through the dorsal vagal complex at the bulbar level rather than through limbic structures. The development of compounds that specifically antagonize CCK-B receptors may be of potential therapeutic activity in the treatment of anxiety disorders.

Evidence of the involvement of CCK-B receptors in the neurobiology of anxiety has been strengthened by the findings that a closely related peptide, pentagastrin, produces dose-related and time-limited symptoms of social anxiety in both control subjects and patients with social phobia undergoing experimental social interactions (Uhde et al. 1993). Pentagastrin is a pentapeptide whose final tetrapeptide is identical to CCK-4.

An interesting link appears to exist in the brain between CCK and 5-HT$_3$ receptors. Activation of 5-HT$_3$ receptors increases CCK release from rat cortical and nucleus accumbens synaptosomes (Raiteri et al. 1993a), suggesting that anxiolytic activity of 5-HT$_3$ antagonists may be mediated through blockade of the CCK system.

Corticotropin-Releasing Factor

Preclinical data demonstrate that CRF administration produces several behavioral effects characteristic of anxiogenic compounds (Britton et al. 1985). In addition, CRF receptor antagonists block the anxiogenic actions of CRF in the rat (Britton et al. 1986). Chlordiazepoxide also attenuates anxiogenic-like effects of CRF (Britton et al. 1985), whereas acute and chronic administration of alprazolam decreases CRF concentration in the locus coeruleus (Owens et al. 1993). These results have led to the hypothesis that administration of benzodiazepines to patients with anxiety and panic disorder may reduce central sympathetic hyperactivity by facilitating the inhibitory action of GABA on the firing of CRF neurons innervating the locus coeruleus (B. E. Leonard 1993).

Neuropeptide Y

The anxiolytic potential of neuropeptide Y, a 36–amino acid peptide with a broad distribution in the central nervous system, has been demonstrated in both animal and human studies (Heilig et al. 1993). The most likely anxiolytic action of neuropeptide Y is mediated through activation of Y1 subtype of neuropeptide Y receptors in the central nucleus of the amygdala and is similar to the action of established anxiolytics (Heilig et al. 1993).

The neuropeptide galanin is functionally related to neuropeptide Y and is present in limbic brain areas important for emotionality. Galanin also has been observed to possess specific anxiolytic-like actions similar to those of neuropeptide Y (Bing et al. 1993).

EXCITATORY AMINO ACID RECEPTORS

Animal research has revealed that antagonists, such as ketamine, phencyclidine, and dizocilpine (MK-801), at the NMDA receptor channel complex are clearly anxiolytic in animal models of anxiety. Because of the risk of abuse with phencyclidine-related drugs, which are thought to act at a site within the channel itself, antagonists at another site associated with the NMDA receptor channel complex—namely, those that act at the glycine-modulatory site on the NMDA receptor—are believed to have promise in the development of future anxiolytics (Hamon 1994).

CONCLUSION

Advances in the neurobiology of anxiety are coming at a rapid pace and are based on improvement in understanding both the biochemical pharmacology and the behavioral pharmacology of neurotransmitters, neuropeptides, and their multiple receptor subtypes. Exploiting these advances is leading to the development of multiple novel pharmacological agents that hold the potential of becoming the next generation of anxiolytic drugs. Specifically, partial agonists for the benzodiazepine receptor; selective agents for 5-HT_{1A}, 5-HT_{2A}, 5-HT_{2C}, and 5-HT_3 receptors; as well as selective agents for neuropeptide receptors such as CCK-B, CRF, and neuropeptide Y1 may prove to be the basis for improved treatments of anxiety in the future.

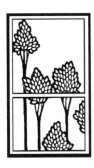

CHAPTER 22

Interactions Between Physiological, Hormonal, and Environmental Determinants: The Anxiety Model

Daniel S. Pine, M.D.,
Jeremy D. Coplan, M.D.,
Laszlo A. Papp, M.D., and
Jack M. Gorman, M.D.

 In current research on anxiety disorders, the potential importance of interactions among physiological, hormonal, and environmental factors has been demonstrated in at least four investigative lines. First, be-

This work was supported by National Institute of Mental Health Center Grant MH-43878 to the Center to Study Youth Depression, Anxiety and Suicide; National Institute of Mental Health Mental Health Clinical Research Center Grant MH-30906; National Institute of Mental Health Research Training Grant MH-16432; Research Scientist Development Award MH-00416 to J.M.G.; Research Scientist Development Award MH-00858 to L.A.P.; Research Scientist Development Award MH-01039 to J.D.C.; and a grant from the Lowenstein Foundation.

havioral genetic studies show that environmental factors are major contributors to anxiety disorders. In fact, Kendler et al. (1987, 1995) suggested that, among individuals at risk for emotional psychopathology, clinical phenotype results from unique environmental factors interacting with common genes predisposing for either anxiety or depression. Second, one specific anxiety disorder, posttraumatic stress disorder, results directly from an environmental event that exerts profound effects on both behavior and the hormonal and physiological milieu (Charney et al. 1993; Yehuda et al. 1995). Third, various manipulations of the environment, including changes related to psychotherapeutic strategies, produce clinical improvement in anxious individuals (Barlow 1988; Marks 1987). Finally, current developmental conceptualizations recognize that anxiety disorders are the end result of complex interactions between biological and environmental factors (Biederman et al. 1995; D. F. Klein 1993; Pine et al. 1996a).

In this chapter, we discuss some of the evidence in this final investigative line. We focus on panic disorder, the anxiety disorder with perhaps the most extensive biological research base, and outline the manner in which environmental factors may interact with biology during human development to produce the pattern of physiological abnormalities found in adulthood. This chapter is not intended to be an exhaustive review of this topic, and readers are referred elsewhere for further discussion (Barlow 1988; Coplan et al. 1992a; Gorman and Papp 1990; D. F. Klein 1993). Rather, in an effort to illustrate the potential processes involved in environmental-biological interactions, we describe evidence consistent with environmental effects on two biological systems implicated in panic disorder: the respiratory and noradrenergic nervous systems.

RESPIRATORY SYSTEM

Extensive research implicates the respiratory system in panic disorder. As shown by our group and others (Barlow 1988; Gorman et al. 1988; D. F. Klein 1993; Papp et al. 1993; Perna et al. 1994; Stein et al. 1995), the most consistently supportive findings include the high rate of respiratory symptoms during panic attacks, the results from respiratory *challenge* studies, and research on the association between panic and pulmonary physiology. In our focused review of these findings, we discuss the influence of both proximal environmental and developmental factors on pulmonary profiles in human anxiety states.

Respiratory Findings in Adults With Panic Disorder

Panic disorder is associated with abnormalities in respiratory physiology both at rest and in response to biological challenges with respiratory stimulants. In our laboratory, the most consistent prechallenge abnormality has been an increased variance in tidal volume, suggesting dysregulation in the central control of respiration (Papp et al. 1993). This finding is unlikely to be simply an effect of anticipatory anxiety, as it also occurs during sleep (Stein et al. 1995). Besides this baseline finding, a number of abnormalities are found across studies during a *respiratory challenge* phase. Panic disorder, but not other anxiety disorders, is associated with a distinct set of respiratory symptoms that are inducible by respiratory challenges with biological "suffocation indicators," including carbon dioxide and lactate (Cowley and Arana 1990; Gorman and Papp 1990; Gorman et al. 1988; Papp et al. 1993). Challenges with such substances in psychiatrically healthy subjects or patients with other anxiety disorders do not produce these symptoms to the same degree (Papp et al. 1993). Furthermore, from a physiological standpoint, panic disorder is associated with an enhanced respiratory response to these challenge agents. This enhanced response has been found with both carbon dioxide and lactate (Gorman and Papp 1990; Papp et al. 1993). As with baseline ventilatory abnormalities, these findings are unlikely to be a reflection of elevated state anxiety, as they are also demonstrable in challenge tests during sleep (Koenigsberg et al. 1994).

The validity of the respiratory challenge model is supported by other findings. Psychopharmacological agents clinically effective in panic disorder successfully block lactate or carbon dioxide–induced panic (Gorman and Papp 1990; Papp et al. 1993). Agents that are effective in other anxiety disorders, but not panic disorder, in contrast, do not block the response to these challenge agents (Liebowitz et al. 1995). Further, the physiological alterations seen during lactate or carbon dioxide–induced panic closely resemble the alterations seen during placebo-induced panic attacks (Goetz et al. 1993). Finally, evidence suggests that behavioral sensitivity to suffocation cues is transmitted within families as a biological diathesis for panic-related anxiety (Perna et al. 1995).

Beyond results using standardized respiratory challenge paradigms, other extensive evidence points to pulmonary dysfunction in panic disorder. For example, respiratory diseases that induce sensations of smothering are associated with a high rate of panic disorder (Karajgi et al. 1990; Yellowlees et al. 1987), whereas panic disorder is associated with subtle abnormalities in pulmonary mechanics that are suggestive of subclinical airway disease (Perna et al. 1994). In summary, when one considers the wealth of data implicating respiratory abnormalities in panic disorder, it becomes clear that there is an important relationship between respiration and panic anxiety. In an effort to integrate the findings, our group has suggested that a biological abnormality in neural systems that regulate respiration (Gorman and Papp 1990; Gorman et al. 1988; Papp et al. 1994) or that monitor cues of suffocation (D. F. Klein 1993) predispose individuals to panic disorder.

Proximal Environmental Effects on Panic and Respiration

Although physiological and clinical studies of sleep-related panic show that respiratory-induced panic attacks clearly can occur independent of any environmental cue (Koenigsberg et al. 1994), a number of studies suggest that proximal environmental manipulations can alter the behavioral and biological susceptibility to respiratory challenges in panic disorder. Our group has been particularly interested in the effects of social stress on panic susceptibility. In naturalistic experiments, stressful changes in the social environment are tied to the development of prominent respiratory symptoms that can result in both acute paniclike syndromes and full-blown panic disorder (Jacobs et al. 1990; D. F. Klein 1993; G. W. Small et al. 1991). As in biological challenge studies, which specifically tie respiratory abnormalities to panic-related states but not generalized anxiety or obsessive-compulsive symptoms (Cowley and Arana 1990), the association between social stress and anxiety appears specific to disorders that involve panic attacks (G. W. Brown and Harris 1993).

An effect of environmental conditions on panic susceptibility is also found in the laboratory. Although laboratory-based research most consistently has included studies using manipulations of perceived threat (Rapee 1995) or control (Sanderson et al. 1989), evidence implicates social stress in the susceptibility to respiratory challenges. For example, as part of a standard 5% carbon dioxide challenge paradigm, Carter et al. (1995) randomly assigned patients with panic disorder to either a control condition or a "safe person condition," where the challenge was conducted in the presence of a supportive friend or therapist. Interestingly, not only did the safe person appear to attenuate the response to the challenge, but the effect of separation from a safe person also appeared to sensitize patients to the effect of the challenge. This finding suggests that the social environment can moderate panic susceptibility, with the effect of social separation appearing particularly important.

Developmental Effects of the Environment

Beyond studies examining the proximal effect of social separation on panic, there is a long history of research on the developmental association between social separation and panic disorder. As discussed by our group elsewhere

(R. G. Klein 1995; Pine et al. 1994, 1996a), extensive evidence suggests that separation anxiety disorder may predispose to panic disorder. This includes results from retrospective studies of panic disorder (R. G. Klein 1995), prospective follow-up studies and psychopharmacological trials in school-refusing children (Gittelman-Klein and Klein 1971; R. G. Klein 1995), as well as family studies in panic disorder accompanied by depression (Warner et al. 1995; Weissman et al. 1984). Drawing on research examining the relationship between social stress and panic susceptibility, D. F. Klein (1993) argued that the association between separation anxiety and panic disorder arises through an interaction between the stress of separation and a subtle underlying respiratory abnormality. Namely, separation experiences may "activate" a biological abnormality by "lowering a suffocation false alarm threshold."

We recently used a naturalistic experiment to test the idea that environmental factors may interact developmentally with the biology of respiration to shape susceptibility to panic disorder. Two diseases of children, severe asthma and congenital central hypoventilation syndrome (CCHS), are associated with a series of stressful experiences, including social separations from primary caretakers during hospitalizations, a risk of sudden death due to respiratory failure, and frequent stressful medical procedures (Mrazek 1992; Pine et al. 1994). These types of environmental stressors have been implicated in the development of panic disorder and have been shown to lead to clinical anxiety disorders among children (G. A. Bernstein and Borchardt 1991; Goodyear et al. 1988; Offord et al. 1989; Velez et al. 1989). Children with these two diseases, however, differ in one crucial aspect: only children with asthma, but not CCHS, may activate a biological substrate potentially implicated in the development of panic disorder. Children with CCHS congenitally lack the ability to perceive rising levels of carbon dioxide, an ability that is felt to be central to the theoretical suffocation alarm (D. F. Klein 1993). In contrast to children with CCHS, children with asthma experience dyspnea and sense the elevations of carbon dioxide that occur during the respiratory exacerbations that are common to the two diseases. Consistent with the idea that environmental stress interacts with the respiratory system to produce panic-related anxiety, children with asthma, but not children with CCHS, were shown to exhibit high rates of anxiety, particularly separation anxiety disorder (Pine et al. 1994).

Summary

In concluding our discussion of respiratory physiology, the extensive research implicating pulmonary dysfunction in panic disorder should be emphasized.

Some of the most supportive research includes studies of pulmonary physiology and response to respiratory challenges. Evidence exists that proximal socioenvironmental factors may interact with an underlying respiratory abnormality. From a developmental perspective, the evidence suggests that social separation may be one particularly important environmental factor in this regard.

NORADRENERGIC NERVOUS SYSTEM

Evidence of noradrenergic involvement in panic disorder includes results from studies on the growth hormone axis, the cardiovascular system, and the homeostatic control of the noradrenergic axis. A review of these three areas is presented below. To illustrate the manner in which the environment may interact with the noradrenergic axis, the review of these three areas integrates research on panic disorder with research on children who may be at risk for panic disorder and with research on nonhuman primate models of human anxiety states.

Growth Hormone Axis

Abnormalities in the noradrenergic nervous system in panic disorder are demonstrable through pharmacological challenge strategies, and these abnormalities clearly relate to the neuroendocrinology of growth. The panic attack has been viewed as a direct result of discharge by the brain stem noradrenergic neurons (Abelson and Cameron 1995). This view is consistent with challenge studies showing that the α_2 antagonist yohimbine induces panic attacks among adults with panic disorder (Charney et al. 1990) and studies in nonhuman primates using electrodes directly implanted in the locus coeruleus (Redmond 1988). Repeated discharges of noradrenergic neurons during panic attacks are thought to downregulate receptor sites distal to the locus coeruleus, producing some of the neuroendocrinological hallmarks of panic disorder. For example, human growth hormone (HGH) secretion is mediated by noradrenergic stimulation of hypothalamic α_2 receptors, which results in an acute rise in HGH releasing factor and subsequent pituitary release of HGH. Consistent with the concept of downstream adaptation to repeated locus coeruleus firing, adults with panic disorder consistently exhibit a blunted HGH response to challenges with the α_2 agonist clonidine (Abelson and Cameron 1995; Brambilla et al. 1995; Coplan et al. 1995c).

Although a blunted HGH response to challenge represents perhaps the best-replicated biological abnormality in panic disorder, this finding remains incompletely understood. For example, Brambilla et al. (1995) found an elevation in somatomedin-C levels in panic disorder, which could account for the blunted HGH response through negative feedback inhibition at the hypothalamus. Nevertheless, if central noradrenergic overactivity is the primary deficit in panic disorder, one might expect to see reduced, rather than elevated, somatomedin-C levels as a result of a chronically downregulated growth hormone system. Similarly, there is some inconsistency across studies using the α_2 antagonists as opposed to the α_2 agonists. Although the panicogenic effect of yohimbine appears to be specific to panic disorder, the same is not true for the blunted HGH response, which is also found in depression and generalized anxiety disorder, to clonidine (Abelson and Cameron 1995; Glue and Nutt 1988).

Evidence suggests that noradrenergic abnormalities arise early in the life of individuals at risk for panic disorder. The blunted HGH response to clonidine, for example, may be a "trait marker," as clinically improved adults with panic disorder continue to exhibit a blunted HGH response to this challenge agent (Coplan et al. 1995c; Uhde et al. 1992). Consistent with the idea of a "trait" abnormality in the noradrenergic system, evidence suggests that children at risk for panic disorder also posses abnormal central noradrenergic activity. This evidence derives from studies of noradrenergic metabolites among behaviorally inhibited or separation anxious children and from research on temperament in children of adults with panic disorder (Biederman et al. 1995; Kagan et al. 1990; Rogeness et al. 1992). Research in animal-based models is also consistent with the concept of a noradrenergic trait abnormality (Kagan et al. 1990; LeDoux 1992). These findings, when integrated with the research on HGH blunting in panic disorder, support the hypothesis that intrinsic noradrenergic overactivity may disrupt the growth of anxious children (Uhde et al. 1992).

In considering the plausibility of an association between childhood anxiety and an alteration in growth, it is important to draw on four areas of research examining the associations among environmental stressors, neuroendocrinological markers, and clinical anxiety disorders in children. First, it has been recognized for more than 25 years that extreme social stress in the form of maternal deprivation can produce profound effects on the growth hormone axis, even to the point of disrupting growth (G. F. Powell et al. 1967). Interestingly, the effect on the growth hormone axis produces a physiological phenocopy of the abnormal HGH response seen in panic disorder (G. M. Brown 1975). Second, with regard to behavior, it is well-known that social stress often produces clinical anxiety disorders in children. Girls appear particularly susceptible to this effect, whereas boys are either less vulnerable or more likely to show signs of disruptive rather than emotional psychopathology (Buchanan et al. 1992; Ge et al. 1994). Third, this differential behavioral susceptibility to the effects of stress across genders may relate to biological effects. Emotional psychopathology in girls may be more closely related to the biological abnormalities found in anxious adults than is emotional psychopathology in boys (Fergusson et al. 1995; Ryan and Dahl 1994; E. J. Sussman and Chrousos 1991). This may reflect an underlying gender-specific vulnerability in the neuroendocrinological systems related to emotional disorders (Buchanan et al. 1992). Finally, such gender-specific associations between stress and anxiety in children may be relevant for adult anxiety disorders, relating to the fact that anxiety in girls appears more chronic over time than does anxiety in boys (Costello and Angold 1995).

Integrating this research examining the effects of environmental stressors on both the neuroendocrinology of growth and the behavior of children across genders, we reasoned that an association between anxiety and stature might arise only in females. We examined the association between childhood anxiety and stature in an epidemiological sample of 712 children who had been selected from upstate New York and followed longitudinally over 9 years from ages 13 to 22. Consistent with our hypothesis, we found that girls with anxiety disorders, particularly separation anxiety disorder, grew up to be nearly two inches shorter than girls without anxiety disorders (Pine et al. 1996a). This study suggested that anxiety disorders in girls may indeed disrupt the neuroendocrinology of growth and that this disruptive effect may be partially mediated by female susceptibility to psychosocial stressors. In future studies, we plan to focus on gender differences while directly examining the relationship between environmental stress and the growth hormone response to challenge in children and adults.

Cardiovascular Activity

An intrinsic abnormality of central noradrenergic activity in panic disorder might produce abnormalities beyond those seen in the hypothalamic-pituitary-somatotropin axis. For example, areas of the central nervous system with profound noradrenergic enervation play a crucial role in the regulation of cardiovascular activity. Hence, noradrenergic dysregulation in panic disorder may be observable in the activity of the cardiovascular system.

The autonomic regulation of cardiac activity can be monitored through entirely noninvasive techniques. These methods are ideal for large-scale epidemiological studies as well as developmentally based research. Autonomic signals to the heart produce oscillation of the R-to-R interval period (i.e., heart period variability [HPV]). By using Fourier analysis to decompose these oscillations, estimates can be generated of parasympathetic activity in the high-frequency component of the HPV power spectrum (0.15–0.50 Hz), baroreceptor functions in the low-frequency component of the HPV power spectrum (0.05–0.15 Hz), and sympathovagal balance in the ratio of these components.

A number of studies have examined HPV patterns or related constructs in panic disorder (Hayward 1995; Yeragani et al. 1993). The two most consistent findings are a reduction in high-frequency power, suggestive of reduced "vagal tone," and an elevated "low-to-high" frequency ratio, suggestive of sympathovagal imbalance.

Research on sudden cardiac death suggests that these autonomic abnormalities may be important when considering the effects of environmental stressors on the cardiac system. The association between stress and sudden cardiac death has been noted for many years. One of the more recent studies demonstrating this association found an increase in sudden death following the SCUD missile attacks in Israel (Meisel et al. 1991). This association, in turn, has been attributed to the effect of stress on an autonomically vulnerable heart. Biologically predisposed individuals with underlying autonomic abnormalities such as reduced vagal tone or sympathovagal imbalance may experience cardiac events, particularly malignant arrhythmias, in the face of stress. Studies describing an association between cardiac events and panic disorder or "phobic anxiety," probably a related condition, are consistent with the idea that the autonomic abnormalities seen in panic disorder may impart cardiac vulnerability in the face of environmental stress (Hayward 1995; Kawachi et al. 1995). Research in children resonates with research describing cardiac correlates of panic disorder in adults. Studies of autonomic regulation in children with behavioral inhibition (Kagan et al. 1987; Snidman et al. 1995) and children with clinical anxiety disorders (Pine et al. 1996b) found evidence of reduced vagal tone and sympathovagal imbalance, consistent with that found in studies of panic disorder. This suggests that there may be a degree of developmental stability in the autonomic correlates of panic-related conditions across the life span. Parenthetically, this may carry implications for the risk of sudden death in children during pharmacological treatment (Walsh et al. 1995).

Some have suggested that cardiac autonomic profiles may classify children with respect to their adaptability to the environment (Porges 1991). In contrast to studies of stature in anxious children, where environmental factors are offered as a potential mediator of the associations found between biology and anxiety, Kagan et al. (1990) suggested that cardiac measures may identify children who are relatively insensitive or maladaptive to a certain class of environmental factors. Although behavioral inhibition is a relatively common feature in infancy, many inhibited infants are no longer inhibited at follow-up, possibly as a result of the shaping effects of the environment on temperament (Kagan et al. 1990). Abnormalities in HPV among inhibited infants are believed to identify those infants who are impervious to these environmental affects. Infants who are inhibited and show a reduction in HPV are more likely to remain inhibited over time than are inhibited infants with normal HPV profiles (Kagan et al. 1990).

Dysregulation of the Noradrenergic System

In much of the research on panic disorder, a relatively simple defect in the noradrenergic system is assumed. Thus, both the growth hormone and the cardiac abnormalities in panic disorder have been attributed to overactivity of the noradrenergic system. As mentioned above, however, the inconsistencies in this research preclude the adoption of a simple "overactivity" model (Abelson and Cameron 1995). Beyond the inconsistencies in the growth hormone findings, other inconsistencies include the facts that normal peripheral noradrenergic profiles are found in many individuals with panic disorder and that the clinical pharmacological response in panic disorder is not consistent with a simple noradrenergic overactivity model. These inconsistencies have led to the theory that the noradrenergic nervous system is "dysregulated," rather than simply overactive, in panic disorder.

Noradrenergic dysregulation can be found in panic disorder by examining the relationship between the noradrenergic axis and the hypothalamic-pituitary-adrenal (HPA) axis. There is a well-described coordination between these axes in humans and nonhuman primates (Chrousos and Gold 1992), and using the clonidine challenge paradigm, we showed that this coordination may be lost in panic disorder (Coplan et al. 1995b). In psychiatrically healthy adults, we found a series of correlations between resting markers of noradrenergic and HPA activity as well as correlations between markers of noradrenergic and HPA sensitivity to clonidine (Coplan et al. 1995b). Furthermore, these correlations were replicated in repeat challenge tests on psychiatrically healthy subjects conducted 3 months after the initial study. Suggestive of a tightly controlled homeostatic system, associations *across* the noradrenergic/HPA axes were found over the 3-month interval. These associations, in contrast, were absent in panic disorder.

We also found evidence of noradrenergic dysregulation that was independent of the HPA axis in subsequent analysis of the noradrenergic response to clonidine in this sample. Although psychiatrically healthy control subjects exhibited stable declines in the levels of 3-methoxy-4-hydroxyphenylglycol (MHPG) during a clonidine challenge, adults with panic disorder exhibited a chaotic MHPG response. Interestingly, whereas fluoxetine treatment had no effect on the dysregulated noradrenergic/HPA relationship, fluoxetine treatment effectively normalized the chaotic MHPG response to clonidine. Hence, these results suggest that the noradrenergic abnormality in panic disorder may be characterized as a loss of the normal homeostasis rather than a simple overactivity. Some aspects of this abnormality may be state-related and normalize following changes in the serotonergic system; other aspects may be impervious to these changes (Coplan et al. 1995a, 1995b, 1995c).

Studies on the noradrenergic axis in nonhuman primates provide evidence that early environmental stressors may provoke biological and behavioral "phenocopies" of human clinical anxiety states. We have used the primate model of developmental psychopathology pioneered by Rosenblum et al. (1991) to explore this issue. Nonhuman primates who were reared as infants by mothers undergoing environmental stress induced by unpredictable or variable foraging demand (VFD-reared) conditions were compared with nonhuman primates reared as infants by mothers exposed to predictable (either low [LFD-reared] or high [HFD-reared]) foraging demand conditions.

VFD-reared but not LFD- or HFD-reared (non–VFD-reared) primates subsequently exhibited clinging behaviors to mother in a novel room test and were more likely to develop depressive-like "despair" responses when maternally separated. Such anxiety and affective traits in the VFD-reared primates resemble high-reactive rhesus (Suomi et al. 1978) and behaviorally inhibited children (Biederman et al. 1995); each entity is hypothesized to predispose to pathological adult anxiety states. Indirect evidence for noradrenergic alterations in young adult VFD-reared subjects has previously been provided by blind behavioral observations of primate affective response, including inhibited behaviors, to pharmacological probes. VFD-reared nonhuman primates exhibited behavioral hyperresponsivity to the noradrenergic probe yohimbine and an associated behavioral hyporesponsivity to the serotonergic probe *m*-chlorophenylpiperazine (Rosenblum et al. 1991). Isolate-reared nonhuman primates exhibited blunted behavioral responses to yohimbine (Coplan et al. 1992c), suggesting a progression of noradrenergic dysregulation with increasing level of stressor.

In addition, biochemical alterations are detectable in cisternal cerebrospinal fluid (CSF) samples obtained from ketamine-anesthetized unpredictably reared grown primates. CSF corticotropin-releasing factor, CSF somatostatin, and CSF 5-hydroxyindoleacetic acid concentrations were elevated, but CSF cortisol concentrations were decreased, in the VFD-reared primates in comparison with levels in non-VFD-reared subjects (Coplan et al. 1994). Although CSF MHPG was not different between rearing groups, a greater degree of between-subject variability in unpredictably versus predictably reared animals was found.

The data provide support for the view that adverse, unpredictable early rearing may lead to persistent behavioral effects manifested as anxiety- and depressive-like behaviors. This VFD-rearing effect is accompanied by noradrenergic abnormalities occurring within a context of synchronized neuropeptidergic and monoaminergic abnormalities. Consistent with the posttraumatic stress disorder but not panic disorder literature (Yehuda et al. 1995), HPA axis function, as reflected by CSF cortisol, appears reduced in the VFD-reared subjects despite increased CSF corticotropin-releasing factor concentrations, and, unlike in panic disorder, a significant positive CSF cortisol–MHPG correlation was observed in both rearing groups (Coplan et al. 1994).

Summary

The relationship between noradrenergic activity and panic disorder draws consistent interest. Recent studies reviewed above suggest that panic disorder may be associated with a loss of the normal homeostasis in the noradrenergic system. Such dysregulation may account for results in noradrenergic challenge studies as well as in cardiovascular challenge studies. Research in children and in nonhuman primates suggests that environmental stressors may play a role in the association between noradrenergic dysregulation and panic disorder.

CONCLUSION

The abnormalities in both the respiratory and the noradrenergic systems among adults with panic disorder are among the most consistent findings in research on human emotional disorders. For respiratory measures, these abnormalities include baseline abnormalities in ventilatory profiles, susceptibility to challenge-induced panic states, and physiological abnormalities during challenge. For noradrenergic measures, these abnormalities include abnormal neuroendocrinological responses to challenge agents, dysregulation of cardiac activity, and dysregulation in noradrenergic axis homeostasis. Research among children and nonhuman primates suggests that these biological abnormalities can be viewed in a developmental context. The reviewed evidence in this chapter suggests that both proximal and developmental factors in the environment may affect these biological systems as they relate to panic disorder in adults.

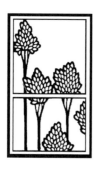

CHAPTER 23

Serotonin-Specific Anxiolytics: Now and in the Future

Jelena L. Kunovac, M.D., and
Stephen M. Stahl, M.D., Ph.D.

Serotonin neurons have been implicated in the regulation of a wide variety of physiological and behavioral processes. The cell bodies of serotonergic neurons arise in the brain stem raphe nuclei and, through several projection pathways, innervate structures as diverse as cortex, hypothalamus, thalamus, basal ganglia, and the limbic system (importantly, the septo-hippocampal system and the amygdala) (Kahn et al. 1988). Consistent with the anatomy of the serotonin system, this neurotransmitter is involved in anxiety, panic, arousal, vigilance, aggression, suicidal behavior, mood, impulsivity, regulation of food intake, and obsessive-compulsive behavior (M. S. Eison 1989).

At least 18 different serotonin receptors, divided into numerous families,

This work was supported in part by National Institute of Mental Health Research Grant 5 R01 MH45787–02 and by a Veterans Administration Merit Review Award to S.M.S. This work was also supported in part by Mental Health Clinical Research Center Grant MH30914 and General Clinical Research Center Grant M01-RR00827 to the University of California, San Diego.

have been identified to date in the mammalian central nervous system. Among them, two groups can be distinguished with regard to their respective affinities for 5-hydroxytryptamine (serotonin; 5-HT) (Miquel and Hamon 1992). The receptors in the first group have a high in vivo binding affinity for serotonin (K_d in the nanomolar range) and can therefore be directly labeled by 5-[^{3}H]HT. Specifically, 5-HT$_1$, 5-HT$_6$, and 5-HT$_7$ receptors have high affinity for serotonin (between 1 and 100 nM) (Miquel and Hamon 1992). 5-HT$_1$ receptors have been further subclassified (5-HT$_{1A}$, 5-HT$_{1B}$, 5-HT$_{1D}$, 5-HT$_{1E}$, 5-HT$_{1F}$) to distinguish pharmacologically defined subgroups. 5-HT$_1$ receptors generally appear to mediate inhibitory actions of serotonin. The 5-HT$_{1B}$ receptor is found in rats and mice, but not in abundance in humans, whereas an analogue of this receptor, called 5-HT$_{1D}$, is found in primates, including humans (Harrington et al. 1992).

In contrast, receptors in the second group have a low affinity (micromolar range) for serotonin and have been divided into three different classes—named 5-HT$_2$, 5-HT$_3$, and 5-HT$_4$—with specific pharmacological properties (Miquel and Hamon 1992). The 5-HT$_2$ receptor (with subgroups 5-HT$_{2A}$, 5-HT$_{2B}$, and 5-HT$_{2C}$) mediates facilitatory effects of serotonin, whereas the 5-HT$_3$ receptor is the only serotonin receptor that directly activates an ion channel and therefore provides rapid activation of target cells.

SEROTONIN AND ANXIETY

The discovery that buspirone, a 5-HT$_{1A}$ receptor partial agonist, possesses anxiolytic properties has generated major interest in serotonin as a neurotransmitter involved in the neurobiology of anxiety. Two seemingly opposing theories attempt to explain a connection between anxiety and the serotonergic system. The older theory addresses generalized anxiety disorder and suggests that increased anxiety is related to increased activity of serotonergic neurons (Iversen 1984). It follows from this theory, therefore, that decreasing serotonin activity causes a decrease in generalized anxiety symptoms. Development of serotonin reuptake inhibitors and their effectiveness in the treatment of obsessive-compulsive disorder, panic disorder, and social phobia has led, however, to an opposing view suggesting that an increase in central serotonergic activity actually diminishes anxiety, especially anxiety associated with obsessive-compulsive disorder, panic disorder, and social phobia (Eriksson 1987).

These two theories may actually be more consistent than they appear on the surface. The short-term increase in central serotonergic activity caused by selective serotonin reuptake inhibitors does not correlate with the onset of therapeutic action because selective serotonin reuptake inhibitors relieve anxiety only in the long term, presumably as a result of their ability to cause diminished sensitivity, that is, downregulation of serotonin receptors on chronic administration. In fact, the initial increase in serotonin activity caused by selective serotonin reuptake inhibitors when treating patients with panic disorder, for example, may initially worsen symptoms, until chronic treatment causes adaptation in serotonin receptors and a delayed diminution of anxiety symptoms.

Animal Studies

Manipulation of the serotonergic system in animal models can be implemented with several strategies: inhibition of serotonin synthesis, destruction of serotonin neurons, use of serotonin antagonists, and increase of serotonin function.

The most frequently used animal models of anxiety are the novel environment model, conflict paradigm, and X-maze anxiety model. The first, the novel environment model, involves placing the animal in a large, ceilingless, brightly lit box. In this situation, animals tend to show decreased exploratory behavior and decreased social interaction, both of which are regarded as indicative of anxiety (Kahn and Moore 1993). The second, the conflict paradigm, is based on a conditioned emotional response model developed by Estes and Skinner (1941) and later modified by Geller and Seifter (1967) and by J. R. Vogel et al. (1971). In conflict models, the animal is faced with the conflict situation between reward and punishment, and, as a result of increased anxiety, "behavioral suppression" follows. The release from behavioral suppression is assumed to be related to anxiety reduction; and the quantity of release, a measure of the anxiolytic effect. A modification of the novel environment model, called the X-maze anxiety model, appears to overcome one important limitation of these two models, namely, a lack of adequate measurement of increased anxiety (Kahn and Moore 1993).

The anxiolytic effects associated with a decrease in serotonin function through the inhibition of serotonin synthesis have been observed in several conflict paradigms and in the novel environmental model (Kahn and Moore 1993). Less consistent data have been observed when serotonin function is diminished using destruction of serotonin neurons or when serotonin antagonists are used (Kahn and Moore 1993). Buspirone, a $5\text{-}HT_{1A}$ partial agonist, and methysergide, a nonselective $5\text{-}HT_{2A}/5\text{-}HT_{2C}$ antagonist, both show anxiolytic effects in the conflict paradigm, whereas ipsapirone, a $5\text{-}HT_{1A}$ partial agonist, shows anxiolytic action in a social interaction model and a staircase model (A. Eison and Eison 1994). 5-HT$_3$ antagonists are consistently effective in reducing anxiety in the novel environment model and in the social interaction model (Kahn and Moore 1993). By contrast, increasing serotonin function by numerous pharmacological means is anxiogenic in nearly all animal models of anxiety (Kahn and Moore 1993).

Human Studies

Findings from peripheral marker studies, challenge studies, and treatment studies provide evidence for serotonin dysfunction in panic disorder, generalized anxiety disorder, and obsessive-compulsive disorder. As also observed in animal studies, 5-HT$_{1A}$, 5-HT$_{2A}$, 5-HT$_{2C}$, and 5-HT$_3$ receptors are all implicated in human disorders of anxiety. However, the question remains as to which anxiety disorder subtype is related to which serotonin abnormality or receptor. Although frequently discussed by basic scientists as a unitary hypothesis linking anxiety in general to serotonin functioning in general, the *serotonin excess hypothesis of anxiety* does not make it at all clear whether the various specific subtypes of anxiety disorders in psychiatric patients share a common serotonin abnormality related to a unitary psychopathological dimension of the symptom of anxiety (Van Praag et al. 1990).

The anxiolytic activity of several compounds in some, but not all, animal models of anxiety in fact suggests that different receptor subtypes may modulate different types of anxiety as discussed below. It would not be surprising if the specific serotonin links to disorders of anxiety also differ among the various disorders of anxiety such as generalized anxiety versus obsessive-compulsive disorder versus panic disorder versus social phobia versus mixed anxiety depression. Such studies are in progress, and much further research is necessary to clarify the potential links between subtypes of anxiety and subtypes of serotonin receptors.

DRUGS ACTING ON 5-HT$_{1A}$ RECEPTORS

5-HT$_{1A}$ Receptor Characteristics

The 5-HT$_{1A}$ receptor was first described in 1981 and is perhaps the best characterized of the serotonin receptors. 5-HT$_{1A}$ receptors have been implicated in the regulation of aggression, affect, anxiety, appetite, sexual behavior, and in the control of stress-related disorders (Dourish et al. 1987). Also, these receptors play a major role in modulating serotonergic transmission.

Structurally, the 5-HT$_{1A}$ receptor belongs to the G protein–coupled family of neurotransmitter receptors. 5-HT$_{1A}$ receptors are located both presynaptically (on cell bodies and/or dendrites) and postsynaptically (Radja et al. 1992). Presynaptic (or somatodendritic) autoreceptors are most dense in dorsal raphe nuclei and are in part responsible for the pacemaker function of raphe neurons, providing the baseline discharge rate of serotonin neurons. Somatodendritic autoreceptors are coupled to the opening of K$^+$ channels in the cell membrane, which in turn leads to an increase in the hyperpolarization across the membrane and a reduction in cell firing rate (Aghajanian and Lakoski 1984). Postsynaptic 5-HT$_{1A}$ receptors are highly expressed in the hippocampus, lateral septum, hypothalamus, and frontal cortex (Verge et al. 1986). In addition to its localization on serotonin neurons, the 5-HT$_{1A}$ receptor is found on a number of other neuronal cell types, where its general function also appears to be inhibition of neuronal activity (Sprouse and Wilkinson 1995).

The second-messenger linkage of postsynaptic 5-HT$_{1A}$ receptors has been connected in various neurons with either inhibition of adenylate cyclase, stimulation of adenylate cyclase, or inhibition of phosphoinositide turnover (Harrington et al. 1992).

Azaperones. Many selective 5-HT$_{1A}$ anxiolytics are pyrimidinyl-piperazine compounds, called azapirones, which share a number of pharmacological properties. Buspirone, a 5-HT$_{1A}$ agonist, was the first serotonin-acting antianxiety drug approved in the United States for the treatment of generalized anxiety disorder. Today, several similar compounds, including gepirone, ipsapirone, and tandospirone, are under clinical development as putative anxiolytics.

These drugs are conceptualized as full agonists at 5-HT$_{1A}$ somatodendritic autoreceptors as well as partial agonists at postsynaptic 5-HT$_{1A}$ receptors. As full agonists at somatodendritic 5-HT$_{1A}$ autoreceptors, these compounds are theoretically capable of producing a complete suppression of neuronal activity at relatively low doses, whereas the capacity of these drugs to activate postsynaptic 5-HT$_{1A}$ receptors is low. Thus, full activation of the postsynaptic 5-HT$_{1A}$ receptor is not thought to be achieved even at doses higher than those needed to influence presynaptic receptors (Sprouse and Wilkinson 1995). In the absence of endogenous serotonin (e.g., in depression), as partial agonists at 5-HT$_{1A}$ receptors, azaperones are conceptualized as net agonists, whereas in the presence of high synaptic serotonin concentrations (e.g., in anxiety), they act as net antagonists.

Overall, azaperones may decrease serotonin neurotransmission through two mechanisms: 1) direct inhibition of raphe cell firing by stimulating presynaptic somatodendritic autoreceptors and 2) as net antagonists, therefore blocking postsynaptic receptors when high synaptic serotonin concentrations are present. The latest results from animal experiments indicate that postsynaptic 5-HT$_{1A}$ receptors may not be responsible for the anxiolytic response to azaperones (Jolas et al. 1995).

Psychopharmacologists have been trying to explain the existence of heterogeneous 5-HT$_{1A}$ receptors. Because measures of the pharmacodynamic properties of presynaptic and postsynaptic 5-HT$_{1A}$ receptors have not revealed any striking differences (Radja et al. 1992), the concept of receptor reserve has emerged. According to this concept, the region of the raphe nuclei has a large receptor reserve (R. F. Cox et al. 1993; Meller et al. 1990), whereas serotonin projection areas, such as the hippocampus, have a low receptor reserve (Yocca et al. 1992). In areas with a large receptor reserve, buspirone-like compounds appear to be full agonists by partially activating many receptors, the sum of which gives full response (Sprouse and Wilkinson 1995). In a region with low receptor reserve, however, a partial agonist such as buspirone should produce a submaximal effect on these cells even when receptors are saturated (Sprouse and Wilkinson 1995).

Buspirone.   Several comparative studies of buspirone and benzodiazepines have reported comparable efficacy in reducing symptoms of anxiety. However, in contrast to benzodiazepines, buspirone is devoid of significant sedative or euphoric effects. Treatment with buspirone and other azaperones, such as gepirone, ipsapirone, and tandospirone, does not result in abuse, addiction, dependence, or withdrawal symptoms (Keppel Hesselink 1992). Buspirone also spares both cognitive and psychomotor performance (N. Sussman 1994).

Several studies (cited in N. Sussman 1994) suggest a preferential effect of buspirone on psychological symptoms of anxiety. Buspirone promotes a greater decrease in symptoms (e.g., anger, hostility, worry, difficulty in concentration) indicative of cognitive and interpersonal problems, whereas diazepam and clorazepate favor somatic symptoms of anxiety (e.g., muscle tension, insomnia).

Feighner and Cohen (1989) performed a pooled-data analysis of six studies of buspirone in the treatment of generalized anxiety disorder. Buspirone was observed to improve all symptom groups on the Hamilton Anxiety Scale (M. Hamilton 1959). Onset of anxiolytic therapy was evident within 1 week, whereas continued improvement was evident until the 4-week end point. The psychic symptoms of anxiety, such as anxious mood, tension, irritability, and aggression, improved earlier than the somatic symptoms of anxiety.

The major disadvantage of buspirone and buspirone-related compounds is slower onset of action, requiring approximately 2–4 weeks of treatment to fully develop (N. Sussman 1994). Also, their short half-lives require dosing several times a day. Once-daily controlled-release formulations are under clinical testing.

In summary, buspirone is an effective generalized anxiety treatment that differs from conventional antianxiety drugs in speed of symptom reduction and types of symptoms affected. Although buspirone might seem to be the drug of choice for treatment of chronic anxiety, it has not displaced the use of benzodiazepines in the treatment of anxiety, perhaps because of its side-effect profile (dizziness, sedation, nausea), slow onset of action, and the opinion of some clinicians that its anxiolytic efficacy is less robust than that of benzodiazepines. Buspirone is accepted as an anxiolytic treatment much more widely in the United States than in most other countries (Kunovac and Stahl 1995).

Gepirone. Gepirone is a chemical analogue of buspirone and also acts as a partial agonist at 5-HT$_{1A}$ receptors. It is active in animal models predictive of anxiolytic action and also shows antidepressant activity in preclinical studies. With long-term administration, gepirone downregulates 5-HT$_2$ receptors, which is a property common to nearly all antidepressant drugs (Stahl 1994). This dual action, suggesting both anxiolytic and antidepressant effects, is typical of many compounds acting at 5-HT$_{1A}$ receptors and may indicate that such compounds may be useful in the treatment of mixed anxiety and depression (Stahl, in press).

Preliminary phase II clinical data have shown that gepirone is an effective anxiolytic that significantly reduces both psychic and somatic symptoms of generalized anxiety disorder. Like buspirone, gepirone does not impair memory, verbal fluency, or psychomotor performance (Harto and Branconnier 1988).

Ipsapirone. Results of a phase II United States multicenter trial of ipsapirone, another azaperone 5-HT$_{1A}$ partial agonist, in the treatment of generalized anxiety disorder have shown that ipsapirone is effective in reducing anxiety as measured by the Hamilton Anxiety Scale (Keppel Hesselink 1992). Ipsapirone is effective at 5 mg three times a day, and significant results are seen after only 1 week of treatment (Borison et al. 1990; Boyer and Feighner 1993). Adverse effects, such as dizziness, nausea, light-headedness, and headache, are dose related. Phase II studies also suggest efficacy of ipsapirone in major depressive disorder. Side effects are apparently much reduced by once-daily controlled-release administration of ipsapirone, and further testing of this formulation in depression is ongoing.

Tandospirone.   Tandospirone is another 5-HT$_{1A}$ receptor agonist under development by Sumitomo Pharmaceutical Co., Ltd., in Japan and Pfizer in the United States. Results of phase II and phase III clinical trials show that tandospirone is effective for the treatment of anxiety neurosis. Significant improvement is also observed in patients with psychosomatic disease, phobia, and depersonalization (Murasaki 1995). The results have shown that initial treatment should be started at 30 mg daily, and the dose should be increased up to 60 mg daily according to symptoms (Murasaki 1995). A double-blind comparative study with diazepam revealed that tandospirone tends to be superior to diazepam in patients with depressive neurosis, whereas diazepam may be more effective than tandospirone in severely ill patients (Murasaki et al. 1992).

Nonazaperone/novel second-generation 5-HT$_{1A}$ agonists.   Several new compounds belonging to the second generation of 5-HT$_{1A}$ receptor–acting drugs are in phase II and III clinical trials throughout the world.

Flesinoxan.   Flesinoxan is a new heterobicyclic-aryl-piperazine, chemically different from buspirone-like compounds. In vitro, flesinoxan is a highly selective 5-HT$_{1A}$ receptor agonist and has much weaker affinity for α_1-adrenergic, dopamine 2, and dopamine 3 receptors compared with buspirone (Duphar, unpublished data). The highest density of flesinoxan binding sites in brain is observed in the hippocampus, dentate gyrus, lateral septum, and entorrhinal cortex (Duphar, unpublished data). In several animal paradigms of anxiety, flesinoxan is more potent in reducing anxiety than are buspirone and ipsapirone (Duphar, unpublished data). Phase II studies have shown that flesinoxan is clearly effective in relieving symptoms of generalized anxiety disorder and better than placebo (Duphar, unpublished data). Generally, a low dose (0.4 mg) of flesinoxan is well tolerated. Higher doses (4.0 mg) are associated with treatment emergent adverse events, such as nausea, vomiting, nervousness, dizziness, and headache (Duphar, unpublished data). Currently, flesinoxan is under clinical development as a treatment both for generalized anxiety disorder and for major depressive disorder.

CP-93,393–1.   CP-93,393–1 is a selective and potent serotonin autoreceptor agonist also under clinical development for the treatment of both anxiety and depression.

DRUGS ACTING ON 5-HT₂ RECEPTORS

5-HT$_{2A}$ Receptor Characteristics

The 5-HT$_{2A}$ receptor is labeled in high concentration in the prefrontal cortex, claustrum, neocortex (in human cortex mainly in layer III and V), tuberculum olfactorium, nucleus accumbens, and the posterolateral extension of the caudate nucleus. In the neocortex, 5-HT$_{2A}$ receptors have been also detected on pyramidal cells and on γ-aminobutyric acid (GABA)-ergic and somatostatin-containing neurons (Araneda and Andrade 1991).

Although pharmacological and pathophysiological roles for 5-HT$_{2A}$ receptors have been identified, their role under normal physiological conditions remains enigmatic (J. E. Leysen 1992). It is possible that 5-HT$_{2A}$ receptors have very low activation under normal physiological conditions and that they are activated only during short periods of the day-night cycle, in emergencies, or in pathological conditions, such as dysthymia, anxiety, or social withdrawal (J. E. Leysen 1992). Leysen has hypothesized that, as a result of a normal low-activation state, 5-HT$_{2A}$ receptors may normally exist in a supersensitive state, which makes them "resistant" to upregulation and susceptible to rapid desensitization and downregulation after agonist stimulation. A most interesting observation relevant to anxiolytic actions is the finding that 5-HT$_{2A}$ receptors are sensitive to heterologous desensitization, such as by 5-HT$_{1A}$ receptor stimulation (J. E. Leysen 1992).

5-HT$_{2C}$ Receptor Characteristics

Recent nomenclature of serotonin receptors (TIPS Receptor Nomenclature Supplement 1994) reclassifies the 5-HT$_{1C}$ receptor as a 5-HT$_{2C}$ receptor because of structural and pharmacological similarities to the 5-HT$_{2A}$ receptor. 5-HT$_{2C}$ receptors have been also implicated in anxiety, as well as in appetite, depression, learning, aversion, and psychosis (Dubovsky 1994). Stimulation of the 5-HT$_{2C}$ receptor, similar to stimulation of the 5-HT$_{2A}$ receptor, leads to activation of phospholipase C and increased phosphoinositide hydrolysis. 5-HT$_{2A}$ and 5-HT$_{2C}$ receptors share an overall amino acid sequence identity of 50%. In fact, in the transmembrane regions the sequence identity is 80%. This observation in large part led to a reclassification of the 5-HT$_{1C}$ receptor as a member of the 5-HT$_2$ receptor family (Dubovsky 1994).

The 5-HT$_{2C}$ receptor has highest density in the choroid plexus on epithelial cells associated with production of cerebrospinal fluid (Pazos and Palacios 1985). 5-HT$_{2C}$ receptors are also found in the cingulate cortex, hippocampus, hypothalamus, thalamus, and several subcortical regions with large monoaminergic cell groups (substantia nigra, the raphe, the reticular nuclei, and the locus coeruleus) (Julius et al. 1988).

As most of the currently available 5-HT$_2$ receptor antagonists for human testing (e.g., amesergide and ritanserin) act at both 5-HT$_{2A}$ and 5-HT$_{2C}$ receptors, it is not always easy to separate the actions of these two receptor subtypes.

m-Chlorophenylpiperazine (mCPP) is a metabolite of antidepressants trazodone and nefazodone and binds 5-HT$_1$, 5-HT$_2$, and 5-HT$_3$ receptors, with the greatest affinity for the 5-HT$_{2C}$ receptor subtypes. Short-term administration of mCPP in humans and laboratory animals causes anxiety (Kennett et al. 1994). The anxiogenic effects of mCPP are blocked by nonselective 5-HT$_{2C}$/5-HT$_{2A}$ receptor antagonists metergoline, methysergide, and ritanserin. Furthermore, preclinical testing of several nonselective 5-HT$_{2C}$/5-HT$_{2A}$ receptor antagonists, including mianserin, *l*-naphthyl piperazine, ICI 169369, and LY 53857 also exhibit an anxiolytic profile in two rat models of anxiety, whereas selective 5-HT$_{2A}$ receptor antagonists have no effect (Kennett et al. 1994). These observations have led to the hypothesis that the anxiogenic effects of mCPP and the anxiolytic effects of nonselective 5-HT$_{2C}$/5-HT$_{2A}$ antagonists may be mediated through 5-HT$_{2C}$ receptors in the hippocampus, a brain region where high levels of 5-HT$_{2C}$ receptor mRNA have been identified (Kennett et al. 1994). Further evaluation of this hypothesis awaits the development of more selective 5-HT$_{2C}$ antagonists. However, the clinical findings that the nonselective 5-HT$_{2A}$/5-HT$_{2C}$ antagonist mianserin possesses anxiolytic properties and that ritanserin is also effective in the treatment of generalized anxiety disorder support results from animal models of anxiety implicating a role of 5-HT$_2$ receptors in anxiety.

FG 5893 is a novel compound with high affinity for 5-HT$_{1A}$ and 5-HT$_{2A}$ receptors, but low affinity for 5-HT$_{2C}$ receptors. Preclinical pharmacology indicates that FG 5893 is a potent stimulator of presynaptic 5-HT$_{1A}$ receptors, but is less active at postsynaptic 5-HT$_{1A}$ sites (Albinsson et al. 1994). In two rat anxiety models, this compound has shown anxiolytic activity comparable to that of known anxiolytics.

DRUGS ACTING ON 5-HT$_3$ RECEPTORS

5-HT$_3$ Receptor Characteristics

The 5-HT$_3$ receptor differs from other monoamine receptor subtypes in constituting a multiunit ion channel analogous to nicotinic acetylcholine, GABA$_A$, and glycine receptors (Derkach et al. 1989). Therefore, responses to serotonin at these receptors are faster compared with serotonin actions at other receptor sites.

5-HT$_3$ receptors are located exclusively on neurons and are widely distributed throughout the peripheral and central nervous systems. In the periphery, 5-HT$_3$ receptors are found on autonomic, sensory, and enteric neurons (Fozard 1984). In the central nervous system, 5-HT$_3$ receptors are labeled in cortex, hippocampus, caudate hypothalamus, brain stem, midbrain, and cerebellum, with the highest density in discrete nuclei of the lower brain stem (e.g., dorsal vagal complex and spinal trigeminal nucleus), the area postrema, and substantia gelatinosa at all levels of the spinal cord (Palacios et al. 1991; Waeber et al. 1989).

Activation of 5-HT$_3$ receptors elicits prominent pharmacological responses from the cardiovascular and respiratory systems and from the gastrointestinal tract (Fozard 1992). Several 5-HT$_3$ receptor antagonists have been marketed for the treatment of nausea and vomiting associated with cancer chemotherapy and radiotherapy (Bunce et al. 1991).

5-HT$_3$ receptor antagonists exhibit anxiolytic profiles in animal models such as the light-dark box and social interaction test and in marmosets and cynomolgus monkeys during encounters with humans (Costall and Naylor 1992a). The preclinical profile of 5-HT$_3$ antagonists suggests that they do not cause sedation, do not have addictive liabilities, do not cause withdrawal symptoms, and are effective anxiolytics when administered following benzodiazepine withdrawal (Costall and Naylor 1992b; Nevins and Anthony 1994).

Ondansetron.   The 5-HT$_3$ antagonist ondansetron has been reported to be effective in the treatment of generalized anxiety disorder, with efficacy comparable to that of diazepam (Lader 1991). Sedation and rebound anxiety during withdrawal from ondansetron were not observed (Lader 1991). Ondansetron has been considered for phase III clinical trials for the treatment of social phobia and panic disorder.

Tropisetron.   The 5-HT$_3$ antagonist tropisetron has also been reported to be effective in the treatment of patients with generalized anxiety disorder (Lecrubier et al. 1993). The anxiolytic effect of tropisetron develops quickly, is dose dependent, and is accompanied by satisfactory tolerability and safety. The incidence of adverse events, including headache, nausea, constipation, and nervousness, is low and the severity is generally mild. The most typical adverse effects of benzodiazepine anxiolytics, such as fatigue, muscle relaxation, and disturbances of attention and memory, are not generally observed (Lecrubier et al. 1993). After withdrawal of tropisetron, there is no rebound anxiety (Lecrubier et al. 1993).

Zacopride.   Pecknold et al. (1991) reported that another 5-HT$_3$ antagonist, zacopride, showed anxiolytic effects in a 4-week double-blind, placebo-controlled study.

BRL 46470A is a highly potent, selective, and long-acting 5-HT$_3$ receptor antagonist that showed anxiolytic-like activity in two animal models, that is, the elevated X-maze and social interaction model in rats, predictive of antianxiety effects. In both models, BRL 46470A showed significant activity over a wide dose range following both oral and systemic administration (Blackburn et al. 1986) and was 100-fold more potent than the 5-HT$_3$ receptor antagonist ondansetron.

CONCLUSION

Recent years have witnessed a rapid escalation in the discovery of serotonin receptor subtypes, complete with agents increasingly selective for a single receptor subtype. Both the behaviors of animals in preclinical models of anxiety and the symptoms in psychiatric patients with anxiety disorder subtypes are modified by pharmacological agents acting at one or more serotonin receptor subtypes. Most emphasis is currently being given to the anxiolytic potential of agents acting at 5-HT$_{1A}$ receptors, with increasing interest in agents acting at 5-HT$_{2A}$, 5-HT$_{2C}$, and 5-HT$_3$ receptors as well. Indeed, some of the newest agents exhibit "intramolecular polypharmacy" in that they act at two or more serotonin receptor subtypes simultaneously (Preskorn 1995). Current research is clarifying the role of each serotonin receptor subtype, not only in anxiety in general, but also in anxiety disorder subtypes such as panic disorder, obsessive-compulsive disorder, social phobia, and mixed anxiety depression. Because of the unique pharmacological mechanisms for agents selective for serotonin receptor subtypes, it is unlikely that they will replicate the exact therapeutic actions of benzodiazepines, tricyclic antidepressants, or selective serotonin reuptake inhibitors. This presents a challenge to the clinical psychopharmacologist to unlock the therapeutic potential of novel agents that have much greater selectivity than earlier generation anxiolytic agents.

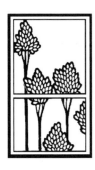

CHAPTER 24

Serotonergic Treatments for Panic Disorder

Herman G. M. Westenberg, Ph.D., and
Johan A. Den Boer, M.D.

Panic disorder is becoming better recognized and under-stood as a chronic and debilitating, but treatable, psychiatric condition. Because panic disorder was first recognized as a specific type of anxiety disorder in the DSM-III classification (American Psychiatric Association 1980), both the condition and its treatment have been the subject of burgeoning interest in the psychiatric community. Subsequent editions of the DSM classification have been progressively adapted to reflect an increasingly refined appreciation of panic (American Psychiatric Association 1987, 1994). As awareness of the various clinical manifestations of panic grows, so does its reported prevalence. Whereas some early studies based on DSM-III criteria suggested a lifetime prevalence for panic disorder as low as 1.4% (Robins et al. 1984), using DSM-III-R criteria, later studies of 1,306 adults found lifetime prevalence rates of 3.8% for panic disorder, 5.6% for panic attacks, and 2.2% for limited-symptom attacks (Katterndahl and Realini 1993). Using the same criteria, a more recent survey of 8,098 patients puts the lifetime prevalence of panic disorder at 4.2% and that for one or more panic attacks as high as 15.0% (W. W. Eaton et al. 1994).

Effective pharmacological treatment of panic disorder began with the antidepressant imipramine, but today a variety of efficacious agents are available for treating the symptoms of panic disorder. The four primary classes of drugs for panic disorder are the tricyclic antidepressants, the serotonin (5-HT) reuptake inhibitors, the monoamine oxidase inhibitors, and the high-potency benzodiazepines. In this chapter, we provide a brief review of the place of selective serotonin reuptake inhibitors (SSRIs) in panic disorder. Issues such as comorbidity, length of treatment, discontinuation, and relapse are discussed briefly. In addition, some information is provided regarding recent developments on the role of selective serotonin receptor agonists and antagonists.

COMORBIDITY

Comorbidity is an important factor influencing the choice of drug treatment. Depression is the most frequent and significant comorbid condition in patients with panic disorder.

A number of epidemiological studies (including several reviewed in May and Lichterman 1993) have shown that panic disorder and unipolar depression occur more commonly together than could be explained by chance. Some 50%–70% of patients with panic disorder also have major depression (J. Johnson et al. 1990; Volrath and Angst 1989). The association also holds true for seasonal depression (Halle and Dilsaver 1993) and to some extent for bipolar disorders (Savino et al. 1993).

Although such a strong association might suggest a single underlying disorder encompassing both depression and panic, family studies suggest that panic disorder and depression are in fact clearly separate entities, with substantial co-occurrence in individuals, and not a single disorder (Weissman et al. 1993). The presence of both conditions concomitantly predicts a less favorable outcome (Albus and Scheibe 1993). Recurrent major depression, in particular, may represent a more serious condition in patients with panic disorder (Maddock et al. 1993), and panic attacks are a statistically significant predictor of suicide in patients with depression (Fawcett 1992). Some evidence suggests that the pattern of panic symptoms in individuals with either present or past depression is distinguishable from the pattern in patients with no history of depression (B. J. Cox et al. 1993b).

Although depression is the most prominent comorbid illness, a variety of other psychiatric conditions may be associated with panic disorder, for example, agoraphobia (60% of patients with panic disorder), other anxiety disorders (20%), and drug and alcohol abuse (15%) (Klerman 1992).

The presence of comorbid depression in patients with panic disorder is associated with an increased prevalence of agoraphobia and suicide attempts.

One analysis (Angst and Wicki 1993) showed agoraphobia in 2.6% of control subjects, 2.8% of subjects with major depression, 7.4% of subjects with pure panic, and 28.0% of subjects with both panic disorder and major depression. Similarly, the attempted suicide rate was 3.5% among control subjects, 5.0% in subjects with pure panic, 13.0% in subjects with depression without panic, and 28.9% in patients with both panic disorder and major depression. These data underline the importance of recognizing and treating comorbid depression in patients with panic disorder.

SEROTONIN REUPTAKE INHIBITORS

Imipramine was first shown to be effective as long ago as 1962 in what would now be classified as panic disorder (D. F. Klein and Fink 1962). Its efficacy has since become well established in many placebo-controlled studies, with approximately 70%–80% of patients experiencing marked-to-moderate improvement (Ballenger 1993; Tesar and Rosenbaum 1993). Among the other tricyclic antidepressants, clomipramine is the most extensively studied for its potential utility in panic disorder, and it is widely used in Europe for this condition. Studies comparing clomipramine with imipramine indicate that these two agents are broadly equivalent in efficacy, assessed after 6–10 weeks in terms of reducing panic attacks and improving phobic avoidance and anxiety (McTavish and Benfield 1990), although it has been suggested that clomipramine has a faster onset of action (Cassano et al. 1988). Modigh et al. (1992), who compared the efficacy of clomipramine and imipramine in a 12-week placebo-controlled trial, found clomipramine superior to imipramine in reducing panic attacks. The major pharmacological difference between clomipramine and imipramine is that the former is more potent in blocking the serotonin uptake transporter. This led Den Boer and Westenberg (1988) to compare the efficacy of maprotiline, a potent and selective norepinephrine reuptake inhibitor, with fluvoxamine, an SSRI, in a double-blind, 6-week treatment study at doses averaging 150 mg/day. Fluvoxamine was effective in significantly decreasing panic attacks and anxiety symptoms. Maprotiline was able to reduce depressive and anxiety symptomatology to a minor degree, but was unable to reduce the frequency of panic attacks. Patients in this study were carefully selected to provide a pure panic disorder sample by excluding those with concomitant depressive symptoms. This study therefore supports the view that the antipanic efficacy of antidepressants is specific and not secondary to their antidepressant effects. This study also provides circumstantial evidence for the idea that the efficacy of tricyclic antidepressants probably entails alterations of the serotonergic system in the brain. This notion has obvious significance for the clinical potential of serotonin reuptake inhibitors in panic disorder.

It is reasonable to hypothesize that SSRIs may have efficacy in panic disorder with fewer and less troublesome side effects than tricyclic antidepressants, including anticholinergic effects (such as dry mouth, blurred vision, constipation), weight gain, memory difficulties, and orthostatic hypotension. In keeping with this notion, an early study comparing the efficacy of clomipramine and fluvoxamine already demonstrated comparable efficacy with both drugs and showed that fluvoxamine was better tolerated (Den Boer et al. 1987). In addition, some early open-label studies with the SSRIs zimeldine and fluoxetine had also demonstrated beneficial effects in patients with panic disorder, most of whom also had agoraphobia (L. Evans et al. 1980; Gorman et al. 1987; Koczkas and Weissman 1981). The results of several controlled trials with SSRIs have now confirmed the efficacy of this class of compounds in panic disorder (Table 24–1). A study of 75 patients with panic disorder compared fluvoxamine, placebo, and cognitive therapy in an 8-week trial (D. W. Black et al. 1993). The patients in the fluvoxamine group were clinically superior to the cognitive therapy group on several measures. Several placebo-controlled studies have confirmed the efficacy of fluvoxamine in panic disorder. The antipanic efficacy of fluvoxamine began as early as week 3, and the authors concluded that fluvoxamine is a well-tolerated and potent antipanic agent with a rapid onset of action.

de Beurs et al. (1995) reported on a study in which patients were randomly allocated to a double-blind, placebo-controlled fluvoxamine trial followed by exposure in vivo, psychological panic management (PPM) and exposure in vivo, and exposure in vivo alone. Exposure in vivo therapy was added to the drug or PPM treatments after 6 weeks of therapy. The combination of fluvoxamine plus exposure in vivo appeared to be superior to placebo plus exposure in vivo, PPM and exposure in vivo, and exposure in vivo alone. No other group differences were found. The fluvoxamine plus exposure group had a twice as large effect size on self-reported agoraphobic avoidance than the other groups.

A meta-analysis (Boyer 1995) has compared some serotonin reuptake inhibitors (paroxetine, fluvoxamine, zimeldine, and clomipramine) with imipramine and alprazolam in the alleviation of panic attacks in patients with DSM-III or DSM-III-R panic disorder. Although all three classes of drugs were shown to be significantly more effective than placebo, the serotonin reuptake inhibitors were also significantly superior to both imipramine and alprazolam. The findings of this meta-analysis highlight the importance of

TABLE 24–1. Controlled studies with selective serotonin reuptake inhibitors in the treatment of panic disorder

Reference	Dx	N	Rx	Results
L. Evans et al. 1986	PD	25	ZIM, IMI, PLA	ZIM > PLA PLA = IMI
Kahn et al. 1987	PD GAD	35 7	5-HTP, CLO, PLA	CLO, 5-HTP > PLA
Den Boer et al. 1987	PD GAD OCD	20 2 4	CLO, FLU	CLO = FLU
Den Boer and Westenberg 1988	PD	44	FLU, MAP	FLU > MAP
Cassano et al. 1988	PD	59	CLO, IMI	CLO = IMI CLO more rapid onset
D. G. Johnston et al. 1988	PD	108	CLO, PLA	CLO > PLA
Den Boer and Westenberg 1990	PD	60	FLU, RIT, PLA	FLU > RIT = PLA
D. W. Black et al. 1993	PD	75	FLU, PLA, CT	FLU > CT > PLA
Hoehn-Saric et al. 1994	PD	84	FLU, PLA	FLU > PLA
Woods et al. 1994	PD	188	FLU, PLA	FLU > PLA
Gorman and Wolkow 1994	PD	320	SERT, PLA	SERT > PLA
Oehrberg et al. 1995	PD	120	PAR + CT PLA + CT	PAR + CT > PLA + CT
Lecrubier et al. 1997	PD	367	PAR, CLO, PLA	PAR, CLO > PLA PAR more rapid onset
de Beurs et al. 1995	PD	96	FLU + EXP PLA + EXP PPM + EXP EXP	FLU + EXP > PLA + EXP, = PPM + EXP, EXP
Bakish et al. 1996	PD	54	FLU, IMI, PLA	FLU > IMI > PLA
Van Vliet et al. 1996a	PD	30	FLU, BROF	FLU + BROF
Lecrubier and Judge 1997	PD	167	PAR, CLO, PLA	PAR, CLO > PLA PAR better tolerated

(continued)

TABLE 24-1. Controlled studies with selective serotonin reuptake inhibitors in the treatment of panic disorder *(continued)*

Reference	Dx	N	Rx	Results
Wade et al. 1997	PD	475	CIT, PLA	CIT > PLA
				Lower doses more effective
Ballenger et al. 1998	PD	425	PAR, PLA	PAR > PLA
				Minimum effective does 40 mg/day
Pohl et al. 1998	PD	168	SERT, PLA	SERT > PLA
Pollack et al. 1998	PD	160	SERT, PLA	SERT > PLA
Londborg et al. 1998	PD	178	SERT, PLA	SERT > PLA
Michelson et al. 1998	PD	243	FLUOX, PLA	FLUOX > PLA
				Most effective dose 20 mg/day

Note. BROF = brofaromine; CIT = citalopram; CLO = clomipramine; CT = cognitive therapy; Dx = diagnosis; EXP = exposure in vivo; FLU = fluvoxamine; FLUOX = fluoxetine; GAD = generalized anxiety disorder; 5-HTP = 5-hydroxytryptophan; IMI = imipramine; MAP = maprotiline; OCD = obsessive-compulsive disorder; PAR = paroxetine; PD = panic disorder; PLA = placebo; PPM = psychological panic management; RIT = ritanserin; Rx = drugs administered; SERT = sertraline; ZIM = zimeldine.

serotonin neuronal systems in the mechanism of action of antipanic agents, evidence for which is also provided in a review by M. R. Johnson et al. (1995).

Extensive databases (see Table 24–1) have now shown that paroxetine and sertraline can reduce panic attacks to zero and prevent relapse. Paroxetine studies constitute the largest data set: more than 700 patients have been treated for periods ranging from 10 to 36 weeks. In the placebo-controlled comparisons with clomipramine, paroxetine had an earlier onset of action and was better tolerated than clomipramine. Paroxetine was significantly better than placebo from week 4 onward, whereas no separation was seen between clomipramine and placebo until the end of the study. Fewer withdrawals occurred as a result of adverse events with paroxetine (7.3%) than with either clomipramine (14.9%) or placebo (11.4%). The minimum dose shown to be superior to placebo was 40 mg/day.

The efficacy and tolerability of paroxetine increased during long-term treatment, with 85% of the patients becoming panic-free after 36 weeks (Lecrubier and Judge 1997). Paroxetine also was effective in preventing relapse: a placebo-controlled study in 105 responders showed that continued treatment with paroxetine prevented relapse for at least 6 months in most patients (Judge and Steiner 1996). Similarly, sertraline has shown significantly superior efficacy when compared with placebo. Sertraline was well tolerated, and doses of 100 and 200 mg/day were no more effective than 50 mg/day (Londborg et al. 1998).

Citalopram and fluoxetine also have been studied in panic disorder (Michelson et al. 1998; Wade et al. 1997). Citalopram was compared with clomipramine. At the most effective citalopram dose (20–30 mg/day), approximately 58% of patients were panic-free compared with 50% of patients receiving clomipramine and 32% of placebo patients. All rating scales suggested that 20 or 30 mg/day of citalopram was more effective than 40 or 60 mg/day of citalopram. Finally, data support the efficacy of fluoxetine in panic disorder. In a study comparing 10 and 20 mg/day of fluoxetine and placebo, fluoxetine treatment, particularly the 20-mg daily dose, was associated with more improvement than placebo across multiple measures, including functional impairment.

SEROTONIN AND ANXIETY

In treatment studies with serotonin reuptake inhibitors, an initial period of symptom exacerbation has been observed by many investigators (Den Boer and Westenberg 1990; Den Boer et al. 1987; Gorman et al. 1987). This transient increase of anxiety, referred to as *jitteriness syndrome*, has also been reported in patients with panic disorder during the first week of treatment with tricyclic antidepressants (Pohl et al. 1988) and monoamine oxidase inhibitors (Van Vliet et al. 1993). Lower doses can reduce this problem but also increase the lag time for efficacy (Alexander 1991). This "biphasic response," in which improvement in symptoms follows an initial period of symptom exacerbation, was first reported in an open pilot study of patients with panic disorder treated with *l*-5-hydroxytryptophan in combination with the peripheral monoamine decarboxylase inhibitor carbidopa (Kahn and Westenberg 1985). It is unlikely that this effect involves the norepinephrine system because it was not seen with the norepinephrine reuptake inhibitor maprotiline (Den Boer and Westenberg 1988). This biphasic profile appears to be unique to patients with panic disorder because it has not been reported in the multitude of studies using antidepressants, including the serotonin reuptake inhibitors, in patients with depression and patients with obsessive-compulsive disorder and in some studies of patients with social phobia. We have hypothesized that this phenomenon might be the result of a hypersensitive serotonin neuronal system in patients with panic disorder.

Challenge studies with the serotonin receptor agonist, *m*-chlorophenylpiperazine support the notion that acute stimulation of the serotonergic systems in the brain might be panicogenic. m-Chlorophenyl-piperazine (0.25 mg/kg) induced anxiety in subjects with panic disorder only (Kahn et al. 1988), suggesting an enhanced sensitivity of patients for this serotonin receptor agonist. Challenge studies using fenfluramine produced comparable results (Targum and Marshall 1989). These studies suggest that patients with panic disorder are sensitive to stimulation of some postsynaptic serotonin receptors and that blockade or desensitization of these receptors could possibly have therapeutic potential.

SEROTONIN RECEPTOR ANTAGONISTS

Following this view, Den Boer and Westenberg (1990) conducted a comparison study of fluvoxamine and ritanserin. The investigators reasoned that, because ritanserin blocks the postsynaptic $5\text{-}HT_2$ receptors, it would work more quickly than fluvoxamine in patients with panic disorder. In an 8-week trial, the efficacy of fluvoxamine again was demonstrated, with further evidence that phobic avoidance also improved progressively. However, ritanserin had no effect on any of the measures in these patients. This would suggest that desensitization of the $5\text{-}HT_2$ receptors, which is thought to take place after repeated administration with some antidepressants, is not central to the antipanic effects of antidepressants. It is interesting to note that patients with generalized anxiety disorder seem to benefit from treatment with ritanserin (Ceulemans et al. 1985), whereas it seems to attenuate the effects of serotonin reuptake inhibitors in patients with obsessive-compulsive disorder (Erzegovesi et al. 1992). Controlled clinical studies with more potent receptor antagonists are required to confirm these apparent differential effects of ritanserin in generalized anxiety disorders, panic disorder, and obsessive-compulsive disorder.

Little is known also about the effects of $5\text{-}HT_3$ antagonists in panic disorder. To the best of our knowledge, there is only one controlled study with ondansetron showing that this $5\text{-}HT_3$ antagonist is superior to placebo in reducing symptoms of panic anxiety in patients with panic disorder (Metz et al. 1994). Further studies are needed to substantiate this preliminary finding.

SEROTONIN RECEPTOR AGONISTS

Substantial preclinical evidence exists that $5\text{-}HT_{1A}$ receptor agonists possess anxiolytic activity in animal screens of anxiety. Clinical studies with the

5-HT_{1A} agonist buspirone have confirmed the efficacy of this compound in patients with generalized anxiety disorder (Böhm et al. 1990; Feighner 1987; A. F. Jacobson et al. 1985; Olajide and Lader 1987; Rickels et al. 1982; Schuckit 1984; Strand et al. 1990). However, placebo-controlled studies with buspirone in panic disorder are either inconclusive or negative (Pohl et al. 1989; D. R. Robinson et al. 1989; Schweizer and Rickels 1988; Sheehan et al. 1988). An open study with gepirone suggests the possible efficacy of this 5-HT_{1A} receptor agonist in panic disorder, but a large proportion of the patients in this study had comorbid generalized anxiety disorders (Pecknold et al. 1993). Buspirone and gepirone are partial 5-HT_{1A} receptor agonists and their major metabolite, 1-(2-pyridiminyl)piperazine (1-PP), has α_2-adrenoreceptor antagonistic properties.

Flesinoxan is a potent 5-HT_{1A} receptor agonist surpassing buspirone and gepirone in affinity and selectivity. In generalized anxiety disorder, flesinoxan has been shown to possess anxiolytic activity in doses ranging from 0.4 to 1.2 mg/day (Bradford and Stevens 1994). Recently, Van Vliet et al. (1996b) investigated the efficacy of this compound in patients with panic disorder. In a small double-blind, placebo-controlled trial with 0.6 and 1.2 mg of flesinoxan, no significant effects were observed on measures of anxiety and panic. However, in the single-blind placebo crossover pilot study, which preceded the double-blind trial, a worsening of anxiety symptoms was seen in all subjects on 2.4 mg of flesinoxan/day. The symptoms abated during the subsequent placebo period. It cannot be excluded that the doses of flesinoxan in these studies have been too high to ascertain efficacy in panic disorder, because recent studies in patients with generalized anxiety disorder disclosed that the lower doses of flesinoxan are more effective on all primary and secondary efficacy variables than the higher doses (Bradford and Stevens 1994). These findings hint at a bell-shaped dose-response curve for flesinoxan in patients with generalized anxiety disorder.

The mechanism of action of 5-HT_{1A} receptor agonists in anxiety and panic disorders is complex and not fully understood. 5-HT_{1A} receptors are abundant in limbic regions, but a high density of receptors has also been observed in the raphe nuclei, where they function as autoreceptors to inhibit the serotonergic activity (Briley et al. 1991). Therefore, long-term administration of 5-HT_{1A} receptor agonists would result in a global reduction in serotonin release in all serotonin terminal fields, as well as in a selective stimulation of those postsynaptic receptor sites that belong to the class of the 5-HT_{1A} receptors. A confounding factor is, however, that most 5-HT_{1A} receptor agonists act as full agonists at the presynaptic autoreceptors, whereas the same compounds are partial agonists at the postsynaptic receptors. Because they are less effective than a full agonist, they can be either net incomplete receptor agonists in the absence of endogenous serotonin, or net incomplete receptor antagonists that compete with high levels of endogenous serotonin at the synapse. Because short-term administration of these drugs reduces serotonin release, they most likely act as incomplete receptor agonists at the postsynaptic receptors following short-term administration. However, sustained treatment with these drugs progressively restores serotonin release through an adaptive desensitization of the autoreceptors located on the cell bodies (Briley et al. 1991).

The gradual recovery of serotonin neuronal activity parallels the onset of clinical action of these drugs in generalized anxiety disorders. It may be postulated, therefore, that long-term administration of these drugs results in a partial antagonistic effect at the postsynaptic 5-HT_{1A} receptors in the presence of the higher levels of serotonin. Evidence to support this hypothesis might be provided by the clinical assessment of selective 5-HT_{1A} receptor antagonists. The complex pharmacological effects of these compounds also implies that the therapeutic effects may depend on the functional status of the serotonin neurotransmission; it may be dampened when excessive and heightened when inadequate. Differences in functional status of a particular serotonin neuronal system may also explain the differential therapeutic effects of these compounds among psychiatric conditions. The anxiogenic effects of high doses of flesinoxan in patients with panic disorder may therefore give a clue to the pathophysiology of the disorder.

SEROTONIN REUPTAKE INHIBITORS AND PINDOLOL

The delay in onset of anxiolytic and antipanic effects of serotonin reuptake inhibitors and related compounds is still an issue of much speculation. It appears paradoxical that serotonin reuptake inhibitors block serotonin uptake immediately, whereas it takes weeks before their therapeutic effects become apparent. Recently, the idea was advanced that the tentative enhanced serotonin neurotransmission caused by short-term administration of serotonin reuptake inhibitors is offset by negative feedback in the raphe nuclei (Artigas 1993; Blier and de Montigny 1994). The increased level of serotonin in the somatodendritic area, resulting from serotonin uptake inhibition, reduces serotonin neuronal firing through activation of the 5-HT_{1A} autoreceptors. Alterations in the feedback regulation upon repeated administration may progressively restore the normal firing rate, resulting in an enhanced serotonin release after chronic treatment. Support for this hypothesis came from microdialysis studies in rodents, demonstrating that short-term administration of antidepressants had little or no effect on extracellular serotonin levels in cortical areas (Bel and Artigas 1992; R. Invernizzi et al. 1992a). Others found that citalopram, when given short-term, significantly decreased the firing rate of the serotonin neurons in the dorsal raphe (Arborelius et al. 1995). This effect could be antagonized by pretreatment with a 5-HT_{1A} receptor antagonist. These findings suggest that 5-HT_{1A} receptor antagonists can augment the effects of serotonin reuptake inhibitors on serotonin neurotransmission. This finding led Artigas et al. (1994) to study the effects of the 5-HT_{1A} receptor antagonist pindolol as an add-on medication in patients with depression treated with serotonin reuptake inhibitors. The results of this preliminary open-label study suggest that pindolol might augment the effects of serotonin reuptake inhibitors in patients with depression.

We recently conducted a study with a similar design in patients with panic disorder (I. M. Van Vliet et al., manuscript submitted for publication). In this open-label study, patients with panic disorder were randomly allocated to a treatment with fluvoxamine or to the combination of fluvoxamine plus pindolol. No differences between the treatment groups were observed on any of the rating scales; neither the effect size nor the onset of action was different among the groups. Although preliminary, this finding does not support the idea that the late onset of action of serotonin reuptake inhibitors in panic disorder can be accounted for by a delayed increase in serotonin release in terminal regions.

CHOLECYSTOKININ AND SEROTONIN REUPTAKE INHIBITORS

Studies have shown that the cholecystokinin tetrapeptide (CCK-4) possesses anxiogenic properties in humans (Bradwejn et al. 1991b; de Montigny 1989; van Megen et al. 1996). Intravenous administration of low doses (25–50 μg) of this peptide to patients with panic disorder results in a full-blown panic attack in most of the subjects. Although similar responses can also be elicited in psychiatrically healthy control subjects, patients with panic disorder appear to be more sensitive to this pharmacological challenge. Pretreatment with a CCK_B antagonist dose-dependently reduced the propensity of CCK-4 to induce panic attacks in patients with panic disorder (Bradwejn et al. 1994c), suggesting that these effects are specific and mediated through the CCK_B receptor. Recently, van Megen et al. (1997) studied the ability of serotonin reuptake inhibitors to attenuate the CCK-4–induced panic attacks. Twenty-six patients with panic disorder were treated with fluvoxamine or placebo in a double-blind design. Before and after 8 weeks of treatment, subjects were challenged with 50 μg of CCK-4. The results demonstrated a significant reduction in the ability of CCK-4 to induce panic attacks after treatment with fluvoxamine. Of the patients who responded to treatment, 83% no longer experienced a panic attack when challenged with CCK-4 versus 28% in the nonresponder group. These findings underscore the panicolytic effects of serotonin reuptake inhibitors.

FACTORS AFFECTING TREATMENT OUTCOME

A prospectively conducted 7-year follow-up study of outcome in panic disorder by Noyes et al. (1993) has been published. Data were analyzed on 69 subjects, with a mean follow-up interval of 83 months (range 74–91 months). Only 13% were completely free of symptoms, and almost two-thirds were still taking medication.

The illness variables that were predictive of poor outcome all reflected severity of illness. They included more severe panic and agoraphobic symptoms, psychiatric hospitalization, and longer duration of illness. The best prognostic indicators were the severity of the illness and its duration at the time of first assessment. Comorbid depression was also associated with poorer outcome. A number of environmental variables were also predictive of poor outcome: separation from a parent by death or divorce, high interpersonal sensitivity, low social class, and unmarried marital status.

ISSUES CONCERNING LONG-TERM TREATMENT

As might be suggested by the treatment outcome studies referred to above, anxiety disorders such as panic disorder have a chronic clinical course. A retrospective survey that reviewed literature on the course of depression and anxiety disorder before effective treatment became available (Keller and Baker 1992) showed that a high proportion of patients had little or no improvement in their condition over a number of years. Roughly half of 300 patients with panic disorder who received no active treatments showed no improvement over a 20-year period, for example. Like depression, panic disorder may therefore be considered as inherently chronic by nature. Comorbid panic disorder and depression is likely to have a still poorer prognosis in this respect.

Being a chronic condition, panic disorder is likely to require long-term treatment. Current clinical practice tends to favor a trial of medication for at least 3 months, with continuation for 6–12 months if there is a good clinical response. However, the most appropriate time to discontinue therapy has not yet been determined, and more data from long-term follow-up studies are needed (Ballenger 1992). Clinical experience indicates that 40% of patients with panic disorder may need treatment for a year, and some 20%–40% may require continued maintenance treatment thereafter (Keller and Hanks 1993).

Long-term efficacy and tolerability is of considerable clinical importance for any medication proposed for the treatment of panic disorder. Tricyclic antidepressants, in particular, are associated with side effects such a weight gain and anticholinergic effects, which may make them difficult for patients to tolerate long-term.

Although the long-term efficacy of the serotonin reuptake inhibitors has not been widely examined, and extension study with paroxetine has shown that patients continue to improve during long-term therapy. Treatment with paroxetine ($n = 70$), clomipramine ($n = 64$), or placebo ($n = 46$) for 9 months following the initial 12-week study referred to above (Lecrubier et al. 1997) showed that paroxetine was more effective than placebo and equivalent in efficacy to clomipramine during this time (Lecrubier and Judge 1997). At the end of 9 months, 85% of patients were panic-free, a significant difference from those given placebo.

Paroxetine and placebo had similar tolerability, whereas clomipramine was less well tolerated, with more patients withdrawn from treatment as a result of emergent adverse events. Holland et al. (1994) reported on the effects of long-term treatment with fluvoxamine in patients who had completed a double-blind study. Patients who were transferred from placebo to fluvoxamine and those who continued taking fluvoxamine showed continued improvement in efficacy parameters.

A second issue relating to long-term medication is the effect of withdrawing medication at the end of a period of treatment. Benzodiazepines are associated with discontinuation symptoms, and their repeated use may foster the development of true physiological dependence. In a study of discontinuation of treatment for panic disorder (Rickels et al. 1993) with either alprazolam ($n = 27$), imipramine ($n = 11$) or placebo ($n = 10$), a withdrawal syndrome was observed in almost all patients treated with alprazolam but in few patients treated with imipramine or placebo. One-third of alprazolam patients were unable to discontinue their medication regimen successfully (judged on predefined symptom-based criteria during tapering of the dose). Severity of initial symptoms, rather than daily dose of alprazolam, predicted difficulty of tapering down the alprazolam dose. Holland (1994) compared the effects on patients with panic disorder discontinuing placebo and fluvoxamine following a double-blind study. Most patients were seen 1 or 2 weeks after being withdrawn from medication. During this period, minor increases in anxiety were seen in most patients, but none of the patients experienced a withdrawal reaction. It is imperative for serotonin reuptake inhibitors that medications be tapered gradually and slowly.

DISCUSSION

Panic disorder is emerging from decades of comparative neglect as an apparently intractable and poorly understood condition to become the focus of intensive interest in epidemiological, pharmacological, and clinical research. Panic disorder is a chronic and distressing condition with a profound effect on the quality of life, similar to or even worse than the effect of major depression (Markowitz et al. 1989; Weissman 1991). Effective and well-tolerated treatment that can be used safely in the long term is badly needed.

Alprazolam, imipramine, and clomipramine are well established as effective antipanic agents but have disadvantages in tolerability and safety. The data currently accumulating concerning the use of serotonin reuptake inhibitors in this condition show that these drugs are the drugs of first choice. They are probably somewhat faster acting and certainly better tolerated than the tricyclic antidepressants and do not carry the problems of dependence and discontinuation syndromes associated with benzodiazepines. The benign cardiovascular profile of the serotonin reuptake inhibitors also makes them a more attractive therapeutic option for patients with cardiac problems. However, like any effective treatment, they are not free of unwanted side effects. Typical side effects associated with serotonin reuptake inhibitors are gastrointestinal distress, headaches, and sleep disturbance; overall, however, these drugs are well tolerated by most patients.

The initial long-term data are promising; however, further long-term studies are needed to confirm the initial promise of serotonin reuptake inhibitors in the treatment of panic disorder, and comparative studies of agents within this class of drugs are needed to clarify their relative profiles.

Although originally developed as selective pharmacological agents, SSRIs are relatively nonselective regarding the serotonin system, given the complexity of this system in terms of receptor heterogeneity. Moreover, the consequence of increased serotonin in the synaptic cleft is not unidimensional; both decreased and increased neurotransmission has been observed, depending on the effect of the drugs on negative feedback mechanisms. In addition, long-term treatment may cause adaptive changes in serotonin neurotransmission and beyond.

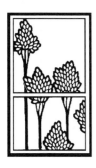

CHAPTER 25

New Treatments for Social Phobia

Cherri M. Miner, M.D., M.B.A.,
Katherine M. Connor, M.D., and
Jonathan R. T. Davidson, M.D.

Social phobia was first described as a unique, diagnosable disorder in DSM-III (American Psychiatric Association 1980). From a historical perspective, the disorder has been recognized since the middle of the 19th century, when Casper described erythrophobia (Casper 1902). Marks (1970) separated social phobia from other types of anxiety, including agoraphobia and simple phobia; thus, he described a clinical picture very similar to the disorder known today as social phobia. W. S. Tseng et al. (1992) described a transcultural variant of social phobia, common in Japan, named *taijiu-kyofu* (meaning anthropophobia), in which the individuals had anxiety related to the fear of causing discomfort in those around them. Although acknowledgment of the social phobia syndrome has been present for this extended period, it was not until the last decade that a true research interest peaked. Thus, from a historical perspective, all the pharmacological treatments of social phobia are relatively new. In this chapter, we review the major pharmacological studies and clinical trials involving social phobia as a target disorder (Table 25–1).

TABLE 25-1.   Drugs studied in the treatment of social phobia

Benzodiazepines
  Alprazolam
  Bromazepam[a]
  Clonazepam
β-Blockers
  Atenolol
  Propranolol
Monoamine oxidase inhibitors (MAOIs) (irreversible)
  Phenelzine
  Tranylcypromine
MAOIs (reversible)
  Brofaromine[b]
  Moclobemide[a]
Novel agents
  Ondansetron[c]
  Buspirone
  Clonidine
Serotonin reuptake inhibitors
  Fluoxetine
  Sertraline
  Paroxetine
  Fluvoxamine

[a]Not available in the United States.
[b]Now unavailable worldwide.
[c]Currently not available in oral form in the United States.

DEFINITION OF SOCIAL PHOBIA

The core features of social phobia center on the intense, irrational fear of scrutiny of others and the anticipation of humiliation (Table 25–2). Individuals with this disorder avoid or endure with marked distress the phobic situations. They realize that their fear is unreasonable or excessive. The disorder has been divided into subtypes. Individuals who have anxiety in well-circumscribed situations (e.g., public speaking) have been designated as having a *performance* subtype; those who experience anxiety in a broader spectrum of interpersonal social situations are designated as having a generalized subtype of social phobia. As social phobia has become better character-

TABLE 25–2. DSM-IV diagnostic criteria for social phobia

A. A marked and persistent fear of one or more social or performance situations in which the person is exposed to unfamiliar people or to possible scrutiny by others. The individual fears that he or she will act in a way (or show anxiety symptoms) that will be humiliating or embarrassing. **Note:** In children, there must be evidence of the capacity for age-appropriate social relationships with familiar people and the anxiety must occur in peer settings, not just in interactions with adults.

B. Exposure to the feared social situation almost invariably provokes anxiety, which may take the form of a situationally bound or situationally predisposed panic attack. **Note:** In children, the anxiety may be expressed by crying, tantrums, freezing, or shrinking from social situations with unfamiliar people.

C. The person recognizes that the fear is excessive or unreasonable.
Note: In children, this feature may be absent.

D. The feared social or performance situations are avoided or else are endured with intense anxiety or distress.

E. The avoidance, anxious anticipation, or distress in the feared social or performance situation(s) interferes significantly with the person's normal routine, occupational (academic) functioning, or social activities or relationships, or there is marked distress about having the phobia.

F. In individuals under age 18 years, the duration is at least 6 months.

G. The fear or avoidance is not due to the direct physiological effects of a substance (e.g., a drug of abuse, a medication) or a general medical condition and is not better accounted for by another mental disorder (e.g., panic disorder with or without agoraphobia, separation anxiety disorder, body dysmorphic disorder, a pervasive developmental disorder, or schizoid personality disorder).

H. If a general medical condition or another mental disorder is present, the fear in Criterion A is unrelated to it, e.g., the fear is not of stuttering, trembling in Parkinson's disease, or exhibiting abnormal eating behavior in anorexia nervosa or bulimia nervosa.

Specify if:

Generalized: if the fears include most social situations (also consider the additional diagnosis of avoidant personality disorder)

Source.   Reprinted from American Psychiatric Association: *Diagnostic and Statistical Manual of Mental Disorders*, Fourth Edition. Washington, DC, American Psychiatric Association, 1994. Used with permission.

ized, interest in this disorder and its treatment has increased. Although initial research focused on psychotherapeutic interventions, in the 1980s formal psychopharmacological studies began. Prior pharmacological research was flawed by many factors: the use of nonpatient populations, the lack of use of control groups, and the lack of defined efficacy variables. As notice of the disorder has increased, better designed studies have been implemented. Rating scales, to be used as efficacy variables, have been developed for diagnosing and evaluating change in the disorder. These scales include the Liebowitz Social Anxiety Scale (Liebowitz 1987) and the Duke Brief Social Phobia Scale (Davidson et al. 1991a). These scales focus on the anxiety, avoidance, and physiological features of the disorder. Through measurement of the core symptoms and behavior patterns related to them, these scales aid in the measurement of change of the disorder with treatment.

PHARMACOLOGICAL STUDIES

β-Blockers

The earliest pharmacological treatment of social phobia involved the use of β-blockers in performers with stage fright. This is thought to be comparable to targeting a performance subtype of social phobia. The use of β-blockers in the treatment of this type of social anxiety was intuitively based on the symptom profile of the disorder. Given the *activated* state (e.g., palpitations, tremors, sweating) during an episode of anxiety, the use of an agent that would block symptoms mediated by the sympathetic nervous system might address a very distressing component of the disorder.

Although early anecdotal reports suggested the usefulness of this class of agents, overall studies of β-blockers in clinical populations have not been supportive of their efficacy in social phobia. Falloon et al. (1981) compared propranolol and placebo, both used in conjunction with social skills training. This study failed to find any difference between the two treatment groups. However, the study was compromised by small sample size and failure to select subjects using specific diagnostic criteria for social phobia.

The β-blocker atenolol has received the most attention in studies of social phobia. Various reasons have pointed to using this agent over propranolol, which was the main drug used in the early trials with nonclinical populations. Because atenolol is a polar, hydrophilic compound, it has a relatively poor ability to penetrate the blood-brain barrier. Thus, it is thought to have less potential to cause the depressogenic effects thought to be caused by more centrally acting agents, such as propranolol.

Gorman et al. (1985) first reported the use of atenolol in an open trial of 10 patients with social phobia. Using doses ranging from 50 to 100 mg/day, the drug demonstrated good efficacy. Using patient rated questionnaires, 50% reported a marked reduction in symptoms, 40% endorsed a moderate reduction, and one subject was a nonresponder. This initial, promising study was followed by controlled studies that proved to be less supportive of the efficacy of atenolol in social phobia. Liebowitz et al. (1992) found phenelzine to be more effective in the relief of social phobia symptoms than atenolol or placebo. An interesting subanalysis of this study looked at the response of symptoms in the different subtypes of social phobia, generalized and performance. Although the number of subjects in this study was not sufficient to compare the two subtypes in each treatment arm, the differences between atenolol and phenelzine were less clear in the analysis of the subject group with the performance subtype. Thus, although the effects of atenolol have been moderate at best, they may be more pronounced in the performance subtype.

S. M. Turner et al. (1994) compared the uses of atenolol, flooding, and placebo in social phobia. Atenolol was used with a dose range of 25–100 mg/day. In this study, atenolol was shown to be the least effective treatment in terms of symptomatic improvement. Only 27% of atenolol-treated subjects displayed improvement, but the flooding and placebo groups, respectively, demonstrated 89% and 44% response rates. Weaknesses of this study included a high rate of comorbid disorders and dramatic placebo response rates. Additionally, the difference between response rates of the subtypes of social phobia was not addressed.

In summary, overall the data are not supportive of the efficacy of β-blockers in the treatment of social phobia. However, given the early findings in nonclinical populations and the Liebowitz study, there may still be a role for the sole or adjunctive use of these drugs in the treatment of "performance anxiety," or the performance subtype of social phobia. These agents may provide relief of the physiological symptoms present in specific anxiety-provoking situations. This effect may be sufficient to control the disorder for some individuals. By controlling the physiological symptoms, the drugs may block the triggers of the cognitive symptoms (i.e., palpitations may stimulate or exacerbate a sense of panic). Thus, the continued popular use of these agents on an as-needed basis may be supportable in the performance subtype of social phobia. However, further investigation into the use of these agents in this specific subtype of social phobia is warranted.

Nonselective and Irreversible Monoamine Oxidase Inhibitors

Monoamine oxidase inhibitors (MAOIs) have been historically the most extensively studied class of medications directed against social anxiety. Early studies documented relief of symptoms in mixed populations of individuals with social phobia and agoraphobia (Mountjoy et al. 1977; Solyom et al. 1973; Tyrer et al. 1973). These early studies unfortunately did not address the responsiveness specifically in social phobia as the disorder is defined today, and thus these findings are difficult to generalize to this precise population.

Recently, studies have addressed the use of MAOIs in clinically defined populations. Liebowitz et al. (1984) studied phenelzine and imipramine in atypical depression, characterized by social rejection sensitivity similar to that seen in social phobia. Phenelzine was found to be superior to imipramine in the symptomatic relief of this interpersonal sensitivity. This finding led to subsequent studies of MAOIs in populations with social phobia.

Liebowitz et al. (1992) conducted a double-blind, placebo-controlled study of 74 subjects meeting DSM-III-R (American Psychiatric Association 1987) criteria for social phobia with phenelzine, atenolol, or placebo for 8 weeks. Phenelzine daily doses were 60–100 mg. Phenelzine was found to be superior to both atenolol and placebo, and atenolol was not significantly different from placebo in measures of responsiveness of social phobia symptoms.

Tranylcypromine, another MAOI, has also been shown to be effective in the treatment of social phobia. Versiani et al. (1988) implemented a 1-year, open trial of tranylcypromine in 32 subjects. Daily doses ranged from 40 to 60 mg. Twenty-nine subjects met criteria for completion of this study. Marked improvement was noted in 62% of patients (18/29), and moderate improvement was shown in 17.2% (5/29). Six of the 29 subjects were deemed nonresponders (20.6%). The most commonly cited side effects were orthostatic dizziness (75.5%), insomnia (44.7%), and daytime sleepiness (41.3%).

Phenelzine and tranylcypromine are both effective in the treatment of social phobia. Many practitioners continue to be hesitant to use this class of medications, given the dietary restrictions required of patients and the potential risk of hypertensive crises when combined with dietary tyramine and sympathomimetic medications. However, the proven effectiveness of this class makes it an important option in the treatment of social phobia.

Selective and Reversible Monoamine Oxidase Inhibitors

Two drugs belonging to the selective and reversible class of MAOIs, moclobemide and brofaromine, have been studied for use in the treatment of social phobia. Both agents are selective inhibitors of monoamine oxidase-A, the enzyme responsible for the deamination of biogenic amines. Thus, these agents will increase levels of 5-hydroxytryptamine (serotonin; 5-HT), noradrenaline, and, to a lesser extent, dopamine. Although this effect is similar to that of the traditional MAOIs, these agents are selective only for this particular isoenzyme and are quickly reversible. Thus, potential risks associated with the irreversible class of MAOIs can be reduced. Given the effectiveness of phenelzine and tranylcypromine, the usefulness of these agents in social phobia would seem consistent.

Moclobemide was compared with phenelzine and placebo (Versiani et al. 1992). Patients were randomly assigned to each treatment arm of this study. Those patients not deemed to be responders were dropped from the study at week 8. Responders were continued for an additional 8 weeks. At week 16, the moclobemide group demonstrated an 82% response rate (14/17); the phenelzine group, a 91% (19/21) response rate; and the placebo group, a 43% (3/7) response rate. At week 8, moclobemide was significantly less effective than phenelzine, but by week 16, a significant difference between the two groups no longer existed. Also, patients in the moclobemide group reported fewer side effects than those treated with phenelzine.

Studies by Schneier et al. (F. Schneier, personal communication, June 1994) and two large, unpublished, multicenter international collaborative trials involving several hundred patients have yielded more modest effects, with less striking but still clinically meaningful superiority of moclobemide over placebo.

A second reversible MAOI, brofaromine, was studied in a double-blind, placebo-controlled fashion by Den Boer et al. (1994). Thirty patients with symptoms meeting DSM-III-R criteria for social phobia were studied for 12 weeks. Those individuals deemed as having a positive response were continued for an additional 12 weeks. Brofaromine was found to be superior to placebo in the reduction of both anxiety and avoidance behaviors by week 8.

The reversible, selective MAOIs are an effective and relatively safe treatment alternative for social phobia. Moclobemide is currently not available in the United States, although it is available and widely used in other countries. Brofaromine has been discontinued entirely for commercial reasons.

Serotonin Reuptake Inhibitors

The selective serotonin reuptake inhibitors (SSRIs) have received increased attention in the treatment of anxiety disorders. With the recent Food and Drug Administration (FDA) approval of fluoxetine and fluvoxamine in the treatment of obsessive-compulsive disorder, it has been made clear that this class of drugs has utility reaching beyond its primary indication of depression.

The agents in this class demonstrate the common feature of specific inhibition of serotonin reuptake without significant effects on norepinephrine and dopamine reuptake. These agents also lack direct agonist or antagonist activity on any neurotransmitter receptor.

Fluoxetine.   Fluoxetine has been the subject of four reports addressing its utility in the treatment of social phobia since 1990. The first report by Sternbach (1990) was a case report of two individuals successfully treated with fluoxetine. The first patient demonstrated improvement at the 3-week treatment mark on a dose of 40 mg/day. The second patient reported a "90%" decrease in his level of anxiety "within days" of starting fluoxetine treatment at 20 mg/day.

Subsequently, Schneier et al. (1992) reported a retrospective review of 12 outpatients with a diagnosis of social phobia meeting DSM-III-R criteria, who had received open-label treatment with fluoxetine. Because of the retrospective nature of the study, limitations in the design were present. Besides being open label and retrospective, many individuals had comorbid disorders and may have displayed symptom overlap. Such individuals might be rated as globally improved, if, for example, their symptoms related to obsessive-compulsive disorder responded over those of their social phobia. Subjects may have also received concomitant medications or psychotherapy. Despite these limitations, the results of this study suggest the probable efficacy of fluoxetine in social phobia. Of the 12 subjects, 10 were diagnosed with the generalized subtype of social phobia; and 2, with the performance subtype of social phobia. Five of the 10 subjects with generalized subtype and both of the subjects with performance subtype showed moderate to marked improvement. The mean maximal daily dose for responders was 25.7 mg (range 20–80 mg). Of the 5 nonresponders, 1 was rated as much improved at week 4 of treatment but lost this benefit as the treatment continued. This subject refused dose escalation beyond 40 mg because of concerns of adverse effects. Another nonresponder discontinued treatment after 2 weeks because of "fear of potential side effects." The remaining 3 nonresponders received adequate trials of at least 5 weeks' duration.

This study suggests efficacy of the agent in social phobia and highlights some important variables that must be addressed in determining efficacy of an agent, that is, dose range and duration of treatment.

In another study, B. Black et al. (1992) reported an open trial of fluoxetine in 14 subjects, all with a primary diagnosis of social phobia, generalized subtype. Ten of the subjects were treated with only fluoxetine. Four subjects had fluoxetine added to anxiolytic medication that had demonstrated some clinical benefit, but still left the subject moderately to severely symptomatic. The daily dose was started at 20 mg and titrated upward until side effects intervened, complete or nearly complete symptom remission occurred, or a maximum daily dose of 100 mg was reached. Seventy-one percent of subjects (10/14) had a moderate or marked improvement. One subject was minimally improved. Two subjects showed no change, and one experienced worsening related to adverse effects. The authors of this study cited the variability in the onset of response, noting that the improvement was "delayed" in some individuals. Also the "effective" dose was variable among the subjects, with responders receiving a dose range of 10–100 mg/day.

Another open trial of fluoxetine was reported by Van Ameringen et al. (1993). In this study, 16 subjects with a primary diagnosis of social phobia were entered into a 12-week clinical trial. Treatment started at a dose of 20 mg/day and was increased every 4 weeks, according to clinical response and side effects, to a maximum daily dose of 60 mg. Of the 16 subjects, 10 were considered responders, 3 were nonresponders, and 3 dropped out of the trial as a result of adverse effects related to the medication. The response rate of the different subtypes of social phobia was not reported in this study.

Fluoxetine has been the subject of four reports in the treatment of social phobia. However, no double-blind, control studies have been reported. Preliminary results suggest that fluoxetine is effective in social phobia. Doses ranged from 10 to 100 mg/day. The onset of symptom resolution was variable among subjects. A justifiable approach to treatment with fluoxetine would be to implement an approach similar to that in the treatment of depression. One would start with a dose of 10–20 mg/day and titrate slowly upward over a period of several weeks. A duration of at least 6 weeks would be recommended as a minimum trial of this agent, with 12 weeks perhaps affording a better opportunity to assess the full measure of improvement.

Sertraline.   Sertraline, the second SSRI to receive FDA approval for depression, has also been suggested as a treatment for social phobia. Katzelnick et al. (1994) carried out a double-blind, placebo-controlled, crossover study comparing sertraline and placebo. Twelve subjects were randomized to either sertraline or placebo for 12 weeks. The agent was then tapered and the subjects received no treatment for 2 weeks. They were then switched to the other treatment arm for an additional 12 weeks. Using the Liebowitz Social Anxiety Scale, analysis revealed statistically significant improvement with sertraline treatment but not with placebo. Forty-two percent of patients were rated as moderately or markedly improved while receiving the sertraline therapy, and 17% had a positive response while taking placebo.

Although the response rate with sertraline was more modest than that cited in the fluoxetine reports, it must be considered that this study was double blind, whereas the fluoxetine studies were open label. This study supports the effectiveness of sertraline in the treatment of social phobia.

Paroxetine.   Paroxetine, also a serotonin reuptake inhibitor, has been the subject of a case report in two subjects. Ringold (1994) reported the effective treatment of two individuals who had not responded to prior therapy with fluoxetine and sertraline. Both individuals had comorbid psychiatric problems. Subject A demonstrated both social phobia and dysthymia. Although her symptoms of dysthymia were clinically responsive to fluoxetine therapy, her social phobia symptoms were resistant. Subject B had body dysmorphic disorder, obsessive-compulsive disorder, and social phobia. His obsessive-compulsive disorder symptoms benefited from fluoxetine therapy, but his social anxiety was resistant. Sertraline therapy was attempted in both subjects. Subject A required discontinuation because of adverse effects. Subject B experienced a worsening of both obsessive-compulsive disorder and social phobia symptoms. Both subjects demonstrated a positive response in their symptoms when switched to paroxetine (20 mg/day).

Paroxetine has been reported to be of benefit in a case report of two individuals with social phobia. Both individuals responded to paroxetine (20 mg/day).

Fluvoxamine.   The second placebo-controlled study of a serotonin reuptake inhibitor in the treatment of social phobia to date involved fluvoxamine (Den Boer et al. 1994). Thirty subjects with social phobia according to DSM-III-R criteria were randomly selected in a double-blind fashion in this 12-week study. At the end of this period, subjects who judged themselves as clinically improved were allowed to continue for an additional 12 weeks. Fourteen of 16 subjects in the fluvoxamine group opted to continue. No subjects in the placebo group proceeded into the follow-up phase of treatment. Fluvoxamine showed superiority to placebo on nearly all psychometric measures.

Of interest was the continued improvement in the subjects' symptoms during the extension phase of this study. Symptoms of general anxiety, social anxiety, and social avoidance demonstrated continued clinical improvement during this phase of treatment. This evidence suggests that patients treated with the serotonin reuptake inhibitors may require treatment of 12 weeks or longer to receive an adequate clinical trial of these agents.

Fluvoxamine has shown good therapeutic benefit in the treatment of social phobia in the one study to date. This small but controlled study demonstrated superiority of fluvoxamine over placebo.

Buspirone

Buspirone, the novel anxiolytic, has also been studied in the treatment of social phobia. This drug's proposed site of pharmacological activity is the 5-HT$_{1A}$ receptor, where it functions as an agonist. In prior studies, buspirone has shown efficacy in the treatment of generalized anxiety disorder (Rickels et al. 1982). Given its effectiveness in generalized anxiety disorder, investigators have started to look at buspirone's utility in social phobia. Two trials have been reported looking at this drug in the treatment of social phobia.

Munjack et al. (1991) conducted a pilot study of buspirone in the treatment of social phobia. Subjects meeting DSM-III-R criteria for social phobia were entered into an 8-week, open-label trial. Buspirone was started at 5 mg twice a day and increased by 5 mg every 2–3 days to a maximum dosage of 60 mg/day, or until side effects prevented further dose escalation. Of the 17 subjects entered in this study, 11 completed it. The 6 dropouts resulted from lack of responsiveness, adverse effects, inability to attend appointments, and a loss to follow-up. At week 6, of the 11 subjects completing the trial, 5 reported "a little" and 6 endorsed "moderate" change in their symptomatology. At the end of week 8, two subjects reported "a little," 5 noted "moderate," and 4 endorsed "marked" improvement. Although the global measures demonstrated the above results, instruments used to measure the features specific to social phobia demonstrated mixed results.

The use of buspirone in social phobia has also been investigated by Schneier et al. (1993). In this 12-week open trial, 21 patients who met DSM-III-R criteria for social phobia and did not display a response during a 1-week placebo run-in, went on to receive buspirone. The drug was initiated at 5 mg three times a day and was increased by 5 mg/day every 3 days to a maximum dosage of 60 mg/day or until side effects prevented further dose increases. Seventeen patients completed the trial. At the end of week 12, 8 (47%) of the 17 subjects were rated as "much" to "very much" improved on the Clinical Global Impression Scale (Guy 1976). Of those subjects tolerating doses of 45 mg/day or more, 67% (9/12) were at least "much improved."

The results of these two open trials suggest that buspirone may at best have modest efficacy in the treatment of social phobia. These studies were limited by the open-label format and duration, given the findings of studies of other agents. Further studies are warranted to investigate the use of this agent in a controlled, blinded fashion. However, given the modest results and limited side-effect profile, some clinicians may want to add buspirone to their list of drugs given trials with patients with social phobia. Recommendations for use would be based on the similar study designs of the reported two trials, suggesting that buspirone should be started at 5 mg two to three times a day and increased by 5 mg/day to a dose of 45–60 mg.

Benzodiazepines

Benzodiazepines, the most commonly used anxiolytic drugs in the treatment of chronic anxiety states, have also been investigated in the treatment of social phobia. These agents have been shown to be effective in the treatment of other anxiety disorders, including panic disorder and generalized anxiety disorder. Three benzodiazepines, all in the "high-potency" class of benzodiazepines have been investigated in the treatment of social phobia.

Alprazolam.   The triazolo analogue alprazolam has been shown to be effective in the treatment of generalized anxiety disorder and panic disorder. Subsequent to this, alprazolam has been cited in three reports in the treatment of social phobia. In the first report, Lydiard et al. (1988) described the open treatment of four patients with alprazolam with a daily dose of 3–8 mg. All subjects were identified as having a positive response in their social anxiety symptoms. The specific details of the treatment (e.g., duration of the trial) were not described. Reich and Yates (1988) detailed another open trial of 14 subjects with social phobia treated with alprazolam. Patients received alprazolam with a daily dose of 1–7 mg. The mean dose was 2.9 mg/day, with most patients receiving 3 mg/day or less. In this report, patients showed a rapid onset of clinical improvement, with all efficacy variables except the Hamilton Anxiety Scale showing clinical improvement. At the end of the 8-week trial, all subjects were rated as responders, with 10 being very much improved and 4 described as much improved on the Clinical Global Improvement Scale. However, at 1 week follow-up after alprazolam discontinuation, the scores on rating scales reverted to being similar to baseline scores. Yet, although not statistically significantly different from baseline scores, these follow-up scores tended to be better.

Gelernter et al. (1991) compared phenelzine, alprazolam, placebo, and cognitive-behavior therapy in social phobia. In those patients receiving alprazolam, only 38% improved, based on the Marks Fear Questionnaire (Marks and Matthews 1982) scores. In this study, the mean daily dose for alprazolam was 4.2 mg. At 2-month follow-up, after discontinuation of the drug, the improvement in the alprazolam group was no longer measurable.

Bromazepam. Another benzodiazepine, bromazepam, which is not currently available in the United States, was the subject of an open trial by Versiani et al. (1989). In this study, 10 subjects with social phobia received the agent over an 8-week period, with a mean dose of 26.4 mg/day. All efficacy variables demonstrated statistically significant improvement at week 8 compared with baseline scores. However, all subjects reported sedation as a side effect, and 4 of 10 subjects reported memory disturbance.

Clonazepam. The most extensively studied benzodiazepine in social phobia has been clonazepam. This agent, which received its primary FDA indication as an anticonvulsant agent for Lennox-Gastaut syndrome, akinetic and myoclonic seizures, has been widely used as an anxiolytic. Because of the agent's long half-life (18–50 hours), it has been suggested as a good agent for the treatment of chronic anxiety states. The characteristic of a long half-life is favorable to avoid the distress of interdose or morning rebound of anxiety symptoms that has been suggested of some shorter-acting agents in other anxiety disorders (Herman et al. 1987).

The initial study of clonazepam in social phobia conducted by Versiani et al. (1989) showed an overall benefit of the drug. This 8-week, open trial of 40 subjects displayed statistically significant lowering of scores on the efficacy variables, which included the Clinical Global Improvement and Severity Scales (Guy 1976), Liebowitz Social Anxiety Scale (Liebowitz 1987), Hamilton Anxiety Scale (M. Hamilton 1959), and the Sheehan Disability Scale (D. V. Sheehan 1986). The mean dose of clonazepam was 3.9 mg/day (SD ± 0.5 mg). Subjects in this study reported high rates of side effects, including sleepiness (67.5%), loss of libido (67.5%), and memory problems (35%).

Subsequent open trials of clonazepam in social phobia have all demonstrated strong symptomatic relief in most of the subjects entered into the trial (Munjack et al. 1990; S. R. Reiter et al. 1990). In these trials, at least 80% of subjects were rated as receiving marked benefit in their social anxiety.

Davidson et al. (1991b) conducted a longer open trial of clonazepam in 26 subjects, with the average duration of treatment being 11.3 months (range 1–29 months). The daily dose range was 0.5–5.0 mg, with a mean daily dose of 2.1 mg. A total of 84.6% of subjects showed good improvement. Notable is the fact that subjects requiring doses in excess of 1.5 mg/day during the initial phase of treatment were able to reduce their daily dose and maintain clinical improvement.

The prior study by Davidson et al. was followed by a placebo-controlled study of clonazepam in 75 patients (Davidson et al. 1993). Prior studies had been strongly supportive of the efficacy of the agent in social phobia but had all been limited by the open-label format. This blinded, placebo-controlled study of 10 weeks' duration demonstrated a 78% response rate with clonazepam and a 20% placebo response rate. The dose of clonazepam initiated at 0.25 mg and was escalated over the first 6 weeks to a maximum of 3.0 mg, with a mean dose at week 10 of 2.5 mg/day. As early as week 2, a relative difference between the clonazepam and the placebo groups could be observed. Subjects were believed to exhibit a full or maximal response to a given dose by week 6, although onset of improvement was noted much earlier. In addition to demonstrating improvement on both the fear and the avoidance subscales of the Liebowitz Social Anxiety Scale, a treatment effect was also measurable on the Sheehan Disability Inventory (D. V. Sheehan 1986), with the clonazepam group showing a marked improvement in work function.

Overall, the studies of benzodiazepines are strongly supportive of the efficacy of this class of drugs in the treatment of social phobia. Still, questions remain. The Davidson study identified that the onset of benefit can be identified as early as the second week of treatment. However, adequate duration of dosage trials remains unclear. Overall duration of treatment is also a question. The long-term open trial by Davidson indicated that a significant number of subjects continued to have symptom relief after their clonazepam was tapered to a lower daily dose. Besides the dose and duration of treatment issues, the general issue of use of benzodiazepines remains a question. Many practitioners remain hesitant to use benzodiazepines in chronic anxiety states. Concern often develops over the physical dependence and withdrawal syndromes associated with these agents. Additionally, in individuals with social phobia, given the high incidence of comorbid alcohol disorders, often thought to be a form of "self-medication," practitioners may understandably be reluctant to use these agents. However, Davidson's study suggests that patients were actually taking less medication with increased duration of trial. The treating practitioner must also weigh the theoretical chance of abuse of these agents against the theoretical benefit to the individual patient. Some psychopharmacologists feel that the depressogenic effects of clonazepam and the benzodiazepines are greater than other medications, especially β-blockers. Careful monitoring of the patient's pattern of medication use and strong patient education can reduce impact of these issues.

Other Agents

Bupropion. A brief case report by Emmanuel et al. (1991) describes one patient with depression and social phobia who responded to bupropion, an aminoketone antidepressant with noradrenergic and dopaminergic effects. We are unaware of any further studies with this drug, which could shed light on the utility of this drug in the treatment of social phobia.

Ondansetron. Ondansetron, a 5-HT$_3$ antagonist, was the subject of a multicenter, double-blind, randomized, placebo-controlled clinical trial. Two hundred seventy-five subjects, meeting DSM-III-R criteria for social phobia and completing a 1-week, single-blind placebo run-in trial, were treated with ondansetron 0.25 mg twice a day or placebo for 10 weeks. On the primary efficacy variable, the Duke Brief Social Phobia Scale, the ondansetron treatment group demonstrated a statistically significant difference from the placebo group. Supportive efficacy variables also displayed statistical trends in favor of ondansetron over placebo (DeVeaugh-Geiss and Bell 1994). The effect size was nonetheless small, and it is unclear whether this drug has competent therapeutic activity in social phobia. However, if the drug is proven to be effective, its unique 5-HT$_3$ antagonist effect could help us understand the pathophysiology of the disorder.

Clonidine. As with the rationale for β-blockers in the treatment of social phobia, clonidine hydrochloride, an α-adrenergic agonist, has been used in an attempt to target the physiological symptoms of the disorder. In a case report by Goldstein (1987), one subject with social phobia who experienced a primary symptom of blushing was treated with clonidine 0.1 mg twice a day after trials with alprazolam, phenelzine, and propranolol failed to provide symptom relief. The patient reported a dramatic decrease in the frequency and intensity of blushing episodes after 1 week of treatment. At 4-month follow-up, his symptoms remained well controlled and he denied any side effects.

SUMMARY: QUESTIONS FOR TREATMENT AND RESEARCH

Pharmacotherapy can effectively and rapidly reduce the symptoms and enable the individual with social phobia to function more effectively. However, several issues remain, including the algorithm by which treatment sequence is determined. Our experience suggests that clonazepam is a particularly effective drug, but the concerns of benzodiazepine use make many people uncomfortable. We do not know yet whether the much-used SSRIs or the selective and reversible MAOIs are as good. How long should pharmacotherapy be continued, and is relapse lower as cognitive-behavior therapy is added? More complex cases of social phobia, comorbid with depression, other anxiety disorders, alcohol abuse, or severe avoidant features are harder to treat and do not fare as well long term. How can such individuals be helped? To these practical questions, we can add the questions of mechanism: how do treatments work, can magnetic resonance studies illuminate their effects, and can some selective, effective, and better-tolerated drugs be developed? To current researchers in anxiety and clinicians we pose these questions.

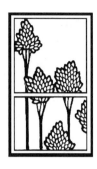

CHAPTER 26

Why a Peptide as an Anxiolytic?

Gary D. Tollefson, M.D., Ph.D.

Despite the numerous advances in psychopharmacology over the past 20 years, novel additions to the anxiolytic armamentarium have lagged. The cornerstone of drug therapy for primary anxiety states continues to be the benzodiazepines. Although benzodiazepines show efficacy, this class of drugs is beset with several safety concerns, for example, sedation, abuse potential, drug interactions, and cognitive impairment. Alternatively, evidence supporting the serotonergic mediation of anxiety (Kahn et al. 1988) has led to trials of select agonist/antagonists and reuptake inhibitors. Although the latter demonstrate symptom attenuation in obsessive-compulsive disorder (OCD), panic disorder, and posttraumatic stress disorder, a general anxiolytic profile has been less distinct.

An improved anxiolytic is needed, but where will it come from? Recent drug development targets for anxiolysis have principally been modulators of conventional neurotransmitters. Examples include the γ-aminobutyric acid $(GABA)_A$ (benzodiazepines), serotonin type 1A receptor (5-HT_{1A}; buspirone), and noradrenaline (β-blockers/α_2 antagonists) binding sites. Neuropeptides offer a refreshing alternative. Because neuropeptides are found throughout the central nervous system (CNS), are behaviorally active, serve as markers of neuronal pathology, and influence the activity of other classical neurotransmitters, they represent an intriguing and alternative target for future drug development.

Neuropeptide candidates for anxiolysis are not bound by their regional site density in brain. These small peptides can readily diffuse from the interstitial space along intraparenchymal vasculature and into the cerebroventricular system (Rennel et al. 1985). From there, the potential targets of influence are many.

Strategies employed to test neuropeptide hypotheses in patients with anxiety disorder have included 1) receptor characterization in postmortem brain, 2) cerebrospinal fluid (CSF) concentration studies, 3) direct challenge with known agonists or antagonists, and 4) observed neuroendocrine links to relevant psychiatric disorders. The main obstacle to a wider number of neuropeptide candidates in clinical development at present has been the technical challenge of identifying not only safe but pharmacokinetically and dynamically attractive options. Despite the lack of more dramatic progress, the use of neuropeptide modulators for CNS disorders continues to represent one of the most promising areas for new CNS drug development.

NEUROPEPTIDE Y

Neuropeptide Y (NPY) is a 36–amino acid peptide. The function of NPY, one of the most abundant peptide transmitters of the mammalian brain, remains unclear because of a lack of specific receptor antagonists. NPY meets many of the criteria of a neurotransmitter itself. NPY is costored and interacts with several monoaminergic neurons within the CNS (Lundberg et al. 1982), for example, noradrenergic afferents from the nucleus solitary tract to the amygdala. Both somatostatin and NPY colocalize at GABA interneurons within the amygdala, neocortex, and striatum. NPY also selectively modulates N-methyl-D-aspartate–induced hippocampal activation (pyramidal neurons) via σ receptors (Debonnel et al. 1994).

Evidence that NPY mediates anxiety is accumulating (Wahlestedt and Reis 1993). The behavioral profile of centrally administered NPY includes stimulation of appetite and anticonflict prominence (B. G. Stanley and Leibowitz 1985). Gehlert (1994) suggested that NPY functioning as a putative endogenous anxiolytic is mediated at the Y1 receptor subtype.

In rats, intracerebroventricular administration of NPY has been associated with an attenuation in ambulation, grooming, and defecation associated with a novel or "open-field" environment (B. E. Leonard and Song 1994). However, in an elevated plus-maze, this group reported that NPY effects were negligible. NPY-associated behavioral changes were also accompanied by changes in homovanillic acid and 5-hydroxyindoleacetic acid and by the suppression of lymphocyte proliferation. Further evidence of anxiolytic effects has been reported using the Vogel punished drinking model and, in contrast to B. E. Leonard and Song (1994), in the elevated plus-maze (Heilig et al. 1993). Heilig and colleagues (1993) employed the Geller-Seifter anxiety model for punished responding and reported that the microinjection of NPY into the amygdala produced an anticonflict/anxiolytic-like effect. In comparison, a selective NPY-1 agonist appears more active than a selective NPY-2 counterpart. Wahlestedt and colleagues (1993) reported an antisense oligo-deoxynucleotide corresponding to the NH_2 terminus of the rat Y1 receptor that was constructed and added to cultures of rat cortical neurons. This treatment resulted in a reduced density of Y1 (but not Y2) receptors and diminished the decrease in cyclic adenosine 3',5'-monophosphate (cAMP) usually seen after Y1 receptor activation. Repeated injection of the same oligodeoxynucleotide into the lateral cerebral ventricle of rats was followed by a similar reduction of cortical Y1 (but not Y2) receptors. Such antisense-treated animals displayed behavioral signs of anxiety. Thus, specific inhibition of neurotransmitter receptor expression can be accomplished in the living brain and demonstrates that altered central NPY transmission produces an anxiety-like state.

In human trials, reduced CSF concentrations have been observed among patients with depression. Upon their stratification into high or low levels of comorbid anxiety, the former demonstrated the most dramatic reductions in NPY (Widerlöv et al. 1988). Wahlestedt and colleagues (1993) have employed an innovative methodology to test the validity of this relationship by compromising brain NPY receptors via an antisense oligonucleotide. This "knock-out" resulted in an escalation of anxiety among test animals.

The control nucleus of the amygdala, dense in NPY-ergic innervation, has been identified as one potential target of interest. Based on this information, it is plausible that a targeted agonist to the NPY-1 binding site in the amygdala might be anxiolytic without adversely influencing consummatory behaviors. Whether such an effect would be direct or through the modulation of other neurotransmitters is unknown.

GALANIN

Human galanin is composed of 30 amino acids and is widely distributed in the CNS. A primary residence is within sensory and selected forebrain cholinergic interneurons; a detailed map of galanin distribution is available (Kordower et al. 1992). Based on several models, galanin appears to be an endogenous analgesic (Wiesenfeld-Hallin et al. 1992) and an inhibitor of acetylcholine release (Fisone et al. 1987). Direct infusion into the medial septum of rats disrupts working memory. The most probable neuropsychiatric application for galanin modulators may be in Alzheimer's dementia, in which galanin-containing neurons have been shown to hypertrophy and hyperinnervate remaining cholinergic (especially Ch4) neurons (see Mufson et al. 1993).

M35, a galanin antagonist, has been shown in rats to facilitate spatial learning in the Morris swim maze (Ogren et al. 1992). A possible secondary effect on anxiety (as it might relate to learning) cannot be excluded. However, any possible contribution of galanin in anxiety-based disorders may be limited to facilitation of behaviorally based learning paradigms and/or via secondary comodulations. Studies by Gabriel and Harsutunian (1994) have suggested that a substantial portion of cerebral cortical galanin may derive from noradrenergic neurons (e.g., double lesioning of the nucleus basalis of Meynert decreases galanin concentrations).

Lastly, in reference to the preceding section, galanin may modulate NPY Y1 receptors, which are subsequently downregulated in small neurons and upregulated in large neurons (Hokfelt et al. 1994).

OXYTOCIN

The general view on oxytocin has been its role in lactation and uterine contraction. However, Kovacs (1986) detailed an interesting series of behavioral and physiological effects attributable to central oxytocin. Pathways originating in the anterior hypothalamus project to multiple central sites, including limbic terminations involved in affect, and basal forebrain sites, involved in parenting, sexual and social behaviors, and feeding. Buijs et al. (1985) suggested that the oxytocin pattern of brain distribution may indicate a regulatory role on several ascending monoamine systems. Possible examples include increased postsynaptic dopamine receptor sensitivity (but decreased presynaptic affinity) and altered utilization of norepinephrine and serotonin (5-HT) in hypothalamus, limbic, and midbrain sites (Pedersen 1991). The major behavioral effects of oxytocin have centered around learning/memory, tolerance to addictive substances, sexuality, and affect. Several lines of evidence suggest that a net deficiency in oxytocin may contribute to depression. Behavioral models, as reviewed by Pedersen (1991), supporting this link include antagonism of immobility in the Porsolt swim test and reversal of learned helplessness. The administration of the C-terminal tripeptide of oxytocin reportedly enhanced mood among patients with major depression (Ehrensing and Kastin 1978).

The belief that oxytocin may be a stress hormone is strengthened by the animal literature (Gibbs 1986), in which oxytocin release accompanied placement in aversive conditions (e.g., immobilization, cold, suspension). However, stress paradigms where behavioral adaptation is possible (e.g., novel milieu) do not seem to elicit a similar response. To explore dose relationships for effects of oxytocin on spontaneous motor activity in the rat, Uvnäs-Moberg et al. (1994) studied oxytocin in doses from 1 to 1,000 µg/kg given subcutaneously to male Sprague-Dawley rats. Spontaneous motor behavior was measured by photocell-operated open-field observations. In the rats treated with low doses of oxytocin (1–4 µg/kg), a decrease in peripheral locomotor activity was found. With increasing doses (250–1,000 µg/kg), clear signs of sedative effects were demonstrated, as indicated by a suppression of locomotor activity and rearing. This spectrum of effects caused by oxytocin was similar to that of midazolam, but different from that induced by raclopride, suggesting an anxiolytic effect in male mice. The possible extension to the anxiety disorders was made by Ansseau and colleagues (1987), who reported that oxytocin improved the symptoms of OCD. However, an investigation of 12 patients administered oxytocin intranasally failed to show any reduction in their obsessive ideation or compulsive behaviors relative to results with placebo (Den Boer and Westenberg 1992a, 1992b). Regardless, a reciprocal role in adrenocorticotropic hormone (ACTH) release and its possible role as an "endogenous coping factor" in response to unmanageable stressors have made this nonapeptide a candidate for the coordination of appropriate neurotransmitter, endocrine, and autonomic response in stress.

CORTICOTROPIN-RELEASING FACTOR

A role for corticotropin-releasing factor (CRF) in coordinating the behavioral response to stress has been well documented (Nemeroff 1991a). Repeated exposure of animals and humans to stress induces adaptive changes in the CRF-modulated stress-response system. Stress-responsive systems, such as those localized to the paraventricular nucleus of the hypothalamus, may play a key role in hypothalamic-pituitary-adrenal regulation. Daily exposure to stress has been shown to increase release of the ACTH secretagogue vasopressin from corticotropin-releasing hormone terminals. This suggests a shift in the hypothalamic drive of stress-induced ACTH secretion from a corticotropin-releasing hormone–dominated to a vasopressin-dominated mode (Tilders et al. 1994). Stress-responsive corticosteroids also interact at the 5-HT$_{1A}$ receptor (Chalmers et al. 1994) and exhibit delayed elevations in homovanillic acid, the major dopamine metabolite (Posener et al. 1994).

The direct infusion of CRF into the locus coeruleus (rat) increases an anxiety response; conversely, administration into the parabrachial nucleus decreases it (J. M. Weiss et al. 1994). Nemeroff (1992) described that several of the effects of centrally administered CRF are reminiscent of certain signs and symptoms of anxiety disorders. CRF exerts clear anxiogenic effects in classic animal models of anxiety such as the conflict test (Britton et al. 1986), and these effects are blocked by both clinically efficacious benzodiazepines, and by the CRF-receptor antagonist α-helical CRF_{9-41}. The direct bilateral injection of CRF into the locus coeruleus of rats, in doses as low as 0.5 ng per side, produces anxiogenic effects in a naturalistic anxiety paradigm. This behavioral effect of CRF was associated with increased norepinephrine turnover in terminal projection areas of the locus coeruleus (Butler et al. 1990). In addition, short-term treatment with alprazolam or adinazolam, two anxiolytic triazolobenzodiazepines, produces effects on CRF concentrations in the locus coeruleus (a decrease) that are opposite to those of stress (an increase). These effects of a single dose of alprazolam persist for up to 3 hours. There is no tolerance to these effects after long-term drug administration. Furthermore, after abrupt withdrawal, marked CRF release occurs with resultant downregulation of pituitary CRF receptors. Thus, CRF release may mediate certain physiological and behavioral effects of benzodiazepine withdrawal.

Andreatini and Leite (1994) have evaluated the anxiolytic effect of corticosterone. Corticosteroid receptor mediation was evaluated by using a dose-response analysis of the effect of corticosterone and by the action of dexamethasone. Male Wistar rats (3 months old) were injected subcutaneously with vehicle ($n = 38$); corticosterone 1.25 mg/kg ($n = 18$), 2.5 mg/kg ($n = 13$), and 5.0 mg/kg ($n = 24$); or dexamethasone 5.0 mg/kg ($n = 19$) and 10.0 ($n = 17$) mg/kg and tested in the elevated plus-maze 2 hours later. The group that received the highest dose of corticosteroid (5.0 mg/kg) showed a significant increase in percentage of open arm entries as well as in percentage of time spent in open arms when compared with the vehicle-treated rats. These data corroborate previous findings of the anxiolytic effect of corticosterone and suggest that inhibition of ACTH/CRF release and corticosteroid receptors does not play a major role in the anxiolytic effect of corticosterone. Administration of a CRF antagonist diminishes exploratory and operant behaviors produced by CRF or stress exposures (A. J. Dunn and Berridge 1990). In an effort to understand the specificity of this response, Heinrichs et al. (1994) used exploration on the elevated plus-maze following exposure to social, swim, or restraint stressors. Like chlordiazepoxide, 1 µg of the CRF antagonist (α-helical CRF_{9-41}) reduced stress-in-duced inhibition of exploratory behavior regardless of the type or intensity of the stressor (ACTH secretory response).

In contrast to the compelling story of CRF hypersecretion/CRF receptor downregulation in depression (Nemeroff 1991a), the role of CRF in human anxiety disorders has not been well elucidated. Roy-Byrne and colleagues (1986) have observed blunted ACTH responses to exogenously administered CRF in patients with panic disorder. This is of particular interest because such patients exhibit suppression in the dexamethasone suppression test and may, therefore, have a subtle form of hypothalamic-pituitary-adrenal axis dysregulation. M. A. Smith et al. (1989) reported that patients with another DSM-III-R (American Psychiatric Association 1987) anxiety disorder, posttraumatic stress disorder, also exhibit blunted ACTH responses to exog-enously administered CRF. Levels of CRF have also been reported to be ele-vated in OCD (Altemus et al. 1993). Uhde and colleagues observed blunted ACTH responses to CRF challenge in patients with panic disorder (T. W. Uhde, personal communication, May 1993). Clinical trials with the synthetic $ACTH_{4-9}$ analogue ORG 2766 in subjects with anxiety disorder (panic disor-der, generalized anxiety disorder, social phobia) have failed to provide evi-dence of robust anxiolysis (Den Boer et al. 1992). DeWied and Jolles (1992) speculated that the true property of this analogue may relate to the motiva-tional aspects of behavior rather than to anxiety. Menzaghi et al. (1994) re-ported that two CRF analogues antagonized CRF and stress-induced behavioral changes in rats. Dose-dependent improvements in locomotor and social stress-induced anxiogenesis within the elevated plus-maze were ob-served. Evidence for the effect of putative CRF antagonists within human subjects is relatively scant and does not permit conclusions to be drawn. The availability of potent and selective CRF antagonists offers the chance to ex-plore the functional role of CRF in anxiety/stress—and ultimately a possible new therapeutic approach.

SOMATOSTATIN

Somatostatin is a 14–amino acid peptide that induces arousal and behavioral stereotypes resembling OCD (Pitman 1989). Somatostatin is synthesized in disparate regions, including the paraventricular nucleus of the hypothalamus, the cerebral cortex, striatum, and hippocampus. When administered cen-trally, somatostatin delays extinction of avoidant behaviors (Vecsei and Widerlov 1988). Altemus and colleagues (1993) determined CSF somatostatin concentrations among 15 unmedicated patients with OCD. In comparison with 27 psychiatrically healthy subjects, mean CSF levels were significantly higher in the OCD cohort independent of CSF volumes. This elevation, in concert with arginine vasopressin and CRF, suggests a disease-related covariance and, in turn, a potential neuroregulatory abnormality in OCD. Evidence suggests that somatostatin is likely derived from extra-hypothalamic brain areas (Berelowitz et al. 1981).

In light of the induction of OCD-like behaviors in animals that were centrally administered somatostatin and the elevation of somatostatin that is reported among humans with OCD, it is tempting to speculate on a somatostatin role in the pathophysiology of OCD. More compelling is evidence that selective serotonin uptake inhibitors, unlike other antidepressants not effective in OCD, produce a consistent and substantial reduction in somatostatin (Kakigi et al. 1990). A similar observation accompanies the dopamine antagonists sometimes used as therapeutic adjuncts in OCD (Zorilla et al. 1990). Such observations tempt those engaged in drug development to explore the utility of a selective somatostatin antagonist in OCD.

CHOLECYSTOKININ

Cholecystokinin is the most widespread and abundant peptide in the brain, with only the mature cerebellum possibly devoid of representation. Interest in this peptide also stems from its potency, prominent colocalization with dopamine, nonsynaptic associations influencing neuronal excitability and cerebral blood flow, and putative links to several neuropsychiatric disorders (Rehfeld 1992a, 1992b). (A detailed account of this peptide is given in Bradwejn et al., Chapter 27, in this volume.)

To date, evidence suggests that cholecystokinin-B activation may trigger a cascade of neurochemical events culminating in both the psychic and the somatic features of anxiety. In summary, these data continue to suggest an interesting opportunity to qualitatively broaden the clinician's armamentarium against one or more of the anxiety disorders.

DIAZEPAM BINDING INHIBITOR

Diazepam binding inhibitor (DBI) is a 10-kd peptide prominently identified among glial cells specializing in steroidogenesis (E. Costa and Guidotti 1991). DBI, and its putative link to anxiety, was deduced on the basis of its ability to displace ligands from the benzodiazepine recognition site associated with the

GABA$_A$ receptor. Specifically, DBI was shown to displace high-affinity ligands from benzodiazepine binding sites located in the outer mitochondrial membrane of glial cells (Guarneri et al. 1992). Indirect evidence suggests that DBI may be a physiological modulator of mitochondrial steroidogenesis. At the level of the adrenal gland, DBI may signal ACTH-induced steroidogenesis. Swerdlow and Britton (1994) reported that CRF-potentiated startle was inhibited by alfaxalone, a pregnane steroid anesthetic believed to act via the GABA/benzodiazepine receptor complex. However, the effects of alfaxalone on CRF-potentiated startle may not be generalized to all CRF-stimulated behaviors because alfaxalone failed to disrupt CRF-stimulated locomotor activity. CRF-potentiated startle is a useful assay for studying the effects of novel anxiolytic agents, and alfaxalone appeared to be a steroid anesthetic with anxiolytic properties in this assay. Similarly, DBI may regulate neurosteroidogenesis within glial cell populations. Interest in turn in the neurosteroids stems from their interaction with both fast-acting, transmitter-gated ion channels and classic cytoplasmic sites. The former reportedly modulate GABA-ergic or glutaminergic neurotransmission—a direct link to potential anxiolytic therapies. The ring–A-reduced progesterone derivative tetrahydroprogesterone is synthesized under normal physiological conditions in the brain and is a potent modulator of the GABA receptor. This neurosteroid reportedly has significant sedative and anxiolytic properties.

Patchev et al. (1994) investigated the effect of tetrahydroprogesterone on corticotropin-releasing hormone–induced anxiety, the basal and methoxamine-stimulated release of corticotropin-releasing hormone from hypothalamic organ explants in vitro, and adrenalectomy-induced upregulation of the gene expression of corticotropin-releasing hormone in the hypothalamic paraventricular nucleus in rats. At doses of 5 and 10 µg administered intracerebroventricularly, tetrahydroprogesterone counteracted the anxiogenic action of 0.5 µg of corticotropin-releasing hormone. Measurements of the steady-state levels of mRNA coding for corticotropin-releasing hormone by quantitative in situ hybridization histochemistry revealed that tetrahydroprogesterone was equipotent with corticosterone in preventing adrenalectomy-induced upregulation of peptide gene expression. These results demonstrated that tetrahydroprogesterone has anxiolytic effects that are mediated through interactions with hypothalamic corticotropin-releasing hormone in both genomic and nongenomic fashions. Although a DBI-based or other steroidomimetic therapeutic is neither a reality nor an absurdity, the proposal that DBI or a relative, perhaps via regulation of neurosteroid production, may provide a means to modulate fast neurotransmission within the CNS is certainly plausible.

OPIOID PEPTIDES

The role of endogenous opioid peptides in mood and anxiety is relatively unknown. However, their existence in large concentrations within relevant limbic structures supports the hypothesis (M. S. Gold et al. 1982a). Direct opioid effects reportedly include anxiolysis and mood enhancement. The selective involvement of the opioids alone is unlikely because their activity is interdigitated with several conventional monoamines such as dopamine, serotonin, and norepinephrine.

In general, therapeutic trials with opioid peptides have been of limited value because of bioavailability problems. However, enkephalins are active in behavioral reinforcement (deWitte et al. 1989). Tejedor-Real and colleagues (1993) have shown that a mixed inhibitor of enkephalin catabolism (RB 38A) induced an "imipramine-like" effect in reducing learned helplessness behaviors in the rat. Whether these effects on behavioral despair reflect on an anxiolytic potential is uncertain. In the study of 23 children admitted to the hospital for elective surgery, a statistically significant increase in plasma β-endorphin was observed 5 minutes before surgery (Constantopoulos et al. 1995). The authors speculated that the elevation, in contrast to levels obtained 24 hours earlier, reflected preoperative anxiety. Schedlowski and colleagues (1995) studied 47 inexperienced tandem parachutists 2 hours before, immediately after, and 1 hour after a jump. Anxiety levels and control attributes were also assessed. A transient but significant increase in β-endorphin levels occurred immediately after jumping. The magnitude of the response was dependent on subjective control attributions. Finally, in a study of 46 women with premenstrual syndrome as defined by DSM-III-R, anxiety and physical discomfort symptoms were correlated with a significant decline in plasma β-endorphin (Giannini et al. 1994). Such observations do little to establish a direct anxiolytic property of β-endorphin but do establish the opioid peptides as yet another potential target for anxiolytic drug development.

CONCLUSION

This brief overview highlights some of the more promising peptide-based relationships to the anxiety disorders from the more than 50 neuropeptides identified. Investigations into the role of peptides in human states of anxiety have included localization, animal modeling, postmortem receptor assays,

CSF or plasma concentration, and challenge testing. Progress made in this field over the past decade has been impressive. As the design of peptide mimetics becomes more sophisticated in providing probes that are specific, bioavailable, and capable of crossing the blood-brain barrier, the likelihood of even greater advances in novel therapeutics will increase substantially. The future is challenging but, in the same token, hopeful.

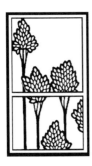

CHAPTER 27

Cholecystokinin Antagonists in Panic and Anxiety Disorders

Jacques Bradwejn, M.D., F.R.C.P.C.,
Diana Koszycki, Ph.D.,
Eero Vasar, M.D., Ph.D.,
Roberta Palmour, Ph.D., and
Franco Vaccarino, Ph.D.

CHOLECYSTOKININ PEPTIDES ARE FOUND IN THE CENTRAL NERVOUS SYSTEM

Cholecystokinin (CCK) belongs to a class of neuropeptides named "brain-gut" peptides, which are found in mammalian gastrointestinal and central nervous systems. Originally discovered in the gastrointestinal tract, CCK was identified in the brain in the late 1970s. Unlike most brain-gut peptides, which are expressed in discrete regions of the brain and in low concentrations, CCK is expressed in a number of regions and in large concentrations in the central nervous system (CNS). It is also unique in its distribution in the brain because of its concentrations in the cerebral cortex (for review, see Rehfeld and Nielsen 1995).

CCK peptides are synthesized in neurons and are encoded by a single gene consisting of three exons, which, after encoding by mature mRNA, leads to a prepro-CCK of 115 amino acids. This peptide chain is then truncated to pro-CCK, which generates a bioactive form of CCK of varying lengths (Deschenes et al. 1984; Y. Takahashi et al. 1985). The biosynthesis of CCK peptide takes place sequentially in several structures of the neuron: from endoplasmic reticulum to Golgi apparatus to synaptic vesicles (Eng et al. 1983; Goltermann et al. 1980; Rehfeld and Hansen 1986; Stengaard-Pedersen et al. 1984). This sequential biosynthetic process generates a mixture of pro-CCK and CCK chains of varying lengths; their distribution and release configurations may vary among species (Cantor and Rehfeld 1989; Eysselein et al. 1988; Rehfeld 1994). The predominant molecule released from most neuronal tissues is a chain of eight amino acids (CCK-8) in its O-sulfated and carboxyamidated form (CCK-8S) (Dockray et al. 1978; Marley et al. 1982; Rehfeld 1978). However, other active shorter forms of CCK, such as CCK-5 or CCK-4, can also be found in the CNS, although at much lower concentrations (N. Lindefors et al. 1993; Marley et al. 1984; Rehfeld 1978, 1981; Shively et al. 1987).

Two types of CCK receptors have been identified pharmacologically and are classified as CCK-A and CCK-B receptors. CCK-A (A for "alimentary") receptors are found in the viscera and in some distinct brain regions and have a higher affinity for CCK-8S than for CCK-4 or gastrin. CCK-B (B for "brain") receptors are widely distributed in the brain and have a high affinity for CCK-8S, CCK-4, and gastrin (Hill et al. 1992). Results from recent studies suggest multiple affinity states for CCK-A and CCK-B (S. Huang et al. 1994; Pandya et al. 1994). The distinction between CCK-A and CCK-B receptors, originally made pharmacologically, has been confirmed by cloning (Y. M. Lee et al. 1993; Pisegna et al. 1992; Wank et al. 1992). In rats, most CCK receptors in the CNS belong to the B subtype, although CCK-A receptors are found in the area postrema, nucleus tractus solitarius, and interpeduncular nucleus (Hill and Woodruff 1990; Hill et al. 1987; Moran et al. 1986; Van Dijk et al. 1984).

CHOLECYSTOKININ PEPTIDES FULFILL CRITERIA FOR A NEUROTRANSMITTER

CCK peptides such as CCK-8S fulfill criteria for a neurotransmitter in the CNS. CCK-8S is localized in cell bodies and in nerve endings of CNS neurons, with a higher concentration in nerve terminal (Emson et al. 1980;

Larsson and Rehfeld 1979; Pinget et al. 1978). Substantial in vivo synthesis of CCK-8S in rat cerebral cortex has been demonstrated using radiolabeling with methionine (Goltermann et al. 1980). CCK-8S is released by depolarization (P. R. Dodd et al. 1980; Emson et al. 1980), affects postsynaptic function (J. Dodd and Kelly 1981), and is inactivated by degradation or by reuptake (Deschodt-Lanckman et al. 1981; Goltermann et al. 1980; Stengaard-Pedersen et al. 1984). Finally, the actions of CCK are antagonized by receptor antagonists (see below).

CHOLECYSTOKININ HYPOTHESIS OF PANIC DISORDER: HISTORICAL PERSPECTIVE

The hypothesis that CCK may be a mediator of anxiety originated from electrophysiological experiments of Bradwejn and de Montigny that demonstrated that low doses of benzodiazepines selectively and specifically antagonized CCK-8S–induced excitation of hippocampal pyramidal neurons in rats, an effect that was mediated by benzodiazepine receptors (Bradwejn and de Montigny 1984). This study provided the first evidence that anxiolytic benzodiazepines could antagonize the central action of a neuropeptide, and it was proposed that benzodiazepine-mediated antagonism of CCK-induced excitation might be an important mechanism by which benzodiazepines exert their clinically relevant action and that CCK might be an endogenous anxiogenic compound. Two pilot studies, one in patients with panic disorder and the other in subjects with no personal or family history of panic attacks, were conducted to address this question using CCK-4. The decision to administer the tetrapeptide form to patients with panic disorder was based on anecdotal data presented by Jens Rehfeld at the Neuronal Cholecystokinin Conference in Brussels in 1984. In the course of investigating the neuroendocrine effects of CCK-4 in psychiatrically healthy human subjects, Jens Rehfeld noted that CCK-4 produced a number of "side effects" such as anxiety, dyspnea, and depersonalization (Rehfeld 1992a, 1992b; Vanderhaeghen and Crawley 1985). In our assessment, these side effects were strikingly similar to symptoms experienced by patients with panic disorder during their spontaneous panic attacks.

Bradwejn and colleagues first administered CCK-4 to patients with panic disorder by using a double-blind, placebo-control methodology. Bolus injections of CCK-4 (50 µg) precipitated a panic attack, as defined by DSM-III criteria (American Psychiatric Association 1980) and patient self-report, within 1 minute following administration in 11 patients studied, whereas none of the patients panicked following administration of placebo (Bradwejn et al. 1990). de Montigny first reported that exogenous CCK-4 produced "paniclike" attacks in psychiatrically healthy volunteers and that these effects could be attenuated by pretreatment with lorazepam (de Montigny 1989). Taken together, these preliminary data suggested a potential link between CCK activity and panic disorder.

CHOLECYSTOKININ TETRAPEPTIDE FULFILLS CRITERIA FOR A PANICOGENIC AGENT

The finding of a close analogy between symptoms produced by CCK-4 and those reported to occur during patients' spontaneous panic attacks was intriguing and suggested that CCK-4 might be a suitable paradigm for studying the neurobiology of panic disorder and for anxiety research in general. An important task remained to systematically evaluate the validity of CCK-4 as a model of panic disorder using the seven criteria for an "ideal" panicogenic agent described by Guttmacher et al. (1993) and Gorman et al. (1987). The seven criteria are as follows:

1. *The agent should be safe.* CCK-4 seems safe to administer to human subjects. Our experiments and experiments of other researchers suggest that the peptide is safe for human research. With the exception of a brief vasovagal reaction occurring in less than 3% of subjects, no significant adverse effects have been observed.
2. *The agent should induce affective as well as somatic symptoms of a panic attack.* CCK-4 generates both emotional (e.g., anxiety, fear, apprehension) and somatic (e.g., dyspnea, palpitations, choking, sweating, faintness) symptoms that typically occur during a panic attack (Bradwejn and Koszycki 1992). In our studies, the occurrence of a subjective sense of anxiety, fear, and/or apprehension, as well as at least four DSM-III-R (American Psychiatric Association 1987) somatic symptoms, are important criteria for judging the occurrence of a panic attack.
3. *The agent should provoke attacks that resemble the patient's clinical panic attacks.* The panic attacks induced by CCK-4 have been appraised by patients to be identical or very similar to their spontaneous panic attacks in terms of the type and quality of symptoms (Bradwejn et al. 1991a). This has been an important criterion of panic attack in our studies with patients. Moreover, CCK-4 does not induce a stereotyped response in

patients. Rather it mimics the individual symptom profile usually experienced by each patient. The majority of patients have reported that the main difference between CCK-4–induced panic attack and their clinical attacks is that the symptoms induced with CCK-4 occur more abruptly and are generally of a shorter duration.

4. *The effects of the agent should be specific for patients with a history of panic attacks.* We have found that response to CCK-4 reliably differentiates patients with panic disorder from control subjects with no personal or family history of panic attacks. In a double-blind, placebo-controlled study (Bradwejn et al. 1991a), we noted that patients with panic disorder experienced a greater number of symptoms and more intense symptoms following challenge with two doses (25 and 50 µg) of CCK-4. In addition, the incidence of panic attacks was markedly higher in patients than that in control subjects following injection of 25 µg (91% vs. 17%, respectively) and 50 µg (100% versus 47%, respectively) of the peptide. Our results are corroborated by studies by Abelson and Nesse (1990, 1994) using pentagastrin, a CCK-B receptor agonist that incorporates the identical 4–amino acid sequence of CCK-4, and by van Megen and colleagues (1992, 1994b) using CCK-4 or pentagastrin. These authors found that these CCK-B agonists provoked panic attacks at a higher frequency in patients with panic disorder than in psychiatrically healthy subjects.

5. *The effects of the agent should be reliable.* To determine whether the behavioral effects of CCK-4 could be replicated in the same individual, we administered 25 µg of CCK-4 to 11 patients with panic disorder on two separate occasions in the absence of intervening treatment (Bradwejn et al. 1992c). Although the latency to effect symptoms with CCK-4 was significantly shorter on the second challenge day, the vulnerability of patients to the panicogenic properties of CCK-4 was undiminished with repeated challenge. Panic attack frequency following the initial and subsequent challenge was 82% and 73%, respectively. In addition, the number and intensity of symptoms remained constant with rechallenge. These results were replicated in other studies in panic disorder and in psychiatrically healthy volunteers (Bradwejn et al. 1994c; Koszycki et al. 1996a, 1996b).

The effectiveness of CCK-4 in provoking panic responses also appears to be dose dependent. In a double-blind dose-response study (Bradwejn et al. 1992b) of CCK-4 (0, 10, 15, 20, and 25 µg) in patients with panic disorder, a significant linear relationship was found for the number and sum intensity of symptoms evoked with CCK-4. None of the patients panicked with placebo. The difference between treatments in panic frequency was significantly different, and there was a significant linear dose-response effect. Paralleling the behavioral changes induced with CCK-4, a marked and dose-related increase in heart rate and blood pressure was evident. In another double-blind study (Bradwejn et al. 1991a) with 36 psychiatrically healthy volunteers, CCK-4 (0, 9, 25, and 50 μg) was also found to induce panic attacks in a dose-dependent manner. No panic attacks occurred with placebo injections.

6. *Antipanic agents should block the effects of the agent.* We have demonstrated that the panicogenic effects of CCK-4 can be antagonized by chronic treatment with imipramine (Bradwejn and Koszycki 1994b). It is also notable that patients who consumed higher doses of imipramine experienced fewer and less-intense panic symptoms at rechallenge, suggesting that the decreased sensitivity to CCK-4 following chronic imipramine therapy was most likely attributed to a drug effect rather than to other factors such as spontaneous remission of symptoms. In addition to our study with imipramine, evidence has been found that treatment with another antipanic agent can inhibit the effects of CCK-4 in humans. van Megen and colleagues (1994a) reported that the selective serotonin reuptake inhibitor fluvoxamine decreased CCK-4–induced panic attacks in patients with panic disorder.

7. *The effects of the agent are not antagonized by drugs without antipanic effects.* Indirect evidence indicates that CCK-4 also satisfies this criterion. In the context of investigating the effects of CCK-B receptor antagonists on CCK-4–induced panic symptoms, we observed that pretreatment with placebo failed to antagonize CCK-4–induced panic symptoms in patients with panic disorder (Bradwejn et al. 1994b). In another study that investigated the possible mediating role of benzodiazepine receptors in CCK-4–induced panic symptoms, pretreatment with the benzodiazepine receptor antagonist flumazenil, a compound without any known antipanic activity, failed to diminish response to CCK-4 challenge in psychiatrically healthy volunteers (Bradwejn et al. 1994a).

EFFECTS OF CHOLECYSTOKININ TETRAPEPTIDE ARE COMPARABLE TO THOSE PRODUCED BY CO_2

Another research approach used in evaluating whether CCK-4 is a valid panicogenic agent has been to compare its effects with those produced by another valid pharmacological model of panic disorder. So far, we have compared response to a 25-μg dose of CCK-4 and a single inhalation of 35% CO_2 in patients with panic disorder (Bradwejn and Koszycki 1991) and psychiatrically healthy volunteers (Koszycki et al. 1991). In the study with patients, CCK-4 produced a greater number of symptoms and more intense symptoms than 35% CO_2. CCK-4 was also more effective in inducing panic attacks than was CO_2 (91% versus 45%, respectively), although the profile of symptoms that emerged in response to either agent was similar in patients who experienced a panic attack. Although CCK-4 was found to produce more intense panic symptoms than did CO_2 in psychiatrically healthy volunteers, these concentrations of CCK-4 and CO_2 were equipotent in promoting panic attacks (17% versus 21%, respectively). It will be interesting in future studies to compare CCK-4 with other panicogenic challenges.

PSYCHOLOGICAL ASPECTS OF CHOLECYSTOKININ TETRAPEPTIDE–INDUCED SYMPTOMS

Marked interindividual differences exist in behavioral sensitivity to panicogens such as CO_2, sodium lactate, and yohimbine. Although variation in behavioral sensitivity to panicogens is believed to reflect alterations in the neurochemistry instrumental to the expression of clinical panic attacks, it has been argued that psychological variables including anticipatory anxiety, interoceptive sensitivity, appraisal of threat or harm, perception of control, and panic expectancy, among other variables, play a more salient role in the induction of anxious/fearful feelings. In addition to according a causal role to cognitions in the onset and maintenance of clinical panic attacks, cognitive theorists have postulated that catastrophic appraisal of somatic symptoms induced by panicogenic agents is central to the provocation of fear and anxiety (D. M. Clark 1993; Rapee 1995).

It could be postulated that there is a link between catastrophic thoughts and the emergence of anxious/fearful affect following systemic administration of CCK-4. However, two lines of evidence suggest that this link is weak. First, all subjects who participate in our CCK challenge studies are provided with explicit information about the possible effects of CCK-4. In addition, they are instructed to attribute the somatic symptoms they experience to the transient effects of the peptide. According to cognitive theory, these instructions should markedly attenuate the degree of anxiety experienced (i.e., subjects are provided with a rational and noncatastrophic explanation for their symptoms). However, such a theory does not appear to be supported. The provision of detailed information about the pharmacological effects of CCK-4 has been found to neither detract from the expression of a panic attack nor limit the degree of anxiety experienced in patients with panic disorder or even in psychiatrically healthy volunteers. For instance, systemic administration of a 50-μg dose of CCK-4 provoked panic episodes in 100% of patients with panic disorder and in 47% of psychiatrically healthy volunteers. Moreover, CCK-4 engendered severe or extremely severe fear and anxiety in all of the patients and in 86% of the control subjects in whom a panic attack was transiently induced. Second, we have noted that a subgroup of patients with panic disorder and psychiatrically healthy control subjects who are challenged with CCK-4 experience "noncognitive" panic attacks (Koszycki et al. 1993, 1996b). That is, they experience both the somatic and the affective components of panic anxiety, but none of the associated catastrophic thoughts (e.g., fear of dying, fear of losing control, fear of going crazy).

We compared the effects of CCK-4 challenge in subjects who panicked but experienced no catastrophic cognition (noncognitive panickers) and in those who panicked and experienced at least one catastrophic cognition (cognitive panickers) (Koszycki et al. 1998). In psychiatrically healthy subjects challenged with a 50-μg dose of CCK-4, no significant difference in affective intensity emerged as a function of panic subtype. Further, the correlation between the intensity of affect and the number of cognitive symptoms endorsed was small and nonsignificant. Analysis of somatic symptoms of panic attack revealed that the overall pattern of symptom endorsement was comparable for cognitive and noncognitive panickers. In patients with panic disorder challenged with a 25-μg dose of CCK-4, neither the severity of affective response nor the severity of somatic response to CCK-4 was found to distinguish between cognitive and noncognitive panickers. Thus, the aforementioned data suggest that the cognitive process of self-labeling is not a major causal influence on affective response to systemic CCK-4.

Anxiety sensitivity is a prominent characteristic of patients with panic disorder. It is defined as a stable dimension of personality that consists of fears of physical sensations based on the belief that these symptoms have harmful consequences (Reiss et al. 1986). Anxiety sensitivity is not dependent on a history of panic attacks, but rather, it is hypothesized to be an important cognitive risk factor in the development of panic attacks and panic disorder. This hypothesis is supported by some (Donnell and McNally 1990; Maller and Reiss 1992) but not all (S. H. Stewart et al. 1992) studies with nonclinical subjects.

It has been proposed that anxiety sensitivity is an important psychological variable that mediates response to panicogenic stimuli. That is, individuals who fear the somatic symptoms produced by such stimuli respond to them with greater fear and anxiety. Given that patients with panic disorder have high levels of anxiety sensitivity relative to those of psychiatrically healthy control subjects, it might be expected that they would react more anxiously to the induction of arousal symptoms. Studies that attempt to show a relationship between anxiety sensitivity and behavioral reactivity to panic provocation procedures are few and inconclusive. Holloway and McNally (1987) tested response to voluntary hyperventilation, a relatively minor aversive event, in college students with high and low self-ratings of anxiety sensitivity and found that individuals with high anxiety sensitivity responded more anxiously to the challenge than those with low anxiety sensitivity. However, this finding may have been the result of differences in baseline anxiety. Indeed, adjusting for differences in baseline anxiety scores resulted in a sizable drop in the P value to nonsignificant levels. It should be noted as well that the hyperventilation challenge effected a relatively small increase in self-rated anxiety and none of the subjects panicked while hyperventilating. This suggests that anxiety sensitivity may well be associated with anticipatory anxiety rather than anxiety associated with panic attacks. Rapee and colleagues (Rapee and Medoro 1994; Rapee et al. 1992) reported that anxiety sensitivity emerged as a significant predictor of affective response to hyperventilation and 5.5% CO_2 challenges, although the amount of variance accounted for by anxiety sensitivity was not impressive. For instance, anxiety sensitivity accounted for only 8% of the variance in affective response to CO_2 inhalation in a combined sample of patients with panic disorder and control subjects (Holloway and McNally 1987). This suggests that factors other than anxiety sensitivity are likely to be involved in the mediation of affective response to panicogenic stimuli.

We have addressed the question of whether individual differences in anxiety sensitivity, as measured by the Anxiety Sensitivity Index (Reiss et al. 1986), play a crucial role in mediating behavioral sensitivity to CCK-4 challenge. In a preliminary study of 36 psychiatrically healthy volunteers (Koszycki et al. 1993), systemic administration of a 50-μg dose of CCK-4 provoked a comparable profile of anxiety and panicogenic response in individuals with low, medium (i.e., average), and high levels of anxiety sensitivity, as well as similar increases in heart rate and blood pressure. Interestingly, although subjects with high anxiety sensitivity were not more predisposed to experiencing a panic attack with CCK-4 than the other subjects, they were more likely to report catastrophic thoughts. This suggests that anxiety sensitivity may be related to interpretation of symptoms rather than to mediation of panic.

Although our preliminary data suggest that the frequency of CCK-4–induced panic attacks does not vary with level of anxiety sensitivity, still some question exists as to whether the quality of panic induced by CCK-4 is modified by level of anxiety sensitivity. To address this question, we evaluated the symptom profile associated with CCK-4–induced panic in subjects with low, medium, and high levels of anxiety sensitivity (Koszycki et al. 1996b). Preliminary analysis of data obtained from 64 psychiatrically healthy volunteers in whom a panic attack was transiently induced revealed that the intensity of affective response to CCK-4 was identical for the three anxiety sensitivity groups. In addition, inspection of DSM-IV (American Psychiatric Association 1994) somatic and cognitive symptoms of panic revealed that the symptom endorsement rates were comparable across the three groups. However, intensity ratings for dizziness, chest/pain discomfort, and fear of dying were higher in high-anxiety-sensitivity subjects relative to the other subjects. Interestingly, whereas high anxiety sensitivity was associated with higher symptom rating for fear of dying, low anxiety sensitivity was associated with a higher (albeit nonsignificant) symptom intensity rating for fear of losing control.

We have also examined the extent to which anxiety sensitivity influences the magnitude of response to CCK-4 in patients with panic disorder (Koszycki et al. 1996b). In this study, anxiety sensitivity did not correlate with the intensity of affective response to CCK-4, although it did correlate with the number and severity of cognitive symptoms at a modest level. No association was found between anxiety sensitivity and the number of somatic symptoms endorsed or the sum intensity of somatic symptoms.

In summary, the results from these studies do not provide compelling evidence that patients with panic disorder have an enhanced sensitivity to the panicogenic effects of CCK-4 relative to that of control subjects simply because they possess high levels of anxiety sensitivity. Nevertheless, it remains to be determined whether response to decreasing CCK-4 doses is influenced by self-rated anxiety sensitivity in psychiatrically healthy subjects. Indeed, it is conceivable that differences between low, medium, and high anxiety sensitivity groups may be observed only with lower dosages of CCK-4. Finally, the apparent discrepancy between the results with CCK-4 and those with hyperventilation in psychiatrically healthy volunteers suggests that the association between anxiety sensitivity and behavioral reactivity to challenges may depend, in part, on the nature and potency of the panicogenic stimulus employed. Voluntary hyperventilation has unreliable anxiolytic effects and is considered by some authors to be a poor model of panic disorder (H. Price et al. 1995). In contrast, CCK-4 produces a reliable, dose-dependent profile of symptoms reminiscent of panic attacks and fulfills criteria for an ideal panicogenic agent (Bradwejn and Koszycki 1994a). As noted, the magnitude of behavioral response to systemic CCK-4 administration in patients with panic disorder does not appear to be strongly influenced by individual differences in anxiety sensitivity. However, it is conceivable that other personality traits play a role. Accordingly, we (Koszycki et al. 1996b) determined whether personality traits that presumably underlie anxiety disorders amplify behavioral sensitivity to systemic CCK-4 administration in patients with panic disorder. The standard Minnesota Multiphasic Personality Inventory (MMPI; Hathaway and McKinley 1983) Hypochondriasis, Depression, Hysteria, Psychasthenia, and Social Introversion Scales and the supplemental MMPI Anxiety Scale (Welsh 1965) were used to measure these dispositions.

Correlational analyses failed to detect significant relationships between somatic, cognitive, and affective responses to CCK-4 and scores on the MMPI Hypochondriasis, Depression, Hysteria, and Psychasthenia Scales. By contrast, significant correlations in the moderate range were found between the MMPI Social Introversion Scale and the number and sum intensity of somatic symptoms.

To further clarify the relationship between psychological variables and behavioral response to CCK-4, hierarchical multiple regression analyses were conducted. The predictor variables that were included in the regression analyses included the Anxiety Sensitivity Index, the MMPI Hypochondriasis Scale, and the MMPI Social Introversion Scale. The Anxiety Sensitivity Index, which was entered into the model first, was not found to be a significant predictor of the magnitude of response to CCK-4, as measured by the three anxiety subscales. Further, the addition of the MMPI Hypochondriasis Scale did not add significantly to the model for any of the measures. In contrast, the MMPI Social Introversion Scale, which was entered next, contributed significantly and meaningfully to the predictive value. Indeed, the magnitude of change was greatest for the intensity of affective response to CCK-4, followed by the intensity of catastrophic cognitions, the number of reported catastrophic cognitions, and the intensity of somatic symptoms.

In summary, the aforementioned data suggest that the behavioral consequences of CCK-4 in patients with panic disorder are largely independent of personality variables. The only notable exception is that the MMPI Social Introversion Scale, a measure of neurotic introversion, was a significant predictor of behavioral response to CCK-4. The variables that potentially account for the apparent enhanced sensitivity of socially introverted patients to the behavioral consequences of CCK-4 are not readily available, although some provisional hypotheses may be proposed. It is conceivable that endogenous variations of central and/or peripheral CCK activity may be a neurochemical concomitant of the introversion personality trait. This argument deserves some consideration in view of the recent identification of a negative correlation between plasma gastrin, which binds preferentially to CCK-B receptors, and measures of socialization in patients with functional gastrointestinal disorders (Uvnäs-Moberg et al. 1991) and in women without gastrointestinal disorders (Uvnäs-Moberg et al. 1993). It is also interesting to note in this regard that the social isolation of rats leads to upregulation of CCK receptors in the frontal cortex (Vasar et al. 1993b). Accordingly, it is conceivable that the enhanced sensitivity to CCK-4 observed in socially introverted patients with panic disorder is attributed, at least in part, to variation in CCK receptor function. It may also be considered that a highly tenuous link between CCK and introversion may be found in the demonstration of CCK availability and a CCK receptor distribution in the septohippocampal and ascending reticular activating system. The provisional involvement of these central structures and CCK in introversion are predicated on the speculative neuroanatomical hypothesis provided by Gray (1982) and H. J. Eysenck (1967), respectively. Any conclusions drawn from such an analysis would require elaborate clinical verification.

IS THERE AN ALTERED FUNCTION OF THE CHOLECYSTOKININ SYSTEM IN ANXIETY STATES IN HUMANS?

A counterpart of evidence that CCK agonists are anxiogenic is to answer the question of whether the CCK system is functionally implicated in non-provoked symptoms of panic or anxiety. It is conceivable that endogenous variations of central and/or peripheral CCK activity may be a neurochemical concomitant of anxiety. It is interesting to mention that serum concentrations of gastrin, a CCK-B agonist, fluctuate in correlation with self-reported tension, conflict, and anxiety in psychiatrically healthy men (M. Feldman et al. 1992). Plasma CCK levels were markedly elevated in sportsmen before a competitive marathon run, as compared with CCK levels under control conditions (Phillip et al. 1992). Plasma concentrations of adrenocorticotropic hormone (ACTH), cortisol, and noradrenaline were also elevated and increased extensively after the running performance. However, CCK levels remained at prerun values. Also, a negative correlation has been found between plasma gastrin and measures of socialization in patients with functional gastrointestinal disorders (Uvnäs-Moberg et al. 1991) and in women without gastrointestinal disorders (Uvnäs-Moberg et al. 1993). These studies suggest that the endogenous CCK system might play a role in responses to stress and in anxiety in humans.

Some evidence exists of disturbances of the CCK system in pathological anxiety. For instance, Lydiard and co-workers (1992) reported that patients with panic disorder have significantly lower cerebrospinal fluid concentrations of CCK-8S than do control subjects. The same group measured CCK-8S in patients with bulimia nervosa (Lydiard et al. 1993), who were found to have significantly lower levels of CCK-8 than the comparison subjects. CCK-8 concentrations were inversely correlated with scores on the anger-hostility, anxiety, and interpersonal sensitivity subscales of the Symptom Checklist–90—Revised (SCL-90-R).

In a study by another group, lymphocyte CCK-8S concentrations were measured in patients with panic disorder and psychiatrically healthy control subjects (Brambilla et al. 1993). In patients, CCK-8S levels were measured again after a 30-day course of alprazolam therapy. The CCK-8S concentrations were significantly lower in the patients than in the control subjects but did not change after alprazolam therapy.

Overall, these studies suggest that endogenous CCK might play a role in the neurobiology of stress and that symptoms of anxiety/panic might be associated with alterations in CCK processing or metabolism.

CHOLECYSTOKININ IS ANXIOGENIC IN ANIMALS

Reports appeared as early as the late 1970s describing the behavioral actions of administration of CCK agonists. The behaviors described then were not considered manifestations of anxiety because they were observed in the context of studies of satiety or electrophysiology. Della-Fera and Baile studied the satiety response to intracerebroventricular injections of pentagastrin in sheep and noted behavioral reactions of vocalization and foot stamping. These could be considered an anxiety-like state in these animals (Della-Fera and Baile 1979). Similarly, Ishibashi and colleagues (1979), after performing electrophysiological recordings of intracerebral injections of CCK-peptides, noticed some agitation in rats.

These early studies can in retrospect be interpreted as evidence for the anxiogenic effect of CCK agonists. More recent studies in rodents have supported this view by showing that peripheral or central administration of CCK peptides can induce behaviors equated with anxiety in animal models (Belcheva et al. 1994; Biro et al. 1993; Csonka et al. 1988; Daugé et al. 1989; Harro and Vasar 1991a; Harro et al. 1990a, 1990b; Palmour et al. 1992a, 1992b; Rex et al. 1994a, 1994b; Singh et al. 1991).

Evidence suggests that behavioral manifestations of anxiety in rodents are associated with changes in the endogenous CCK system. For example, social isolation, which is anxiogenic in rats, results in an increased number of CCK receptors in the frontal cortex, but not in the striatum and hippocampus (Vasar et al. 1993b). Housing rats in the close vicinity of a location where other rats are being sacrificed, which constitutes a stressor, leads also to the upregulation of CCK receptor binding in the frontal cortex and to an increase in the CCK levels in the hippocampus (Harro et al. 1994). Rats exposed to the odor of a cat, an ethologically relevant fear paradigm, display anxious behaviors that are associated with increased levels of CCK-4 in several brain regions and increases of CCK-8S only in the ventral striatum (Pavlasevic et al. 1993). Recently, it has also been reported that blocking endogenous CCK-B activity attenuates fear-potentiated startle (Frankland et al. 1997).

Pharmacological induction of anxiety has also been shown to induce change in the CCK system in rats. For example, anxiogenic γ-aminobutyric acid (GABA) negative compounds, such as the β-carboline FG 7142, or picrotoxin cause upregulation of ^{3}H-labeled propionylated CCK-8 binding sites in the rat frontal cortex. Benzodiazepine withdrawal, which is associated with anxiety in humans and with behaviors indicative of anxiety in rodents, results in increased density of CCK receptors in the cortex and hippocampus of rats (Harro et al. 1990b, 1990c).

Rodent models have been used successfully to study generalized anxiety, but, unfortunately, their applicability to the study of panic attacks is doubtful (File 1995). In contrast, nonhuman primate models of both anxiety and panic have been developed in our own group and in other laboratories. These models, which typically involve the administration of a challenge agent to a singly caged animal, have been successful because fear and anxiety occur spontaneously in the primate, typically in response to social or environmental threat, and because monkeys exhibit much the same behavioral repertoire in their natural environment and in captivity (Higley and Suomi 1989; Kalin and Shelton 1989; Sapolsky 1990; Suomi 1982).

Immobilization and freezing reactions are observed in monkeys in reaction to social stress or threat and have been equated to human fear or panic. Specific actions of this type may include retreating, crouching, cowering, and hiding, as well as hypervigilance and frozen immobility, depending on the species and the stimulus. In less intense situations, monkeys display a range of behaviors that are thought to reflect anxiety. These behaviors include defensive behaviors, such as threat or yawn, ear flap, and adoption of bipedal stance, as well as motor behaviors, including scratch, fidget, pace, climb, jump (typically onto perch), and agitated or stereotyped locomotion. These behaviors may be enhanced by peer-rearing (Higley and Suomi 1989), by confrontation with a dominant conspecific or a human (Carey et al. 1992; Kalin and Shelton 1989; Sapolsky 1990), by electrical activation of the locus coeruleus (Redmond and Huang 1979), or by the administration of any of panicogenic agents used in clinical research (Coplan et al. 1992a, 1992b, 1992c; Crawley et al. 1985; Dager et al. 1990; S. Friedman et al. 1987; Lagarde et al. 1990; Masserman and Pechtel 1953; Rosenblum et al. 1991).

As yet, few attempts have been made to study the effects of pharmacological challenge in individual primates that have been socially stressed or that are temperamentally vulnerable. The success of this approach is illustrated by an important study (Insel et al. 1988) in which peer-reared rhesus monkeys were shown to be especially sensitive to a β-CCE challenge and by our own studies using a behavioral test battery as a screening instrument to identify vulnerable and resistant subjects before administration of CCK-4 (Palmour et al. 1992a).

Although there is a wide range of individual personalities within any primate species or population, species-characteristic temperaments have also been described (I. Bernstein et al. 1983; Kaufman and Rosenblum 1966). The rhesus macaque is known to be mean and paranoid; the stump-tailed macaque, amiable; the baboon, aggressive; the chimpanzee, mischievous; and the marmoset, hyperactive. The vervet (*Cercopithecus aethiops*), although evolutionarily successful, is an anxious and stress-responsive species. In social colonies, subordinate animals can literally be harassed to death, and documentation exists of collapse following adrenal exhaustion and of death following rupture of an acute stress ulcer.

Within this framework, individual vervet monkeys can be characterized as calm ("laid-back") or anxious ("uptight") on the basis of baseline social behavior and the response to standard behavioral challenges as originally suggested by Suomi (1976). In particular, the response to threat by a dominant male monkey (cower, submit, or return threat), the response to presentation of limited quantities of a highly desirable food (compete or avoid competition), and the response to threat by a novel human observer (cower, ignore, or return threat) were important in making this distinction. In a large captive population, approximately 15% of young adult males were anxious.

The behaviors of calm and anxious monkeys differ both intrinsically and in response to varying doses of CCK-4 (Palmour et al. 1992b). In the social group, calm monkeys explored more actively, were groomed more often, and competed more effectively for food, drink, and desired sitting and sleeping places. Anxious monkeys were more isolated, more frequently lost confrontations, and typically adopted crouched or cowering postures. In a single cage, anxious monkeys often crouched on the floor of the cage, paced stereotypically, or exhibited bizarre postures, whereas calm monkeys typically sat quietly or attended to external stimuli.

A dose of 2.5 μg of CCK-4, given intravenously to a 4- to 6-kg monkey, stimulated behaviors thought to reflect anxiety in both calm and anxious monkeys. In calm monkeys, higher doses of CCK-4 increased the frequency and especially the duration of arousal behaviors, but we have not been able to elicit a full panic attack, even with a 10-fold excess (150 μg) of the dose that engenders panic in anxious monkeys. Preliminary data suggest, however, that vigilance and irritability persist for many hours following administration of these doses. An evaluation of these animals in a social group environment, though technically difficult, would be of great interest.

By contrast, 15–20 μg of intravenous CCK-4 in anxious monkeys evoked 1–5 minutes of frozen immobility, self-clasping, cowering, and huddling. During this period, some monkeys appeared to be tremulous and dizzy. Behaviors of this type are seen in this species in the wild under conditions of extreme stress or danger and can be inferred to represent intense fear and panic.

One behavior that is particularly useful in quantifying the behavioral effects of CCK agonists and antagonists is the "yawn" or "threat"—the mouth is opened wide with the object of displaying the long canines. This behavior appears in two forms. A full threat as illustrated in a social context is a display of dominance. In social groups, this behavior also appears as a forme fruste, with mouth open but teeth covered. We have termed this behavior *covert threat*. It would appear socially, for example, when a clearly subordinate male wants to express irritation with a larger and dominant male who cannot be beaten in a fight. The distinction between panic and anxiety is also illustrated by the relative frequencies of these two related behaviors. In monkeys given small doses of peptide or in calm monkeys given larger doses of CCK-4, full or overt threat increases, peaks, and declines. Few covert threats appear. By contrast, in anxious monkeys given large (10- to 20-μg) doses of peptide and monitored over a longer time, covert threat predominates during the first 5–15 minutes and is gradually replaced by full threat.

As in the human studies, CCK-4 and other peptides must be given to primates intravenously to compensate for the short half-life, but the behavioral stress of short-term administration would confound behavioral observations. The implantation of an indwelling venous catheter that is protected by a jacket and swivel assembly allows administration of peptide or placebo without handling or alerting the animals. Behavioral observations may be made both immediately and from videotape records; habituation and daily observations minimize nonspecific behavioral effects. In our own studies, monkeys typically receive placebo, CCK-4, or an analogue intravenously every second or third day but are often videotaped every day.

These results support the contention that CCK-4 can serve as a candidate for provoking both panic attacks and behaviors thought to reflect anxiety in vervet monkeys. In addition, anxious monkeys appeared to be hyperresponsive to the behavioral effects of exogenous CCK-4, but the biochemical or physiological basis of this difference is not yet known. This monkey model can serve for the study of interactions of the CCK system with other neurotransmitter systems in eliciting anxiety/panic by pharmacological dissection with agents not available for human use and as a screening tool for anxiolytic or antipanic agents.

INTERACTION BETWEEN CHOLECYSTOKININ AND OTHER NEUROTRANSMITTER SYSTEMS

The mechanism and site of action of CCK-4 in inducing panic symptoms are still largely unknown. Several investigations using animal models of anxiety have revealed that the anxiogenic effects of CCK-4 are blocked by selective CCK-B receptor antagonists, suggesting that CCK-B receptors are an important site of anxiogenic action of exogenous CCK-4 (for review, see Harro et al. 1995). These animal studies have been supported by clinical studies (Bradwejn et al. 1994b, 1995). As it is most likely that CCK-4 affects several neurotransmitter systems, pharmacological dissection of its effects by using agonists or antagonists of candidate targets is needed to determine likely interactions between CCK-4 and other neurotransmitter systems. So far, candidate systems for study have been the benzodiazepine-GABA, serotonin (5-HT), noradrenaline, and dopaminergic systems.

γ-Aminobutyric Acid

As indicated earlier, benzodiazepine receptor agonists selectively and specifically antagonized CCK-8S–induced excitation of rat hippocampal neurons. It was subsequently demonstrated that neuronal responsiveness to CCK-8 in rats decreases following long-term administration of benzodiazepine agonists (Bouthillier and de Montigny 1988). Additional studies using neurochemical, binding, and behavioral approaches suggest a functional interaction between the CCK and GABA systems. However, the specific involvement of CCK receptor subtypes is not clear, and the nature and direction of interaction between the CCK and GABA systems is not consistent over paradigms (Harro et al. 1990b, 1990c; Perez de la Mora et al. 1993; Rattray et al. 1993; M. Sheehan and de Belleroche 1983). Evidence also suggests that benzodiazepine receptor agonists attenuate the anxiogenic effects of exogenous CCK-4 in nonhuman primates (Palmour et al. 1992b) and psychiatrically healthy volunteers (de Montigny 1989), although such data do not establish that benzodiazepine receptors invariably contribute to the panicogenic effects of CCK-4.

To further explore the role of benzodiazepine receptors in CCK-4–induced panic symptoms, by using a double-blind, placebo-controlled crossover design, we determined whether pretreatment with the benzodiazepine receptor antagonist flumazenil could influence response to CCK-4 in psychiatrically healthy volunteers. In investigating the potential interaction between CCK and benzodiazepine receptors in CCK-4–induced panic response, we proposed a model that was based on the premise that exogenous CCK-4, through actions on CCK-B receptors, interacts with benzodiazepine receptors in eliciting symptoms by indirectly acting like a benzodiazepine receptor inverse agonist. In other words, we postulated that CCK-4 might act as an endogenous "virtual" inverse agonist of benzodiazepine receptors. To support this hypothesis, it was necessary to determine whether flumazenil could antagonize the panicogenic effects of CCK-4. We found no discernible difference between flumazenil and placebo pretreatment for the number of symptoms induced with CCK-4, sum intensity of symptoms, and panic attack frequency (Bradwejn et al. 1994a). Our findings indicate that benzodiazepine receptors are not mediators of CCK-4–induced panic symptoms in psychiatrically normal subjects.

Serotonin

Interactions between CCK and serotonin in animal brain have been studied. The nature and direction of these interactions are not yet well defined because of the differences in effects induced by different CCK fragments, the variety of approaches used, and the range of sites examined. It seems useful to review the effects of CCK-8S and CCK-4 separately.

CCK-8S has excitatory effects on dorsal raphe serotoninergic neurons, primarily mediated by a CCK-A receptor subtype (Boden et al. 1991). In the substantia nigra, it was shown that intraperitoneal injection of CCK-8S in rats causes a release of serotonin (Kaneyuki et al. 1989). Injection of high doses of CCK-8S into the ventral tegmental area was shown to significantly decrease levels of the serotonin metabolite, 5-hydroxyindoleacetic acid (5-HIAA) in the nucleus accumbens, olfactory tubercles, and striatum (Widerlöv et al. 1983). Fekete and colleagues (1981a, 1981b) reported that intracerebroventricular administration of CCK-8S decreases serotonin content in the hypothalamus and mesencephalon. The same authors have shown that intracerebroventricular administration of the same peptide decreased serotonin turnover only in the hypothalamus but not in the mesencephalon, amygdala, septum, striatum, and cerebral cortex in rats (Fekete et al. 1981b). Vasar and colleagues (1985) also observed a decrease in serotonin turnover after CCK-8S intraventricular administration to rats, but the changes were seen in several brain regions. These studies seem to indicate that the overall effects of CCK-8S in most brain regions are in the direction of increasing serotoninergic activity.

Itoh and colleagues (1988) evaluated the effect of intracerebroventricular administration of CCK-4 on serotonin and 5-HIAA in various regions of rat brain. After CCK-4 administration, the ratio of 5-HIAA to serotonin increased significantly in most regions of the brain, except in the striatum and the olfactory tubercle. On the other hand, treatment with a CCK-4 analogue, BOC-CCK-4, was shown to potentiate the rise in serotonin in the guinea pig cerebral cortex, but only during performance in the elevated plus-maze task, an animal model of anxiety, but not in home cage conditions (Rex et al. 1994a). Both the rise in serotonin and the anxiogenic effect of the CCK-4 analogue could be reversed by the CCK-B antagonist L-365,260.

In summary, these studies might point to a modulating effect by CCK peptides on the serotonin system in resting and stressful situations. The CCK-A system, activated partly by CCK-8S, might increase serotonin content in resting conditions only, whereas the CCK-B system would increase serotonin content only during stressful conditions.

So far we have discussed the effect of CCK peptides on serotonin brain concentrations. Some evidence also exist on the action of serotonin on the CCK system. Raiteri and colleagues (1993a) looked at the effects of serotonin on the release of cholecystokinin-like immunoreactivity (CCK-LI) in synaptosomes prepared from rat cerebral cortex and nucleus accumbens. In both areas, serotonin increased the calcium-dependent depolarization-evoked CCK-LI release in a dose-related fashion. This effect was antagonized by 5-HT$_3$ receptor antagonists but not by 5-HT$_1$ or 5-HT$_2$ antagonists. Moreover, the CCK-releasing effect of serotonin was mimicked by a 5-HT$_3$ receptor agonist. It was concluded that serotonin can act as a potent releaser of CCK-LI in rat cerebral cortex and nucleus accumbens through the activation of 5-HT$_3$ receptors on CCK-releasing terminals (Gourch et al. 1990; Paudice and Raiteri 1991). A behavioral study suggested that 5-HT$_3$ receptors are mediators of CCK-induced anxiety in the rat. In this respect, Vasar and his associates (1993a) reported that the anxiogenic effect of caerulein, a CCK agonist, was prevented by prior treatment with the 5-HT$_3$ receptor antagonist ondansetron.

Our study, which showed that chronic treatment with imipramine, which inhibits noradrenaline and serotonin reuptake, could antagonize the panicogenic effects of CCK-4 in patients with panic disorder, argued that these monoamines may be instrumental in interacting with CCK in promoting symptoms of panic. Accordingly, we investigated the effect of lowering plasma tryptophan to the elicitation of behavioral, cardiovascular, and hormonal changes in psychiatrically healthy volunteers challenged with CCK-4 (Koszycki et al. 1996a). Forty males without personal or family history of psychiatric disorders were randomly assigned to either a tryptophan-free amino acid mixture, which decreases central serotonin by decreasing the rate of tryptophan hydroxylation, or a control mixture. Five hours after administration of the amino acid mixture, all subjects received a single intravenous injection of CCK-4. Tryptophan depletion did not alter behavioral or cardiovascular sensitivity to CCK-4 despite depletion of plasma tryptophan by 92%. By contrast, tryptophan depletion potentiated the stimulatory action of CCK-4 on prolactin and ACTH/cortisol secretion. Although these findings suggest that at least part of the neuroendocrine action of CCK-4 is mediated through the serotonin system, the locus of the serotonin-CCK interaction and the specific serotonin receptor subtype involved remain to be determined. In addition, a disruption or underactivity of serotonin may contribute to a dysregulation of neurotransmitter systems involved in stress or anxiety regulation.

Norepinephrine

Some information is available on the relationship between the CCK and the noradrenergic systems. In the lateral hypothalamus of satiated rats, perfused CCK-8S by push-pull perfusion enhanced the efflux of noradrenaline. However, in fasted animals, CCK-8S often suppressed the catecholamine's release. Perfused in the lateral hypothalamus, CCK exerted opposite effects, typically augmenting noradrenergic output when the rat was fasted but not affecting the amine's activity during the sated condition (R. D. Myers et al. 1986). Kaneyuki and colleagues (1989) have shown that CCK-8S, injected intraperitoneally into rats, resulted in increases in noradrenaline levels in the dorsal amygdala and in the septum. Intracerebroventricularly administered CCK-8S increased noradrenaline content in the hypothalamus and mesencephalon. In the amygdala, a biphasic action was observed on noradrenaline content in the amygdala and septum, depending on the time and doses used. In the striatum, the noradrenaline level first increased and then decreased. The data indicate that CCK-8S is able to modify the activity of noradrenaline in different brain regions in a time- and dose-dependent manner, with a local specificity (Fekete et al. 1981a). Beresford and colleagues (1988) studied the interaction between CCK-8S and noradrenaline by investigating the effect of the peptide on potassium-stimulated release of ^{3}H-labeled noradrenaline from superfused hypothalamic slices. CCK was found to produce a significant but small inhibition of ^{3}H-labeled noradrenaline release. Intracerebroventricular administration of CCK-8S was evaluated for effects on noradrenaline turnover of the hypothalamus, mesencephalon, amygdala, septum, striatum, and cerebral cortex in rats. CCK-8S increased the noradrenaline turnover in the hypothalamus and amygdala but decreased it in the striatum (Fekete et al. 1981a). Another study (Olenik et al. 1993) looked at the mediatory effect of the noradrenergic system on response of the CCK system to injury. A knife cut injuring the meninges and the upper layers of rat neocortex transiently increased the levels of preprocholecystokinin-mRNA in the whole ipsilateral cortex. The β-adrenoceptor antagonists alprenolol and propranolol, given prior to the injury, reduced this increase, an effect not seen after α-adrenergic blockade. These results suggest that noradrenergic neurons can contribute via stimulation of β adrenoceptors to the initiation of the injury-induced increase in CCK gene expression.

Harro and colleagues (1992b) used *N*-(2-chloroethyl)-*N*-ethyl-2-bromobenzylamine (DSP-4), a neurotoxin that selectively destroys noradrenaline-containing nerve terminals originating from the locus coeruleus, administered to rats intraperitoneally 7 days before decapitation to study the action of the noradrenergic system on the CCK system. CCK receptor density was significantly higher in the frontal cortex and hippocampus of DSP-4–treated rats. If desipramine (25 mg/kg) was administered before DSP-4 treatment, the DSP-4–induced changes in both noradrenaline uptake and CCK receptor binding were not present, suggesting that both effects were exerted after uptake of the neurotoxin by the nerve terminals. The time course of the development of changes in CCK-8 binding paralleled with some time lag to the development of changes in noradrenaline uptake. These findings demonstrate that the noradrenergic system of the locus coeruleus affects CCK neurotransmission.

In monkeys, evidence exists that the behavioral effects of CCK-4 might in part be mediated by the noradrenergic system. Indeed, the behavioral effects of CCK-4 can be reduced by pretreatment with the β-adrenergic antagonist propranolol (R. Palmour, unpublished data). Indirect evidence suggests a link between the adrenergic and noradrenergic systems and the panicogenic effect of CCK-B agonists in humans. Administration of pentagastrin is associated with acute and brief increases in plasma adrenaline in psychiatrically healthy volunteers (Abelson et al. 1994). In another study (Boulenger et al. 1994), also in psychiatrically healthy volunteers, intravenous administration of 25 μg of CCK-4 caused a significant increase in platelet noradrenaline concentrations starting approximately 4–5 minutes after the panicogenic effect.

Dopamine

The mesolimbic and cortical dopamine systems are known to be critical for the establishment of behaviors conditioned by emotional events (Talalaenko et al. 1994). It is also known that individual differences in mesolimbic dopamine sensitivity are associated with differences in stress sensitivity (Piazza et al. 1989). These findings are important to consider in the context of anxiety and, particularly, anticipatory anxiety. Studies suggest that CCK-A and CCK-B receptors may play opposing roles in modulating dopamine function. CCK and dopamine are colocalized in mesolimbic and mesocortical networks. Thus, efforts have been spent in understanding the relationship between these two neurotransmitter systems. This has not been easy because of the differences in experimental approaches used, functional heterogeneity of anatomical structures studied, and different effects of CCK-A and CCK-B receptor activation on dopamine function. For example, current evidence suggests that activation of CCK-B and CCK-A receptors in the nucleus accumbens (a major projection site for mesolimbic dopamine neurons) produces an attenuation and potentiation, respectively, of dopamine-mediated behaviors (Crawley 1992; Vaccarino 1994).

SITE OF ACTION OF CHOLECYSTOKININ TETRAPEPTIDE

A question of central importance concerns the site(s) of action of CCK-4 in humans. Until recently, no available evidence existed that CCK-4 does or does not cross the blood-brain barrier. Merani and colleagues injected iodin-ated CCK-4 into the tail vein of rats; the animals were decapitated a few min-utes after the injection, and various brain regions and peripheral tissues were assessed for the presence of iodinated CCK-4. To control for background ra-dioactivity, the same amount of free iodine was injected in a group of control animals. Iodinated CCK-4 was detected at moderate concentrations in sev-eral brain regions including brain stem, limbic, and cortical structures. The re-sults suggested that CCK-4 could cross the blood-brain barrier.

Even if CCK-4 or pentagastrin does not cross the blood-brain barrier, the possibility exists that CCK-4 affects CCK receptors in brain regions that are not fully protected by this barrier. Knowledge of cardiovascular neuro-physiology, as well as studies on the behavioral and cardiovascular effects of CCK-4, permit some speculation as to the possible site of action of CCK-4. Some investigators have suggested that brain stem regions ordinarily function to monitor sympathetic nerve discharge and vasomotor tone. Increases in blood pressure and heart rate have been observed following electrical or pharmacological stimulation of the nucleus tractus solitarius (Jordan and Spyer 1986), the medullary nuclei (Dampney et al. 1982; Pilowsky et al. 1985), and the parabrachial nucleus (Marovitch et al. 1982).

These brain-stem regions are interrelated by diverse neuronal projections and are connected to adrenergic structures (Dampney et al. 1977; Marovitch et al. 1982), such as the locus coeruleus, which are postulated to play a role in panic attacks (Gorman et al. 1989). Further, experimental evidence sug-gests that CCK interacts with these brain stem mechanisms in modulating respiratory and cardiovascular functions. Microiontophoretic application of CCK-8S to neurons of the nucleus tractus solitarius in cats decreased both neuronal firing and respiratory frequency, effects that were reversed by ad-ministration of CCK-4 (Denavit-Saubié et al. 1985).

Our clinical investigations (Bradwejn et al. 1992b) have demonstrated that exogenous CCK-4 produces robust and dose-dependent increases in heart rate and blood pressure. Moreover, pretreatment with the CCK-B an-tagonist L-365,260 significantly decreased CCK-4–induced increases in heart rate. It might be argued that increases in cardiovascular activity in re-sponse to CCK-4 challenge may be the result of direct or indirect stimulation of CCK receptors in brain stem structures such as the nucleus tractus solitarius. It is also conceivable that the evocation of emotional and psy-chosensorial symptoms following CCK-4 challenge results from an action of CCK-4 on brain stem structures and a subsequent activation or inhibition of higher CNS regions mediated by neuronal projections. As these brain stem structures are not fully shielded by the blood-brain barrier, CNS penetration by CCK-4 might not even be necessary for this action. This might also explain the rapid (in less than 1 minute) appearance of symptoms observed in both patients with panic disorder and psychiatrically healthy control subjects following CCK-4 challenge.

Imaging techniques might help identify the neuroanatomical correlates associated with administration of CCK agonists, although these techniques might not be informative as to the primary site of action of the peptides. One recent report addressed the functional neuroanatomy of CCK-4–induced anxiety in psychiatrically healthy volunteers using $[^{15}O]H_2O$ positron-emission tomography (Benkelfat et al. 1995). Increases in regional cerebral blood flow were seen in the anterior cingulate gyrus, the claustrum-insular-amygdala region, and the cerebellar vermis. This implies that limbic regions might be directly or indirectly implicated in the panicogenic effect of CCK-4. Further imaging studies might help elucidate the interplay of brain regions associated with the panicogenic effects of CCK-4.

BRAIN CHOLECYSTOKININ ANTAGONISTS AND THERAPEUTIC IMPLICATIONS

A number of CCK receptor antagonists have been developed for both receptor subtypes (for review, see Woodruff and Hughes 1991). Dibutyryl cyclic guanosine monophosphate was the first competitive antagonist to be discovered. This compound was shown to antagonize the functional action of CCK in the periphery, but failed to act as a specific inhibitor of CCK binding in mouse cortical preparations. Following the discovery of dibutyril cyclic guanosine monophosphate, several classes of CCK antagonists have appeared that included amino acid derivatives (proglumide, benzotript, lorglumide, loxiglumide, spiroglumide), peptide derivatives (CCK-27–32-NH2, CCK-JMV-180), benzodiazepine derivatives (asperlicin, L-364,718, L-365,260), dipeptoids (CI-988, CAM-1028), pyrazolidinones (LY 262691, LY 288513), and ureidoacetamides (RP 69758, RP 72540).

The nonselective CCK receptor antagonist proglumide and the selective CCK-B receptor antagonists L-365,260, CI-988, and LY 262691 show anxiolytic effects in several animal anxiety tests (Harro and Vasar 1991a, 1991b; Woodruff and Hughes 1991). However, the most robust effects are observed with tests of exploratory behavior and are not generally seen in models that use punishment or conflicts and are dependent on the baseline state of the animal (Hughes et al. 1990; K. R. Powell and Barrett 1991). Thus, it could be that CCK-B antagonists decrease anxiety related to the exploration of novel environment, but do not alleviate fear of punishment.

CI-988 has been found to reduce the behavioral stress in marmosets exposed to a human threat (Hughes et al. 1990). L-365,260 can antagonize the behavioral effects of exposition to the odor of a cat in rats and suppress the behavioral reaction of mice to the calls of an owl, an effect also found with LY 288513 (Hendrie and Dourish 1994). Thus, evidence suggests an anxiolytic activity of CCK-B antagonists. The activity seems more evident in ethologically based models of anxiety than in conflict-based tests and does not follow a linear dose-dependent relationship but rather a bell-curve one. Also, most studies point to a selectivity of CCK-B antagonists, but not CCK-A antagonists, for anxiolytic effects.

A question not considered so far about CCK-B antagonists is whether they possess any "intrinsic" activity. It seems that some of these antagonists behave like mixed agonist-antagonists. In "normal" rats, they do not have an action of their own, but, if the sensitivity of CCK receptors is increased, they start to act like agonists. Therefore, a possible mixed agonist-antagonist activity of CCK antagonists should be taken into account for long-term studies.

We have completed two studies that suggest that CCK-B receptors are also important mediators of the behavioral and cardiovascular changes during CCK-4 challenge in humans. In one study (Bradwejn et al. 1994b), we investigated whether the selective brain cholecystokinin (CCK-B) receptor antagonist, L-365,260, could antagonize the panicogenic effects of CCK-4 in patients with panic disorder. Only the difference between the effects of the 50-mg dose and placebo was statistically significant. Increases in heart rate following CCK-4 injection were markedly reduced with both the 50-mg and the 10-mg doses compared with the heart rate with placebo. In the other study (Bradwejn et al. 1995), we have evaluated the effects of another CCK-B antagonist, CI-988 (100 mg), on CCK-4–induced panic symptoms in 30 psychiatrically healthy males in a placebo-controlled, double-blind design. A modest but significant decrease was found in sum intensity scores and panic attack frequency following CI-988 treatment. These studies suggest that CCK-B receptors are mediators of the panicogenic effects of CCK-4 in humans.

The panicogenic effects of CCK-B agonists and the ability of CCK-B antagonists to block this effect raise the question of therapeutic efficacy of CCK-B antagonists on spontaneous panic attacks. Thus far, the only clinical trial carried out is inconclusive. Kramer and colleagues (1995) used a multicenter, placebo-controlled, double-blind trial to investigate the efficacy of L-365,260 (30 mg four times a day) in patients with panic disorder with or without agoraphobia. At the dose tested, no clinically significant differences were found between L-365,260 and placebo in global improvement ratings, anxiety rating scale scores, panic attack frequency, panic attack intensity, or disability measures.

SUMMARY AND FUTURE DIRECTIONS

The data summarized indicate that CCK-4 satisfies previously established criteria for an ideal panicogenic agent and that it compares well to at least one widely accepted pharmacological model of panic disorder. It is important to mention that of all pharmacological agents known to provoke panic attacks in humans, including sodium lactate, CO_2, caffeine, yohimbine, isoproterenol, and m-chlorophenylpiperazine, CCK-4 is the only one that fulfills criteria for a neurotransmitter. CCK is well characterized in the CNS and is abundant in brain regions, including the brain stem, hippocampus, amygdala, and cerebral cortex, implicated in the promotion of panic attacks. Moreover, biochemical and electrophysiological data suggest interactions between CCK and multiple neurotransmitter systems. As a panicogenic agent, therefore, CCK-4 provides an important opportunity to identify endogenous anomalies associated with panic disorder and to enhance our understanding of the multiple neurotransmitter systems that potentially contribute to the neural network generators of panic attacks.

An important feature of CCK-4 is that it is simple to administer in a low-volume intravenous bolus infusion (in less than 5 seconds). This method of administration has considerable advantage over the slow infusion procedures required to induce symptoms of panic with other panicogens, particularly sodium lactate. The relatively protracted infusion interval has been associated with physiologic alterations, such as volume overload, and metabolic changes that can introduce nonspecific psychological effects (Margraf et al. 1986). Another technical advantage is that the latency to effect symptoms of panic with CCK-4 is rapid and predictable, permitting measurement of central and peripheral nervous system activity during the interval associated with peak panic symptoms. Considered together, the technical advantage of the administration of CCK-4 and its presence in the CNS commends its use for research into the pathophysiology of panic disorder.

The data generated from validation studies also highlight some of the usefulness of CCK-4 as a panicogenic challenge for research in anxiety. For instance, demonstrating that the effects of CCK-4 are reproducible in the same patient has important implications in relation to testing the effectiveness of antipanic drugs in blocking CCK-4–induced panic symptoms. In addition, the dose-response study in patients indicated that a 20-μg dose of CCK-4, which produced panic attacks in 75% of patients, might be suitable for efficacy studies. In particular, this dose promotes noticeable changes in behavior and other indices of anxiety without being excessively potent to mask the effectiveness of potential antipanic drugs to block the effects of CCK-4.

Unanswered questions remain about the role of the CCK system in anxiety and panic. It is still unknown whether CCK plays a role in panic disorder exclusively or whether it is involved in the pathogenesis of other anxiety disorders. Additional provocation studies will help answer this question and might be useful not only for the understanding of the neurobiology of anxiety and panic but possibly in their diagnosis.

The enhanced sensitivity of patients with panic disorder to the effects of CCK-B agonists might be the consequence of an aberration of the CCK system. This aberration could exist at any level of production of CCK, spanning from gene encoding to synthesis, release, and metabolism, or at the receptor level. Molecular biology and biochemistry approaches are needed for further investigations.

Concerted human and animal research strategies will be useful in locating sites of action of CCK-B agonists and in elucidating the neurotransmitter network subserving anxiety and panic. Last but not least, research will be needed to determine whether CCK-B antagonists have therapeutic efficacy in the treatment of anxiety and panic. A demonstration of efficacy could provide major support for the role of the CCK system in anxiety. Fortunately, compounds with pharmacokinetic profiles superior to L-365,260 and CI-988 exist and are targeted for clinical trials. However, it should be emphasized that, even if results of clinical trials are negative, the CCK-4 challenge paradigm could nevertheless remain a practical research tool that might enhance our knowledge of neurobiological mechanisms involved in anxiety disorders and of their treatment.

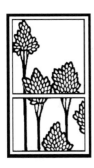

CHAPTER 28

Neurosteroids

Isabella Heuser, M.D.

The term *neurosteroid* was introduced in 1981 (Baulieu 1981). Evidence that the brain can be a steroidogenic tissue was derived from the finding that substantial quantities of pregnenolone, dehydroepiandrosterone (DHEA), their sulfate esters, and their fatty acid esters were found in the central nervous system (CNS) of mice, rats, pigs, guinea pigs, monkeys, and humans (Mathur et al. 1993). Concentration of these steroids in the brain exceeded their plasma concentration and were estimated to be up to 10 times higher, in the order of 10–100 nmol/L (Corpéchot et al. 1981; Robel et al. 1987). Furthermore, these steroids appeared to be independent of gonadal and adrenal synthesis because they were present after adrenalectomy and gonadectomy (Baulieu and Robel 1990; Corpéchot et al. 1993). In addition, incubation of primary cultures of rat forebrain glial cultures with a precursor of cholesterol led to the formation of cholesterol, pregnenolone, 20-OH-pregnenolone, and progesterone (Jung-Testas et al. 1989). These findings from animal studies are supplemented by results from postmortem human brains, in which high concentrations of neurosteroids far exceeding plasma concentrations have also been detected in all CNS regions (Lacroix et al. 1987; Lanthier and Patwardhan 1986). Of special interest from a neuropsychobiological perspective are neuroactive steroids, which include those steroids that act via neuronal cell surface receptors (S. M. Paul and Purdy 1992).

I am gratefully indebted to Andreas Hartmann, M.D., and Rainer Rupprecht, M.D., for their critical comments in the preparation of this manuscript.

439

BIOCHEMISTRY AND PHARMACOLOGY OF NEUROSTEROIDOGENESIS

In adrenal tissue and other steroidogenic tissues including glial cells—in particular, oligodendrocytes (Hu et al. 1987)—conversion of cholesterol into pregnenolone is catalyzed by cytochrome P450scc, located in the inner mitochondrial membrane (E. Costa et al. 1994; Le Goascogne et al. 1987; Mellon and Deschepper 1993). Further synthesis of neurosteroids probably proceeds through different pathways than those used in adrenals, gonads, and placenta (Mellon 1994). The brain contains enzymes that metabolize pregnenolone, progesterone, and 11-deoxycorticosterone (DOC) into a variety of neuroactive compounds. The major metabolites of progesterone include allopregnanolone (3α-hydroxy-5α-pregnan-20-one, 3α-5α-tetrahydroprogesterone; THP). DOC is metabolized to 3α,21-dihydroxy-5α-pregnan-20-one, allotetrahydro-DOC (allo-THDOC), indicating that these neural tissues contain 5α-reductase and 3α-hydroxysteroid oxidoreductase (Figure 28–1). Pregnenolone (3α-hydroxy-5β-pregnan-20-one, 3α-5β-tetrahydroprogesterone, 3α-5β-THP) and THDOC (3α,21-dihydroxy-5β-pregnan-20-one, 3α-5β-tetrahydroDOC) are synthesized via 5β-reductase instead of 5α-reductase activity and further by 3α-hydroxysteroid oxidoreductase.

Whereas 5α-reductase shows a significantly higher function in neurons than in glial cells, 3α-hydroxysteroid dehydrogenase, which converts pregnenolone to progesterone, is present mainly in type-1 astrocytes (Melcangi et al. 1994). All enzymes mentioned are found in highest concentrations in the pituitary and the hypothalamus, as well as in the cerebellum, thalamus, midbrain, pineal, medulla, white matter, and peripheral nerves (Celotti et al. 1992; Mensah-Niagan et al. 1994). Because the adult rat brain does not have 17α-hydroxylase activity nor contains 17α-hydroxylase (P450c17) messenger ribonucleic acid (mRNA), the origin of brain DHEA is unknown because it cannot be synthesized from pregnenolone via P450c17, but its concentrations in brain persists long after removal of gonads and adrenals (Mellon and Deschepper 1993).

CLASSIC AND NONCLASSIC EFFECTS OF STEROIDS

Regardless of their source of synthesis, glucocorticoids, mineralocorticoids, androgens, estrogens, and progestins exert their effects on the brain through

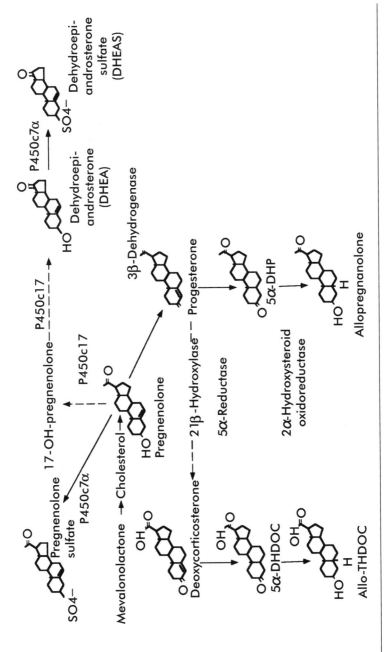

FIGURE 28–1. Biosynthesis and metabolism of neurosteroids. Solid arrows refer to enzyme activities demonstrated in the central nervous system (CNS); dashed arrows refer to enzyme activities not demonstrated in the CNS. allo-THDOC = allotetrahydrodeoxycorticosterone; 5α-DHDOC = 5α-dihydro-deoxycorticosterone; 5α-DHP = 5α-dihydro-progesterone.

high-affinity intracellular steroid hormone receptors, thereby modifying the expression of specific genes (McEwen 1991). Allopregnanolone and allo-THDOC have been shown to regulate neuronal function through effects on gene expression by activating the intracellular progesterone receptor (Rupprecht et al. 1993). However, the major body of work to date has investigated nongenomic effects of neurosteroids on transmitter-gated ion channels. A first description of rapidly mediated steroid effects was given by Selye (1941). He reported on the anesthetic and sedative properties of progesterone and DOC in the rat; this discovery eventually resulted in the development of steroid-based anesthetics, for example, alfaxalone and hydroxydione (Gyermek and Soyka 1975). Electrophysiological and ligand binding studies have shown that pregnenolone and THDOC exert these properties by interacting with the γ-aminobutyric acid type A (GABA$_A$) receptor (Majewska et al. 1986). These neurosteroids act as allosteric agonists of the GABA$_A$ receptor by increasing the frequency and duration of chloride channel openings and further potentiate the inhibitory action of GABA (Majewska 1992). It is important to note that neurosteroid action at the GABA$_A$ receptor is coupled to the presence of a 3α-hydroxyl group (Gee et al. 1988; Harrison et al. 1987; Purdy et al. 1990). Sulfated neurosteroids, for example, pregnenolone sulfate and DHEA sulfate (DHEAS), act as noncompetitive antagonist of the GABA$_A$ receptor and inhibit GABA-induced chloride transport by a reduction in GABA chloride channel opening frequency (Demirgoren et al. 1991; Majewska et al. 1990). They are less selective and have a lower affinity for GABA$_A$ receptors than do allopregnanolone and allo-THDOC (S. M. Paul and Purdy 1992). DHEA also acts as noncompetitive antagonist at the GABA$_A$ receptor, although three to four times less potently than DHEAS (Demirgoren et al. 1991). Neither progesterone nor pregnenolone are active as modulators of the GABA$_A$ receptor and probably display their in vivo effects via formation of their reduced metabolites (Harrison et al. 1987; D. M. Turner et al. 1989).

Whereas benzodiazepines, barbiturates, convulsant channel agonists, and GABA itself bind at the GABA$_A$ receptor ectodomain, neurosteroids most likely bind to a site distinct from the benzodiazepine site of the GABA$_A$ receptor (E. Costa et al. 1994; S. I. Deutsch et al. 1992; Lan et al. 1991; Morrow et al. 1990; Shingai et al. 1991). Although the allosteric modulatory efficacy of benzodiazepines acting in the receptor ectodomain differs according to the structural diversity of GABA$_A$ receptors, neurosteroid modulation is much less dependent on GABA$_A$ receptor structure diversity (Puia et al. 1993). Moreover, neurosteroids can operate GABA$_A$ receptors in the absence of GABA, whereas benzodiazepines and other anxiolytics not only require

GABA for their action, but their maximal modulatory efficacy never surpasses the maximal response elicited by GABA in the same receptor channel (Puia et al. 1990). This explains why neurosteroids do and benzodiazepines do not possess anesthetic properties surpassing their anxiolytic effect.

Another receptor system with which neurosteroids interact is the N-methyl-D-aspartate (NMDA) receptor. Pregnenolone sulfate acts as a positive allosteric modulator of the NMDA receptor, in analogy to GABA-ergic effects, by increasing the frequency and duration of NMDA-activated channel opening (Bowlby 1993; Irwin et al. 1992; Wu et al. 1991).

POSSIBLE CLINICAL EFFECTS OF NEUROSTEROIDS

The precise role of neurosteroids in cognition as well as neurological and psychiatric disorders is currently under investigation. Although data from human studies are sparse, results obtained from in vitro and in vivo experiments show promising leads for future clinical applications of neurosteroids.

Memory

In recent years, memory-enhancing properties have been attributed to pregnenolone and pregnenolone sulfate. This effect is probably related to its agonistic function at the NMDA receptor (Bowlby 1993) because NMDA receptor antagonists impair acquisition and/or retention of various memory tasks in rodents (Flood et al. 1990; Ungerer et al. 1991). Studies investigating the effects of intracerebroventricular administration of pregnenolone and pregnenolone sulfate on performances in avoidance tasks in mice (Flood et al. 1992) and rats (Mathis et al. 1994) have so far yielded positive results. Memory-enhancing properties had previously also been described for DHEA and its sulfate in mice (Flood et al. 1988). In addition, lack of progesterone in aged female rats seems to contribute steroid-mediated neuronal degeneration (H. M. Chao et al. 1994), pointing toward possible application of neurosteroids in the treatment of dementia disorders.

Pain

Increased levels of progesterone are known to be associated with decreases in pain sensitivity (C. A. Frye et al. 1993; Gintzler and Bohan 1990), but the mechanisms by which progesterone exerts its antinoceptive effects are unclear. A first description of analgesic properties of neurosteroids, for example, the progesterone metabolite pregnenolone, was given by Kavaliers and Wiebe (1987). A study investigating the effects of intracerebroventricularly administered neurosteroids showed that progesterone, dihydroprogesterone, pregnenolone, and THDOC decreased pain sensitivity, whereas 17-OH-pregnenolone, pregnenolone sulfate, and DHEAS did not. The speed of action and the substances involved, for example, nonsulfated steroids producing analgesic effects, suggest that pain modulation by neurosteroids occurs via agonistic GABA$_A$ receptor action (C. A. Frye and Duncan 1994).

Stress and Seizure Disorders

Purdy et al. (1991) have reported that allopregnanolone and allo-THDOC rise sufficiently in cerebral cortex of stressed rats to affect GABA-mediated inhibition, a mechanism that has been suggested to increase seizure thresholds (Belelli et al. 1990; Kokate et al. 1994). However, the relation between elevated stress levels with consecutive changes in neurosteroid concentrations and increases in seizure thresholds remains unclear because sulfated neurosteroids, for example, pregnenolone sulfate, may conceivably cause a potent epileptogenic event (Myslobodsky 1993; Wu et al. 1991). It has been proposed that elevated CNS levels of neurosteroids, particularly pregnenolone sulfate, with antagonistic properties inhibit the action of GABA and contribute to the arousal present in the initial phase of stress; in later phases, the secretion of nonsulfated neurosteroids, for example, THDOC, induced by adrenocorticotropic hormone, might protect neurons from overstimulation through a potentiation of the inhibitory effects of GABA (Majewska 1992). Interestingly, a recent study (Brinton 1994) proposed that allopregnanolone protects against seizure activity through inhibition of nerve cell growth because seizure activity is associated with aberrant nerve cell growth.

Pregnancy and Premenstrual Syndrome

It has long been recognized that during pregnancy the risk of developing emotional disease is decreased (Pough et al. 1963). Furthermore, mood and behavioral changes typical of pregnancy, such as somnolence and the sense of well-being, may be dependent on the activation of the GABA-ergic system by steroids because circulating plasma levels of progesterone, DOC, pregnenolone, and allopregnanolone are elevated (M. L. Casey et al. 1985). On the other hand, depression, anxiety, and irritability associated with the premenstrual syndrome (PMS) appear in a phase of the cycle where progesterone levels are decreasing or low (Halbreich 1995). Some claim that the symptoms can be reversed by administration of progesterone (Dennerstein et al. 1985); but most well-controlled studies did not confirm this claim (for review, see Halbreich 1996). A recent study failed to demonstrate that symptoms of PMS are associated with a simple deficiency state of either progesterone or its anxiolytic steroid metabolites (allopregnanolone or pregnenolone) in human plasma; however, no cerebrospinal fluid (CSF) values of these compounds were determined (P. J. Schmidt et al. 1994).

Affective Disorders

THP has been shown to influence neuropeptide secretion by modulation of $GABA_A$ receptors in peptidergic nerve terminals (Zhang and Jackson 1994). GABA is a coregulator of neurohypophysial hormone secretion (Mitsushima et al. 1994; Saridaki et al. 1989), involving inhibition of corticotropin-releasing hormone (CRH) secretion (Plotsky et al. 1987). Because centrally mediated oversecretion of CRH has been implied in the etiology of depressive illness (Holsboer et al. 1992), the possibility is raised that neuroactive steroids could be used as potential therapeutics by modulating GABA-ergic neurohypophysial inputs (Nemeroff 1992). On the other hand, considering that the GABA-ergic system appears not to be critically involved in the pathogenesis of major depression, the use of neurosteroids for the treatment of these disorders remains to be elucidated. Preliminary studies investigating CSF levels of progesterone, pregnenolone, and diazepam binding inhibitor, known to promote steroid biosynthesis (E. Costa and Guidotti 1991), in medication-free patients with depression compared with euthymic control subjects demonstrated significantly lower CSF concentrations of pregnenolone (M. S. George et al. 1994).

NEUROSTEROIDS AS ANXIOLYTICS

The first evidence that neurosteroids might represent endogenous anxiolytic agents was derived from behavioral changes occurring during pregnancy and PMS and from associated circulating plasma progesterone levels (M. L. Casey et al. 1985; Dennerstein et al. 1985). The assumption that progesterone and its neuroactive metabolites possess anxiolytic activity through their action at the $GABA_A$ receptor complex related to the estrous cycle or pregnancy was further supported by findings from animal models (D. Bitran et al. 1991, 1993; Fernandez-Guasti and Picazo 1990; Hansen et al. 1985; Majewska et al. 1989; Qureshi et al. 1987).

Independently from sex-dependent anxiolytic effects, and based on the findings of Majewska et al. (1986), Crawley et al. (1986) investigated the possibility that THDOC might be an endogenous anxiolytic compound. Intraperitoneally injected THDOC showed anxiolytic activity in two rat models of anxiety tested, separable from the sedative dose range (Crawley et al. 1986). After subcutaneous administration of progesterone to rats, D. Bitran et al. (1993) observed anxiolytic effects, which were most probably the result of bioconversion of progesterone to allopregnanolone with subsequent augmentation of $GABA_A$ receptor–mediated function. When administered intracerebroventricularly in rats, pregnenolone and allopregnanolone were also shown to display anxiolytic properties, with sedative effects occurring at the highest doses tested (D. Bitran et al. 1991). Moreover, D. Bitran et al. (1991) provided in vivo evidence that a 3α-hydroxyl group is necessary for neurosteroids to interact with the $GABA_A$ receptor, because the 3β-hydroxy-epimer of allopregnanolone proved to be behaviorally inactive.

Similarly, Wieland et al. (1991) reported that allopregnanolone produced anxiolytic effects in rats when given intraperitoneally and that anxiolytic activity of allopregnanolone was coupled to its 3α-hydroxyl group, further emphasizing the notion that modulation of the GABA/benzodiazepine receptor chloride ionophore complex by pregnane steroids follows stringent structural requirements including stereospecificity, which had already been described in vitro (Gee et al. 1988; Harrison et al. 1987; Purdy et al. 1990). Moreover, Britton et al. (1991) have demonstrated anxiolytic activity of the intraperitoneally administered synthetic pregnane steroid alfaxalone in rats. Interestingly, no tolerance to the antianxiety effect of alfaxalone was observed after 1 week of daily administration in contrast to the well-recognized tolerance following long-term administration of benzodiazepines (Britton et al. 1991). The same group also reported on attenuation of anxiogenic behavioral effects of intracerebroventricularly administered CRH and swim stress following intraperitoneal administration of alfaxalone in rats (Britton et al. 1992). Apart from adult animals, anxiolytic activity of intracerebroventricular allopregnanolone, as well as sedative activity at higher doses, could also be demonstrated in neonate rats (Zimmerberg et al. 1994).

The in vitro results indicating that neurosteroids bind at a different site of the $GABA_A$ receptor complex than do benzodiazepines and barbiturates has been supported by studies investigating drug discrimination in rats, suggesting that allopregnanolone and allo-THDOC might possess a more desirable profile in terms of abuse liability than benzodiazepines and barbiturates (Ator et al. 1993). Similar results have been obtained by S. I. Deutsch and Mastropaolo (1993) concerning the anxiolytic efficacy of peripherally administered allo-THDOC in a drug discrimination paradigm in rats.

Further evidence concerning anxiolytic effects of neurosteroids involves its action on the prefrontal cortical dopamine system. This system has been identified as one of the neuroanatomically involved CNS areas in stress and anxiety responses, where increases in dopamine metabolism are observed following a variety of stressors (A. Y. Deutch and Roth 1990). Grobin et al. (1992) demonstrated that intracerebroventricularly administered allo-THDOC effectively reduced dopamine metabolism in rats, thereby antagonizing stress-induced activation of the prefrontal cortical dopamine innervation.

Conflicting results with regard to previous studies have been obtained by Melchior and Ritzmann (1994b), reporting on anxiogenic responses of mice following intraperitoneal administration of pregnenolone and mixed anxiogenic/anxiolytic responses following administration of pregnenolone sulfate that were dose-dependent. These authors have speculated that both substances that were tested participate in the initial response to stressful stimuli, which is then terminated by the action of pregnenolone and pregnenolone sulfate metabolites with anxiolytic activity. In a further study by the same authors, intraperitoneally administered DHEA and DHEAS both showed anxiolytic activity in mice, with DHEA being effective over a wide range of doses (Melchior and Ritzmann 1994a). Moreover, ethanol enhanced the anxiolytic effect of DHEA, but at 1.0 mg/kg DHEAS blocked the anxiolytic effect of ethanol. Melchior and Ritzmann concluded that DHEA and DHEAS, in contrast to pregnenolone and pregnenolone sulfate, might be involved in the termination of a stress response.

FUTURE PERSPECTIVES

The use of benzodiazepines in anxiety disorders represents a difficult issue because of the well-known addictive properties of this substance class; furthermore, the depressogenic lability of benzodiazepines represents a major problem in the treatment of generalized anxiety disorders, in which concomitant depressive symptoms occur in up to 50% of patients (Gulley and Nemeroff 1993; Rickels and Schweizer 1993). Therefore, a compound mimicking endogenous anxiolytic effects, and that might further possess potential antidepressive properties, is warranted. Neuroactive steroids could represent such a substance class. However, the following issues need to be addressed in this respect:

- Although theoretically lipophilic (nonsulfated) neurosteroids penetrate the blood-brain barrier easily, with plasma and CSF concentrations of these compounds being almost identical (S. Schwarz and Pohl 1994), Corpéchot et al. (1993) reported that brain uptake of intravenously injected allopregnanolone is about 100-fold lower than that of progesterone. In this respect, it is noteworthy that allopregnanolone has failed to display anxiolytic or sedative effects following systemic administration in one earlier study (W. B. Mendelson et al. 1987b). Compared with allo-THDOC though, CNS uptake of the more hydrophobic allopregnanolone is significantly greater; therefore, potential difficulty in brain availability of these compounds resulting from drug penetrance or rapid systemic metabolization requires further clarification (Purdy et al. 1990).

- With regard to the administration of pregnenolone or DHEA, it will be important to take potential sulfation/desulfation of these substances (Iwamori et al. 1976) into consideration to avoid possible GABA agonistic/antagonistic effects. Indirect evidence for this possibility can be derived from first systemic administrations of neurosteroids in human sleep research, with pregnenolone inducing sleep patterns compatible with inverse agonistic $GABA_A$ receptor modulation (Steiger et al. 1993) and DHEA exerting mixed $GABA_A$–agonistic/antagonistic effects (Friess et al. 1995).

- A further issue is raised with regard to dose-dependent effects, suggesting dual or U-shaped psychotropic responses, because recent studies have indicated that neurosteroids may induce anxiogenic or anxiolytic responses in relation to the dosage used and subsequent metabolizing steps involved (Melchior and Ritzmann 1994a, 1994b).

- Gender differences in response to GABA-ergic neurosteroids have also to be taken into consideration. Although many studies cited used male animals (Ator et al. 1993; Britton et al. 1991, 1992; S. I. Deutsch and Mastropaolo 1993; Wieland et al. 1991; Zimmerberg et al. 1994), which were sensitive to the anxiolytic effects of the neurosteroids tested, gender or hormonal status, for example, estrous cycle phase, may influence the metabolization and/or CNS response to neuroactive steroids (G. Fink et al. 1982; Finn and Gee 1993; Kokka et al. 1992; Rodriguez-Sierra et al. 1986; Zimmerberg and Farley 1993; Zimmerberg et al. 1994).

- Finally, neuroanatomical distribution of steroid-sensitive $GABA_A$ receptors in the CNS needs to be further correlated with CNS areas involved in anxiety responses as well as their interaction with other transmitter systems, for example, CRH or dopamine (Grobin et al. 1992; Zhang and Jackson 1994). Such characterization may result in the development of more specific compounds, possibly also involving concomitant antidepressive effects.

In conclusion, neurosteroid-based anxiolytics with low intrinsic toxicity may represent an exciting new pharmacological development with potential advantages over existing classes of anxiolytics with regard to tolerance, dependence, and abuse liability.

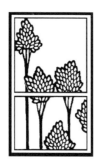

CHAPTER 29

Nonbenzodiazepine Anxiolytics Acting on the GABA Receptor

Caroline Bell, M.R.C.Psych.,
John Potokar, M.R.C.Psych., and
David J. Nutt, D.M., M.R.C.P.,
F.R.C.Psych.

NONBENZODIAZEPINE LIGANDS ACTING AT THE GABA$_A$ RECEPTOR

The γ-aminobutyric acid–A receptor (GABA$_A$) is a macromolecular complex through which a variety of ligands act. Our understanding of this receptor complex and the mechanism of action of these ligands has expanded rapidly over recent years. This is as a consequence of substantial developments in the fields of molecular biology and immunochemistry and has been fueled by the as yet elusive quest for effective anxiolytics that do not have the problems associated with the benzodiazepines, that is, adverse effects, interaction with alcohol, and the related issues of tolerance, dependency, and problems on withdrawal.

STRUCTURE OF THE GABA$_A$ RECEPTOR COMPLEX

The GABA$_A$ receptor is a protein complex that mediates neuronal inhibition throughout the central nervous system. The inhibitory neurotransmitter GABA and various substances, including benzodiazepines, neurosteroids, barbiturates, and alcohol, all have binding sites on it (Figure 29–1).

The receptor complex is made up of five protein subunits that are linked together to form a doughnut-shaped structure that spans the membrane. The center of this doughnut is a chloride channel, which in the closed conformation is impermeable to ions. When GABA binds, the conformation of the receptor complex is altered, the channel opens, and there is a net influx of chloride ions. This causes hyperpolarization of the cell and depression of membrane excitability. Benzodiazepines and benzodiazepine-like drugs have no direct actions on the pore but exert their effects by allosterically modulating the GABA$_A$ recognition site. This enhances the binding of GABA and

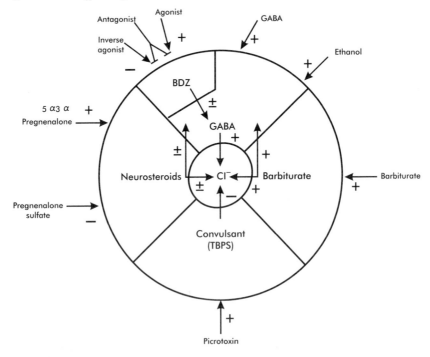

FIGURE 29–1.   Binding sites on the γ-aminobutyric acid type A (GABA$_A$)/benzodiazepine (BDZ) receptor complex.

thereby enhances inhibition. The other drugs mentioned above also act in this way but in high doses can open the channel directly, causing unchecked hyperpolarization and inhibition resulting in severe central nervous system depression and subsequent death. This may well be why these drugs are so dangerous in overdose in comparison with benzodiazepines.

The five protein subunits that form the receptor complex are from four distinct structural classes (α, β, γ, δ). To date, the cDNA and amino acid sequences for six α subunits ($\alpha_1-\alpha_6$), four β subunits ($\beta_1-\beta_4$), three γ subunits ($\gamma_1-\gamma_3$), and a δ subunit have been reported (Burt and Kamatchi 1991). Sixty to seventy percent of GABA$_A$ receptors have been found to be made up of the subunit combination $\alpha_1\beta_2\gamma_2$ (Fritschy et al. 1992), but the potential for different permutations and therefore different subtypes is huge. In vivo, only a fraction of the possible subunit combinations are actually thought to exist, but even this fraction represents considerable receptor diversity. The significance of the different subunit combinations and receptor subtypes is an area that is currently being actively researched. The hypothesis that different receptor subtypes exist in different brain regions and subserve specific functions is attractive, but has yet to be established. Significant advances have been made, however; techniques of immunochemistry have raised antisera to particular subunits, which has given insights into the regional distribution of receptor subtypes; molecular biology has allowed different combinations of subunits to be coexpressed, which has allowed the pharmacology of the subsequent receptor complexes to be determined (Verdoorn et al. 1990); and pharmacological studies have identified some drugs with subtype specificity.

Benzodiazepine Recognition Site

Specific high-affinity binding sites for benzodiazepines were first identified in the rat brain in 1977 (Squires and Braestrup 1977) but have now been visualized in the living brain of humans using positron-emission tomography and single photon emission computed tomography. By using the techniques described earlier, a considerable amount of further information about their structure and function has now been determined.

The benzodiazepine receptor is that portion of the receptor complex to which the benzodiazepines and related drugs bind and is located on the α protein subunit. The γ_2 subunit has also been shown to be important in that its presence appears to be essential for normal responsiveness of the receptor complex to the benzodiazepines (Verdoorn et al. 1990). Benzodiazepine-sensitive receptors also seem to require α, β, and γ subunits to be present in some combination.

Other Ligand Binding Sites

Our knowledge of the binding sites of the other ligands at the $GABA_A$ receptor is more limited. The barbiturates and neurosteroids act through distinct binding sites, but the specific subunits involved have not been clearly determined. Unlike the benzodiazepines, they do not seem to require the γ subunit to function and may just require α and β subunits.

Alcohol is interesting in that its potentiating effects seem to be brain region specific, that is, GABA receptors in the cerebellum, cortex, and spinal cord seem to be more sensitive to alcohol than those in other brain regions. Expression studies have also shown that a specific form of γ_2 subunit appears to be crucial (see below).

BENZODIAZEPINE-RELATED DRUGS

That the benzodiazepine structure was a prerequisite for the characteristic tranquilizer profile and specific binding at the benzodiazepine receptor was a long-held belief. This has now been shown not to be the case by the discovery of a range of different compounds that bind to the benzodiazepine receptor (Figure 29–2). These include the β-carbolines (e.g., abecarnil), the triazolo-pyridazines (e.g., CL 218,872), the imidazopyridines (e.g., zolpidem), the cyclopyrrolones (e.g., suriclone), and the pyrazoloquinolines.

Figure 29–2 also illustrates the important bidirectional action of the benzodiazepine receptor on GABA function. A spectrum of activity exists from full agonism, in which the actions of GABA are increased (anxiolytic, anticonvulsant, sedative), through antagonism to inverse agonism, in which the actions of GABA are reduced (anxiogenic, proconvulsant, alerting).

This section describes the partial agonists and the nonbenzodiazepine drugs that act at the benzodiazepine receptor. What these drugs have in common is that their development has been driven by the search for effective anxiolytics that do not have the adverse effects of sedation, amnesia, ataxia, interaction with alcohol, or the problems of tolerance, dependency, and withdrawal seen with classic benzodiazepines. These problems have been addressed by the development of partial agonists, subtype-selective ligands, and other drugs, the cyclopyrrolones, which do not seem to cause these problems.

Partial Agonists

The effects of agonists and inverse agonists do not represent two distinct states but rather the ends of a spectrum of activity. Compounds that have less

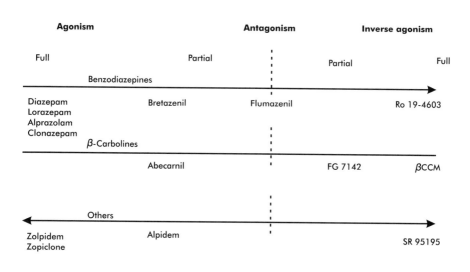

FIGURE 29–2.   Benzodiazepine receptor spectrum.

but not zero agonism or inverse agonism have also been identified. These are called partial agonists/inverse agonists, respectively.

Partial agonists have a number of pharmacological features. In the presence of full agonists, they compete for the receptor and therefore attenuate the effects of full agonists. This could theoretically mean that, in patients who are already taking full agonists, partial agonists may actually precipitate withdrawal.

On their own, partial agonists have lower maximal effects than full agonists and require a greater receptor occupancy to produce the same effect. This is important because it has been suggested that there is a hierarchy both clinically and pharmacologically in relation to receptor occupancy—as receptor occupancy increases there is a gradation of effects from anxiolysis through anticonvulsant, hypnotic, and amnesic effects to sedation and coma. Partial agonists may thus be able to achieve anxiolysis without causing the problems of sedation and ataxia and may well be even safer than the classical benzodiazepines in overdose even when mixed with alcohol or other sedative drugs. The hope is that they will also cause fewer problems of tolerance and dependency.

The one serious question that hangs over the partial agonists is whether they will have enough efficacy to be therapeutic, especially in patients who have previously been treated with full agonists. This query will be answered by clinical studies.

Several partial agonists are currently in development. Some are described in this section, others are described in the sections on subtype-selective drugs and the cyclopyrrolones. The work so far has tended to show the hoped-for features of lack of adverse effects, lack of interaction with alcohol, and reduced liability to cause tolerance, in addition to being effective anxiolytics.

Bretazenil.   Bretazenil is an imidazobenzodiazepine partial agonist and a potent anxiolytic. It is rapidly absorbed and has a half-life of 2.5 hours. Animal work has shown that, even after long-term administration of bretazenil, there are no changes in GABA receptor binding or function, and tolerance does not occur. Studies in humans have also suggested that bretazenil has a low abuse potential (Sellers et al. 1991). In terms of clinical effects, bretazenil has demonstrated anxiolytic efficacy in both generalized anxiety disorder and panic disorder (Katschnig et al. 1991), but no controlled study has compared bretazenil with a classic full agonist.

Abecarnil.   Abecarnil is a β-carboline-3-carboxylic acid derivative that is in development for the treatment of anxiety disorders. Animal work has shown that abecarnil has a low propensity to cause the problems of dependency and abuse and that the drug has marked anxiolytic and anticonvulsant activity but does not appear to have significant effects on motor coordination—a finding in marked contrast to the effects of diazepam (Stephens et al. 1990). This interesting phenomena may be explained by the fact that abecarnil is acting as a full agonist at some receptors that mediate certain effects (potent anxiolytic) and as a partial agonist at others (lack of side effects). One published clinical study compared abecarnil at different doses with placebo in patients with generalized anxiety disorder (Ballenger et al. 1991). This showed that abecarnil was significantly more effective than placebo in terms of anxiolysis. Stopping treatment produced no withdrawal effects in patients on the lower dose, although some effects were seen in those taking higher doses.

Pazinaclone.   Pazinaclone is a nonbenzodiazepine partial agonist. Animal work has shown that it has anxiolytic and anticonvulsant activity. Pazinaclone does not, however, produce the sedative, muscle relaxant, or motor coordination effects seen with diazepam (Waka and Fukada 1991). Phase II clinical trials are currently under way in the United States, Europe, and Japan, which have so far demonstrated that it is well tolerated and seems to cause significantly less sedation than do benzodiazepines (Uchiumi et al. 1992).

Imidazenil.   Imidazenil is an imidazobenzodiazepine with the profile of a partial agonist. Animal studies have shown that it does not produce sedation or ataxia in rats nor does it potentiate the effects of alcohol (Guisti et al. 1993). Imidazenil has a low intrinsic activity at the $GABA_A$ receptor and therefore causes only slight enhancement of GABA-ergic tone. Its efficacy may, however, be increased when GABA tone is reduced, which could lead to its being active only in conditions where GABA tone is altered. This may well make it an ideal treatment for anxiety and epilepsy.

Others. Various other substances from different drug classes have also been found to possess partial agonist properties. So far, most of the work on these has been on animals. Listed here for completeness, they are pipequaline, CGS 9895 and CGS 9896, FG8205, ZK 91296 and ZK 95962, and panadiplon (reviewed in Potokar and Nutt 1994).

Subtype-Selective Ligands

The rationale behind the development of subtype-selective ligands is based on the recognition of the marked heterogeneity of the $GABA_A$ receptor complex and the extrapolation of the hypothesis that specific receptors in specific brain regions are concerned with specific functions. The aim is to target drugs so that they would bind only to the relevant receptors and would therefore bring about only the desired effects. There would be no adverse effects because the receptors involved with these would not be affected. The concept is attractive in theory, but unfortunately in practice has proved more difficult to realize.

CL 218,872. The subtype selectivity of ligands was actually recognized long before purification and molecular cloning studies had demonstrated the heterogeneity of the receptor complex.

The initial observation was based on the fact that the triazolopyridazine CL 218,872 had a significantly higher affinity for receptors in the cerebellum (benzodiazepine type I receptor) than it had for receptors in the hippocampus (benzodiazepine type II receptor) (Klepner et al. 1979). CL 218,872 was also known to be an anxiolytic without sedative effects. The proposal was that anxiolysis was mediated by the receptors in the cerebellum, whereas sedation was mediated by receptors elsewhere. Subsequent work has shown that the case is not as simple as that. With the advent of molecular biology and coexpression studies, it has been established that the $\alpha_1\beta_2\gamma_2$ receptor is equivalent to the type 1 receptor. The type II receptors appear to be a more heterogeneous receptor class as $\alpha_2\beta_2\gamma_2$, $\alpha_3\beta_2\gamma_2$, and $\alpha_5\beta_2\gamma_2$ all seem to display this type of pharmacology. A newer compound, zalaplon, which has similar pharmacology, is undergoing clinical trials.

Zolpidem. Zolpidem is an imidazolopyridine that, like CL 218,872, binds with high affinity to $\alpha_1\beta_2\gamma_2$ receptors. In contrast to CL 218,872, zolpidem differentiates within benzodiazepine type II receptors in that it displays a 20-fold reduced affinity at $\alpha_2\beta_2\gamma_2$ and $\alpha_3\beta_3\gamma_2$ receptors, but shows nearly no affinity to $\alpha_5\beta_2\gamma_2$ receptors (Pritchett and Seeburg 1990). Zolpidem is also unusual in that it has sedative activity at lower doses than those producing anxiolytic, muscle relaxant, and anticonvulsant effects and is consequently marketed for night sedation.

Alpidem. Alpidem is an imidazopyridine partial agonist that also shows relative selectivity for the type I benzodiazepine receptor. Studies have shown an anxiolytic effect comparable with the classic benzodiazepines, but with an improved adverse effect profile (Pancheri et al. 1993). It has also been compared with buspirone in patients with generalized anxiety disorder and shown to be more rapidly effective and again to have a more favorable adverse effect profile (Legris et al. 1993). Longer-term studies with alpidem have shown that tolerance does not occur, and no significant problems of withdrawal on discontinuation were found (Chevalier et al. 1993). Alpidem was licensed in France for the treatment of anxiety but has now been suspended because of recent reports of alpidem-induced hepatic dysfunction. The reason for this is unclear, but it may be a reflection of the fact that alpidem also binds to peripheral benzodiazepine receptors, which are present in high density in the liver.

Cyclopyrrolones

The cyclopyrrolone zopiclone was one of the first compounds other than the benzodiazepines to be shown to bind at the benzodiazepine receptor. More potent compounds have also been developed (e.g., suriclone and pagoclone). The cyclopyrrolones may actually bind to a different domain on the α subunit from the benzodiazepines (Canton and Doble 1992), and this may underlie the pharmacological differences seen in vivo, that is, lack of some side effects and lack of tolerance after long-term dosing.

Zopiclone. Zopiclone is a full agonist that has been shown to have sedative properties in experimental animals and to be a potent hypnotic in humans. It has a short duration of action and minimal effects on sleep architecture, which means that it has few residual effects on waking. It appears to cause less tolerance and problems on withdrawal than the classic benzodiazepines and is currently marketed as a hypnotic.

Suriclone.   Suriclone is one of the most potent of all agents known to act at the benzodiazepine receptor. Its anxiolytic effects have been clearly demonstrated in rodents (Doble et al. 1992). It has also been demonstrated to be efficacious in the treatment of generalized anxiety disorder in humans (Ansseau et al. 1991). Animal work has shown it to have fewer side effects and less potential for interacting with alcohol than do benzodiazepines. These would represent significant advantages if they were also seen in humans. Repeated doses have failed to show tolerance and do not produce the change in "set point" of the $GABA_A$ receptor seen with the benzodiazepines. The reason for this is unclear but may be linked to a difference in the interaction of the cyclopyrrolones with the receptor compared with that of the benzodiazepines.

Pagoclone.   Pagoclone is a new cyclopyrrolone partial agonist. In animal models of antianxiety activity, pagoclone is more potent than benzodiazepines, is less sedating, and has a high therapeutic index (Table 29–1). In clinical studies, pagoclone is well tolerated and does not appear to cause sedation or affect psychomotor or cognitive performance. In studies of volunteers, it has been shown that it does not cause withdrawal symptoms on abrupt discontinuation after 14 days. These factors all suggest that pagoclone may be an important drug for the future. It is currently entering dose-ranging and comparative studies involving patients with anxiety disorders, and in a pilot crossover study, it reduced panic attacks; adverse effects were not different from or more numerous than those reported with placebo (Sandford et al. 1998).

In the next section, we describe the other known main ligands of the $GABA_A$ receptor, that is, neurosteroids, alcohol, and the barbiturates. (The neurosteroid section is only a summary for completeness; for a more comprehensive overview, the reader is referred to Siegfried, Chapter 33, in this volume.)

TABLE 29–1.   Pagoclone versus full agonist benzodiazepines

	Antianxiety (mg/kg)	Sedation (mg/kg)	Therapeutic index
Pagoclone	0.08	375	> 4,600
Alprazolam	0.3	0.05	< 0.1
Diazepam	0.3	1.9	7
Lorazepam	0.5	1.0	2

NEUROSTEROIDS

Steroids have both positive and negative effects on $GABA_A$ chloride ion conductance, and 3α OH ring A reduced steroids are among the most active of ligands at the $GABA_A$ receptor, with affinity equal to or greater than that of the benzodiazepines (S. M. Paul and Purdy 1992). (Neurosteroids are reviewed in Heuser, Chapter 28, in this volume.)

ALCOHOL

Alcohol is one of the most commonly consumed drugs in the world and has been used by humans since the Stone Age. It is anxiolytic; for this reason, it has been used not only for relaxation purposes but also by people with anxiety disorders to suppress their symptoms. Between 10% and 20% of agoraphobic patients are alcohol dependent. Thyrer et al. (1986) reported a 36% prevalence of alcoholism among socially phobic patients entering an anxiety disorders clinic, and (according to population studies) 20%–80% of people with posttraumatic stress disorder (PTSD) are dependent on alcohol. Sierles et al. (1983), in their study of Vietnam War veterans with PTSD, found that 64% were alcohol dependent. Since the Epidemiological Catchment Area study estimated the lifetime prevalence of PTSD to be 1% in the United States population, it is clear that self-medication with alcohol for anxiety symptoms will have a major influence on the development of alcohol dependency (Regier et al. 1990).

It is also clear that anxiety symptoms are common among primary alcoholic patients (although abstinence leads to a reduction in symptoms even without any specific pharmacological or psychosocial treatments [S. A. Brown et al. 1991]). Repeated alcohol withdrawals may result in "kindling" of the limbic system, producing chronic elevation in sympathetic tone (D. T. George et al. 1988). This in turn can result in further anxiety symptoms and hence maintenance of drinking behavior.

The above reflects not only the ubiquity of alcohol but also its short-term effectiveness in reducing anxiety. The latter results (at least in part) from its effects at the $GABA_A$ receptor, which is described in more detail below.

ALCOHOL AND THE $GABA_A$ RECEPTOR

In the past, it was believed that alcohol exerted its effect on the brain by altering membrane fluidity (H. H. Meyer and Gottlieb 1926). It is now clear that alcohol can alter the function of membrane-bound proteins, especially receptor-gated ion channels, including that of the main excitatory amino acid glutamate (via the N-methyl-D-aspartate receptor) and the main inhibitory amino acid GABA. It also has effects on monoamine systems, peptides, and calcium channels.

Its effects on the GABA receptor are interesting and may partially explain why some people are more sensitive to the effects of alcohol than others. Low concentrations enhance GABA-stimulated chloride flux as measured in synaptoneurosomal brain preparations (Allan and Harris 1987; Susdak et al. 1986). However, it appears that this action is genetically determined. In mice that have been selectively bred to be sensitive to the hypnotic effects of alcohol (*long-sleep mice*), alcohol increases chloride ion transport via the GABA-benzodiazepine receptor complex. This does not occur in *short-sleep mice*, who are resistant to the effects of alcohol (Allan and Harris 1986). More recent work suggested that alcohol enhances the $GABA_A$ complex in selective brain regions (Aguayo 1990); this may be because of the molecular heterogeneity of the $GABA_A$ receptor (see earlier). The γ subunit appears to be crucial in conferring sensitivity of the $GABA_A$ receptor to alcohol.

The γ subunit takes two forms, one of which has an intracellular loop that is 8 amino acids shorter than the other form. Alcohol potentiates $GABA_A$ receptors only in cells where the long form is expressed (Wafford 1991). Within the 8–amino acid insertion is a serine residue that is especially important because deletion results in loss of alcohol sensitivity (Wafford et al. 1993). The current view is that this serine residue must be phosphorylated to allow alcohol activity at $GABA_A$ receptors. More recent research has shown that alcohol potentiates GABA chloride flux only in brain regions containing zolpidem-sensitive GABA receptors (i.e., those with the $\alpha_1\beta_2\gamma_2$ configuration) (Criswell et al. 1995). Although this does not exclude binding at other sites, these subtle variations in subunit structure and subunit binding may offer explanations as to why some people are more likely to develop alcohol dependency problems (although clearly alcohol metabolism is also important). Furthermore, the knowledge that the γ subunit is also essential for the expression of benzodiazepine sensitivity in $GABA_A$ receptors helps to explain associations between alcohol and benzodiazepines such as cross-tolerance, cross-dependence, and the fact that benzodiazepine agonists such as chlordiazepoxide are the treatment of choice for alcohol withdrawal.

Chronic alcohol intake changes the functioning of the GABA benzodiazepine receptor complex. For example, chronic alcohol intake increases the binding (Mhatre et al. 1988) and function of benzodiazepine inverse agonists (Lister and Karanian 1987) and attenuates the effect of benzodiazepine agonists. These effects have different time courses. Attenuation of agonist efficacy is (at least in animal models) transient, returning to control levels within 24 hours after alcohol withdrawal. In contrast, the increased inverse agonist sensitivity is prolonged and observable 8 days postwithdrawal (Buck and Harris 1990). These effects may be the result of changes in the coupling between agonist/inverse agonist sites and the chloride channel and may offer some explanation of the time course of the different withdrawal syndromes seen in humans.

Alcohol withdrawal can result in mild symptoms of anxiety through to severe panic attacks and even frank delirium. Frequently symptom relief is achieved by further alcohol use, thus "feeding the cause." It is thought that the $GABA_A$ receptor may be important in mediating at least some of these symptoms, and theories have been proposed in an attempt to explain what is actually happening at the $GABA_A$ receptor during withdrawal. It may be that chronic alcohol intake leads to increases in an endogenous inverse agonist whose effects would compensate for the sedating effects of alcohol. When alcohol is withdrawn, this inverse agonist could act unopposed, producing symptoms of anxiety. Several substances have been proposed as possible endogenous inverse agonists, and one of them (tribulin) has been found in increased amounts in the urine of alcoholic patients undergoing withdrawal (Bhattacharya et al. 1982).

An alternative explanation for the anxiety symptoms of withdrawal is that chronic alcohol intake shifts the "set point" of the $GABA_A$ benzodiazepine receptor, such that agonists act as partial agonists and antagonists act as partial inverse agonists. We tested the above two theories by giving the benzodiazepine antagonist flumazenil to alcoholic patients in withdrawal. If flumazenil was anxiolytic in this group, it would lend support to the first theory (since it would act more as a partial inverse agonist), whereas if it was anxiogenic, the latter theory would seem more likely (since it would prevent binding of endogenous inverse agonist to the receptor). In fact, flumazenil had little effect, which suggests that other factors may prove more important in withdrawal. However, one important conclusion that can be drawn from this work is that alcohol withdrawal and panic disorder (which are clinically similar and are both associated with noradrenergic overactivity) are mediated differently because flumazenil is anxiogenic in panic disorder (Nutt et al. 1990).

BARBITURATES

Barbiturates were first developed at the beginning of the 20th century and, until the advent of the benzodiazepines in the early 1960s, were commonly used for the treatment of anxiety and insomnia, as well as behavioral distur-bance. Their mechanism of action is not well understood. Barbiturates bind to the GABA receptor/chloride channel, but this is not the same site to which benzodiazepines bind because the effect of barbiturates is not blocked by flumazenil. Barbiturates appear to have dual actions to enhance GABA-mediated chloride ion conductance (Scolnick et al. 1981; Study and Barker 1981). At low concentrations, barbiturates augment the affinity of the $GABA_A$ receptor for GABA. They also increase the mean channel opening time induced by GABA. At higher concentrations, they can directly increase channel openings, even when GABA is not present. This effect explains the dangers of barbiturates. Because direct opening of chloride channels can occur (as opposed to the indirect effects of benzodiazepines that modulate channel opening), central inhibition can be profound, leading to coma and death with overdose. It is possible that partial agonist barbiturates could overcome these dangers, but whether they will be developed, given the historical precedent of full agonist barbiturates, seems unlikely.

CONCLUSION

In medication terms, the benzodiazepines represented significant advantages compared with the barbiturates. Our knowledge and understanding of the GABA receptor and the ligands that bind to it has increased considerably since the pioneering work of Squires and Braestrup (1977). It is now clear that this receptor system has a pivotal role in mediating anxiety. The concepts of a receptor spectrum and subtype specificity have been and will continue to be important in the development of anxiolytics with improved profiles. This is perhaps especially important when one considers that stress can both result in altered GABA function through the action of endogenous ligands and lead to self-medication in attempts to quell the resulting anxiety.

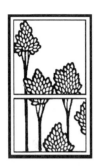

CHAPTER 30

Treatment of Obsessive-Compulsive Disorder: From Theory to Practice

Iulian Iancu, M.D.,

Pinhas N. Dannon, M.D.,

Ornah T. Dolberg, M.D., and

Joseph Zohar, M.D.

Obsessive-compulsive disorder (OCD) is characterized by recurrent, intrusive, and distressing thoughts, images, or impulses (obsessions) and repetitive, seemingly purposeful behaviors that a person feels driven to perform (compulsions).

Until the early 1980s, OCD was considered a rare, treatment-refractory, chronic condition of psychological origins. Treatment strategies included dynamic psychotherapy, which in general was of little benefit, and a variety of pharmacological treatments, which had been tried without much success (Salzman and Thaler 1981). However, several studies in the past decade have found OCD to be a prevalent disorder (Robins et al. 1984; Weissman et al. 1994), and a vast number of reports has appeared concerning various specific and efficient therapies for this disorder. Today, OCD is believed to have psychobiological origins and a specific response to serotonin reuptake inhibitors (SRIs). In this chapter, we present the clinical data supporting the unique response to SRIs and the implications of these well-established clinical findings on the development of the serotonergic hypothesis of OCD.

PHARMACOLOGICAL TREATMENT OF OBSESSIVE-COMPULSIVE DISORDER

The outlook for the treatment of OCD was not very promising in the early 1980s. However, since then, several potent SRIs have been studied extensively in the treatment of OCD. Aggregate statistics for all SRIs suggest that 70% of treatment-naive patients will respond at least moderately (Rasmussen et al. 1993).

Serotonin Reuptake Inhibitors

Among the variety of medications used in the treatment of patients with OCD, clomipramine (CMI) has been the most extensively studied. CMI was first reported to be efficient in OCD in the late 1960s (Fernandez-Cordoba and López-Ibor 1967; Renynghe de Voxrie 1968). Since then, several placebo-controlled studies have clearly shown CMI's effectiveness (Ananth et al. 1981; Flament et al. 1985; Insel et al. 1982a; Marks et al. 1980; S. A. Montgomery 1980; Thoren et al. 1980; Volavka et al. 1985; Zohar et al. 1987).

A large multicenter trial with CMI ($N = 520$), which included 21 centers in two studies, examined the efficacy, safety, and tolerability of CMI up to 300 mg/day (CMI Collaborative Study Group 1991). CMI was significantly more effective than placebo on the Yale-Brown Obsessive Compulsive Scale (Y-BOCS) and the National Institute of Mental Health Global Obsessive Compulsive Scale. After 10 weeks of treatment, 58% of patients treated with CMI rated themselves much or very much improved versus only 3% of patients treated with placebo.

Selective Serotonin Reuptake Inhibitors

Besides CMI, other nontricyclic SRIs, such as fluoxetine, fluvoxamine, paroxetine, and sertraline, are gaining acceptance as effective alternatives for the treatment of OCD.

Fluoxetine. Fluoxetine has been proven to be effective for OCD in open studies as well as in a few controlled trials. In the Lilly European OCD study (Montgomery et al. 1993b), 217 patients with OCD were treated with fixed doses of fluoxetine (20 mg, 40 mg, or 60 mg) or placebo in a double-blind manner for 8 weeks, 161 patients continuing the drug until the 16th week. Fluoxetine at doses of 40 mg and 60 mg was significantly superior to placebo, whereas no significant difference was found between patients treated with fluoxetine 20 mg and those administered placebo. The rate of discontinuation as a result of adverse effects was low and not significantly different among the groups.

Tollefson et al. (1994) reported an American multicenter investigation of fixed-dose fluoxetine in the treatment of OCD. Three hundred fifty-five outpatients participated in two randomized, double-blind, parallel, 13-week trials, receiving fluoxetine or placebo. Fluoxetine (20 mg, 40 mg, and 60 mg) was significantly superior to placebo on the Y-BOCS total score and other efficacy measures. However, a trend was noted suggesting greater efficacy of the 60 mg/day dose. The authors reported few side effects, and most patients (79.2%) completed the study. Similarly to CMI, fluoxetine led to a significant reduction in OCD severity, regarding both obsessions and compulsions.

Fluvoxamine. Another selective serotonin reuptake inhibitor (SSRI) that has been compared with placebo in several studies and has been found superior to it is fluvoxamine (W. K. Goodman et al. 1989a; Jenike et al. 1990; Perse et al. 1987). Westenberg et al. (1992) confirmed these results in 20 outpatients with OCD who were not depressed and treated for 8 weeks with fluvoxamine in a double-blind, placebo-controlled study designed in an incremental dosing fashion, beginning at 50 mg and up to 300 mg, depending on response and emergence of side effects. Two multicenter studies have confirmed fluvoxamine's efficacy in OCD in 320 patients (Greist 1991). Similar efficacy was reported by Mallya et al. (1992) in a double-blind, controlled study. Of 21 patients who continued in an open extension of the controlled study for an additional 2–12 months, 12 (57%) displayed improvement. Seven of nine patients relapsed within a few days of discontinuation of fluvoxamine.

Sertraline. Sertraline was reported to be effective and well tolerated in an 8-week placebo-controlled study with 87 patients with OCD (Chouinard et al. 1990). Sertraline was also compared with placebo in a fixed-dose study with 325 nondepressed patients with OCD who were randomly selected to 12 weeks of double-blind treatment with either placebo or 50 mg, 100 mg, or 200 mg of sertraline (Greist et al. 1993a). Sertraline had significant effectiveness at all doses, although the dose of 100 mg was effective on only one outcome measure. In a recent study, Greist et al. (1995b) reported efficacy for the three sertraline doses in a fixed-dose study (50 mg, 100 mg, and 200 mg), again more for the 50-mg and the 200-mg doses than the 100-mg dose.

Long-term efficacy of sertraline in OCD has been examined in a follow-up study of 40 weeks' duration by the same group (Greist et al. 1993b). Patients continued to improve with time, and the treatment was well tolerated. With the exception of headache, the occurrence of side effects decreased significantly throughout the year of treatment, demonstrating a waning of adverse reactions.

Paroxetine.   Wheadon and associates (1993) reported the results of a 12-week, fixed-dose, multicenter study of 348 patients with OCD. The subjects were randomly selected in a double-blind fashion to receive either 20 mg, 40 mg, or 60 mg of paroxetine or placebo. Statistical analysis revealed improvement for the two higher paroxetine doses as compared with that of placebo. In a further analysis of the results, M. Steiner et al. (1994) reported that male gender, lack of comorbidity, and longer illness correlated with greater improvement with the paroxetine treatment. Patients with moderate OCD responded to 40 mg of paroxetine, whereas patients with severe OCD (Y-BOCS > 26) showed a greater response with the 60-mg dose.

Onset of Treatment Response

It has been suggested that a relatively long period is needed for CMI to be significantly effective. Thoren et al. (1980) reported that only at week 5 did the differences between CMI and other treatments become evident. Volavka et al. (1985) postulated that at least 12 weeks are required for CMI to exceed imipramine's effects.

Altogether, it seems that it might take as long as 10–12 weeks for patients with OCD to arrive at an initial response, and it may take several months, half a year, or even longer to achieve the maximum response.

Long-Term Treatment of
Obsessive-Compulsive Disorder

What the length of maintenance therapy with CMI should be is unclear. It has been demonstrated that the length of treatment should be considerable and that most patients relapse after premature discontinuation. Pato et al. (1988) reported that 16 of 18 patients with OCD relapsed within 7 weeks after stopping CMI, although some had been treated for more than a year (mean = 10.7 months). All patients regained therapeutic effects when CMI was reintroduced. H. L. Leonard et al. (1989, 1991) examined the effect of CMI substitution during a long-term CMI treatment in 26 children and adolescents with OCD (mean duration of treatment was 17 months). Half of the patients were blindly assigned to 2 months of desipramine treatment, and then CMI was reintroduced. Almost 90% relapsed during the 2 months' substitution period in comparison with only 18% of those who continued with CMI treatment.

Further studies are therefore needed to determine the length of maintenance of SRI treatment. It seems, however, that patients with OCD should be maintained on CMI more than a year before a very gradual attempt to discontinue the treatment is carried out.

Obsessive-Compulsive Disorder, Depression, and the Response to Serotonin Reuptake Inhibitors

One of the first controversies regarding the treatment with CMI of patients with OCD was whether the patients benefited from the drug's antidepressant effect or whether the improvement was actually the result of an antiobsessive effect. In an early study, Marks et al. (1980) reported on the efficacy of CMI in depressed patients with OCD. However, subsequent reports demonstrated that the antiobsessive efficacy of CMI is independent of its antidepressant activity (Ananth et al. 1981; Flament et al. 1985; Insel et al. 1982a; Mavissakalian et al. 1985; S. A. Montgomery 1980; Thoren et al. 1980; Volavka et al. 1985; Zohar and Insel 1987). Depression is not a prerequisite for an antiobsessional response to CMI. In this regard, OCD resembles other nonaffective disorders, such as panic disorder, bulimia, enuresis, migraine, and chronic pain syndrome, in which antidepressants are effective in the absence of depression (D. L. Murphy et al. 1985).

Drug Dosage

Higher doses of antidepressants have been used in the treatment of OCD than those used in treatment of depression, although empirical data supporting this practice are scant. Some fixed-dose studies using SSRIs have found some advantage with using higher doses (S. A. Montgomery et al. 1993b; Wheadon et al. 1993), whereas others have not (Greist 1992). The tradition of using high doses of SSRIs must be supported by further research, although it seems reasonable to use higher doses in nonresponders or when only partial relief is attained.

Comparative Studies of Clomipramine Versus Selective Serotonin Reuptake Inhibitors

The introduction of SSRIs has raised the question regarding the comparative efficacy of CMI versus that of the SSRIs. SSRIs are important alternatives to CMI, because their range of side effects is clearly different (e.g., lacking anticholinergic side effects, sedation, weight gain). Although SSRIs may provoke nausea, headaches, and sleep disturbances, these side effects are usually less troublesome to most patients.

Fluoxetine was compared with CMI by Pigott et al. (1990) in 11 patients with OCD in a 10-week crossover study. Although no significant differences were noted regarding the clinical efficacy, the proportion of fluoxetine nonresponders who responded later to CMI tended to be higher in comparison with the CMI nonresponders who were switched to fluoxetine. Patients reported significantly fewer side effects while taking fluoxetine.

C. P. L. Freeman et al. (1994) compared the efficacy of fluvoxamine with that of CMI in a multicenter, randomized, double-blind, parallel-group comparison in 66 patients. Both drugs were equally effective and well tolerated, but fluvoxamine produced fewer anticholinergic side effects and caused less sexual dysfunction and more reports of headache and insomnia than did CMI.

The efficacy and tolerability of paroxetine was examined in a multinational, double-blind, placebo-controlled, parallel-group study with 399 patients with OCD (Zohar et al. 1994). Two hundred one patients received paroxetine (mean dose = 37.5 mg), 99 received CMI (mean dose = 113.1 mg), and 99 received placebo. Paroxetine was of comparable efficacy to CMI, and both were significantly more effective than was placebo.

Greist et al. (1995c) compared the results from the four large multicenter placebo-controlled trials of the SRIs: CMI ($n = 520$), fluoxetine ($n = 355$), fluvoxamine ($n = 320$), and sertraline ($n = 325$). Using the Y-BOCS as the primary outcome measures, the authors of this meta-analysis reported that all four agents were significantly more effective than placebo. Also, Greist et al. (1995c) found that a significantly greater percentage of patients treated with CMI were rated as much or very much improved in comparison with patients on the other treatments. However, the four studies summed in this meta-analysis had different subject characteristics, and this difference might have affected the results, as more treatment-naive patients (who are more likely to respond) participated in the CMI study.

OTHER PHARMACOLOGICAL APPROACHES

Anxiolytics

Because OCD is considered one of the anxiety disorders according to DSM-IV (American Psychiatric Association 1994) (but not according to ICD-10 [World Health Organization 1992]), it is not surprising that anxiolytics have been suggested for its treatment. Thus, alprazolam and clonazepam have been reported as efficient in several uncontrolled studies and case series (Hewlett et al. 1990; Tollefson 1985).

More recently, Hewlett et al. (1992a) reported in a small ($N = 28$), double-blind, randomized, multiple crossover study that clonazepam was as effective as CMI and superior to diphenhydramine (a control drug). However, more studies with large samples of patients with OCD are needed in order to draw substantial conclusions on this topic. Furthermore, because OCD is a chronic disorder, the use of anxiolytics for long periods raises questions of dependency brought about by benzodiazepine use.

Monoamine Oxidase Inhibitors

In an early study, Insel et al. (1983b) compared the efficacy of CMI with that of clorgiline, a monoamine oxidase-A inhibitor, in a controlled crossover study of patients with OCD. Although CMI was effective, patients on clorgiline did not improve at all. Vallejo et al. (1992) conducted a controlled clinical trial of the efficacy of CMI and phenelzine in 30 patients with OCD. The authors reported improvement in both groups; however, the lack of a placebo control and the small size of the study groups limit the applicability of these findings. Further studies on the therapeutic role of monoamine oxidase inhibitors in OCD, especially in OCD with comorbid panic disorder, are warranted.

Other Agents

The role of trazodone and buspirone has been studied in several open studies, as well as in a few controlled trials. Thus, Hermesh et al. (1990) reported improvement with trazodone in nine patients with OCD that was refractory to treatment, whereas Pigott et al. (1992b) did not confirm trazodone's efficacy in a controlled study ($N = 21$). Buspirone's efficacy was reported in only one double-blind study comparing it with CMI (Pato et al. 1991), but this efficacy was not found in another open trial (Jenike and Baer 1988).

PREDICTORS OF TREATMENT OUTCOME IN OBSESSIVE-COMPULSIVE DISORDER

Studies on predictive factors of response to therapy are relatively scarce (Alarcon et al. 1993). DeVeaugh-Geiss et al. (1990) reported that male patients and patients with a longer duration of illness were less likely to respond to CMI treatment. In a predictive study with CMI, Alarcon et al. (1993) studied the characteristics of 45 patients treated for a mean period of 18.6 months. Higher initial Y-BOCS score and cleaning rituals were predictors of poor outcome, based on multiple regression analyses. Other predictors of poor outcome included schizotypal personality disorder (DeVeaugh-Geiss et al. 1990); multiple Axis II diagnoses (Baer et al. 1992); baseline depression, overvalued ideas, and high avoidance (Cottraux 1989); and nonsuppression on the dexamethasone suppression test at baseline (Catapano et al. 1991). However, based on a larger sample (the multicenter CMI study), the abovementioned predictors were not confirmed and no correlation was found between baseline patient characteristics (age, gender, duration, and severity of OCD and depression) and outcome.

In a study of biological predictors of outcome in OCD, Hollander et al. (1993) assessed whether treatment outcome correlated with behavioral or neuroendocrine responses to challenges with the serotonergic probe m-chlorophenylpiperazine (mCPP). In this study, 16 patients underwent biological challenges before receiving CMI or fluoxetine. Worse outcome tended to correlate with increased prolactin blunting and with behavioral exacerbation on mCPP challenge. Thus, measures of serotonergic function may predict the response to SRIs in OCD. Altogether, additional studies on possible predictors of outcome in OCD are of awesome importance, and further research using sound methodology and large samples of patients is warranted.

SEROTONERGIC HYPOTHESIS OF OBSESSIVE-COMPULSIVE DISORDER

The serotonergic hypothesis of OCD is based on three lines of evidence: specificity of drug response, peripheral markers of the function of the serotonergic system, and pharmacological challenge studies with serotonergic agonists or antagonists.

Drug Response Profile

The serotonergic hypothesis of OCD was initially derived from clinical observations that pointed to the preferential response of patients with OCD to medications possessing a serotonergic profile. CMI and other SRIs have been demonstrated to be superior not only to placebo in OCD, but also to other antidepressants, such as the noradrenergic tricyclic antidepressant desipramine (W. K. Goodman et al. 1990b; H. L. Leonard et al. 1991; Zohar and Insel 1987) as well as nortriptyline, amitriptyline, and imipramine, with much of the same results (Ananth et al. 1981; Volavka et al. 1985).

MARKERS OF SEROTONERGIC FUNCTION

Cerebrospinal Fluid Studies

Thoren et al. (1980) reported a trend toward a higher level of 5-hydroxyindoleacetic acid in the cerebrospinal fluid (CSF), and Insel et al. (1985) found higher levels of 5-hydroxyindoleacetic acid in the CSF in patients with OCD compared with levels in psychiatrically healthy control subjects. However, Lydiard et al. (1990) failed to demonstrate significant differences between 23 patients with OCD and 17 psychiatrically healthy control subjects.

Blood Studies

Weizman and coworkers (1986) compared 18 nonmedicated patients with OCD to 18 sex- and age-matched control subjects. These nonmedicated patients had reduced levels of ^{3}H-labeled imipramine binding site density, which is related to the serotonin transport system. These findings were replicated by Marazziti et al. (1992), who also reported on lower ^{3}H-labeled imipramine binding sites in 17 drug-free patients with OCD compared with psychiatrically healthy control subjects. Bastani et al. (1991) compared 20 patients with OCD with 53 psychiatrically healthy control subjects and found significantly reduced affinity for serotonin uptake in the patients with OCD. However, in two large studies, these findings have not been replicated (S. W. Kim et al. 1991; Vitiello et al. 1991).

PHARMACOLOGICAL CHALLENGE STUDIES

Serotonergic Challenges

By focusing on dynamic changes produced by the introduction of serotonergic probes, challenge studies differ from the investigation of biological markers, which examine systems in equilibrium. In the challenge paradigm, the researchers exert a stress test to the desired system and then look for neuroendocrine and behavioral changes.

L-Tryptophan Challenge Studies

Addition of exogenous tryptophan increases endogenous serotonin synthesis (Barr et al. 1992, 1993). However, this does not necessarily mean that there is an increase in the activity of the serotonergic system. Charney et al. (1988) have demonstrated a small but significant rise in prolactin in response to an intravenous administration of tryptophan in 21 patients with OCD compared with 21 psychiatrically healthy control subjects.

L-Tryptophan Depletion

The effects of a short-term tryptophan depletion were examined in 15 patients with OCD who had responded to treatment with various SRIs such as CMI, fluvoxamine, and fluoxetine. These patients underwent tryptophan depletion under double-blind, placebo-controlled conditions. Reduction of tryptophan had no significant effects on either obsessions or compulsions, but mean depression ratings were significantly increased during tryptophan depletion (Barr et al. 1994).

m-Chlorophenylpiperazine

To date, the only serotonergic agonist that was associated with the provocation of brief exacerbations of OCD symptoms in some studies is mCPP, which possesses only weak affinity for dopamine, acetylcholine, and α_1-adrenergic and β-adrenergic receptors (Hamik and Peroutka 1989). The agonistic activity of mCPP is greatest for the 5-hydroxytryptamine (5-HT; serotonin) 5-HT_{2C} and 5-HT_3 receptor subtypes and to a lesser extent to the 5-HT_{1A} and 5-HT_{1D} subtypes (Barr et al. 1992).

The first controlled report on the use of mCPP in OCD patients came from Zohar and Insel (1987). This study found no effect on prolactin levels, but reported a blunted response of cortisol in patients with OCD. As for the behavioral effects, relative to the psychiatrically healthy control subjects, the patients with OCD became more anxious and depressed, and approximately half of the patients reported an acute, transient exacerbation of their OCD symptoms (Zohar and Insel 1987).

Another study that examined the effect of oral mCPP was performed by Hollander in 1992, who also reported on a transient worsening of OC symptoms in a group of 20 patients with OCD compared with 10 psychiatrically healthy volunteers (Hollander et al. 1992). Hollander et al. found no difference between patients and control subjects regarding cortisol, but prolactin response in the patient group was blunted in comparison with that of the control subjects.

Charney and co-workers in 1988 used intravenous mCPP and found no exacerbation in OCD symptoms, but noted a rise in anxiety and depression, significantly more so in the group of patients with OCD. They reported on a blunted prolactin response, but no difference regarding cortisol in female patients with OCD versus female control subjects (Charney et al. 1988).

The third study using oral mCPP was conducted by Pigott and co-workers in 1992. This group compared the effects of oral versus intravenous mCPP (Pigott et al. 1993). The most prominent finding was that, while using oral mCPP, no significant difference was noted between the two groups. In contrast, while using intravenous mCPP, a statistically significant rise in all behavioral measures—OCD symptoms, anxiety, and depression—was recorded.

To evaluate whether mCPP's behavioral effects in patients with OCD might be attributable to activity of serotonergic receptors, pretreatment of participants with a single dose (4 mg) of metergoline, 1 hour before mCPP administration, was performed. Metergoline is a nonselective serotonin receptor antagonist and is known to have an effect on 5-HT_{1A}, 5-HT_{1D}, and 5-HT_{2C} receptors. Indeed, the addition of metergoline abolished the behavioral and endocrine response to mCPP in patients with OCD (Pigott et al. 1991b, 1993). This effect was noted regardless of whether mCPP was administered orally or intravenously. Studies with medicated patients with OCD suggest that the therapeutic effects of SRIs are associated with a development of an adaptive downregulation of the serotonergic subsystems affected by mCPP (Hollander et al. 1991; Zohar et al. 1988a, 1988b, 1988c).

Other Probes

Fenfluramine, a nonspecific serotonin agonist, has been used as a probe with inconclusive results (Hewlett et al. 1992b; Hollander et al. 1992; Lucey et al.

1993). Its administration alone has not influenced OCD symptoms. Other agents, such as ipsapirone (a selective 5-HT_{1A} ligand) and MK212 (with affinity for 5-HT_{1A} and 5-HT_{2C}) have also not been associated with behavioral changes in patients with OCD.

Which Serotonergic Receptor Subsystem Is Implicated in Obsessive-Compulsive Disorder?

Because only mCPP was associated with an exacerbation of OCD symptoms, the differences in receptor affinity between mCPP on one hand and MK212 and ipsapirone on the other might provide us with important clues regarding the receptor subtype that may be associated with provocation of OCD symptoms. mCPP shows affinity for 5-HT_{1A}, 5-HT_{1D}, and 5-HT_{2C}; MK212 has affinities mainly for 5-HT_{1A} and 5-HT_{2C}. The chief difference between mCPP and MK212 is the 5-HT_{1D} receptor affinity. It would therefore suggest that the 5-HT_{1D} receptor subtype merits further investigation as a possible candidate for the mediation of obsessive-compulsive behavior in patients who have OCD.

ELECTROCONVULSIVE THERAPY

The literature regarding the role of electroconvulsive therapy (ECT) in OCD has been conflicting and confusing. Several case reports reported efficacy in individual patients (Mellman and Gorman 1992). In a study of eight patients with OCD who received ECT, only one had a good and sustained antiobsessional response (B. Guttmacher, personal communication, 1993).

Maletzky et al. (1994) reported their 12-year experience in treating patients with OCD who were refractory to treatment. The patients ($N = 32$) had received extensive psychological and pharmacological interventions before the initiation of ECT, but without apparent benefit. After ECT, most subjects showed considerable improvement on OCD rating scales and remained improved up to 1 year after ECT. Eight patients even exhibited short-term remissions (4 months) immediately after ECT. Eighteen patients maintained striking gains even at a 12-month follow-up. However, the patients received other treatments post-ECT, a fact that obscures ECT's role in the long-term improvement. The change in OCD symptoms was independent of changes in measures of depression (Maletzky et al. 1994). Thus, the authors suggested that ECT has a specific anti-OCD action, distinct from its antidepressant effects.

Despite these impressive results, it is important to note several limitations of this study: retrospective design, application of additional therapies after ECT, and lack of ECT measurements and of currently definitive objective instruments in the measurement of OCD and depression. In our opinion, ECT does not have antiobsessive properties, and our experience is in contradiction with that of Maletzky et al. (1994).

The unclear role of ECT, a powerful antidepressant in OCD, lends further support to the hypothesis that the antiobsessive response to treatment is distinct from the antidepressant response.

NEUROSURGICAL TREATMENT

Despite the progress in the treatment modalities, a substantial number of patients treated with drugs and behavioral therapy either do not improve or relapse. Some of these patients are candidates for neurosurgery, especially in cases of intractable disability resulting from the OCD.

Neurosurgical procedures in OCD include cingulectomy (or cingulotomy), anterior capsulotomy, subcaudate tractotomy, and limbic leukotomy (Mindus and Jenike 1992). In a retrospective study, Jenike et al. (1991b) examined the records of 18 patients who underwent a cingulotomy several years previously. The initial number of patients in this study was 33, but 6 were deceased (4 by suicide) and 9 did not agree to participate. Twenty-five percent to 30% seemed to benefit substantially from the procedure. One patient showed a 100% decrease in Y-BOCS score, and some patients showed slight to no improvement at all, and thus underwent a second procedure. Despite the occurrence of seizures (9%) and transient mania (6%), these results support the use of cingulotomy in disabling and refractory OCD.

In a prospective study (Jenike et al. 1991b) of 11 severely ill patients with OCD who underwent bilateral anterior cingulotomy, the researchers assessed the patient's condition before and 6 months after the procedure. Two of the patients improved more than 50%, four improved 25%–50%, and two were unchanged. One of the patients who improved more than 50% was assessed 1 year after the operation, and his improvement level had diminished to 15% from baseline. After the surgical procedure, some patients may gain more relief from the different treatment modalities that were previously ineffective.

Current neurosurgical techniques involve stereotactic surgery and permit a high degree of accuracy with fewer side effects. Thus, these procedures are rapidly gaining acceptance. Understandably, studies done in this field have several methodological drawbacks such as a lack of control patients, and small study groups. The availability of gamma-knife technique makes it possible to start double-blind studies, employing sham procedures. Currently, this controversial mode of treatment is reserved for patients with intractable OCD of several years' duration that has failed to respond to all existing interventions.

SUMMARY

SRIs have proven to be effective in OCD both with and without depression. Other treatment modalities, such as nonserotonergic antidepressants or anxiolytics, do not appear to be consistently effective. Despite the impressive progress achieved in the clinical management of OCD, several issues await clarification, such as the length of maintenance therapy, the role of behavioral therapy and pharmacological therapy alone and in combination, and the approach to patients who are nonresponsive to treatment. Also, further research is needed to differentiate nonresponsive patients into various subgroups and apply specific techniques for each group.

A good deal of the research so far has been on the serotonergic hypothesis of OCD. Results of challenge studies suggest a possible dysregulation in serotonin function, although the precise mechanism has yet to be elucidated. Further refinement in the dependent and independent variables used in probe studies and combining them with treatment and neuroimaging studies may shed light on this intriguing and probably heterogeneous disorder.

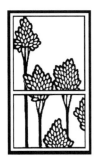

CHAPTER 31

New Approaches to Treatment-Refractory Obsessive-Compulsive Disorder

Wayne K. Goodman, M.D.,
Christopher J. McDougle, M.D.,
Matthew Byerly, M.D.,
Tanya Murphy, M.D., and
Herbert E. Ward, M.D.

Obsessive-compulsive disorder (OCD) is usually chronic, often debilitating, and much more common than previously believed. Not long ago, OCD was widely viewed as untreatable. The 1980s witnessed renewed optimism about the prognosis of OCD as new, more effective forms of pharmacotherapy (i.e., potent serotonin reuptake inhibitors [SRIs]) and behavior therapy (i.e., exposure/response prevention) were introduced and tested. Despite these advances, a substantial number of patients with OCD

This work was supported, in part, by National Institute of Mental Health Grant MH-45803, the state of Florida, and the state of Connecticut. We thank Donna Epting for her expert assistance.

remain symptomatic or show no improvement at all. Although the effectiveness of SRIs is well-established in OCD, between 40% and 60% of patients are nonresponders (Greist et al. 1995a). Even among "responders" to SRIs, the response is usually incomplete, with few patients becoming asymptomatic. In clinical trials, a 25%–35% decrease in mean Yale-Brown Obsessive Compulsive Scale (Y-BOCS) (W. K. Goodman et al. 1989b, 1989c) scores from baseline is often used to define the threshold for a categorical response to treatment. Although this degree of change may represent a clinically meaningful reduction in symptom severity, considerable room for further improvement remains.

In this chapter, we focus on medical approaches to the patient with OCD who is either a nonresponder or a partial responder to treatment with SRIs. (A review of the efficacy and use of SRIs in OCD appears elsewhere in this volume.) The current state of knowledge regarding the efficacy of these approaches is summarized and recommendations are proposed based on empirical evidence and the clinical experience of the authors. The role of behavior therapy alone or in combination with SRIs is mentioned, but a comprehensive discussion of this topic is beyond the scope of this chapter. The place of SRI monotherapy in nonresponders to behavior therapy is not addressed here, nor is evaluation of the adequacy of behavior therapy.

REASONS FOR SEROTONIN REUPTAKE INHIBITOR REFRACTORINESS

Different factors may account for the failure of a patient with OCD to respond to a potent SRI. First, the adequacy of the short-term drug trial must be evaluated. Was the duration of the trial too short or the dose too low? An example of an "adequate trial" would be 10–12 weeks of treatment with clomipramine, with a minimum mean daily dose of 150 mg for at least 6 weeks. Some (Wheadon et al. 1993), but not all (Greist et al. 1995b; Tollefson et al. 1994), fixed-dose trials of selective SRIs indicate that higher doses are significantly superior to lower doses in the treatment of OCD. In most cases, it seems reasonable to increase gradually up to the maximally tolerated dose (not exceeding the recommended daily dose) before declaring an individual patient a nonresponder. The anti-obsessive-compulsive (OC) efficacy of supramaximal (above-recommended) doses of SRIs has not been formally studied.

Some estimate of compliance is helpful in determining whether the trial was adequate, as indicated by drug plasma levels or pill counts. Drug plasma levels may also be useful in identifying patients who are rapid metabolizers. On the other hand, most studies have not found a direct relationship between plasma levels of SRIs and response of OCD.

Evidence indicates that certain comorbid conditions are associated with a lower treatment response rate. Patients with OCD who have Cluster A personality disorders (e.g., schizotypal) appear to have a relatively poor outcome (Baer et al. 1992; Jenike et al. 1986). Patients with OCD who have neurological soft signs may also do less well with SRIs (Hollander et al. 1990b). In contrast, most studies indicate that the response of OC symptoms to SRIs is generally independent of the presence or severity of coexisting depression (R. J. Katz and DeVeaugh-Geiss 1990; Mavissakalian et al. 1985). Another study suggests that the response rate to SRI monotherapy is lower in patients with OCD who have a chronic tic disorder (McDougle et al. 1993a).

By using a retrospective case-controlled design, treatment response to the SRI fluvoxamine was compared in patients with OCD with ($n = 33$) or without ($n = 33$) a comorbid chronic tic disorder. Although both groups of patients demonstrated statistically significant reductions in OC, depressive, and anxiety symptoms with fluvoxamine treatment, the frequency and magnitude of response of OC symptoms was significantly different between the two groups. A clinically meaningful improvement in OC symptoms occurred in only 21% of patients with OCD with comorbid chronic tics compared with a 52% response rate in patients with OCD without chronic tics. Patients with OCD with a concurrent chronic tic disorder showed only a 17% reduction in Y-BOCS scores compared with a 32% decrease in severity of OC symptoms in those patients who have OCD without chronic tics.

A careful differential diagnostic assessment should precede a drug trial. It is especially important to distinguish between OCD and the Axis II condition of OC personality disorder because little evidence indicates that the latter responds to pharmacotherapy. In devising a treatment plan, one should make the distinction between OCD as a primary disturbance and OC-like symptoms as part of the clinical picture of another disorder, such as autism (McDougle et al. 1992), mental retardation (McNally and Calamari 1989; Vitiello et al. 1989), or schizophrenia (Bark and Lindenmayer 1992; Fenton and McGlashan 1986). It is noteworthy that OC-like symptoms may indeed respond to SRIs in the presence of autism (Gordon et al. 1992; McDougle et al. 1990a, 1992) or mental retardation (Cook et al. 1992). Because it is unrealistic to expect all the primary and associated symptoms of the underlying disorder to respond equally well to SRI treatment, it is important to indicate which symptoms are being targeted for treatment.

The influence of an OCD patient's family environment on treatment outcome or long-term course has only recently become the subject of formal study. A family member's reaction can range from complete compliance with the patient's rituals to total opposition to the symptomatic behaviors (Livingston-Van Noppen et al. 1990). Clinicians have reported that either extreme response may contribute to an exacerbation of OC symptoms, posing a formidable countervailing force to otherwise effective treatment. In most instances, family members are advised to encourage the patient to resist his or her OC symptoms, but discouraged from extreme reactions to the patient's behaviors (i.e., either hostile opposition or performing compulsions on his or her behalf). The possible contribution of family factors to treatment resistance was explored in studies performed at Yale (Calvocoressi et al. 1995).

In one study (Mawson et al. 1982), the anti-OC effects of clomipramine were partially neutralized by instructing patients not to expose themselves to situations that would elicit OC symptoms. These antiexposure instructions contrast with the usual practice of advising patients to confront feared situations without performing compulsions. The impact of antiexposure instructions on outcome is more a theoretical than a clinical issue because most patients conduct self-exposure despite instructions to the contrary (Cottraux et al. 1989).

Even patients with apparently classic and uncomplicated OCD demonstrate a variable response to SRI monotherapy. Variability in drug response raises the possibility that OCD is heterogeneous with respect to pathogenesis. Accidents of nature furnish direct evidence for this premise. Numerous clinical reports document that injury to structures of the basal ganglia can be associated with the development of OC symptoms (Cummings and Cunningham 1992; W. K. Goodman et al. 1990a; Wise and Rapoport 1989). At present, however, one cannot rely on putative clinical subtypes of OCD to predict whether an individual patient will respond to SRI treatment.

SWITCHING TO ANOTHER POTENT SEROTONIN REUPTAKE INHIBITOR OR DIFFERENT CLASS OF ANTIDEPRESSANT

Although there is debate in the literature regarding the value of prescribing a different potent SRI after a patient with OCD has not responded to clomipramine (Pigott and Murphy 1991; Tamimi and Mavissakalian 1991), numerous anecdotal examples show therapeutic success with one SRI following failure with a different SRI, including clomipramine. Several different authors of literature reviews on the pharmacotherapy of OCD have advocated changing to a different SRI if there has been no improvement at all following an adequate trial with one SRI; if there have been partial gains, a combination treatment approach is generally recommended instead. However, we are unaware of any controlled data substantiating this intuitively appealing approach: whether partial responders do better than nonresponders to SRIs during a subsequent combination treatment trial has yet to be formally examined. A multicenter collaborative study should investigate this question to obtain the necessary sample size to achieve enough statistical power. Naturally, if the patient does not tolerate one SRI, it is advisable to try a different one, selected on the basis of expected side-effect profile.

Based on some intriguing case reports (Jenike et al. 1983), a trial with a monoamine oxidase inhibitor (MAOI) may be an option in OCD patients who have comorbid panic disorder. In a double-blind trial, both phenelzine and clomipramine were found to be effective in reducing symptoms in OCD, as reflected on two of four OC measures (Vallejo et al. 1992). None of the patients in this study had panic disorder. This study suggests that MAOIs may be helpful in some patients with OCD even in the absence of panic disorder. However, in an earlier comparison trial, clomipramine, but not the MAOI clorgiline, resulted in significant reduction in OC symptoms (Insel et al. 1983b). Additional studies are needed to evaluate the place of MAOIs (including the newer reversible inhibitors of monoamine oxidase A [RIMAs], such as moclobemide) in the pharmacotherapy of OCD.

Recently, several novel medications have been introduced for the treatment of depression, but their value in the treatment of OCD has not been established. Venlafaxine inhibits the reuptake of both serotonin and norepinephrine without affinity for muscarinic, histaminergic, or noradrenergic receptors (Nierenberg et al. 1994b) In an 8-week double-blind study of 30 patients with OCD, venlafaxine failed to show a significant advantage over placebo (Yaryura-Tobias et al. 1994). Nefazodone is structurally related to trazodone but has a somewhat different pharmacological profile and less propensity for inducing sedation (R. Fontaine et al. 1994). Early pilot studies of nefazodone in OCD were suspended because of apparent lack of efficacy (T. Pigott, W. K. Goodman, S. A. Rasmussen, unpublished data, 1991).

COMBINATION STRATEGIES: ADDING ANOTHER TREATMENT TO THE SEROTONIN REUPTAKE INHIBITOR

The patient who has had a partial response to SRI monotherapy or failed to show any improvement following two consecutive trials with different SRIs is a candidate for combination treatment.

Serotonin Reuptake Inhibitor Plus Behavior Therapy

It is believed that a combination of an SRI and exposure/response prevention is the most broadly effective treatment for OCD (W. K. Goodman et al. 1994), but support from double-blind, placebo-controlled studies is still sparse (see recent meta-analyses for review) (B. J. Cox et al. 1993a; M. A. Stanley and Turner 1995; van Balkom et al. 1994). In fact, few studies have adequately addressed the question of whether a potent SRI plus behavior therapy is superior to either treatment alone. The studies that have examined this question either have methodological shortcomings that hamper data interpretation or do not show clear advantages of combined SRI–behavior therapy over SRI therapy alone. For example, a leading group from England (Marks et al. 1980) studied the combination of clomipramine and behavior therapy in 40 patients with OCD who received 4 weeks of drug or placebo, followed by 3 weeks of behavior therapy for all patients, while clomipramine or placebo was continued. The authors found a large behavior therapy effect and a small additive effect of drug and behavior therapy. The brief drug-only period (4 weeks) may have resulted in an underestimation of the efficacy of drug therapy alone. Moreover, drug and behavior therapy were compared after 7 weeks of treatment, when the maximum effect of medication may still not yet have occurred. A study by a French and British team (Cottraux et al. 1989) found only a minimal anti-OC advantage of combined fluvoxamine–behavior therapy over fluvoxamine alone.

It is anticipated that the findings from a National Institute of Mental Health (NIMH)–sponsored study being conducted by investigators at the Medical College of Pennsylvania and Columbia University will shed light on the comparative efficacy of clomipramine plus behavior therapy, clomipramine alone, and behavior therapy alone. Apart from considerations of short-term treatment efficacy, other advantages to the combination of an SRI and behavior therapy may be found. For example, clinical experience suggests that concomitant behavior therapy may decrease the likelihood of relapse in OCD patients after drug discontinuation. Although our emphasis in this chapter is on biological approaches to OCD, behavioral therapy should be integrated into the overall treatment plan. For additional discussion of combined drug and behavior therapy, see the review by Greist (1992).

Serotonin Reuptake Inhibitor Plus Agents That May Affect Serotonin Function

To date, the rationale for most drug combination strategies has been to add to ongoing SRI therapy agents such as tryptophan, fenfluramine, lithium, or buspirone, agents that may modify serotonergic function. The addition of clonazepam, pindolol, or another SRI is also discussed in this section.

Adding tryptophan. Addition of tryptophan, the amino acid precursor of serotonin, has been reported helpful in a patient with OCD who was taking clomipramine (Rasmussen 1984), but ineffective in patients with OCD who were taking trazodone (Mattes 1986). Trazodone is a selective, but weak, inhibitor of serotonin reuptake (Marek et al. 1992). Adverse neurological reactions resembling the serotonin syndrome seen in laboratory animals have been reported when tryptophan is used in combination with fluoxetine (W. Steiner and Fontain 1986). At present, oral tryptophan supplements are not available in the United States because of evidence linking some of these preparations to the eosinophilia-myalgia syndrome, a serious and potentially fatal hematological/connective tissue illness (Hertzman et al. 1990).

Adding fenfluramine. Fenfluramine is marketed in the United States as an anorectic under the trade name Pondimin. In an open-label study, a research group from New York City (Hollander et al. 1990a) reported that addition of the serotonin releaser and reuptake blocker *d,l*-fenfluramine to ongoing treatment with various SRIs led to improvement in OCD symptoms in six of seven patients. Subsequently, other investigators (Judd et al. 1991) reported that two patients with OCD who were treated with clomipramine improved after addition of *d*-fenfluramine. *d*-Fenfluramine is thought to have more specific effects on serotonin transport and release than the racemic mixture, but only *d,l*-fenfluramine is marketed in the United States. Clinicians should be aware that administration of fenfluramine (particularly *d*-fenfluramine) was neurotoxic to 5-hydroxytryptamine (5-HT; serotonin) neurons in some studies of laboratory animals, including nonhuman primates (Kleven and Seiden 1989; McCann et al. 1994). Although there is no evidence that fenfluramine is neurotoxic in humans, this may reflect the difficulty in assessing subtle neurological changes in the living human. In animal studies, preadministration of an SRI appears to prevent fenfluramine-induced neurotoxicity by blocking entry of fenfluramine into serotonin nerve terminals (Clineschmidt et al. 1978). This suggests that SRI-fenfluramine cotherapy may be safer than fenfluramine monotherapy with respect to serotonin neuronal damage. Nevertheless, until the anti-OC efficacy of SRI-fenfluramine treatment is confirmed in controlled trials, we are reluctant to recommend this combination except in seriously ill patients with OCD with well-documented treatment resistance. A major side effect of fenfluramine is pulmonary hypertension and valvular disease, which were documented in patients using fenfluramine as a diet pill (Abenhaim et al. 1996). The patient should be advised about potential risks of fenfluramine before it is prescribed.

Adding lithium.   Coadministration of lithium is a proven method for enhancing the thymoleptic action of antidepressants in patients with depression (Heninger et al. 1983). Lithium has been hypothesized to potentiate antidepressant-induced increases in serotonin neurotransmission by enhancing presynaptic serotonin release in some brain regions (Blier and de Montigny 1992). The success of lithium augmentation in depression and the hypothesized role of serotonin in OCD has prompted studies of the anti-OC efficacy of this approach.

Lithium has been reported in individual cases to augment the anti-OC effect of chronic treatment with imipramine (T. A. Stern and Jenike 1983), clomipramine (Feder 1988; Golden et al. 1988; Rasmussen 1984), desipramine (Eisenberg and Asnis 1985), and doxepin (Golden et al. 1988) in patients with OCD. In a small open-case series, the addition of lithium to ongoing fluoxetine treatment reportedly led to an improvement in OC symptoms in three of four patients with OCD (Ruegg et al. 1990). In contrast, no significant improvement in OC symptoms was observed by researchers from NIMH (Pigott et al. 1991a) following 4 weeks of double-blind addition of lithium to ongoing clomipramine treatment, and only 2 of 11 patients with fluvoxamine-refractory OCD responded to a 2-week, double-blind, placebo-controlled trial of lithium addition to ongoing fluvoxamine treatment. In the latter study (McDougle et al. 1991), lithium was no better than placebo. Thus, on the basis of controlled trials, the efficacy of lithium addition in patients with OCD does not appear to approach the rate or quality of response that is typically observed when this strategy is employed in patients with treatment-resistant depression (L. H. Price et al. 1986). Although the overall yield is low in OCD, individual patients, particularly those with marked depressive symptoms, may benefit from lithium augmentation. In both the NIMH (Pigott et al. 1991a) and the Yale (McDougle et al. 1991) studies, there was some improvement in depression ratings with addition of lithium. That lithium augmentation seems useful in depression, but not in OCD, may reflect regional brain differences in lithium's effects on serotonin neurotransmission (Blier and de Montigny 1992).

Adding buspirone. In two open-label studies (Jenike et al. 1991a; Markovitz et al. 1990), addition of the 5-HT$_{1A}$ agonist buspirone to ongoing fluoxetine treatment in patients with OCD led to greater improvement in OC symptoms than did continued treatment with fluoxetine alone. These initially encouraging findings have not been corroborated by three subsequent double-blind trials (Grady et al. 1993; McDougle et al. 1993b; Pigott et al. 1992a). Together, these controlled studies suggest that addition of buspirone to SRI therapy is not an effective treatment strategy for most patients with OCD. It should also be noted that addition of buspirone to fluoxetine produced a paradoxical worsening of OC symptoms in one case report of a patient with OCD (Tanquary and Masand 1990). Although the SRI-buspirone combination is generally well-tolerated, there is a case report of a patient with OCD who experienced a seizure when buspirone was added to fluoxetine (Grady et al. 1992).

Despite these rather discouraging efficacy data, it appears that a minority of patients do experience some improvement in OC symptoms with combined SRI-buspirone treatment (Pigott et al. 1992a). It is the clinical impression of one of the authors (W. K. G.) that buspirone addition may occasionally be helpful in reducing OC symptoms in OCD patients with comorbid generalized anxiety disorder. Controlled studies with sufficient numbers of OCD patients with comorbid generalized anxiety disorder would be required to test the validity of these observations.

Adding clonazepam. The benzodiazepine clonazepam is not generally considered a serotonergic agent. However, evidence from studies in both animals and humans indicates that clonazepam may possess serotonergic properties not shared by other benzodiazepines (Wagner et al. 1986). For example, unlike diazepam, clonazepam will induce certain animal behaviors that are blocked by serotonergic agents but not by benzodiazepine antagonists (Pranzatelli 1989). In humans, the antimyoclonic effects of clonazepam are blocked by serotonin antagonists (Hwang and Van Woert 1979).

A number of clinicians maintain that addition of clonazepam to ongoing SRI therapy is helpful in reducing symptoms of OCD, but substantiation by published reports is scarce (Jenike 1990). In a single case of an adolescent with refractory OCD, a combination of fluoxetine and clonazepam produced a marked improvement (H. L. Leonard et al. 1994). Although existing literature furnishes limited support for the anti-OC efficacy of adjuvant clonazepam, it seems worthwhile to conduct additional studies with longer durations of combined treatment.

A controlled trial (Hewlett et al. 1992a), in which clonazepam alone was as effective as clomipramine alone, gives further impetus to investigating the role of clonazepam in OCD. However, apart from this study, most other evidence for the anti-OC efficacy of benzodiazepine monotherapy is limited to case reports (Bacher 1990; Bodkin and White 1989; Hewlett et al. 1990). Furthermore, this study (Hewlett et al. 1990) was subject to several design limitations. Treatment duration was brief (6 weeks), and high doses of clonazepam (mean = 6.85 mg/day) were used. It is not known whether patients would have begun to lose their response to clonazepam over a longer trial or if the marked side effects (which seemed to resemble intoxication) produced by high-dose clonazepam created only an apparent improvement in OCD. It is also likely that the efficacy of clomipramine was underestimated as a result of the trial's relatively short duration.

Until further studies of clonazepam alone or as an adjunct in OCD are conducted, the physician should use benzodiazepines sparingly in this condition. In our clinical experience, benzodiazepines may help secondary anxiety, but are rarely useful for the core symptoms of OCD; when they do seem to work, the anti-OC benefit is rarely sustained. Furthermore, a theoretical, albeit unproven, disadvantage of benzodiazepines is that they may impede the therapeutic effects of behavior therapy (H. H. Jensen et al. 1989).

Adding trazodone. In addition to weakly inhibiting serotonin reuptake, the antidepressant trazodone and its major metabolite *m*-chlorophenylpiperazine are active at a number of different neuroreceptors, including several serotonin receptor subtypes and α-adrenergic receptors (Marek et al. 1992). Several open-label reports suggested that trazodone may reduce symptoms of OCD when used either alone (L. R. Baxter et al. 1987; Haresh et al. 1990; S. W. Kim 1987; Lydiard 1986) or in combination (Swerdlow and Andia 1989) with an SRI. However, a placebo-controlled, double-blind trial failed to confirm the efficacy of trazodone monotherapy (Pigott et al. 1992b). In clinical practice, low-dose trazodone is often used as a sedative-hypnotic in conjunction with activating SRIs such as fluoxetine (Nierenberg et al. 1994a). Whether this combination confers any direct anti-OC benefit remains to be established in controlled studies.

Adding pindolol. Response to an SRI may be delayed by 10–12 weeks. To date, no approaches have been developed that hasten SRI response in OCD. To develop a rational strategy for accelerating or augmenting the effects of SRI monotherapy in OCD, one needs to consider recent preclinical evidence for why response to SRIs may be delayed. Studies in laboratory animals suggest that antidepressant-induced enhancement of serotonin neurotransmission does not occur immediately because of serotonin autoreceptor–mediated inhibition of firing rate and release. As these autoreceptors desensitize during chronic antidepressant administration, both firing rate and release recover, leading to a net increase in serotonin neurotransmission.

A research group from Spain (Artigas et al. 1994) hypothesized that addition of an agent, such as pindolol, that blocks somatodendritic 5-HT_{1A} autoreceptors might accelerate or augment the action of antidepressants in humans. (A general discussion of the pindolol strategy is found in Montgomery, Chapter 12, in this volume.) Pindolol is a nonselective β-adrenergic antagonist that binds with high affinity to the 5-HT_{1A} receptor (Hoyer 1988) and antagonizes the actions of 5-HT_{1A} agonists in animals (Tricklebank et al. 1984) and humans (I. M. Anderson and Cowen 1992; Coccaro et al. 1990b). Artigas et al. (1994) conducted an open-label study on the effects of pindolol augmentation of either SRIs or MAOIs in patients with major depression. They found that patients with major depression that was not treatment resistant ($n = 7$) responded rapidly, with latency periods of between 3 and 6 days in four patients with complete remission, 5 days in one patient with partial remission, and no response in two patients after 2 weeks of treatment. Patients with major depression that was treatment resistant ($n = 8$) were also studied. Five patients responded completely and one responded partially within 1 week, with two patients showing no improvement after 2 weeks.

In a recent report, pindolol (2.5 mg tid) was added to ongoing SRI treatment of nine patients with OCD who had not responded to SRIs alone (Blier et al. 1995). Four weeks of combined pindolol-SRI treatment had a clear antidepressant effect in patients with depressive symptomatology, but did not reduce severity of OC symptoms as reflected on the Y-BOCS. The authors posit that the observed dissociation between the effects of pindolol augmentation on depression versus OCD might be explained by regional brain differences in 5-HT_{1A} autoreceptor regulation of serotonin function. Neuroimaging studies have implicated the orbitofrontal cortex in OCD. That pindolol augmentation did not appear effective in treatment-refractory OCD is consistent with preclinical data showing that administration of pindolol does not inhibit serotonin release in guinea pig frontal cortex (Blier et al. 1995). Despite this negative preliminary study, further study of pindolol addition to hasten (rather than augment) response to SRIs in OCD seems warranted.

Combining Serotonin Reuptake Inhibitors

In clinical practice, a number of patients with SRI-resistant OCD receive simultaneous treatment with two potent SRIs. Apart from encouraging case reports of coadministering fluoxetine and clomipramine in adolescents (Simeon et al. 1990) and adults (Browne et al. 1993) with OCD, the efficacy and safety of this approach have not been subjected to rigorous examination. Because of the risks associated with fluoxetine-induced elevations in plasma levels of tricyclic antidepressants, caution should be exercised when these drugs are used concurrently (Rosenstein et al. 1991). Clomipramine's potential for lowering seizure threshold is of particular concern, making it advisable to measure clomipramine plasma levels before and after addition of another SRI.

Assuming that a therapeutic advantage of a combination of clomipramine and a selective SRI could be demonstrated, what mechanisms might be involved? It could be a pharmacokinetic effect: in that case, just increasing the dose of clomipramine (or selective SRI) should achieve the same net effect. It could also be related to some of clomipramine's pharmacological properties other than its effects on serotonin transport. The most likely possibilities include either the norepinephrine reuptake blocking effects of its metabolites or the mild dopamine (DA)-blocking effects (L. S. Austin et al. 1991). It is much more difficult to understand how a combination of two selective SRIs would act synergistically except to increase the degree of serotonin transport inhibition. Increasing the dose of a single selective SRI should achieve the same end as combining two selective SRIs. In the absence of new data, the only sound rationale for adding a selective SRI to clomipramine is the presence of side effects that prohibit further dose escalation of clomipramine in a patient experiencing some benefit on clomipramine alone (Simeon et al. 1990). Even so, side effects should be monitored carefully because interactions with the selective SRI may lead to increases in clomipramine levels.

Serotonin Reuptake Inhibitor–Antipsychotic Combinations

Conventional neuroleptics.   Conventional neuroleptics alone do not appear effective in OCD (C. J. McDougle, W. K. Goodman, L. H. Price: "The Role of Neuroleptics in the Treatment of Obsessive Compulsive Disorder," unpublished manuscript), but emerging evidence suggests that conjoint SRI-neuroleptic treatment may be beneficial in some cases of OCD (Delgado et al. 1990a; McDougle et al. 1990b). To date, the putative subgroup that has received the most attention has been OCD with a comorbid chronic tic disorder. This research has been based on the phenomenological, family/genetic, neurochemical, and neuroanatomical overlap between OCD and Tourette syndrome (TS) and the extensive preclinical literature documenting anatomical and functional interactions between the serotonin and DA systems in the brain (W. K. Goodman et al. 1990a; Leckman et al. 1995; Pauls et al. 1986). TS is a chronic neuropsychiatric disorder of childhood onset that is characterized by multiple motor and phonic tics that wax and wane in severity and by an array of behavior problems, including symptoms of attention-deficit/hyperactivity disorder and OCD. Conventional neuroleptics (dopamine-2 [DA_2] antagonists) such as haloperidol and pimozide have been the mainstay of treatment for TS (Shapiro et al. 1989).

M. A. Riddle et al. (1988) reported on the anti-OC benefits of adding an SRI to a neuroleptic in two cases of concomitant TS and OCD. Subsequently, Delgado et al. (1990a) reported on a young man with coexisting TS and OCD who showed marked improvement in his OC symptoms as well as tics when pimozide was added to fluvoxamine. Of interest, OC symptoms returned and tics remained suppressed when fluvoxamine was discontinued and the patient was left on pimozide alone. This case was followed up with an open-case series in which low-dose neuroleptic (primarily pimozide) was added to ongoing treatment in nonpsychotic patients with OCD who were unresponsive to fluvoxamine (McDougle et al. 1990b). Nine of 17 (53%) patients were judged as responders after combined SRI-DA antagonist treatment. Seven of 8 patients with comorbid tic-spectrum disorders or schizotypal personality disorder were responders, whereas only 2 of 9 patients without these comorbid diagnoses were responders.

Results from a double-blind, placebo-controlled study of haloperidol administration to patients with fluvoxamine-refractory OCD lend further support to the efficacy of this combination treatment strategy (McDougle et al. 1994). The fluvoxamine-haloperidol combination was significantly superior to the fluvoxamine-placebo combination on the basis of both stringent categorical response criteria and mean change in weekly Y-BOCS scores. Eleven of 17 (65%) of the patients who received haloperidol were responders, whereas none of the placebo-treated group showed a response. No significant differences were seen in plasma fluvoxamine levels between the fluvoxamine-haloperidol and fluvoxamine-placebo groups at the end of the 4-week trial. Thus, it is seems unlikely that the therapeutic action of haloperidol addition was mediated through pharmacokinetic effects.

The aforementioned study had insufficient power to determine whether patients with SRI-resistant OCD with comorbid schizotypal personality show a significant improvement after addition of neuroleptic. Despite the widespread clinical impression that neuroleptics are useful in treating OCD with psychotic symptoms, no controlled trials have been performed with this population. Further controlled studies with other SRIs are needed to confirm the findings of McDougle et al. (1994) and to better define the appropriate target population for neuroleptic addition. The prescribing physician should be wary about exposing patients unnecessarily to the risks of chronic neuroleptic treatment.

Atypical neuroleptics. Because of the limited effectiveness and safety of conventional neuroleptics in TS, clinicians have turned to a new generation of neuroleptics that have been introduced for the treatment of schizophrenia. Risperidone, a member of a class of antipsychotics that blocks both DA and serotonin receptors, has been established as superior to placebo and equal, or superior, to haloperidol in the treatment of schizophrenia (Chouinard et al. 1993; Marder and Meibach 1994). Risperidone has a more favorable side-effect profile than that of conventional neuroleptics and may have less potential for producing tardive dyskinesia. Compared with haloperidol, fewer extrapyramidal side effects are observed with risperidone in doses of 6 mg/day or less. As encouraging reports appear in the literature (Lombroso et al. 1995; Stamenkovic et al. 1994; van der Linden et al. 1994), risperidone is currently being widely used by clinicians to treat tic disorders.

Might risperidone earn a place in the treatment of OCD, particularly, TS-related OCD? Several brief reports suggest that risperidone might alleviate OC symptoms when added to ongoing SRI therapy. In a study at Yale (Tucker et al. 1996), one of three children with TS with comorbid OCD showed substantial improvement in OC symptoms when risperidone was added to paroxetine. McDougle et al. (1995), also of Yale, recently reported that three of three patients with primary OCD who were unresponsive to fluvoxamine alone showed marked improvement after risperidone was added to fluvoxamine. In a separate report of five cases with SRI-refractory OCD, addition of risperidone was associated with a 44% decrease in mean Y-BOCS scores (Jacobsen 1995). It is less clear whether risperidone reduces OC symptoms when given alone. A group from the Netherlands reported that three of five patients with TS experienced improvement in their OC behavior during risperidone (Lombroso et al. 1995). A shortcoming of this study, however, is the absence of OC-specific rating scales.

The prototypic "atypical" neuroleptic clozapine appears ineffective in both TS (Caine and Polinsky 1979) and OCD (McDougle et al. 1995). There is a positive case report in one adult with treatment-resistant OCD (C. R. Young et al. 1994), but negative findings in an open-label study of 12 patients with treatment-resistant OCD (McDougle et al. 1995). Clozapine, like risperidone, antagonizes both DA and serotonin receptors (Breier 1995), but it has a much lower affinity for D_2 receptors, a property that may be critical to tic suppression, and perhaps alleviation of OC symptoms in some cases of OCD as well. It is noteworthy that clozapine and, to a lesser extent, risperidone have been associated with exacerbation or induction of OCD in patients with schizophrenia. At present, 12 cases from six independent centers have been reported in which OC symptoms emerged during the course of clozapine treatment of patients with schizophrenia (Allen and Tejera 1994; R. W. Baker et al. 1992; Cassady and Taker 1992; Eales and Layeni 1994; B. Patel and Tandon 1993; Patil 1992). One case was reported of risperidone-induced OC symptoms in a 56-year-old man with schizophrenia who had initially presented with OCD at age 25 (Remington and Adams 1994). It has been suggested that emergence of OC symptoms in patients with schizophrenia who are treated with clozapine may be related to withdrawal from chronic D_2 blockade (R. W. Baker et al. 1992). Indirect evidence suggests that increased DA_2 activity may produce OC-like behavior in animals or humans (for review, see Goodman et al. 1990a). Alternatively, it has been suggested that blockade of $5\text{-}HT_2$ receptors might be involved (Dursun and Reveley 1994). It is of interest that coadministration of an SRI has been shown to reverse OC symptoms in cases of clozapine-induced (Allen and Tejera 1994; Cassady and Taker 1992; Kopala and Honer 1994; B. Patel and Tandon 1993) or risperidone-induced (Kopala and Honer 1994) OC symptoms—although some authors have had more variable success (Steingard et al. 1993). A 10-week open-label trial of clozapine monotherapy was conducted in 12 adults with treatment-refractory OCD (McDougle et al. 1995). None of the 10 completers was a responder. This study does not address whether conjoint SRI-clozapine treatment might be effective in some cases of OCD.

Novel and experimental drug treatments. A variety of alternative drug treatments have been used in OCD. Of those considered here, intravenous clomipramine is the only treatment supported by a reasonable degree of empirical evidence. Several open-label trials suggest that intravenous administration of clomipramine may be helpful in patients with OCD that is refractory to oral clomipramine (Fallon et al. 1992; Thakur et al. 1991; Warneke 1989).

Preliminary results from a double-blind, placebo-controlled trial indicate that intravenous clomipramine is safe, but helpful in only approximately 20% of patients (Fallon et al. 1995). A disadvantage of this experimental technique is its limited availability.

The α_2-adrenergic agonist clonidine has been found effective in suppressing motor tics, and an early report suggested that clonidine was helpful for treating OC symptoms in patients with TS (Leckman et al. 1991). One investigative group reported that a single dose of intravenous clonidine reduced symptoms of OCD, but cautioned that the apparent anti-OC effect might have been the result of clonidine-induced sedation (Hollander et al. 1988a, 1988b). Except for a few case reports of successful treatment of OCD with oral clonidine alone (Knesevich 1982) or in combination with clomipramine (Lipsedge and Prothero 1987), most published evidence points to the ineffectiveness of clonidine for OCD when used alone (Hewlett et al. 1992a; Hollander et al. 1988a, 1988b) or in combination with other medications (Jenike 1990). Moreover, clonidine seems to be poorly tolerated, with sedation prompting discontinuation in many patients (Jenike 1990).

Support is scant for the efficacy of anticonvulsant agents in the treatment of OCD (Jenike 1990; Joffe and Swinson 1987). If there is a role for carbamazepine in OCD, it may be in patients with clinical or electroencephalographic evidence of a seizure disorder (Jenike and Brotman 1984; Khanna 1988). The anti-OC efficacy of combined SRI-carbamazepine treatment has not been adequately studied. Sodium valproate was found ineffective in two cases of OCD (McElroy and Pope 1988; McElroy et al. 1987). However, one author has suggested that sodium valproate may be a useful pretreatment for patients with OCD who might otherwise tolerate SRIs poorly (Deltito 1994). The anticonvulsant clonazepam is discussed earlier in this chapter.

A paucity of empirical data exists on psychostimulants as a possible treatment for OCD. What does exist consists mostly of pharmacological challenge findings or anecdotal reports. An early report states that single doses of d-amphetamine induced transient improvement in obsessional symptoms in a group of 12 patients with OCD (Insel et al. 1983a). Another group, also using a challenge paradigm, confirmed that single doses of oral d-amphetamine reduced OC symptoms (Joffe et al. 1991), but found that oral methylphenidate had no overall effect (Joffe et al. 1991; Swinson and Joffe 1988). Another group of investigators found that intravenous administration of methylphenidate produced a worsening of OC symptoms in three of five patients with OCD (Lemus et al. 1991). In a study of hyperactive boys, a trial with dextroamphetamine was associated with production of compulsive behaviors (Borcherding et al. 1990). Numerous anecdotal reports suggest that recreational use of stimulants can exacerbate OC symptoms (Goodman et al. 1990a; Koizumi 1985), in some cases permanently (P. E. Frye and Arnold 1981). Discrepancies in the literature regarding the effects of psychostimulants on OC symptoms may be related to differences in dosing, route of administration, or clinical characteristics of the subjects. To our knowledge, the effects of chronic administration of psychostimulants on OC symptoms in patients with OCD have not been evaluated in a controlled trial.

An open-label case series described a significant reduction in OC and depressive symptoms during long-term treatment with the DA receptor agonist bromocriptine (12.5–30 mg/day) in three of four adults with OCD and comorbid depression (Ceccherini-Nelli and Guazzelli 1994). Controlled studies of bromocriptine in OCD are needed to determine the efficacy of this approach.

The possible role of hormones and neuropeptides in the treatment of OCD has begun to be explored, but preliminary findings are not encouraging. Four weeks of adjuvant triiodothyronine treatment was ineffective in 16 patients with OCD who had a partial response to clomipramine (Pigott et al. 1991a). Preclinical studies suggest that the neuropeptide oxytocin mediates a number of behavioral effects that may be related to OCD (Leckman et al. 1994), including inhibiting the acquisition of aversive conditioning (Insel 1992). Ansseau et al. (1987) reported a case of OCD in which 4 weeks of intranasal administration of oxytocin led to improvement in OC symptoms, but the side effects were profound, including memory disturbances, psychosis, and osmotic abnormalities. In a more recent publication, oxytocin was ineffective in reducing symptoms of OCD (Den Boer and Westenberg 1992a). In a small study of females with OCD, the antiandrogen cyproterone acetate seemed to exert an anti-OC effect, but it was not sustained (Casas et al. 1986). An attempt by another group to replicate this finding in a woman with severe OCD was unsuccessful (J. D. Feldman et al. 1988). Given the small sample sizes involved, further investigations of antiandrogen therapy may be warranted.

Addition of the steroid suppressant aminoglutethimide to treatment with fluoxetine led to significant improvement in a case of treatment-refractory OCD (Chouinard et al. 1995). The rationale for this approach was based on evidence that steroids contribute to the maintenance of the depressed mood state and that steroid-suppressant agents may be useful in cases of treatment-resistant depression.

It has been proposed that some cases of childhood-onset OCD may be related to the development of antineuronal antibodies triggered by a group A β-hemolytic streptococcal infection (Swedo et al. 1994). More than 75% of cases of chorea, the model for this putative subtype of OCD, have OC symptoms (Swedo et al. 1989). The Child Psychiatry Branch at the NIMH has collected a cohort of cases with a clinical profile that is compatible with an autoimmune process: abrupt childhood-onset of OC symptoms that are accompanied by adventitious movements, preceded by a streptococcal infection and followed by an episodic course. Various protocols with immunosuppressant agents or antimicrobial prophylaxis are under way. Preliminary data suggest encouraging experience with some of these approaches (Swedo et al. 1989). This exciting new avenue of research will undoubtedly be the subject of intense investigation over the next few years. Even if the efficacy of these approaches can be established in selected cases, it will be important to establish what proportion of patients with OCD have an autoimmune-related form of the illness.

NONPHARMACOLOGICAL BIOLOGICAL APPROACHES

Nonpharmacological biological treatments of OCD have included electroconvulsive therapy (ECT), neurosurgery, sleep deprivation, and phototherapy. ECT, regarded as the gold standard for treating depression, is generally viewed as having limited benefit in OCD (Jenike et al. 1996), despite sporadic reports of its success in treatment-resistant cases (Beale et al. 1995; D. A. Casey and Davis 1994; Husain et al. 1993; Khanna et al. 1988; Mellman and Gorman 1984). In some instances, the favorable response to ECT was short-lived (D. A. Casey and Davis 1994; Khanna et al. 1988). In a retrospective review, the authors examined the response to ECT in 32 patients with treatment-refractory OCD (Maletzky et al. 1994). Comparison of pre-ECT and post-ECT measures of OC symptom severity (as measured by the Maudsley Obsessional-Compulsive Inventory) revealed a significant improvement in OCD. As noted by the authors themselves, limitations of this report include its retrospective design, the shortcomings of the outcome measures, and the application of "unevenly applied and diverse behavioral, cognitive, and chemotherapies" during the post-ECT evaluation period. ECT should certainly be considered in the treatment of depressive symptoms in the patient with treatment-refractory OCD who is at risk for suicide. A sham-controlled trial of ECT in OCD (with and without depression) seems long overdue.

Past abuses of neurosurgery (sometimes euphemistically called psychosurgery) should not be forgotten (Stagno et al. 1994), but data emerging from the application of modern stereotactic surgical methods to patients with OCD should not be summarily ignored. Recent evidence suggests that stereotactic lesions of the cingulum bundle (Baer et al. 1995; Jenike et al. 1991b) or anterior limb of the internal capsule (Mindus et al. 1994) may produce substantial clinical benefit in some patients with OCD without causing appreciable morbidity. Nevertheless, stereotactic psychosurgery should be viewed as the option of last resort in the gravely ill patient with OCD who has not responded to well-documented adequate trials with at least two potent SRIs, exposure and response prevention, two combination strategies (including combined SRI and behavior therapy), and ECT (if depression is present).

Sleep deprivation had no overall beneficial effect on OC symptoms or mood in 16 patients with OCD (Joffe and Swinson 1988). Likewise, in one report, bright light therapy was ineffective in reducing severity of OC symptoms in a small group of patients with OCD (Yoney et al. 1991).

SUMMARY

In summary, despite advances in the pharmacotherapy and behavior therapy of OCD, a number of patients experience minimal or no clinical gains. The first step in approaching the treatment-resistant case of OCD is to determine whether an adequate SRI trial has actually taken place and to evaluate what factors may have contributed to treatment resistance. Options in dealing with the patient with SRI-resistant OCD include switching to a different SRI, combining another medication (or behavior therapy) with the SRI, considering novel or experimental drug treatments, or employing nonpharmacological biological approaches. A discussion of behavior therapy is beyond the scope of this chapter, but there is reason to believe that, in many cases, combined SRI and behavior therapy may be the most broadly effective treatment for OCD. How much more effective the combination is than SRI therapy alone or behavior therapy alone remains an active area of study and the subject of considerable debate.

Unfortunately, none of the SRI-drug combination approaches to treatment-resistant OCD can be viewed as firmly established. In the case of SRI plus lithium or SRI plus buspirone, encouraging open-label reports have been followed up by mostly negative controlled trials. The lack of a mean between-group difference should not completely overshadow the observation that some individual patients do seem to benefit from lithium or buspirone addition. Potential clinical indicators for adding lithium or buspirone to an SRI are, respectively, prominent depressive symptoms or generalized anxiety disorder. The proposed predictor for buspirone needs to be evaluated prospectively in a controlled trial. Both an open-label and a double-blind trial have shown that a combination of fluvoxamine and a neuroleptic is effective in reducing OC symptoms in patients with fluvoxamine-refractory OCD with comorbid tic disorders. The addition of a neuroleptic to an SRI should also be considered if delusional ideation is present. Addition of fenfluramine or clonazepam to SRI therapy may be worthy of consideration, but cannot be enthusiastically endorsed until more controlled trials appear. Several reports over a number of years suggest that intravenously administered clomipramine may have a place in the management of treatment-resistant OCD. ECT may have a role in the severely depressed patient with OCD who has been nonresponsive to pharmacological and behavioral approaches. The physician should be cognizant of current evidence regarding the possible role of stereotactic neurosurgery in severe refractory OCD.

Identification of meaningful subtypes of OCD and clinical or biological markers of those subtypes presents an important challenge for the future. Subtype markers may serve as predictors of treatment response and help in the selection of appropriate treatment. At present, years can be lost before the best fit is found between the patient and the treatment. Future research is needed to develop new and better approaches to the patient with treatment-refractory OCD.

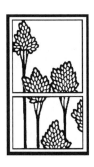

SECTION V

Cognition and Dementia

Juan J. López-Ibor Jr., M.D.,
Section Editor

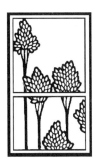

CHAPTER 32

Pharmacological Strategies for Cognitive Disorders: An Overview

Juan J. López-Ibor Jr., M.D.,
Pedro Gil Gregorio, and
Alfredo Calcedo-Barba Jr.

Cognitive disorders are part of the organic mental disorders. In ICD-10 (World Health Organization 1992), those are

> grouped together on the basis of their common, demonstrable etiology in cerebral disease, brain injury or other insult leading to cerebral dysfunction. The dysfunction may be primary, as in diseases, injuries, and insults that affect the brain directly or with predilection; or secondary, as in systemic diseases and disorders that attack the brain only as one of the multiple organs or systems of the body involved.

The spectrum of clinical manifestations of organic mental disorders consists of two main clusters. The first includes the decline in the various cognitive functions (e.g., attention, memory, abstract thinking, judgment). The second cluster is related to symptoms that are found in other psychiatric disorders and that also appear in patients with organic mental disorders. Table 32–1 shows organic mental disorders included in sections F00–F09 of ICD-10.

TABLE 32–1.   Organic mental disorders included in ICD-10

F00	Dementia in Alzheimer's disease
F01	Vascular dementia
F02	Dementia in other diseases classified elsewhere
F03	Unspecified dementia
F04	Organic amnestic syndrome, not induced by alcohol and other psychoactive substances
F05	Delirium, not induced by alcohol and other psychoactive substances
F06	Other mental disorders due to brain damage and dysfunction and to physical disease
F07	Personality and behavioral disorders due to brain disease, damage, and dysfunction
F09	Unspecified organic or symptomatic mental disorder

Source.   World Health Organization 1992.

To deal with the different disorders included in this section would be excessive; therefore, we focus on dementia in Alzheimer's disease (AD). Nevertheless, the less specific treatment options for AD are also complementary options to the usual treatment approaches for other forms of dementia or cognitive deficits in which etiological or more specific treatments may be useful (e.g., dementia in normal pressure hydrocephalus).

Cognitive deficits are only part of the symptoms of AD. Patients present other symptoms in different stages of the evolution of the disease: mood and behavior disturbances in early stages, paranoid and hallucinatory symptoms in middle stages, and predominantly full-blown dementia in the latter stages (Manzano et al. 1994). These various stages of symptoms should be considered when treating AD and patients with cognitive deficits. Therefore, in this chapter, we consider first the treatment of cognitive deficits and then the management of behavioral disturbances and other manifestations related to symptoms not related to cognitive deficits.

A specific drug for treatment of AD has unfortunately not yet been found in spite of the significant efforts carried out. The lack of knowledge of the main etiological and pathogenic mechanisms of AD and the lack of a sensible, specific, and easily accessible biological marker that could simplify the performing of clinical trials are the main determinants for the lack of an adequate specific therapeutic strategy. Therefore, the alternatives that we consider include (Gottfries 1992) 1) empirical pharmacological trials, which include currently available and possible future substitute and pathogenic therapies based on present knowledge, and 2) complementary psychopharmacological treatment to control accompanying behavioral symptoms. Other strategies are oriented to enhancing the psychosocial support of the patient.

SUBSTITUTE TREATMENTS

Substitute treatments are based on research that has found a metabolic reduction of several neurotransmitters in the brain.

Cholinergic Enhancers

Acetylcholine is the best studied neurotransmitter regarding its relation to memory and learning capability deficits. Cholinergic precursors and agonists have been used with poor results. A group with a large representation are the anticholinesterase drugs, mainly tacrine (Maltby et al. 1994; Roger et al. 1998; Rösler et al. 1999; Winker 1994). Another chapter of this book is largely dedicated to all aspects related to cholinergic enhancers.

Monoaminergic Enhancers

Noradrenergic neurons at the locus coeruleus and serotonergic neurons at the raphe dorsalis complex project to the brain cortex and may play a role in AD. Drugs that raise serotonin levels, such as imipramine or zimeldine or a noradrenaline such as clonidine or guanfacine, have been used in AD (Mohr et al. 1989). Again, another chapter of this book deals with this aspect.

The involvement of *dopaminergic neurotransmission* in AD has led to the use of agonists such as bromocriptine, lisuride, and pergolide, with poor results. A selective monoamine oxidase B inhibitor (MAO-B) such as deprenyl has also been employed. Little solid information exists on the effects of deprenyl on AD. Unfortunately, all information available comes from small studies. In a double-blind study, Tariot et al. (1987) observed that, with a daily dose of 10 mg in 17 patients with AD, a significant reduction in the scores for anxiety, depression, tension, and excitement was achieved. Burke et al. (1993), in a study of more than 20 patients with AD during a period of 15 months, found no behavioral changes in the progression of the illness nor in its scores.

L-Deprenyl selectively inhibits MAO-B and increases activity in the catecholaminergic system. In an initial placebo-controlled study, no cognitive improvement was found, but studies have shown an improvement in the performance in neuropsychiatric batteries in patients taking deprenyl. More studies are needed because milacemide, an MAO-B inhibitor, did not show any improvement in any of the psychometric batteries employed during a double-blind study of 225 patients with AD (Dysken et al. 1992).

Neuropeptide Enhancers

The alterations in the peptidergic neurotransmission present in AD are considered to be an epiphenomenon of the illness. An almost constant somatostatin deficit is observed.

Agents with a selective central action, an average long life, and easy trespassing of the blood-brain barrier are being developed so that the new neuropeptides may have a specific use for the treatment of AD. To date, vasopressin, adrenocorticotropic hormone, thyrotropin-releasing hormone, growth hormone–releasing factor, and somatostatin have shown no clear therapeutic benefits (Mouradian et al. 1991).

Opioid antagonists such as naloxone or naltrexone have also been used. In a double-blind study, patients with AD showed no significant improvement in the performance of tests or in neuropsychological batteries after receiving intravenous administration of 1–10 mg of naloxone. Consequently, there is no reason to use this drug in AD (Henderson et al. 1989).

PATHOGENIC THERAPIES

During the 1990s, several compounds have been developed whose actions on AD are based on pathogenic aspects such as the loss of neurons and peptides, the amyloid protein deposits, and immune reaction present in AD.

Action Over β-Amyloid Protein

AD is accompanied by the deposit of β-amyloid protein from the β-amyloid protein precursor (β-APP). Consequently, a pathogenic therapeutic action would be to act over the deposit of this protein. The present stage of our knowledge suggests four large intervention areas: 1) APP gene regulation, 2) modulation of APP turnover through interactions that stabilize the normal protein conformation, 3) development of strategies directed at the mechanism of the βA4 proteolytic release, and 4) the ability to block the aggregation and spread of the βA4 monomer or to solubilize the aggregated forms of βA4 (Whyte et al. 1994).

A change in expression of APP messenger ribonucleic acid (mRNA) has been shown to be affected by a number of potential pharmacologically active agents, including interleukin-1, phorbol esters, tissue plasminogen activator, nerve growth factor (NGF), fibroblast growth factor, retinoic acid, and phytohemagglutinin (Buxbaum et al. 1990; Yoshikai et al. 1990).

The βA4 peptide and an excessive amount of APP have proved to be neurotoxic. The accumulation of the βA4 peptide between synapses may be responsible for neuronal dysfunction and death (Schubert et al. 1991). βA4 could also modify the N-methyl-D-aspartate (NMDA) receptor, making possible the presence of neurotoxicity via the excitotoxin and calcium pathways (Mattson et al. 1992). Drugs that interfere with these pathways or alter calcium homeostasis have a potential therapeutic role.

The protease (APP secretase) responsible for the normal cleavage of APP through the βA4 segment is unknown, but a number of proteases, including calpain (D. H. Small et al. 1992), a serine protease, and cathepsin B (Cataldo et al. 1991), have been proposed. It remains to be determined whether therapy should be directed at enhancing the function of the secretase to accelerate the breakdown of the βA4 segment or at inhibiting the enzyme to reduce APP turnover.

Neurotrophic Agents

Neurotrophic factors responsible for neuronal survival, dendritic proliferation, and the activation of the different neurotransmission systems are present in the central nervous system (CNS). The most well-known one is the NGF, a peptidergic complex of 140 kd and with a sedimentation coefficient of 7s. NGF has three subunits, α, β, and γ. Subunit β is the active part of the molecule. Other neurotrophic factors (F. Hefti 1994) include 1) brain-derived neurotrophic factor (BDNF), 2) neurotrophin 3, 3) neurotrophin 4/5, and 4) ciliary neurotrophic factor.

The response to neurotrophin is the result of its capacity to stimulate specific receptors, protein kinase of the *trK* gene family, and the receptors with low-affinity NGF (p75 NGFR). Three specific genes compose the tr K family (*tr kA, tr kB,* and *tr kC*), which differ in their selectivity through individual neurotrophins.

tr kA receptor is linked to NGF and mediates the functional response of NGF. tr kB is linked to BDNF, neurotrophin 4/5, and less selectively to neurotrophin 3. tr kC is linked only to neurotrophin 3 (M. V. Chao 1992). p75 NGFR needs a previous signal of transduction (K. F. Lee et al. 1992).

In brains without AD, mRNA NGF is detected in granular cells of the gyrus dentatus and in pyramidal CA cells, as well as in diverse cortical neurons and glial cells. The cholinergic neurons of the basal ganglia not only require NGF for their development, but also all through their existence continue to express affinity for NGF receptors. These regions are also the main production areas of NGF in the CNS.

BDNF has a large distribution in the CNS but above all in the cholinergic and dopaminergic neurons. BDNF stimulates the differentiations of cholinergic basal neurons during development in a way similar to that of NGF. The mRNA of the BDNF in the hippocampus is present in a concentration 50 times higher than the mRNA NGF. The expression of tr kA is limited in cholinergic basal neurons, whereas tr kB is largely distributed in cortex and hippocampus (Hofer et al. 1990).

With age, the total number of NGF receptors in the brain are reduced in animals and humans. They are also slightly altered in patients with AD. The postmortem examination of cerebral tissue has shown a diminution of BDNF mRNA in the hippocampus of patients with AD. Several findings suggest that BDNF is able to protect some cholinergic neurons from degeneration, but this factor is specifically unable to regulate the specific cellular proteins. NGF increases strongly the acetylcholinesterase and the tr kA expression, which suggests that this factor not only prevents the loss of cells caused by damage, but also induces a hypertrophy of the cholinergic cells through the stimulation of specific cell protein synthesis (Knusel et al. 1992).

The loss of synapses and the formation of plaques and tangles are important factors in the pathogenesis of AD. A clear correlation between the synapse loss and cognitive performance has been observed. Some authors such as R. D. Terry (1985) have proposed that the physical basis for cognitive alterations in AD is the synapse loss observed in the neocortex.

If the functional deficit in AD is the result of neuronal and synapse loss, the ideal strategy would be to use techniques to reestablish neuronal and synaptic viability. In this sense, trophic factors are very promising. The positive results obtained in animal models of AD with brain tissue implantations with NGF and the memory enhancement and learning from laboratory animals treated with NGF have opened new windows to the possibility of the clinical use of NGF to treat AD. However, the potential benefits of the NGF may be counterbalanced by its capacity to increase the β-APP synthesis, consequently having an adverse effect in the progression of the illness. The increase of the APP synthesis may not necessarily affect all APP isoforms equally. The possibility of aberrant synapses and of alterations in the metabolism of the t- and β-amyloid protein exists (F. Hefti et al. 1995).

The administration of NGF not only prevents the retraction of cholinergic terminals in experimental models, but also expands its extensions with a concomitant increase in the number of cholinergic terminal varicosities.

Electromicroscopy of the presynaptic terminals of injured cortex treated with NGF shows a slight hypertrophy with an increase in synaptic differentiations of the membrane. The synaptic changes are larger and more pronounced in the cerebral cortex than in the cholinergic system. Biochemical changes have also been observed that indicate an improvement in the presynaptic functions of the cholinergic projections in the hippocampus and cerebral cortex.

Research in mice in which NGF receptor genes were altered through knockout techniques confirms a clear correlation between cholinergic neurons and NGF (Smeyne et al. 1994). Several animal studies indicate that the NGF administration could counteract the cholinergic atrophy and increase resistance to experimental insults. Hypertrophy increases the ability of cholinergic neurons to influence postsynaptic cells. NGF may attenuate the degenerative stage of surviving cholinergic neurons in brains with AD and improve their functioning. It has been shown that NGF has positive behavioral effects in older animals.

As a result of the poor penetration of the growth factor through the blood-brain barrier, an administration method for it has not been clearly established. Pumps have been employed for a direct release to cerebral spaces, but these pumps need invasive surgery. with associated risks and complications, which lead to ethical and medical problems (F. Hefti et al. 1989). Other approaches, such as the implantation of genetically altered cells that overexpress growth factors and the development of agonists or drugs that stimulate the production of the growth factor, are being explored.

AD produces changes in the olfactory mucus in initial stages of the illness, and the degeneration of the olfactory bulb produces a loss of the olfactory sense. The olfactory neuroepithelium is the only area of the body in which an extension of the CNS gets in contact with the environment (Hilger 1989). Some authors have demonstrated that biomolecules and small colloidal particles can be directly carried to the brain through the olfactory neurons avoiding the blood-brain barrier (M. T. Shipley 1985). It has also been shown that some proteins can be released through the olfactory pathway without its losing its biological activity (Thorne et al. 1992).

Receptor-mediated endocytosis may be possible because receptors have a high affinity for BDNF (Deckner et al. 1993). A linear relation between intranasal administration of ^{125}I-labeled NGF and brain concentrations of the compound suggest that this transportation is not mediated by receptors and that this releasing method of agents to the brain via olfactory nerves may be effective for many therapies (Frey et al. 1995). BDNF and the insulin-type growth factor (IGF-1) are currently used in clinical studies (Appel 1997).

In summary, this method is able to

- Overcome the need of the medication to go through the blood-brain barrier
- Direct the release of agents to specific brain areas affected by AD
- Decrease the systemic effects of drugs because a lower dose is needed
- Reach a high security level with few side effects
- Reduce the cost of the pumps and implantation surgery

Stress Oxidative-Antioxidant Agents

Free radicals (FRs) are highly reactive compounds generated in normal and abnormal metabolic mechanisms. Defense systems neutralize their toxic effects. FRs derived from oxygen are also formed during various physiological and pathological processes. One of the most active FRs is the hydroxyl radical formed from the superoxide and the peroxide of hydrogen by the Haber-Weiss reaction or originated from hydrogen peroxide in the presence of the cofactor (Fe^{2+}, Cu^{2+}) by the Fenton reaction. The main enzymes of the cerebral antioxidant systems are superoxide dismutase, glutathione peroxidase, glutathione reductase, glucose-6-phosphate dehydrogenase, and 6-phosphogluconate dehydrogenase.

It has been proposed that FRs influence the aging process and that they are implicated in neurodegeneration, which is present in senile AD. Increased levels of FRs in frontal areas and an increase of the oxidative stress in brains of patients with AD have been found (C. D. Smith et al. 1991). Although the role of FRs in the pathogenesis of AD remains unclear, the antioxidant or specific therapies directed to neutralize the toxic effects of these products may be beneficial, especially if the microglia is, as it seems, a great FR source.

A new line of drugs, the lazaroids, or 21-aminosteroids, seem to be a promising therapeutic alternative, interfering with the stage of propagation of the lipidic peroxidation (Braughler et al. 1989). The average life of a 21-aminosteroid is 90–120 minutes, with a total elimination in 4–5 days and a good penetration in the CNS. The positive effects of these drugs are the facilitation and recuperation of the cerebral blood flow and its neuroprotective effect against neurodegenerative processes.

Excitatory Amino Acids

An imbalance of excitatory amino acids and of calcium homeostasis or both have been implied in the etiopathogenesis of a large number of neuropsychiatric illnesses including senile AD. Glutamate is an excitatory amino acid of the

CNS but has excitotoxic effects also on the neurons. Glutamate has been implicated in the normal functioning of learning and memory and is significantly affected in cerebral regions and neurons that are severely affected in diverse neurovegetative illnesses. Glutamate receptors are of four types: 1) NMDA, 2) α-amino-3-hydroxy-5-methyl-isoxazolpropionate, 3) kainate receptors (KA), and 4) l-AD receptors.

Various exogenous or endogenous factors may act in different ways on glutamate through 1) activation of the different glutamate receptors, 2) increase in glutamate synthesis or in its release, 3) inhibition of glutamate reuptake, and 4) interference with glutamate-linked ion channels or enhancement of glutamate-linked second messenger systems (Horowski et al. 1994).

Several toxins may also alter the mechanisms that need the excitatory action of glutamate. Neurotoxicity mechanisms by excitatory amino acids can be of two types:

1. Sodium inflow and acute excitotoxicity. Neurotoxicity of excitatory amino acids is a direct consequence of the excessive excitatory depolarization—may be related to a loss of the ionic homeostasis and/or to a depletion of the energetic stocks of the cell (Olney et al. 1986). Neuronal damage could depend on the extracellular presence of sodium accompanied by a passive flow of chlorine and water (Hablitz and Langmoen 1982). Some considerations suggest that the acute excitatory swelling does not explain completely the damages induced by excitatory amino acids (Pulsinelli et al. 1982).

2. Calcium and late neuronal damage. Some toxins cause neuronal damage by medication by an excessive calcium entrance to the cell (Eimerl and Schramm 1994; Krieger et al. 1994). This mechanism has also specifically been involved in the neurotoxicity caused by excitatory amino acids. Calcium entrance occurs through receptor-operated ionic channels or indirectly by channels depending on voltage activation by the depolarization of the membrane. All subtypes of excitatory amino acid receptors open permeable sodium channels, provoking the opening of the membrane to voltage-dependent calcium channels. Only the NMDA receptor also opens channels highly permeable to calcium (McDermott et al. 1986); however, AMPA and KA receptors seem to do this, but less so, although studies reject this entrance way (i.e., Schousboe et al. 1994). In any case, neuronal damage mediated by glutamate mainly occurs in two ways: 1) rapid excitotoxic release resulting from a brief but intense stimulation of a high number of NMDA receptors and 2) slow excitotoxic release induced by a prolonged stimulation of AMPA and KA receptors (P. J. Shaw and Ince 1994).

Increase of free cytosolic calcium is toxic for various reasons. Among them are the diminution of ATP levels (Tsuji et al. 1994), the protease and lipase activation, and the FR production that causes a peroxidation of lipids. The inflow of calcium in the terminals could also increase the release of endogenous excitatory amino acids and propagate neuronal damage through positive feedback (Choi and Hartley 1993). Glutamic neurotoxicity mediated by calcium follows three stages:

1. *Induction:* Calcium, sodium, chlorine, water, inositol 1,4,5-triphosphate, and diacylglycerol levels are increased, which at the same time activate later processes (L. G. Costa 1994).
2. *Amplification:* Enzymatic groups such as protein kinase C, calmodulin, and calpaine-regulating enzymes (e.g., phospholipase) are activated. These changes give way to the long-term activation of neuronal circuits, which increase excitotoxicity.
3. *Expression:* The sustained high calcium concentrations pave the way for destructive cascades causing neuronal degeneration. Phospholipase, proteases, and FRs are activated, degrading neuronal membranes and causing cellular death (Babu et al. 1994).

The increase in glutamate activity may not necessarily be caused by neurotoxins and may be of metabolic or genetic origin. Other amino acids, such as those containing aspartate or sulfur, can also produce an excitotoxic effect. The hypothesis of the role of the excitotoxicity of glutamate in chronic neurodegenerative illnesses has been analogous to physiological events occurring during brain differentiation, in which a transitory increase of the postsynaptic glutamate activity plays an important role in promoting plasticity but can lead also to cellular death.

The relations between AD and excitatory amino acids such as glutamate are based on diverse findings:

- A marked and initial loss of long pyramidal neurons in layer II has been observed in the brain cortex. These neurons are predominantly involved in the corticocortical connections and probably use aspartic and glutamic acid as neurotransmitters (Maragos et al. 1987).
- Glutaminergic neurons are also found in large numbers in the hippocampus and entorhinal neocortex, where modified glutaminergic receptors are found.
- A reduction of the total number of NMDA receptors in the neocortex has also been observed, presumably related to pyramidal cell loss (Francis et al. 1992).

- β-Amyloid protein increases toxic effects of glutamate in neuron cell growth.
- A number of glutamate agonists including NMDA, kainate acid, quisqualic acid, and ibotenic acid, when applied locally, are able to destroy the cholinergic system.

It has been proposed that the agonists of the glutamate receptor can improve cognitive deterioration in AD. This idea is based on the high incidence of senile plaques and tangles in regions of glutaminergic innervation.

The noncompetitive antagonists of glutamate include phencyclidine, ketamine, *N*-allylnormetazocine, dextromethorphan, and dyzolcipine. The action of these compounds depends on the previous opening situation of the channel. Unfortunately, some of these useful NMDA antagonists have a narrow therapeutic margin. This could explain the contradictory results of studies.

In animal studies, NMDA antagonists have shown a capacity to deteriorate the long-term potentiation development in hippocampal neurons. On the other hand, drugs that facilitate the NMDA transmission have induced the long-term enhancement and improved learning.

D-Cycloserine is a central partial agonist of NMDA receptors in place of β-glycine, which in low doses has shown an antagonism of cognitive deterioration induced by scopolamine. Confusion, disorientation, and memory loss have been observed at high doses. D-Cycloserine can provide a symptomatic treatment of AD at low dosage (Bowen et al. 1992; B. L. Schwartz et al. 1996).

AMPA receptors are bound to the neurotransmitter glutamate, which prompts them to open a channel into the cell on the far side of the synapse, allowing sodium ions to flow into it. These charge-carrying ions produce an electrical current. If this electrical stimulation is high enough, it will enhance the opening of another channel by neighboring molecules, called NMDA receptors, whose effect is the long-term modification of the synapse found in long-term enhancement. By increasing the excitatory signal from AMPA receptors, aniracetam immediately became a candidate for boosting long-term potentiation in learning (Service 1994).

Anti-Inflammatory Drugs and Microglia

The proposed use of anti-inflammatory drugs to modify the course of AD is based on research of two kinds:

- *Epidemiological.* A study has described a reduced incidence of AD in patients with rheumatoid arthritis who were presumably treated with nonsteroidal anti-inflammatory drugs (NSAIDs) (McGeer et al. 1990). In another study, patients with leprosy showed a low incidence of AD when taking dapsone-type NSAIDs (McGeer et al. 1992). It is possible that the immune response and NSAIDs are able to affect the progression of AD when altering the APP production, induced by interleukin (Goldgaber et al. 1989).

- *Neuropathological.* Mature senile plaques are formed by dystrophic neurites and microglia cells. These microglia cells are phenotypically related to monocytes and express leukocytic markers and high levels of class I and II glycoproteins. They are also able to generate FRs, which may induce protease release. A large variety of plasma proteins are associated with an immune response strongly related to senile plaques. Although these data may be an epiphenomenon, it has been suggested that the presence of complexes attacking the membrane are evidence of a possible causal role of immune mechanisms (McGeer and Rogers 1992).

Rogers et al. (1988) found several antigens (HDL A-DR, a histocompatibility complex class II antigen) in AD associated with neuritic plaques. Other authors have detected C1–C4 compounds of the protein complements in senile plaques, neuritic dystrophy, and some neurofibrillary tangles. These inflammatory changes can be involved in the development of AD or can be a secondary response. The cells apparently involved in the antigenic expression are the reactive microglia associated with phagocytosis of immune complexes. Reactive microglia was the predominant inflammatory cell in the CNS.

NSAIDs may award a protective function in AD for their primary anti-inflammatory properties. Another potential mechanism involves the radicals. The salicylates, NSAID prototypes, reduce inflammation through the suppression of FRs such as hydroxil (Udassin et al. 1991). In a recent study (J. B. Rich et al. 1995), treatment with indomethacin showed a lower reduction in cognitive parameters, especially orientation, verbal fluency, and space recognition, after a year of treatment. Other drugs involved in the treatment were ibuprofen and naproxen; however, aspirin and paracetamol were not effective (W. F. Stewart et al. 1997). Celozib is an anti-inflamatory compound that selectively inhibits type 2 cyclooxygenase in the brain and is currently undergoing clinical tests to be used as a treatment of AD.

MISCELLANEA

L-Acetylcarnitine

L-Acetylcarnitine is a endogenous substance, synthesized in the mitochondria, that increases cellular oxidative metabolism and cholinergic activity. It has a good penetration in the CNS when administered orally and intravenously, and no side effects have been observed. L-Acetylcarnitine has a large variety of interesting pharmacological properties:

- It is a cholinergic agent because it promotes the synthesis and freeing of acetylcholine.
- It reduces oxidation processes, thus reducing lipofuscin deposits in the brain.
- It acts on the hypothalamic-hypophyseal-adrenal axis, antagonizing the existing downregulation (Carta and Calvani 1991).

In a 1-year study of 130 patients with AD (63 in treatment with L-acetylcarnitine and 67 with placebo), an improvement in the cognitive decline measured through neuropsychiatric batteries was observed (Spagnoli et al. 1991).

Nootropics

Nootropics facilitate the brain metabolism or neurotransmission by mechanisms not yet well-known. Nootropics may act on the transmembrane ionic flow as well as through an increase of the brain flow. Among other effects are an increase of glucose consumption in positron-emission tomography and an increase in phospholipid and RNA synthesis. Some nootropics also have a homeorologic and antiaggregate plaquetary effect. Piracetam, aniracetam, and oxiracetam among others belong to this group. Oxiracetam crosses the blood-brain barrier and fixes itself to the septum, hypothalamus, and hippocampus. Preliminary studies indicate that oxiracetam increases alertness and, as a side effect, produces anxiety (Itil and Itil 1986).

Drugs That Alter the Permeability of the Membrane

Included among drugs that alter the permeability of the membrane are phosphatidylserine, S-adenosylmethionine, and ganglioside extracts. Phosphatidylserine, produced from purified extracts of bovine brain cortex, alters the permeability and functionality of the neuronal membrane. A study with phosphatidylserine has shown a slight improvement in cognitive deficits in AD (Klinkhamer et al. 1990). The use of gangliosides as enhancers of the cholinergic activity has been postulated. Gangliosides seem to reduce the effects of damage in the entorhinal cortex and increase the cholinergic dendritic proliferation in the septum-dentate pathway.

Calcium Antagonists

The increase of intraneuronal calcium is related to degeneration and cellular death. Excitatory amino acids have been associated with calcium levels. In this sense, the blocking agents of the inflow of calcium to the neurons, which also produce a vasodilation, could have a therapeutic use in AD. Nimodipine, a dihydropyridine with a selective action on the vascular brain territory, has shown improvement in some psychometric batteries of patients with AD at 90–180 mg/day (Jarvik 1991). However, more studies with this drug are needed.

PHARMACOTHERAPY FOR NONCOGNITIVE SYMPTOMS

The great majority of patients with AD present symptomatologies that are not the direct expression of intellectual functioning but are similar to noncognitive symptoms observed in other mental diseases. Noncognitive symptoms that can be present in patients with AD include depressive episodes, psychotic symptomatology, and anxiety, as well as multiple disruptive behaviors. However, it is not clear if the moody behavior and psychotic symptoms present in AD are the manifestation of the same disorder present in psychiatric patients without a dementia (Raskind 1995). Affective and psychotic symptoms may be manifestations of comorbid processes with a common psychopathology, which could support the use and explain the effect of psychotropic medication to relieve the symptoms. However, as pointed out by Raskind (1995), it has still not been proven with sufficient reliability that the pharmacological treatments that we now have are as effective with noncognitive symptoms as with psychiatric disorders we use as reference. We now analyze the noncognitive symptoms that most frequently appear in dementia.

Depression

The main problem in the context of depression is to differentiate the symptoms as being from either the expression of dementia or the mood disorder itself. Psychomotor retardation, concentration difficulties, memory failures, and so on are frequent findings in patients with depression. This has to be taken into account in a careful differential diagnosis.

The studies carried out to measure the prevalence of depressive disorders in patients with dementia provide contradictory results; prevalence ranges between 0% (Reifler et al. 1986) and 80% (Wragg and Jeste 1989). This discrepancy can be explained, first, because it is known that the prevalence of depression in the elderly is not higher than that in the younger population. However, approximately 10% (Blazer 1994) of the elderly living in the community do present depressive symptoms, although generally these symptoms do not meet the criteria for a major depressive disorder. Second, it has been described that, in patients with dementia, a reaction of demoralization logically takes place because the patient is aware that the deterioration progresses irremediably. Whatever the cause, the prevalence of depression in dementia patients is very high (S. C. Newman 1999).

Studies of the treatment response raise more doubts. Reifler et al. (1989) studied a sample of patients with diagnoses of dementia and major depressive disorder. The sample was divided into two groups, and through a double-blind design the response to tricyclic antidepressants and to placebo was studied. A great improvement was achieved in both groups, but it was surprising to discover that no remarkable differences arose. The authors concluded that the improvement in both groups was not due to the therapeutic effect of tricyclic antidepressants. Other studies have shown that both tricyclic and newer antidepressants are effective in the treatment of depression in patients with dementia (Burke et al. 1997; Katona et al. 1998).

Psychotic Symptoms

Point prevalence of psychotic symptomatology in AD fluctuates between 30% and 40% (Cummings et al. 1987; Wragg and Jeste 1989). Psychotic symptoms may appear at different points in the course of the illness. Longitudinal studies (Drevets and Rubin 1989) have found that 50% of the patients with AD presented psychotic symptoms at least at one point in the course of the illness. However, many studies consider disruptive behavior as psychotic symptomatology, in our judgment erroneously, without taking into consideration if delusional symptoms are present. Verbal and physical aggression, wandering, shouting, and incontinence should not be considered psychotic symptoms in the absence of delusional or hallucinatory manifestations.

Devanand et al. (1989) studied the effects of haloperidol (3 mg/day) in a group of patients with AD who presented with delusions and hallucinations. With a double-blind design, these researchers showed that haloperidol was more effective than placebo for the control of psychotic symptoms. However, a worsening of the cognitive performance in patients treated with this neuroleptic was observed, and the extrapyramidal effects were also important.

In a similar study, Petrie et al. (1982) studied the effectiveness of haloperidol and loxapine in the same type of patients. The conclusion was that, although the improvement of the psychotic symptomatology was evident, the global improvement of life quality was not that evident. The authors suggested that the medication response in elderly patients with dementia and psychotic symptoms was much inferior to the one observed in young patients with schizophrenia. R. Barnes et al. (1982) carried out a similarly designed study and found an improvement in only one-third of the treated patients. However, that sample was oriented not only to psychotic symptoms (delusions and hallucinations) but also to disruptive behaviors in general.

In summary, we can conclude that antipsychotic agents are only slightly efficient for the treatment of delusions and hallucinations. The obtained therapeutic responses in studies carried out up to now reveal that the improvement obtained is less than that observed in young patients with schizophrenia with equivalent doses. Another important point, on which the great majority of studies agree, is the greater sensibility of patients with AD to extrapyramidal side effects. Raskind (1995) suggested that this results more from the pharmacodynamic features than from the pharmacokinetics of neuroleptics. It has not been proven that, at similar doses, haloperidol levels in blood are increased in elderly patients compared with levels in younger patients (Aoba et al. 1985; Dysken et al. 1994). In fact, some studies have found lower haloperidol levels in elderly patients (Devanand et al. 1992).

Atypical neuroleptics have a better side-effect profile, and several studies have confirmed their efficacy. Risperidone has been found effective in the treatment of dementia in patients with agitation (N. Hermann et al. 1998; Jeanblanc and Davis 1995; Jeste et al. 1996; I. R. Katz et al. 1999; Lavretsky and Sultzer 1998), in patients with Lewy body disease (Geizer and Ancill 1998), or in patients with L-dopa-induced hallucinations (Meco et al. 1994). Risperidone has better tolerability than classic neuroleptics such as thioridazine and haloperidol (Frenchman and Prince 1997). No studies of the efficacy of olanzapine in the treatment of agitation in patients with dementia have been done, but its use is widely advocated.

Disruptive Behaviors

We have already mentioned that alterations in behavior have been included among psychotic symptoms in many of the studies carried out. This is a questionable practice because it is not acceptable that wandering and agitation should be included in the same category as delusions and hallucinations. Jeste et al. (1998) reviewed the available literature on the treatment of agitation in the elderly. They found 37 studies in 1998 with different classic neuroleptics. Several substances have been used to control disruptive behavior, but none of the obtained improvements have been very significant. Coccaro et al. (1990a) compared the efficacy of haloperidol, oxazepam, and diphenhydramine in the control of aggression, wandering, and motor hyperactivity. The authors did not find significant differences, although they did find that haloperidol and diphenhydramine were slightly superior to oxazepam for the control of disruptive behaviors. In another similar study, Herz et al. (1992) also found that neuroleptics were more efficient than benzodiazepines. Clozapine has shown efficacy in the treatment of agitation in patients with dementia (Oberholzer et al. 1992).

Studies have been carried out with antidepressants, and trazodone is probably the most studied. These studies contained small samples, and no double-blind design was applied. The general conclusion of these works (Pinner and Rich 1988; D. M. Simpson and Foster 1986) is that trazodone at high doses (200–500 mg/day) helps to control disruptive behaviors. Slight improvement with buspirone was obtained in two studies carried out in small samples of patients with dementia and disruptive behavior (N. Hermann and Eryavec 1993; Sakauye et al. 1993).

The results obtained with anticonvulsants are controversial. The utility of valproate (Haas et al. 1997; N. Hermann 1998; Kunik et al. 1998; Mellow et al. 1993; Porsteinsson et al. 1997) and carbamazepine (Chambers et al. 1982; Gleason and Schneider 1990; Lemke 1995; Marin and Greenwald 1989; Tariot et al. 1987) has been studied. The results obtained suggest that carbamazepine can be useful in the treatment of agitation in demented patients.

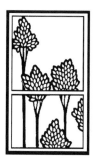

CHAPTER 33

Cholinergic Approaches to Cognition and Dementia

Klaudius R. Siegfried, Ph.D.

The objective of this chapter is to review the current status of research on the role of the cholinergic neurotransmitter system in cognition and dementia. Cognitive processes are central nervous system functions responsible for the acquisition, processing, storing, organization, retention, and retrieval of information or knowledge. Cognitive processes include functions such as perception, attention, learning and various memory processes, concept formation, language comprehension and production, problem solving, and other thinking processes (M. W. Eysenck 1984). Disturbances of cognitive functions represent the core symptoms of a subgroup of organic mental disorders, namely, dementia, delirium, the amnestic syndrome (amnesia), and hallucinosis. Evidence indicates that all of these four syndromes involve a pathology of the cholinergic system.

Cholinergic agents have been found to improve amnesia (Peters and Levin 1977). Both delirium and hallucinations can be produced by scopolamine, an anticholinergic drug, when given in high doses. Delirium has been shown to improve under physostigmine, a cholinesterase inhibitor (Powers et al. 1981). Most research activities dealing with the association of cholinergic function and cognition have been driven by the endeavor to find an effective treatment for dementia of the Alzheimer's type (DAT). Therefore, my focus in this chapter is on the effectiveness of cholinergic approaches in Alzheimer's disease (AD).

BIOCHEMISTRY AND PHARMACOLOGY OF THE CHOLINERGIC TRANSMITTER SYSTEM

Acetylcholine (ACh) has excitatory properties in most of the synapses in the central nervous system (Birbaumer and Schmidt 1991). ACh is synthesized within the nerve terminals from two precursors, choline and acetyl-coenzyme A, by the enzyme choline acetyltransferase (CAT) (Jenden 1987). Choline is of both endogenous and dietary origin (e.g., as lecithin). Acetyl-coenzyme A is derived from glucose and some other intermediates via glycolysis and the pyruvate oxidase system. Two main systems transport choline into the nerve terminal: a high-affinity system, which is dependent on sodium ions and adenosine triphosphate (ATP), and a low-affinity system, which operates by passive diffusion. ATP provides the chemical energy for high-affinity uptake. The high-affinity system controls the rate of the synthesis of ACh. Released ACh is catabolized and inactivated in the synaptic cleft by acetyl-cholinesterase and butyrylcholinesterase. The former is present in the central nervous system; the latter, mainly outside of it.

Two distinct types of cholinergic receptors differ not only in their stereo-chemical structure but also in their pharmacological properties (E. K. Perry 1986; M. Watson et al. 1987). One of these receptor types is stimulated by muscarine and blocked by atropine; the other is stimulated by nicotine and blocked by curare. Accordingly, they are called muscarinic and nicotinic receptors. Both receptor types have been found to consist of further subgroups (Bonner et al. 1987; Hulme et al. 1990; Sargent 1993; M. Williams et al. 1993). So far, five structurally different muscarinic receptor subtypes (M_1 to M_5) have been detected and pharmacologically characterized. They fit the cloned subtype proteins m_1 to m_5 (A. Fisher and Barak 1994). Nicotinic receptors have been classified into N-m and N-n receptors. Molecular biology techniques also have identified and cloned several potential neuronal subtypes of nicotinic receptors (Court and Perry 1994; Sargent 1993).

For the study of the association of the cholinergic system with cognition, two major cholinergic projecting systems are of primary importance. One of these is the rostral cholinergic column of the basal forebrain (nucleus basalis of Meynert, diagonal band of Broca, medial septal nucleus), which projects to neocortical and archicortical areas. The horizontal limb of the nucleus of the diagonal band of Broca provides cholinergic innervations to the bulbus olfactorius; the medial septal nucleus and part of the diagonal band of Broca project to the hippocampus. There are also cholinergic pathways from the nucleus basalis of Meynert to the cerebral cortex (e.g., orbitofrontal and temporal cortex) and the amygdala (Fibiger and Vincent 1987; Lewis and Shute 1967; E. K. Perry 1986). These pathways appear to be involved in memory functions. The second major cholinergic projecting system is the caudal cholinergic column of the mesencephalic and pontine reticular formation, which has projections to the interpeduncular nucleus, tectum, hypothalamus, thalamus, basal forebrain, and the medial prefrontal cortex (Fibiger and Vincent 1987). These pathways are part of the ascending reticular activation system (ARAS) that provides unspecific activation or arousal to the cortex and thus represents the neurophysiological basis of alertness, wakefulness, and attention (Shute and Lewis 1967).

ANIMAL AND HUMAN PSYCHOPHARMACOLOGY FINDINGS ON THE ASSOCIATION BETWEEN CHOLINERGIC FUNCTION AND COGNITION

Long before animal and human psychopharmacology studies had started with systematic investigations of the effects of cholinergic agents, clinicians described the impact of scopolamine on wakefulness and memory (Gauss 1906). When using scopolamine as a premedication for surgical operations, clinicians observed amnesia and an altered state of consciousness called *twilight sleep*. The latter is characterized by reduced alertness and narrowed awareness, that is, a state of impaired attention. Systematic experimental investigations of the effects of cholinergic agents in animals started in the early 1960s. Approximately 10 years later, the first human studies were carried out. Two basic techniques were employed. On the one hand, the effects of a blocking of cholinergic transmission were studied by using cholinergic antagonists, the centrally active muscarinic blocking agents atropine and scopolamine. On the other hand, the impact of enhanced cholinergic function was tested by using cholinesterase inhibitors, mainly physostigmine, or cholinergic agonists such as arecoline. A frequently recurring theme was the question as to whether cholinergic agents have a direct influence on memory processes or on attention.

Animal studies in rats and mice (for survey, see Holttum and Gershon 1992) have consistently shown an impairment in memory acquisition with higher doses of cholinergic antagonists when these were administered *prior to* learning sessions. When cholinergic agents were administered *after* training (learning), scopolamine was found to impair recall; and physostigmine, to improve recall. Effects were observed only when drug administration occurred shortly after memory acquisition. This suggests that the cholinergic system is also involved in initial stages of memory consolidation. No evidence exists for an effect on memory retention. When scopolamine was injected immediately *before* recall, it impaired memory retrieval. The first experimental trials with scopolamine in psychiatrically healthy human subjects confirmed these effects on memory processes. Scopolamine was found to produce an impairment of memory acquisition in recent episodic memory (immediate and delayed recall of supraspan tasks) and, to a lesser degree, also an impairment of category retrieval (i.e., from semantic memory), but had no effect on attention and short-term memory (e.g., digit-span task) (Crow and Grove-White 1973; Drachman and Leavitt 1974). Most of these conclusions were supported by further studies, as demonstrated by a review of 14 published scopolamine studies compiled by Kopelman (1986). Studies with cholinergic enhancers such as physostigmine and arecoline basically confirmed these findings in that they showed improvements of recent memory functions (Davis et al. 1976, 1978; Sitaram et al. 1978).

Although evidence clearly indicates that the cholinergic system is related to recent memory functions, the specificity of its involvement has remained an issue. J. A. Deutsch (1971) suggested the cholinergic synapse to be the site of memory. He assumed that learning and storing of memory traces were linked to increased cholinergic transmission and attributed weaker recall after a longer time interval to a gradual decrease of cholinergic activity. It appears, however, that Deutsch overestimated the specificity of the cholinergic system for memory. First, also other transmitter systems, in particular the noradrenergic and glutaminergic systems, seem to be involved in memory processes (Arnsten and Goldman-Rakic 1985; Zornetzer 1985). Second, evidence indicates that cholinergic agents also affect attention. Contrary to both early trials in human subjects mentioned above, Kopelman's review (1986) indicated that most studies that included measures of alertness and attention found not only memory but also attentional functions are impaired by scopolamine. A similar conclusion came from a review by Rusted and Warburton (1989). According to these authors, the maintenance of both focused attention and selective attention appears to be modulated by cholinergic activity.

More recent studies have not only challenged the early conclusion that the cholinergic system has no relation to attention, but these studies have brought into question the notion that the cholinergic system is not associated with short-term or immediate memory (Kopelman and Corn 1988; Rusted 1988; Rusted and Warburton 1988, 1989). Former studies had used only simple ("mechanic") short-term retention tasks such as the digit-span forward test. Rusted (1988) demonstrated an impairment of immediate memory by scopolamine when more complex short-term retention tasks were used that required a heavier information processing load. Examples are the concurrent performance of two simple tasks, so-called dual-task experiments, which require divided attention, or complex problem-solving tasks. Rusted and Warburton suggested that the differential effects of scopolamine on simple and more complex immediate retention tasks can be adequately explained if the traditional stage-model of memory (Atkinson and Shiffrin 1968) and its conception of short-term memory is replaced by the more complex model of (short-term) working memory (Baddeley 1986, 1992). Working memory is conceived to be composed of a central executive mechanism and slave systems, such as the *articulatory loop* (short-term retention of auditory information) and the *visuospatial scratch pad* (short-term retention of visuospatial information). The central executive mechanism controls the flow of information, maintains ongoing information processing, and allocates (limited) processing resources. It is implicated in tasks of holding, sorting, and processing information and also connects incoming information with retrieved information from semantic memory (in order to identify its meaning). Simple short-term retention tasks are performed solely by the slave systems; the central executive mechanism is involved to the extent that information processing is needed and processing energy has to be divided. Baddeley (1981) considers the central executive mechanism as a complex attentional system linked to short-term retention stores. Ample evidence indicates the involvement of working memory in memory acquisition, encoding, retrieval, language comprehension, reading, problem solving, and other thinking processes (Baddeley 1986).

From their findings of dissociative effects of cholinergic agents on simple short-term memory and complex information processing tasks, Rusted and Warburton (1988) concluded that the cholinergic system is associated only with the central executive mechanism of working memory. This explanation resolves the old issue of attentional versus recent memory effects of cholinergic agents. Additionally, it makes understandable why not only memory input (acquisition, encoding, initial consolidation) but also retrieval processes are associated with central cholinergic activity. For all of these activities, processing energy is required. Because more complex cognitive tasks require combinations of the above-mentioned cognitive processes, the working memory hypothesis of cholinergic function also explains the effect of the cholinergic system on so-called higher mental processes.

Neuroanatomical findings on the localization of memory and attentional functions fit with findings on the distribution of cholinergic pathways. The limbic cholinergic system (Lewis and Shute 1967) originates in the basal forebrain and projects mainly to the hippocampus and the amygdala. It seems to be involved in memory acquisition and consolidation processes. The other major cholinergic projecting system, which is part of the mesencephalic ascending reticular activation system and has projections to the limbic system and the prefrontal cortex (Shute and Lewis 1967), is important for wakefulness and selective attention (Birbaumer and Schmidt 1991). A connection between the hippocampus and the prefrontal cortex is likely to be the basis of working memory (Dunnett et al. 1990; Fuster 1989; Goldman-Rakic 1990; Granon et al. 1995).

CHOLINERGIC HYPOTHESIS OF GERIATRIC MEMORY DYSFUNCTION AND DEMENTIA OF THE ALZHEIMER'S TYPE

The central cholinergic hypothesis of geriatric memory dysfunction and DAT asserts that memory and other cognitive problems associated with aging and DAT are related to significant functional disturbances of the cholinergic neurotransmitter system (Bartus et al. 1982, 1985; Coyle et al. 1983; Davies 1981; Drachman and Glosser 1981; E. K. Perry 1986; Siegfried 1992, 1995a). Drachman and Leavitt (1974) were the first who formally suggested a relationship between cognitive aging and cholinergic dysfunction. When comparing the pattern of cognitive deficits in elderly people to that induced by scopolamine in psychiatrically healthy young subjects, they found considerable similarities. These findings were replicated in monkeys (Bartus 1980, 1981). An age-dependent impairment in recent episodic memory has been clinically described by Kral (1962) in his concept of benign and malignant forms of "senescent forgetfulness," and diagnostic criteria for "age-associated memory impairment" have been formally suggested (Crook et al. 1986). The concept of age-associated memory impairment appears, however, to be too narrow to be broadened into an "age-associated cognitive impairment," which would additionally include attentional and other cognitive deficits, for example, those described as impairments of "fluid intelligence" (Horn 1982). Although age-related reductions in cholinergic activity have been found to go along with cognitive aging, they are unlikely to account for all aspects of cognitive aging. Age-dependent reductions have also been found for the noradrenergic, dopaminergic, serotoninergic, and neuropeptidergic neurotransmitter systems (Carlsson 1981; Samorajski 1977; Zornetzer 1985).

The cholinergic hypothesis of geriatric memory dysfunction also relates DAT to a cholinergic pathology. This relation is supported by both psychopharmacological and pathological evidence, as described below.

Psychopharmacological Findings

A similarity exists between the pattern of cognitive deficits induced by scopolamine (sometimes referred to as *scopolamine dementia*) in psychiatrically healthy young subjects and the pattern of cognitive deficits found in patients with DAT (Davis et al. 1981). It has been suggested above that scopolamine-induced cognitive deficits are best interpreted as an impairment of the central executive mechanism of working memory. Baddeley et al. (1986) demonstrated that patients with DAT indeed showed a disproportionate disruption of the central executive mechanism of working memory compared with that shown by age-matched control subjects. Another finding indicative of an association of DAT with a cholinergic pathology is that scopolamine produces markedly more pronounced recent memory and attentional deficits in patients with DAT than in young psychiatrically healthy subjects (Huff et al. 1988; Sunderland et al. 1985). Several clinical studies showed that physostigmine was able to improve recent memory deficits and other cognitive symptoms in patients with AD. (For a survey of studies, see Thal 1994.)

Pathological Findings

Brain areas mostly affected by AD are the temporal cortex, especially its basal, medial limbic part (hippocampus and amygdala), the postcentral parietal region, and, to a lesser extent, the frontal cortex (Brun 1983). These brain structures are not only known to be associated with memory, attentional processes, and other cognitive functions (e.g., praxis functions) impaired by AD, but have also been found to be rich in cholinergic neurons. Pathology studies in patients with AD detected a selective loss of cholinergic innervations and reductions in cholinergic markers such as cholinesterase activity, the high-affinity uptake of choline into presynaptic nerve terminals, and CAT activity (Bowen and Davison 1986; Davies and Maloney 1976; E. K. Perry et al. 1977). Reductions in CAT activity were in the range of 40%–90% of the levels of age-matched control subjects. The decrease of CAT is likely to be the result of presynaptic degeneration of cholinergic neurons that originate in the nucleus basalis of Meynert (Whitehouse et al. 1981, 1982). Originally, no consistent reduction of muscarinic receptors was found. The picture has, however, become more complex when subclasses of these receptors were differentiated and a selective loss of M_2 receptors was found. M_1-type receptors appear to be largely unaffected (A. Fisher and Barak 1994). Also, the number of nicotinic central nervous system receptors in AD decreases (Court and Perry 1994).

Correlations of Cholinergic Deficits With Clinical and Pathological Findings

The cholinergic deficits described were found to be correlated with both clinical observations and pathological findings. The postmortem reduction of CAT activity correlates not only with measures of the severity of dementia (e.g., the Memory and Information Test and the Blessed Dementia Rating Scale) obtained from patients shortly before their death, but also with the histological hallmarks of AD, that is, the number of senile plaques (Blessed et al. 1968; E. K. Perry et al. 1978; White et al. 1977). Both the selectivity of the cholinergic deficit and its correlation with the severity of dementia were confirmed in vivo by cerebrospinal fluid analyses (Davis et al. 1982, according to Johns et al. 1983). Patients with severer cognitive impairments tended to have lower cerebrospinal fluid levels of ACh ($r = -0.79$, $P < .001$). In contrast, no significant correlations were found with the levels of metabolites of noradrenaline and serotonin.

CHOLINERGIC TREATMENT APPROACHES TO ALZHEIMER'S DISEASE

The consistent findings of cholinergic deficits in AD and their correlations with both pathological and clinical features have suggested cholinergic maintenance and replacement therapies similar to the dopaminergic treatment of patients with Parkinson's disease. Theoretically, an enhancement of cholinergic neurotransmission can be achieved in various ways (Davies 1981):

- Precursor therapy with choline or lecithin
- Treatment with cholinesterase inhibitors (e.g., physostigmine, aminoacridines)
- Treatment with (muscarinic and nicotinic) agonists
- Other types of cholinergic treatment (modulators of cholinergic function, nerve growth factor [NGF])

Precursor Therapy

The cholinergic deficit in AD is primarily the result of a presynaptic pathology that results in a decreased production of ACh. Therefore, it has been logical to try to compensate for that deficit by increasing the supply of choline or lecithin (phosphatidylcholine), one of the precursors of ACh. These attempts have, however, been largely unsuccessful. Bartus and colleagues (1982) found in a review of 17 lecithin or choline studies in AD that 16 had completely negative results. Thal (1994) came to a similar conclusion in a review of nine double-blind, placebo-controlled choline/lecithin studies. Some researchers have argued that the duration of these studies was too short to show a marked effect. However, a 26-week study yielded similarly negative results (A. Little et al. 1985). The reason for this outcome is most likely that not the availability of choline but the deficiency of the high-affinity choline uptake and the reduced CAT activity are the problem underlying a reduced synthesis of ACh in AD.

Treatment With Cholinesterase Inhibitors

The use of cholinesterase inhibitors has become the most successful approach so far. The first compound tested was physostigmine (Davis et al. 1981; see also López-Ibor et al., Chapter 32, in this volume). A review by Thal (1994) of double-blind, placebo-controlled physostigmine trials in patients with AD indicated that 11 of the 17 trials had obtained statistically significant effects on tests and scales of verbal and nonverbal memory tasks, but also, in one study (Muramoto et al. 1984) on a test of constructional praxis. Oral administration brought about more variable effects than individually dosed intravenous or intramuscular application. All of the trials of intravenous administration were short-term treatment studies (single doses). The duration of oral treatment ranged between 2 and 42 days. The results obtained were scientifically interesting but clinically unsatisfactory because the effects were only modest and short-lasting (approximately 1 hour) resulting from problems in the bioavailability of physostigmine and its short elimination half-life (approximately 20–30 minutes). An additional problem has been the small safety margin. Effects can usually be achieved only with doses just below the threshold to massive peripheral cholinergic effects (e.g., nausea, vomiting, stomach cramps).

One way of improving the therapeutic value of physostigmine in the treatment of AD is the use of slow-release forms. Some of these are currently in clinical development. The search for cholinesterase inhibitors with longer half-lives and stronger effects led to the discovery of the aminoacridines, tacrine and its major metabolite, velnacrine maleate (Davis and Powchik

1995; Siegfried 1995a). The results of the first clinical tacrine study published (Summers et al. 1986) looked so promising that the initiation of a large-scale tacrine development program in AD (Diagnosis of "Probable AD") appeared to be justified. The study was later criticized for its methodological weaknesses and biased presentation of results (Division of Neuropharmacological Drug Products 1991). Six ensuing tacrine studies with various methodological problems made their internal validity questionable. Five of these failed to demonstrate efficacy (Chatellier and Lacomblez 1990; Gauthier et al. 1990; Maltby et al. 1994; Molloy et al. 1991; Wilcock et al. 1993), and one had favorable results (Eagger et al. 1991). The findings of the three methodologically adequate tacrine studies (Davis et al. 1992; Farlow et al. 1992; Knapp et al. 1994) were considered sufficient by the U.S. Food and Drug Administration (FDA) to demonstrate efficacy. All of the four velnacrine efficacy studies rendered favorable results, but one of them was only a pilot trial too short for a convincing proof of efficacy (Siegfried 1995b, 1995c; Siegfried and Civil 1994). Efficacy was judged according to the so-called dual outcome criterion proposed by the FDA. This requires statistically significant effects over placebo on both a comprehensive performance-based cognitive assessment (e.g., the cognitive subscale of the Alzheimer's Disease Assessment Scale [ADAS Cog.]) (W. G. Rosen et al. 1984) and a clinical global impression of change rating (Clinician's Interview Based Impression of Change [CIBIC]) (Leber 1991) obtained separately from cognitive performance measures. Secondary outcome measures in the tacrine and velnacrine trials indicated that effects were also observed in everyday life by the patients' caregivers, for example, on caregivers' global ratings, the Brody Instrumental Activities of Daily Living [IADL] Scale (Lawton and Brody 1969), the Physical Self-Maintenance Scale (Lawton and Brody 1969), and the "memory" and IADL subscales of the Nurses' Observation Scale for Geriatric Patients (Spiegel 1989). In the 6-month United States velnacrine study, the time spent for various care services was found to be significantly reduced when the patients were taking velnacrine as compared with that when patients were taking placebo. Although these results are encouraging, the use of the aminoacridines is restricted by both safety and efficacy problems. Most noteworthy has been the occurrence of clinically important elevations of transaminase levels in 20%–30% of patients and of peripheral cholinergic effects (nausea, vomiting, diarrhea, stomach cramps). Although these adverse events have proved to be reversible on discontinuation of treatment, they are nevertheless a matter of concern and require careful and frequent safety checks.

Efficacy has been found to be limited to a subgroup of patients. With an improvement of at least four points on the ADAS Cog. as a response crite-rion, responder rates have been found to range between 40% and 55% ini-tially (i.e., after 3–5 weeks of treatment) and between only approximately 25% and 50% after a 6-month treatment period. When the number of re-sponders to placebo are subtracted from these figures, the proportion of "true biological" responders ranges between approximately 15% and 30%. Skeptics have been pointing out that even these figures give too favorable an impression of the therapeutic value of the aminoacridines because these fig-ures take into account only the study completers and ignore the high rates of premature treatment discontinuations. On the one hand, this seems to be correct, but, on the other hand, the validity of the four-point improvement in ADAS Cog. response criterion for the appraisal of the outcome of long-term treatment of a chronic progressive disease is questionable. A "no change" from baseline after 6 months or longer may in some patients reflect an impor-tant treatment effect.

The conclusion is that the aminoacridines have clinically relevant effects on core symptoms of dementia in a subgroup of patients with the clinical di-agnosis of "probable AD" and mild to moderate degrees of cognitive impair-ment. The effects seem to be of a symptomatic nature. Approximately one-third of the patients showed both a response to and an adequate toler-ance of the drug, but the size of the group with marked sustained effects ap-pears to be smaller, and this remains a controversial issue. Estimations of the size of the group of patients with marked sustained effects range from 5% to 30%. In view of such figures, skeptics of the aminoacridines consider their risk-benefit ratio as questionable; others have found it acceptable, provided that a dense schedule of regular safety assessments is observed. A final evalu-ation of the therapeutic value of tacrine needs more systematically obtained data on sustained effects after 1 or more years of treatment. The safety risks in "real life" need to be evaluated in large-scale postmarketing surveillance studies. The development of new cholinergic agents (see Giacobini and Becker 1994) that are devoid of at least part of the safety problems could help to increase the patient group that profits from cholinergic therapy and has a favorable risk-benefit ratio. Additionally, a marker for identifying po-tential responders to cholinergic treatment (e.g., apolipoprotein E4) would improve this ratio.

Treatment With Cholinergic Agonists

Treatment with cholinesterase inhibitors requires that at least a certain amount of ACh is produced by the presynaptic nerve terminals and released into the synaptic cleft. However, presynaptic cholinergic functions have been found to be compromised by AD, whereas postsynaptic muscarinic receptors in the hippocampus and neocortex are largely spared. Therefore, it makes sense to use compounds that directly act at the cholinergic receptors, muscarinic or nicotinic agonists.

The first muscarinic agonists tested in pilot trials in patients with AD were arecoline, oxotremorine, pilocarpine, bethanechol, and RS 86. With the exception of two studies of intravenous arecoline, which showed some mild but statistically significant effects in specific cognitive tasks (J. E. Christie et al. 1981; Raffaele et al. 1991), the vast majority of double-blind, placebo-controlled studies were unable to demonstrate treatment effects (Enz et al. 1991; Thal 1994). Partly this resulted from severe peripheral cholinergic side effects that led to many premature treatment discontinuations and made an efficacy evaluation impossible; partly this resulted from similar pharmaco-kinetic problems (bioavailability problem and very short elimination half-life) as those encountered with physostigmine. It also has been specu-lated that treatment failures may result from a receptor downregulation be-cause of the constant (tonic) flooding of ACh against receptors. However, the findings of Raffaele and colleagues (1991), who successfully tested the effects of a continuous 14-day infusion of arecoline on verbal memory in pa-tients with AD, cast doubts on this speculation. The unsatisfactory results obtained with the first generation of muscarinic agonists have led several re-search groups to develop agonists with improved properties such as a selec-tive affinity to M_1 receptors (which, in contrast to M_2 receptors, have been found to be spared in AD), a higher degree of lipophilicity (to achieve a greater split between peripheral and central cholinergic effects and thus have cognitive effects at doses that do not yet cause massive peripheral side ef-fects), a longer elimination half-life and longer duration of action, and no im-portant liver enzyme elevations. Some potentially promising candidates have been detected, such as AF102B (A. Fisher et al. 1994), PD 142505 (R. D. Schwarz et al. 1994), xanomeline (Bodrick et al. 1994), and milameline (CI-979/RU 35926) (Hoover 1994). These compounds have, indeed, some of the desirable properties listed but none seems to combine all of them. Xanomeline and milameline are currently already in clinical development and seem to have surmounted the first hurdles of clinical testing. If further studies can demonstrate efficacy and a more benign safety profile than the aminoacridines, these candidates could represent a real improvement over tacrine.

Another approach to improve cholinergic treatment could be the use of selective nicotinic agonists. So far, there are only a few studies in humans

(Newhouse et al. 1990; Sahakian et al. 1989). First results indicate that nicotinic agents primarily enhance attention. In some patients, they also have been found to increase anxiety. (For further information, see Newhouse, Chapter 35, in this volume.)

Other Types of Cholinergic Treatment

An enhancement of cholinergic function in patients with AD could theoretically also be achieved by using drugs that influence or modulate cholinergic function indirectly. The idea behind this approach is that these agents may be better tolerated, in particular, by being largely devoid of major cholinergic side effects. Another potential advantage could be that these drugs may prevent cholinergic neurons from an expedited exhaustion by exerting a weaker effect on them. However, the potential downside of this approach is the risk that the modulation of cholinergic function is not strong enough to produce clinically relevant effects. Examples of modulators are neuropeptides such as vasopressin and short-chained adrenocorticotropic hormone fragments (P. A. Berger and Tinklenberg 1981; Jolles 1983; Peabody et al. 1985; Siegfried 1991; Thal 1994). These peptides are known to partly coexist with classic neurotransmitters such as ACh and monoamines. The mentioned peptidergic agents were so far mainly tested in single-dose trials because they had to be administered intravenously because of their low metabolic stability. In general, the effects observed were mild improvements of attention not judged to be of clinical relevance. Another way of "modulating" cholinergic transmission is the use of serotonin subtype 3 or partial benzodiazepine antagonists. These were shown to have effects in animal models of cognition (e.g., Preston 1994). No published results of efficacy in AD are available, but the clinical development of representatives of these classes of agents has been discontinued.

A quite different cholinergic treatment approach is based on the use of neurotrophic factors. Among these, NGF is best characterized and has been demonstrated to affect cholinergic neurons of the medial septal/diagonal band complex, the nucleus basalis of Meynert, and the hippocampus (I. Hefti 1986). These findings have been suggestive of using NGF in the treatment of AD. NGF stimulation could have neuroprotective effects by exerting trophic effects on surviving cholinergic neurons. Because NGF is a large protein molecule that does not pass the blood-brain barrier, intracerebroventricular infusions are required. First clinical trials using this method in patients with AD brought about only very modest effects on cognition (Olson et al. 1992), but experience is so far too limited to justify a final conclusion.

PROSPECTS AND LIMITATIONS OF THE CHOLINERGIC TREATMENT APPROACH

The overall conclusion is that the cholinergic neurotransmitter system plays an important but not exclusive role in cognitive functioning. The cholinergic neurotransmitter system is primarily associated with sustained and selective attention, recent memory acquisition, encoding, and (initial) consolidation processes and is partly associated with retrieval from long-term memory. The multiple cognitive disorders resulting from deficiencies of the central cholinergic system seem to be best explained by the assumption of an impairment of the central executive mechanism of working memory. The latter has been demonstrated to be involved in all complex and demanding cognitive processes. A pathology of the central executive mechanism would therefore result not only in problems of memory acquisition, consolidation, and retrieval, but also in disturbances of language comprehension, speech, judgment, reasoning, and problem-solving processes.

A cholinergic maintenance and replacement therapy in patients with DAT can bring about a clinically relevant improvement or suppression of cognitive core symptoms. However, because of their unfavorable safety profile, the aminoacridines are unlikely to show the full potential of a cholinergic treatment. Therefore, further improvement of cholinergic compounds that cause no liver enzyme elevations and have fewer peripheral cholinergic side effects is needed. However, the cholinergic system is not the only transmitter system associated with cognition, and neuropathological evidence indicates that other neurotransmitters are compromised in AD, in particular the noradrenergic and the serotoninergic systems (Chan-Palay and Asan 1989; Geula and Mesulam 1994). Therefore, even cholinergic agents with more favorable safety profiles than that of tacrine will have a limited efficacy in AD. A larger subgroup of patients is likely to show only a moderate improvement or no response. This group may need simultaneous treatment of several neurotransmitter deficits.

It has been speculated (Nitsch and Growden 1994) that muscarinic M_1 agonists could influence the regulation of β-amyloid protein precursor processing. Provided that the amyloid cascade hypothesis of AD is a correct assumption of the etiology of AD (Cotman and Pike 1994), this would mean that cholinergic compounds have not only symptomatic effects but also an influence on the disease process. So far, however, this has not yet been clinically demonstrated. Unless such effects can be shown, it would be useful to think of a combination treatment of a cholinergic therapy with a drug that can alter the progression of the disease.

Because of the important role of the cholinergic system in cognition, other syndromes of cognitive deficits, including dementias of origins other than AD, may profit from cholinergic treatment. Delirium, the amnestic syndrome, and hallucinosis have already been mentioned as candidates. Because significant reductions of cortical CAT were also found in other types of dementia, such as Down syndrome, Parkinson's disease dementia, Gerstmann-Sträussler-Sheinker syndrome, and alcoholic dementia (E. K. Perry 1986), these also might prove to be alleviated by cholinergic therapy.

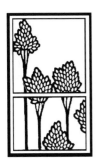

CHAPTER 34

Serotonin Mechanisms and Cognition

Brenda Costall, M.D., and
Robert J. Naylor, M.D.

If serotonin (5-hydroxytryptamine; 5-HT) receptors evolved to mediate the effects of serotonin, then it would appear that serotonin has been in existence from almost the very beginnings of life. In their fascinating commentary on the molecular evolution of G protein–coupled receptors, Peroutka and Howell (1994) suggested that a primordial serotonin receptor commenced its long and tortuous differentiation into numerous receptor subtypes some 800 million years ago. Indeed, on the basis of receptor homology, these researchers went further and suggested that all biogenic amine receptors might be considered direct descendants of the primordial serotonin receptor. In any event, the lowest life form found to possess G protein–coupled serotonin receptors is *Planaria* (Venter et al. 1988), and it is predicted that their subsequent evolution has endowed invertebrates and vertebrates with multiple serotonin receptor subtypes.

Given the pivotal evolutionary role of the serotonin receptor, it is not surprising that the serotonin receptor has evolved numerous and diverse roles, and the mammalian receptors are known to be involved in sleep, mood, sexual activity, temperature, and motor, endocrine, trophic, developmental, and other roles, including cognition. Such functions are not exclusive. Drugs acting on serotonin receptors have a well-established role to moderate hormone release (e.g., growth hormone, prolactin, adrenocorticotropic hormone, cortisol), which may have widespread functions to moderate neuronal activity and cognition and also to regulate serotonin synthesis and release. Such in-

535

teractions are beyond the scope of this chapter (see Cowen 1992; DeKloet et al. 1982; H. Y. Meltzer 1990; D. L. Murphy et al. 1992). Cognitive events also involve developmental and trophic influences exerted by serotonin, and not merely in higher species. It is salutary to consider that the serotonin-induced long-term facilitation of synaptic efficiency in dissociated cell cultures of sensory and motor neurons of Aplysia is accompanied by new synaptic connections and a downregulation in the sensory neuron of cell adhesion molecules (Bailey et al. 1992). Furthermore, in a comparison of the effects of serotonin in juvenile and adult Aplysia sensory neurons, the effects of serotonin were dissociated in two functional classes, those that contribute differentially to short- and long-term synaptic plasticity in adults and those that emerge differentially during development (Emptage et al. 1994). The authors proposed that, early in development, one class of mechanisms mediates structural changes and is retained to subserve long-term memory in the adult, whereas the second mechanism develops late and contributes to short-term memory. The role of serotonin in the development of different forms of memory, neuromodulation, and protein synthesis in memory storage is discussed by K. C. Martin et al. (1997) and Marcus and Carew (1998).

Our understanding of cognitive events has progressed most rapidly in mammals, in which knowledge includes a wealth of activities, including attention and sensory gating; recognition and interpretation; and the encoding, storage, and retrieval of information. The coherence of such activities permits learning and memory. These many and varied processes probably involve numerous neurotransmitters, with the potential for dysfunction in many systems. Therefore, it is not surprising that cognitive disorders in humans arise in an array of illnesses, with presumably different etiologies, for example, depression, anxiety, schizophrenia, Huntington's chorea, subcortical dementias, and Alzheimer's disease. Study of some of these disorders has provided major working hypotheses for brain systems and neurotransmitter mechanisms that may be relevant to cognitive processing. For example, identification of the destruction of the forebrain cholinergic projection in Alzheimer's disease provided a major emphasis of the importance of the cholinergic system in learning and memory and as a site of drug action to attenuate the disorder (Bartus et al. 1982; E. K. Perry 1986).

The basis of any drug treatment for such disorders requires the presence of a residual physiological function that may subserve a site of action. In this chapter, we review the evidence that serotonin systems are important for cognition and that serotonin receptor ligands acting on serotonin receptor subtypes may modify cognitive processing. The serotonergic receptor families are reviewed elsewhere (Hoyer et al. 1994).

INHIBITION OF NEUROTRANSMITTER RELEASE BY PRESYNAPTIC SEROTONIN HETERORECEPTORS

Inhibitory $5\text{-}HT_1$ heteroreceptors have been located on cholinergic and glutaminergic neurons in the striatum, hippocampus, and cerebellum. Dopamine release in the striatum or nucleus accumbens of the rat brain is either inhibited (via an unspecified serotonin receptor) or enhanced via a $5\text{-}HT_3$ receptor stimulation. Serotonin did not inhibit noradrenaline release from rat cortical slices (see review by Göthert 1991). Evidence that serotonin receptor stimulation may reduce acetylcholine (ACh) release in rat striatal, hippocampal, or cortical slices came initially from two observations: that serotonin agonists can reduce release and that inhibition of the synthesis of serotonin or destruction of the serotonin neuron can enhance ACh release (Gillett et al. 1985; Jackson et al. 1988; S. E. Robinson 1983; Vizi et al. 1981). A characterization of the receptor mechanisms mediating the changes in ACh release has revealed a more complex situation. Using slices of rat entorhinal cortex, serotonin or the $5\text{-}HT_3$ receptor agonist 2-methyl-5-HT, when administered alone, failed to modify potassium-stimulated ACh release (J. M. Barnes et al. 1989). However, in the presence of the $5\text{-}HT_{2A/2B/2C}$ receptor antagonist ritanserin, 2-methyl-5-HT reduced ACh release, a reduction that was blocked by cotreatment with the $5\text{-}HT_3$ receptor antagonist ondansetron. Conversely, in the presence of ondansetron alone, 2-methyl-5-HT increased ACh release, the latter increase being blocked by ritanserin. This was interpreted as the potential of serotonin agonists to mediate an increase in ACh release, via a $5\text{-}HT_2$ receptor mechanism, and an inhibition of ACh release, via a $5\text{-}HT_3$ receptor. The latter action may be mediated via the release of an inhibitory neurotransmitter, for example, γ-aminobutyric acid (GABA), from an interneuron.

The presence of a $5\text{-}HT_3$ receptor mediating (indirectly?) an inhibition of ACh release has also been recorded using in vitro brain slices from rat hippocampus (Barnes, personal communication), human cortex (Maura et al. 1992), and guinea pig brain in vivo using the cortical cup technique (C. Bianchi et al. 1990). Consolo et al. (1994) also have recorded a 2-methyl-5-HT–induced increase in ACh in the dorsal hippocampus using an in vivo microdialysis technique. However, R. M. Johnson et al. (1993), using a series of serotonin receptor agonists and antagonists, failed to record any significant change in ACh release from slices of the rat entorhinal cortex. Differences in balance or presence between various serotonin receptor mechanisms may contribute to the different literature findings.

NEUROMODULATORY FUNCTION OF SEROTONIN

Sizer et al. (1992) defined a neuromodulatory response to serotonin as one that should influence the response to an excitatory amino acid without having any detectable effect on the passive electrical properties of the neuron. Some of the earliest studies used rat cerebellar preparations, and serotonin was shown to attenuate the excitation of the cell caused by L-glutamate, quisqualate, aspartate, and N-methyl-D-aspartate (NMDA) (Gardette et al. 1987; Hicks et al. 1989; M. Lee et al. 1986); the last authors found that the neuromodulatory action of serotonin was blocked by methysergide. However, in cat neocortical neurons, serotonin was shown to enhance the response to NMDA, quisqualate, and L-glutamate, a response that was antagonized by cinanserin, but not by methysergide (Nedergaard et al. 1986, 1987).

Subsequently, serotonin was shown to affect responses to excitatory amino acids in rat neocortical neurons, in cells of the ventrobasal thalamus, dorsal horn neurons, and rat locus coeruleus neurons (Aston-Jones et al. 1991; S. A. Eaton and Salt 1989; Murase et al. 1990; Read et al. 1990; J. N. Reynolds et al. 1988). Whether the modulatory effect of serotonin is to enhance or attenuate the effect of the excitatory amino acid appears to depend on the brain region investigated. Also, many of the experiments used extracellular recording techniques, although Sizer et al. (1992) used intracellular current clamp in vitro experiments to investigate neurons of the rat entorhinal cortex and neocortex. In the entorhinal cortex and neocortex, the predominant effects of serotonin were to reduce and enhance, respectively, the response to excitatory amino acids.

The importance of such studies is that the effects elicited by serotonin may be absent or profound, depending on the degree of excitatory amino acid challenge. Furthermore, the ability of serotonin to reduce the neuronal response to ACh may be particularly important in cognition and may broaden the modulatory role (S. A. Eaton and Salt 1989). Future studies are required to establish the serotonin receptor subtype mediating the effects, whether the interaction is physiologically relevant or can be manipulated to secure a change in learning and memory. That noradrenaline can also exert a modulating role (Nicoll et al. 1987) emphasizes the importance of the response.

SEROTONIN AS A TROPHIC FACTOR

In both whole animal studies and tissue culture, evidence suggests that serotonin receptor stimulation is trophic to the development of serotonin neurons (Whitaker-Azmitia and Azmitia 1991). By exposing immature glial cells in culture to serotonin receptor agonists, then adding the glial-conditioned media to serotonin neurons derived from a fetal rat brain, the 5-HT_{1A} receptor was identified as releasing or producing the astroglial specific protein S-100β (Whitaker-Azmitia et al. 1990). This protein is reported to stimulate neurite growth of serotonergic and cortical cells (Azmitia et al. 1990; Kligman and Marshak 1985). Thus, serotonin appears to regulate its own development and plasticity, and this may also occur in the adult brain because transplantation of fetal serotonin neurons into the rat hippocampus of the serotonin denervated animal results in a substantial increase in serotonin content (Azmitia et al. 1990). The expression of S-100β in the astrocytes at an early stage of implantation is critical for fiber ingrowth of serotonergic neurons and expression of 5-HT_{1A} receptors (Ueda et al. 1996) and the number of synaptophysin immunoreactive varicosities in a rat hippocampal culture (Nishi et al. 1996).

A decline in trophic factors may contribute to aging, and a reduced level of hippocampal 5-HT_{1A} receptors in Alzheimer's disease would lead to decreased release of S-100 and increased levels of S-100 within cells (Griffin et al. 1989). The relevance of such changes to neuronal cell loss in the hippocampus and cortex remains to be established. The possibility that other serotonin receptor subtypes may also regulate the release of trophic factors remains to be determined (Whitaker-Azmitia and Azmitia 1991), as does the search for other neuronal growth factors (Zhou and Azmitia 1991). However, such factors and the involvement of serotonin in their release may subsequently be shown to afford a site of drug action to attenuate cell decline and cognitive impairment.

INVESTIGATIONS OF SEROTONIN FUNCTION ON LEARNING AND MEMORY IN ANIMALS

Nonspecific Manipulations of Serotonin Function

Early experiments that attempted to increase serotonin function were necessarily restricted to drug treatments that caused a generalized effect throughout the brain and presumably were influencing all serotonin receptors. Using this approach, the systemic administration of 5-hydroxytryptophan, to increase the synthesis and release of serotonin, and the administration of p-chloramphetamine or electrical stimulation of the raphe nuclei, to increase the release of serotonin, were reported to impair performance in learning or memory tests (Fibiger et al. 1978; D. Joyce and Hurwitz 1964; Ogren et al. 1977). Although all such treatments influence other neurotransmitter systems in addition to serotonin, the importance of serotonin was shown by the impaired performance in a learning/memory and light/dark discrimination test in the rat following the intracerebroventricular injection of serotonin, but not ACh, noradrenaline, or GABA (Taniguti 1980). More recently, the septum has been recognized as important in learning and memory, and the intraseptal infusion of serotonin (but not dopamine, Ach, or glutamate) in the rat impaired retention of footshock avoidance training in the T maze (Flood et al. 1998).

Such results indicate that a raised serotonin function can impair cognitive performance, and, therefore, a reduction in serotonin function would be expected to increase performance. In support of this hypothesis, in young and old rats the depletion of serotonin caused by p-chloramphetamine enhanced performance in a Stone 14-unit T-maze test (Altman et al. 1985; Normile et al. 1986), and a 5,7-dihydroxytryptamine–induced deafferentation of the serotonergic input to the hippocampus similarly enhanced spatial discrimination in the rat (Altmanm et al. 1990). Also, the inhibition of the synthesis of serotonin by parachlorophenylalanine (PCA) facilitated brightness discrimination learning in the rat (Stevens et al. 1967). However, lesions of the serotonergic system have also revealed inconsistencies. Thus, PCA failed to

- Impair or enhance the performance of rats in an active avoidance task (V. Paul et al. 1994; Petkov et al. 1995)
- Affect water maze spatial performance (while exaggerating the effects of scopolamine) (Beiko et al. 1997)
- Affect the performance of rats using a delayed nonmatching-to-position task assessing spatial working memory (Jakala et al. 1993)
- Improve the aversive memory retrieval in rats conditioned in a T maze with appetitive and aversive events (Kumar et al. 1995)

5,7-Dihydroxytryptamine Lesions

- In the fimbria/fornix or cingulate bundle, selectively reduced the concentration of serotonin in the rat hippocampus but had no effect on spatial memory in the Morris water maze or radial arm maze. However, the lesion did augment the reference memory impairment caused by an NMDA lesion (Murtha and Pappas 1994).

- In the dorsal and median raphe nuclei, failed to modify performance in the acquisition of temporal discrimination and memory in a delayed conditional discrimination task in rats (Al-Zahrani et al. 1996) and using a delayed interval bisection task (Al-Zahrani et al. 1997).
- In the olfactory nucleus of the neonate rat pup, selectively depleted serotonin in the olfactory bulb, failed to modify locomotor behavior, but significantly modified the acquisition or expression of an olfactory-based learned behavior (McLean et al. 1993).
- In the raphe nuclei, while transiently impairing nonmnemonic aspects of performance, failed to modify the overall performance of rats trained on a delayed nonmatching-to-position task (Sahgal and Keith 1993).
- Administered in the presence of desmethylimipramine, impaired rat choice accuracy in a T maze with respect to acquisition with a constant and short delay interval, performance with variable delays, and treatment with scopolamine (Ricaurte et al. 1993).
- Following intracerebroventricular injection, slightly impaired choice accuracy of rats in the delayed nonmatching-to-position test (Ruotsalainen et al. 1997) but augmented the effect of scopolamine, although this was nonmnemonic in character.

A study of the behavioral and neurochemical effects of the putative serotonergic neurotoxicant methylenedioxymethamphetamine (MDMA) or dexfenfluramine in rhesus macaques failed to reveal any effects on short-term memory, motivation learning, and color and position discrimination (Frederick et al. 1995, 1998).

p-Chloroamphetamine also failed to impair rat performance in a working memory (delayed nonmatching *p* position) task but aggravated the effects of scopolamine (Ruotsalainen et al. 1998).

These varying effects of neurotoxic or pharmacological lesioning of the serotonergic systems on cognitive tasks may relate to some degree to variations in animal strain, doses of drug, or treatment regimens. It remains an interesting observation that even in those studies in which the lesion failed to overtly modify behavior in its own right, the lesion did exacerbate the effects of scopolamine. In these experiments, the degree of serotonergic disruption was clearly sufficient to compromise the cholinergic tone. The use of scopolamine would afford a valuable control agent in future lesion experiments.

However, another possibility may account for the discrepant results of the lesion experiments. Serotonin may act in a complexity of ways to influence cognitive events via different serotonin receptors, each possibly with a different role. Additionally, serotonin may interact with other neurotransmitter systems. Indeed, in their analysis of morphological aspects of serotonergic innervation, Mamounas et al. (1992) indicated that forebrain innervation is composed of at least two anatomically and functionally distinct systems arising from the dorsal and medial raphe nuclei, which have dissimilar morphological and pharmacological properties and may therefore have different functional consequences. Undoubtedly evidence exists for considerable functional heterogeneity between different serotonin systems and, most important, some with opposing actions on behavior, food intake, and temperature (C. H. K. Cheng et al. 1994; Hjorth 1992; Kosofsky and Molliver 1987).

Such conclusions may also be derived from data obtained using serotonin reuptake inhibitors. Relatively few reports cover the effects of serotonin reuptake inhibitors such as fluoxetine, alaproclate, zimeldine, and FG 7080 to influence cognition, but no reports indicate that in their own right these agents can improve or impair normal basal performance. However, in a study using rats in which olfactory bulbs were removed, the acquisition of a passive avoidance task was disrupted by bilateral ablation. The acquisition rate was restored by short-term treatment with fenfluramine and fluoxetine and partially by quipazine and by long-term treatment with imipramine and mianserin (Broekkamp et al. 1980). The administration of PCA to rats before shock elicited fear conditioning caused a total block of fear retention but had no effect on the acquisition of fear conditioning; the retrograde amnesic effect was antagonized by zimeldine (Archer et al. 1981). In mice, using a one-trial inhibitory avoidance task, both alaproclate and zimeldine were found to facilitate memory retrieval in a dose- and time-dependent manner that was blocked by the serotonin receptor agonist quipazine, but not by cyproheptadine (Altman et al. 1985). The dose-related impairment in avoidance acquisition in rats caused by PCA was blocked by zimeldine and also by inhibiting the synthesis of serotonin (Ogren and Johansson 1985). Also, FG 7080 was found to improve the performance of rats in a radial arm maze task that had been impaired by scopolamine. FG 7080 also reduced the scopolamine-induced acquisition deficits in a passive avoidance task (Miura et al. 1993). In an associative learning task in the rat, in which presynaptic serotonin activity was eliminated by PCA treatment and cognition was impaired by scopolamine and dizocilpine, fluoxetine enhanced learning of the conditioned response in a dose-related manner. The $5\text{-HT}_1/5\text{-HT}_2$ receptor antagonists ketanserin, ritanserin, NAN-190, and mesulergine, and the $5\text{-HT}_3/5\text{-HT}_4$ receptor antagonists MDL 72,222 and SDZ 205-557, prevented the effects of fluoxetine (Meneses and Hong 1995). The consensus view from such studies is that serotonin reuptake inhibitors may enhance cognitive processing in rodents, at least that impaired by pharmacological manipulations, and that many serotonin receptor mechanisms may be involved in the mediation of the effects of serotonin.

There remains the study of Lalonde and Vikis-Freibergs (1985) in which fluoxetine and fenfluramine produced retrograde amnesia in a one-trial appetitive learning task in rats, although the study failed to find consistent effects to treatments with 5-hydroxytryptophan, which can influence all serotonin receptor subtypes. In this respect, the use of serotonin receptor agonists and antagonists with a selectivity of action for the serotonin receptor subtypes is beginning to reveal the role of serotonin function in cognition, and experiments have focused on the role of $5\text{-}HT_1$, $5\text{-}HT_2$, and $5\text{-}HT_3$ receptors.

$5\text{-}HT_1/5\text{-}HT_2$ Involvement in Cognition

Most early studies focused on the use of antagonists because agonists have limited selectivity or poor penetration into the brain and frequently are associated with cardiovascular and other changes. The initial experiments with $5\text{-}HT_1$ receptor antagonists were limited to agents such as cyproheptadine, methysergide, mianserin, and metergoline, an obvious disadvantage being their relative lack of selectivity for the $5\text{-}HT_1$ or $5\text{-}HT_2$ receptor. The results were inconclusive: cyproheptadine, but not methysergide, administered peripherally impaired the retention of a one-trial inhibitory avoidance task in mice (Bammer 1982), and metergoline also administered peripherally did not affect acquisition of a one-way active avoidance task in rats (Ogren 1982). However, Wetzel et al. (1980), using rats trained to avoid the dark alley of a Y maze, found that, when mianserin was injected directly into the hippocampus immediately after training, animals receiving the treatment exhibited significantly greater savings during a retraining session. Single-dose administrations limited an interpretation of some of these findings. In a detailed dose-response investigation using pirenperone, ketanserin, methysergide, metergoline, and mianserin to assess pretest drug administration on the retrieval of a previously learned aversive habituation in the mouse, all five agents caused a dose-dependent increase in the latency to complete drinking after training. This suppression of drinking showed for the first time that blockade of serotonin receptors can enhance retrieval and may allow the brain to more selectively process or access information (Altman and Normile 1986). Yet, notwithstanding the use of agents, such as ketanserin or pirenperone, with a relatively greater selectivity for the $5\text{-}HT_2$ receptor, it could not be excluded that the effects of such agents may have partly reflected a $5\text{-}HT_1$ receptor antagonism or even an action on noradrenaline or histamine receptors. Nevertheless, it is relevant that the release of serotonin by p-chloroamphetamine was found to impair both avoidance acquisition and retention in rats using a one-way active avoidance task. The impairment was blocked by serotonin but not noradrenaline synthesis inhibition (Ogren 1985).

In further development of such studies, p-chloroamphetamine was found to impair memory retrieval in a dose- and time-dependent fashion in a one-way active, but not in a passive, avoidance test (Ogren 1986). Pretraining administration of p-chloroamphetamine produced a progressive loss of passive and active avoidance performance at increasingly longer retention intervals. It was concluded that serotonin has dual effects on processes underlying learning and memory involving effects on both associative and nonassociative learning. The concomitant administration of p-chloroamphetamine and selective serotonin receptor antagonists would provide a useful future approach to delineating the serotonin receptor subtype involvement.

In a different model, an impairment of working memory caused by cerebral ischemia was investigated in the rat using a three-panel runway task. Pirenperone, cinanserin, and ritanserin administered immediately after blood flow reperfusion significantly reduced the increase in errors expected to occur after 24 hours. It was concluded that 5-HT$_2$ receptor blockade may prevent the impairment of working memory following transient forebrain ischemia (Ohno et al. 1991). In an important primate study (squirrel monkeys), serotonin antagonists were evaluated in a delayed matching-to-sample task in one group of animals in which the baseline performance was low and in another in which it was high, but impaired by exposure to hypoxia. Cyproheptadine, ketanserin, and mianserin improved performance in both groups, whereas pirenperone was effective only in the low baseline performance group. It was suggested that serotonin has a major role in cognitive performance (Denoble et al. 1991).

It remains clear from experiments that have used 5-HT$_1$ receptor agonists that the involvement of the 5-HT$_{1A}$ receptor in cognition has received the greatest attention. Most studies have been performed in the rat and mouse using limited dose ranges of drugs; extended dose ranges are precluded by the appearance of sedative or motor side effects at high doses. Nevertheless, a clear picture has emerged that activation of 5-HT$_{1A}$ receptors is to impair performance in the radial maze, the Morris water maze, and one-trial passive and active avoidance tasks using a range of 5-HT$_{1A}$ receptor ligands, buspirone, gepirone, MDL 73,005EF, tandospirone, 8-hydroxy-2-di-n-propylamino tetralin (8-OH-DPAT), and others (Bass et al. 1992; Carli and Samanin 1992; Carli et al. 1992, 1995a; S. D. Mendelson et al. 1993;

Quartermain et al. 1993, 1994; Rowan et al. 1990; Winter and Petti 1987). Also, low doses of gepirone and atropine, which individually fail to modify rat performance in a spatial task, when administered together impair performance (Barrett and Rowan 1990). Similarly, the selection of a single dose of MDL 73,005EF that did not impair the acquisition or recall of a task in the Morris water maze enhanced the deficits caused by gepirone or atropine (Barrett and Rowan 1992).

The ability of agonist action at the $5-HT_{1A}$ receptors to impair cognitive performance appears paradoxical. The potent inhibitory action at the presynaptic autoreceptor in the raphe nucleus could be predicted to cause a decrease in serotonin function throughout the forebrain and to enhance cognitive performance. However, $5-HT_{1A}$ receptors are located throughout the forebrain and in high density in the hippocampus (Pazos and Palacios 1985) where the local injection of serotonin or 8-OH-DPAT in the rat has been shown to impair working memory and retention in a Y-maze brightness discrimination task (Ohno et al. 1993, 1996; Wetzel et al. 1980). That endogenous serotonin may normally exert a similar role is indicated by the facilitated learning of a positive reinforced spatial discrimination task following a 5-hydroxytryptaminergic deafferentation of the hippocampus (Altman et al. 1990). Confirmatory evidence that the hippocampal serotonin receptor actually mediating the inhibitory effects of serotonin and 8-OH-DPAT is the $5-HT_{1A}$ receptor subtype has awaited the development of selective $5-HT_{1A}$ receptor antagonists. (S)WAY-1100135 is the first agent to become available (A. Fletcher et al. 1993) and has been shown to prevent the impairment of spatial learning caused by intrahippocampal scopolamine (Carli et al. 1995b). This provides the first evidence that endogenous serotonin in the hippocampus mediates its effects on cognition via a $5-HT_{1A}$ receptor.

Studies were required to establish the interaction between 8-OH-DPAT and WAY-1100135 to moderate cognition, which has been established in a number of models. In an analysis of the role of $5-HT_{1A}$ receptors in consolidation learning in the rat, 8-OH-DPAT increased the number of conditional responses; the $5-HT_{1A}$ receptor antagonist WAY-100635 (see A. Fletcher et al. 1996), ketanserin (a $5-HT_{2A/2C}$ receptor antagonist), and ondansetron but not the $5-HT_{1B/1D}$ receptor antagonist GR127935 or the $5-HT_{2A}$ receptor antagonist MDL 100907 reversed the effect of 8-OH-DPAT (Meneses and Hong 1999). WAY-100635 also reversed the learning deficit induced by scopolamine. A water-maze navigation task showed that treatment with either scopolamine or 8-OH-DPAT before daily training disrupted spatial navigation at medium doses and cue navigation at high doses but did not impair water-maze performance if given post training. (Riekkinen et al. 1995). It was concluded that the activation of 5-HT$_{1A}$ receptors greatly impairs water-maze learning and performance but does not impair spatial memory.

Similarly, intrahippocampal injections of 8-OH-DPAT induced no change in performance levels of the rat trained to run in a radial maze (Buhot et al. 1995). However, the intrahippocampal injection of the 5-HT$_{1B}$ receptor agonist CP-93,129 [3-(1,2,5,6-tetrahydropyrid-4-yl] pyrrolo [3,2-6] pyrid-5-one] induced a higher frequency of reference memory errors than of working memory. It was concluded that stimulation of 5-HT$_{1B}$ receptors in the CA1 field of the dorsal hippocampus impairs performance of rats in a spatial learning task.

Three 5-HT$_{1A}$ receptor agonists [NDO 008 (3-dipropyl amino-5-hydroxychroman and the enantiomers of 8-OH-DPAT, (R(+)-8-OH-DPAT, and S(-)-8-OH-DPAT)] were studied in a step-through passive avoidance test in the male rat and produced a dose-dependent impairment in passive avoidance retention. The impairment was blocked by WAY-1100135 but not by the mixed 5-HT$_{2A/2C}$ antagonists ketanserin and pirenperone. A PCA treatment failed to modify passive avoidance retention or the inhibitory effects of the 5-HT$_{1A}$ agonists (Misane et al. 1998). It was concluded that the 5-HT$_{1A}$ receptor interferes with learning processes operating at both acquisition and retrieval.

Glutamate is required for neuroplastic changes in animals that are associated with place learning and the NMDA antagonist MK801 in blocking the effects of glutamate in the hippocampus impairs spatial memory (Butelman 1990). Serotonin appears to exert an inhibitory effect on the glutamate neuron, which may be the site of action of 5-HT$_{1A}$ agonists to impair rat performance in the water-maze task following infusion of 8-OH-DPAT into the CA1 region of the dorsal hippocampus (Carli et al. 1992). Researchers are now interested in the possibility that 5-HT$_{1A}$ receptor antagonists, in blocking the inhibitory actions of serotonin, may enhance cognition.

The role of other forebrain sites in the mediation of 5-HT$_{1A}$ receptor-induced changes in cognition remains to be investigated, and the establishment of dose-related responses is important. Thus, Winter and Petti (1987), while recording that 8-OH-DPAT (0.3–3.0 mg/kg) reduced performance in the rat radial maze, noted, in an observation of at least equal importance, that a lower dose of 0.1 mg/kg enhanced performance by 173%. The inhibitory and facilitatory effects may reflect a presynaptic action in the raphe nuclei followed by a postsynaptic receptor activation in the forebrain, respectively. In any case, 5-HT$_{1A}$ receptor agonist potential must be carefully examined to eliminate or reveal opposing roles.

Involvement of 5-HT$_3$ Receptors in Cognition

The first report that a 5-HT$_3$ receptor antagonist could enhance performance in cognition came from the use of ondansetron in the mouse. Mice, when placed daily into the light compartment of a black and white test box, habituate to the system, moving more rapidly into the dark compartment. This pattern of habituation was impaired by scopolamine, lesions of the nucleus basalis magnocellularis, and aging, the impairment being prevented by ondansetron (J. M. Barnes et al. 1990). The researchers also showed that ondansetron and arecoline attenuated a scopolamine-induced impairment in a T-maze reinforced alternation test in the rat. Furthermore, the studies were extended to the primate in an object discrimination and reversal test using the marmoset. Ondansetron decreased the number of trials to criteria in both an object discrimination and a reversal learning task.

Subsequently, Altman and Berman (1990) reported that zacopride and dazopride facilitated learning and memory in mice. Chugh et al. (1991) also reported that ICS 205–930 in the mouse produced a dose-dependent increase in the retrieval of a previously learned aversive habit and attenuated a scopolamine-induced impairment. In experiments on rats using passive avoidance with punishment reinforcement, ondansetron was shown to improve retention when tested after training as compared with control rats and where 5-HT$_1$ and 5-HT$_2$ receptor antagonists impaired performance (Petkov and Kehayov 1994). In a different paradigm, using the Morris water maze as a spatial learning task, the 5-HT$_3$ receptor antagonist DAU 6125 was shown to attenuate a scopolamine-induced behavioral deficit in the rat (Pitsikas et al. 1994). Also, using the Morris water maze, Hodges et al. (1995) reported that the 5-HT$_3$ receptor antagonist WAY-100289 improved performance over a wide dose range in retention and relearning after lesioning the cholinergic projections to cortex and hippocampus using ibotenic acid lesions to the nucleus basalis and medial septal brain regions. Interestingly, nicotine and arecoline were more effective than WAY-100289 in the retention measurements and also improved the initial acquisition.

Rats lesioned with excitotoxic challenge (S-AMPA) to the nucleus basalis and medial septum showed substantial impairment in spatial learning in the water-maze test. The lesioned animals showed marked improvement in response to the 5-HT$_3$ receptor antagonists ondansetron and WAY-100579 (Hodges et al. 1996). In an associative learning task in the rat, both ondansetron and tropisetron improved the retention of a conditioned response; *p*-chloroamphetamine blocked the effects of the 5-HT$_3$ receptor antagonists (E. Hong and Meneses 1996). In the aged rat given a multiple-choice avoidance behavioral task, treatment with low doses of the 5-HT$_3$ receptor antagonist itasetron twice daily for 3 weeks significantly improved retentional abilities (Pitsikas and Borsini 1996). In adult rats, both ondansetron and physostigmine enhanced performance in the Morris water-maze test that had been impaired by atropine. In aged rats impaired with atropine, ondansetron (but not physostigmine) enhanced performance, but neither ondansetron nor physostigmine improved performance in aged nonimpaired rats (Fontana et al. 1995).

In a passive avoidance procedure in the rat, low doses of ondansetron reversed the scopolamine-induced memory deficit, whereas tropisetron was ineffective. However, in the Morris water-maze test, tropisetron but not ondansetron counteracted the learning and memory impairment caused by scopolamine (Pitsikas and Borsini 1997).

Aged rhesus monkeys were assessed in several cognitive and motor tasks, acquisition of a visual object discrimination, reversal of a visual object discrimination, a delayed response task, a spatial working memory task, and a fine motor task. The 5-HT$_3$ receptor antagonists ondansetron and SEC-579 at very low oral doses selectively enhanced acquisition of a visual object discrimination task but not the reversal or delayed tasks (Arnsten et al. 1997).

However, in macaques, the R and S isomers of the potent 5-HT$_3$ receptor antagonist RS-56812 enhanced certain aspects of task performance in a delayed matching-to-sample task. The differential sensitivity of the isomers paralleled the higher 5-HT$_3$ receptor affinity (A. V. Terry et al. 1996).

In an examination of the effects of low doses of ondansetron on acquisition of responding for a conditioned reward and on the response-potentiating effect of amphetamine in the rat, ondansetron had no effect on the learning of stimulus reward relationships but caused a small attenuation of the amphetamine effect, suggesting a possible modulatory role for 5-HT$_3$ receptors in this process (P. J. Fletcher and Higgins 1997).

Ondansetron also produced a dose-dependent blockade of conditioned taste aversion induced by apomorphine (McAllister and Pratt 1998).

The hippocampus is regarded as a key structure in learning and memory, and serotonergic brain-stem projections are thought to increase, via 5-HT$_3$ receptors, the excitability of interneurons that regulate GABA$_B$-mediated inhibition of pyramidal cells. The GABA$_B$ inhibitory postsynaptic potentials are thought to play a significant role in controlling the strength of long-term potentiation induced with σ burst stimulation. Staubli and Xu (1995) hypothesized that 5-HT$_3$ receptor blockade should enhance learning by reducing the hyperpolarization caused by slow GABA$_B$-mediated inhibitory postsynaptic potentials, and thereby enhance the frequency of the σ rhythm and the induction of long-term potentiation, which is considered an important basis of learning. When injected in the freely moving rat, ondansetron reliably and significantly increased the frequency of the hippocampal σ rhythm, significantly increased the magnitude and duration of long-term potentiation, and improved retention in an odor matching problem task and a spatial task.

The injection of scopolamine into the dorsal hippocampus of the rat impaired choice accuracy in a two-platform spatial discrimination task. The subcutaneous injection of ondansetron antagonized the effect of scopolamine but had no effect when administered alone (Carli et al. 1997). A working memory task with a three-panel runway arrangement showed that the concurrent infusion of the 5-HT$_3$ receptor antagonist Y-25130 and scopolamine into the dorsal hippocampus of the rat significantly attenuated the impairment induced by scopolamine. Y-25130 administered alone had no effect and failed to block the impairment induced by the NMDA receptor antagonist ($\pm$)-3-(2-carboxypiperazin-4-yl) propyl-1-phosphonic acid (Ohno and Watanabe 1997).

Therefore, considerable and increasing evidence indicates that 5-HT$_3$ receptor antagonists can attenuate an impaired cognitive processing in the rodent and primate. It is also an important observation that no reports indicate that any 5-HT$_3$ receptor antagonist can improve a response to above basal control levels. Therefore, an abuse potential would not be predicted.

Involvement of 5-HT$_4$ Receptors in Cognition

The role of 5-HT$_4$ receptors in cognition has received little attention. In a mouse passive avoidance test, the administration of the 5-HT$_4$ receptor antagonists SDZ 205557 and GR 125487 immediately after the training session produced an amnesic effect. The 5-HT$_4$ receptor agonists BIMU1 and BIMU8 administered before the training session prevented the amnesia induced by the 5-HT$_4$ receptor antagonists. The intracerebroventricular injection of BIMU1 and BIMU8 also prevented a scopolamine-induced impairment. Ondansetron failed to modify the effects of scopolamine (Galeotti et al. 1998).

A social olfactory recognition test in rats determined that the 5-HT$_4$ receptor agonist/5-HT$_3$ receptor antagonist BIMU1 enhanced short-term memory (a recognition of a juvenile after 2 hours), whereas ondansetron had no effect. The effect of BIMU1 was antagonized by GR 125487 (Letty et al. 1997).

These preliminary studies offer encouragement to the design of further studies with more selective 5-HT$_4$ receptor agonists to firmly establish the role of the 5-HT$_4$ receptor in cognition.

ROLE OF SEROTONIN IN COGNITIVE DISORDERS IN HUMANS

The treatment of obsessive-compulsive disorders provides the clearest evidence of a role for serotonin in cognition. The subject is discussed in detail in another chapter and reviewed elsewhere (Insel 1992; Insel et al. 1983b; S. A. Montgomery 1992b; D. L. Murphy et al. 1992).

LEARNING AND MEMORY DISORDERS: NEUROCHEMICAL PATHOLOGY IN DEMENTIA

It was to be expected with the many events contributing to cognition that an involvement of numerous neurotransmitter mechanisms could be demonstrated, for example, cholinergic, dopaminergic, and noradrenergic excitatory amino acids and peptides (see reviews by E. M. Joyce 1987; Rossor 1987). However, the consistent finding of a reduced choline acetyltransferase activity within the cerebral cortex of patients with Alzheimer's disease has focused attention on the pivotal role of ACh in memory and learning and their disorders (see Bartus et al. 1982; E. K. Perry 1986). The loss of the enzyme in Alzheimer's disease is related to a degeneration of the cholinergic system arising from the nucleus basalis of Meynert, the medial septal nucleus, and diagonal band of Broca (Mesulam et al. 1984). This has given rise to the search for cholinergic agents to ameliorate impairments in humans (Giacobini and Becker 1988), but with little success. Side effects of peripheral parasympathetic overactivity or toxicity have limited drug usefulness and efficacy. Therefore, attention has turned to other ways to enhance cholinergic and/or other functions to improve cognitive performance.

ROLE OF SEROTONIN

The first neurochemical evidence of a disturbed serotonin function in cognition came from the changes in serotonin and/or 5-hydroxyindoleacetic acid (5-HIAA) levels in a number of forebrain nuclei, the temporal and cingulate cortex, hippocampus, and other areas of the brain taken at autopsy from patients with senile dementia of the Alzheimer's type (Adolfsson et al. 1978; Arai et al. 1984; D. M. Bowen et al. 1979, 1983; A. J. Cross et al. 1983; Winblad et al. 1982). The depletions are regionally selective: reductions in serotonin and 5-HIAA in the hippocampus are not mirrored by changes in the substantia innominata (G. B. Baker and Reynolds 1989). The use of autopsy material has obvious limitations to an understanding of neurotransmitter release potential during disease. Therefore, it is particularly important to note that significant reductions were found in serotonin/5-HIAA taken from the cerebrospinal fluid of patients with senile dementia of the Alzheimer's type (Argentiero and Tavolato 1980; Gottfries and Roos 1976; Gottfries et al. 1974; Tohgi et al. 1995).

Reduced levels of serotonin suggest adverse changes in the raphe nuclei, and considerable evidence suggests that cells in the dorsal and medial raphe nuclei of patients with senile dementia of the Alzheimer's type contain dense neurofibrillary tangle formations (Ishii 1966) and that there is cell loss and the presence of senile plaques in dorsal raphe nuclei (Yamamoto and Hirano 1985). These findings have been confirmed in a detailed study of raphe pathology, using Nissl staining techniques of raphe neurons, immunohistochemical analysis of the number of serotonin-synthesizing neurons, and the number of neuritic plaques and neurofibrillary tangles in brain stem tissue. Based on such analyses taken from control subjects and patients with Alzheimer's disease, the patients could be divided into two groups: those with (AD[+]) and without (AD[-]) raphe pathology. A significant correlation was found between the number of large raphe neurons and serotonin-synthesizing neurons in control material (i.e., all the large neurons were serotonergic), which are not present in the AD[+] group, in which the number of serotonin-synthesizing neurons correlated with the number of neurofibrillary tangles. In brief, the serotonin neurons were found to be selectively and adversely affected in this group. No immediate correlation was found between raphe and cortical pathology, or age, or minimum mental scores. However, a trend was seen for raphe pathology to correlate with age at onset of the disease and its rate of progression and duration. Most of the patients with AD[+] with severe raphe lesions had clinical dementia only, whereas the other patients had additional features (G. M. Halliday et al. 1992).

Similar results were obtained from material taken from patients with senile dementia of the Alzheimer's type (Chan-Palay et al. 1992). A loss of tryptophan hydroxylase immunoreactive neurons in the raphe nuclei, which was most pronounced in the lateral division, was correlated with both age and cortical pathology. Furthermore, tyrosine hydroxylase reactive neurons were also found to be reduced in the locus coeruleus, even more so than the tryptophan hydroxylase reactive neurons. The same was also found for material taken from brains with Parkinson's disease.

The summary of all the above findings indicates a seriously impaired serotonin neurotransmission in a significant proportion of patients with dementia. The neurochemical changes are all the more impressive in the perspective that no consistent changes were found in brain concentrations of serotonin or 5-HIAA in the mouse, rat, or humans during aging (McEntee and Crook 1991).

Although 5-HT$_3$ receptors appear not to be reduced in Alzheimer's disease (N. M. Barnes et al. 1990), reports consistently indicate regional reductions in 5-HT$_{1A}$ and 5-HT$_2$ receptors (Briley et al. 1986; A. J. Cross et al. 1984, 1988; Middlemiss et al. 1986; E. K. Perry et al. 1984). Such studies were conducted using autopsy material, but have more recently been confirmed in vivo using positron-emission tomography. Using the selective 5-HT$_2$ receptor ligand [^{18}F]setoperone in patients with Alzheimer's disease, a decrease of cortical 5-HT$_2$ receptor density of 35%–65% was recorded (Blin et al. 1993). Clearly, the imaging technique has major capabilities of recording receptor presence and change during disease progression, a landmark advance. This is exemplified by a preliminary study of serotonin S2 binding in patients with stroke (P. L. P. Morris et al. 1993). In uninjured regions of the cortex in 26 patients, left frontal cortex serotonin binding was correlated positively with a Mini-Mental State Exam (Folstein et al. 1975) total score and concentration, writing, and copying tasks and also tests of orientation and repetition of difficult phrases. The findings indicated that cognitive performance after stroke may be influenced by alterations in the serotonergic system.

EFFECT OF DRUGS INFLUENCING SEROTONIN FUNCTION ON COGNITIVE IMPAIRMENTS IN HUMANS

Notwithstanding the substantial and increasing preclinical evidence indicating a role for serotonin in cognition, the influence of drugs affecting serotonin function on learning and memory disorders in humans has received little attention. It was inevitable that the initial experiments had to use pharmacological probes with limited specificity of action. For example, the administration of 5-hydroxytryptophan and serotonin reuptake inhibitors would inevitably affect all serotonergic process, and such treatment had no significant or consistent effects to improve cognitive performance in Alzheimer's or senile dementia (Cutler et al. 1985; Dehlin et al. 1985; J. S. Meyer et al. 1977). Similarly, such agents have no effect to modify the memory impairments produced by ethanol (Weingartner et al. 1983). Such studies fail to offer any support for the use of 5-hydroxytryptophan or serotonin reuptake inhibitors to improve cognitive performance, at least in the conditions proscribed, but offer limited comment as to the involvement of serotonin. Thus, either 5-hydroxytryptophan or the serotonin reuptake inhibitors would be predicted to influence presynaptic inhibitory mechanisms in the midbrain and presynaptic/postsynaptic serotonin receptors in the forebrain; the indiscriminate actions may oppose each other. Also, the nonselective actions on different serotonin receptor subtypes may seriously complicate the effects of drug action.

More selective serotonin receptor agonists are required to differentially activate discrete serotonin receptor subtypes, but such agents generally remain as experimental compounds for use only in preclinical studies. However, *m*-chlorophenylpiperazine is an exception, having a relatively selective action on serotonin receptors (Kennett et al. 1989), and this agent has been shown to diminish performance on tests of recent memory in elderly control subjects and also patients with Alzheimer's disease (Lawlor et al. 1989a, 1989b). This result is in broad agreement with the preclinical data indicating that a raised serotonin function at the 5-HT$_2$ receptor may predispose to an impaired performance in cognition. However, it is interesting that cognitive impairments in schizophrenia are shown readily in tests involving attention, memory, and executive function and appear to be an enduring and core feature; the patient has a major inability to manipulate available information. Cognitive impairments reflected in the negative symptoms retard psychosocial performance and delay reintegration into society (Weinberger and Gallhoffer 1997).

Evidence is increasing that antipsychotic treatment with 5-HT$_2$ receptor–blocking drugs such as clozapine and olanzapine improves cognitive performance better than the traditional neuroleptic therapy. 5-HT$_2$ receptors are significantly reduced in prefrontal cortex samples from schizophrenic patients (Arora and Meltzer 1991; Laruelle et al. 1993; Mita et al. 1986). Ohouha et al. (1993) reviewed the role of serotonin in schizophrenia and hypothesized that alterations in the serotonergic systems in the prefrontal cortex render the cortex incapable of subcortical inhibition. The use of selective serotonin receptor antagonists would be required to establish the precise serotonin receptor subtype mediating such effects, and such experiments remain to be performed. In this respect, the administration of the 5-HT$_{1/2}$ receptor antagonist methysergide alone has been shown to lead to improved performance in a visual memory task in a group of patients with Korsakoff's amnesia (McEntee and Mair 1980).

However, another pharmacological model to study the involvement of the serotonergic system in cognitive impairment is to reduce central serotonin synthesis through L-tryptophan depletion. In healthy volunteers with or without a family history of depression, tryptophan depletion specifically impaired long-term memory performance (delayed recall, recognition sensitivity, recognition reaction times) but did not change short-term memory or perceptual or psychomotor functions (Riedel et al. 1999). This may reflect a generalized effect on all serotonin systems.

Evidence from both animals and humans indicates that the repeated (recreational) use of MDMA ("Ecstasy") produces long-lasting decreases in serotonergic function (see above). This may produce a fortuitous insight into the role of serotonergic processes in cognition. Morgan (1999) used the Rivermead Behavioural Memory test to investigate both immediate and delayed recall and obtained the first evidence that deficits in memory performance in both the immediate and the delayed recall conditions in recreational users are primarily associated with past exposure to MDMA. This finding supported a previous study showing that a greater use of MDMA was associated with a greater impairment in immediate verbal memory and delayed visual memory (Bolla et al. 1998). Lower concentrations of 5-HIAA in the cerebrospinal fluid also were associated with poorer memory performance. Again, such administrations will inevitably affect all serotonin systems, and the specificity of MDMA action to the serotonin pathway remains to be determined.

Notwithstanding the clinical use of many 5-HT_{1A} receptor ligands for the treatment of anxiety, only one report was found that has investigated the potential to influence cognitive performance. In patients with a generalized anxiety disorder, Lucki et al. (1987) compared the effect of buspirone (at 5 and 10 mg) with that of diazepam (5 mg). Diazepam impaired performance; buspirone was without effect.

A number of studies have commenced to investigate the effect of 5-HT_3 receptor antagonists on cognition. First, it should be noted that no reports indicate that, following the use of ondansetron, granisetron, and tropisetron as antiemetics in patients with cancer, such treatments can cause overt changes in behavior. Millions of doses have been administered over a period of days, and the doses employed have been among the highest used in any of the clinical studies. Certainly, sedation and endocrine or autonomic changes that are readily observed with the use of other antiemetic treatments are absent. Although, for obvious reasons, no controlled measures exist of changes in cognitive performance during antiemetic treatment, any dramatic increases or decreases in cognitive performance would probably have become self-evident. In particular, no evidence of abuse potential that could result from a social or other inappropriate use of an agent with "cognitive-enhancing" potential has been reported. Similar comments would apply to the use of ondansetron in postoperative nausea and vomiting, although the duration of treatment is short. Such results agree closely with the preclinical findings.

To reveal the cognition-enhancing potential of the 5-HT$_3$ antagonists, studies in age-related memory impairment have been carried out with psychiatrically healthy subjects impaired with scopolamine and patients with dementia. In a randomized double-blind, double-dummy, four-way crossover study in a small number of subjects, each psychiatrically healthy male subject received placebo, scopolamine (0.4 mg im), scopolamine plus alosetron (10 μg iv), or alosetron (250 μg) (Preston 1994; Preston et al. 1991). Assessments of verbal and spatial memory, sedation, and sustained attention were performed before and after treatment. The main results from the study were that scopolamine induced robust deficits on all primary variables measured, the reduction in verbal and spatial memories being attenuated by 10-μg and 250-μg doses of alosetron, respectively. No effects on the sedation or on changes in attention were noted.

In a study designed to measure the modulation of anticholinergic effects on cognition and behavior in elderly humans, 10 elderly psychiatrically healthy subjects received, by infusion, placebo, ondansetron (0.15 mg/kg iv), scopolamine (0.4 mg iv), scopolamine plus ondansetron, and scopolamine plus *m*-chlorophenylpiperazine (0.09 mg/kg iv), the 5 study days being separated by at least 72 hours (J. T. Little et al. 1995). Cognitive measures examined episodic and semantic memory, lexical search and retrieval, and processing speed. Behavioral ratings were also undertaken. Scopolamine caused impairment in a host of tests, and such impairments were exacerbated by the serotonin receptor agonist *m*-chlorophenylpiperazine in areas of letter fluency and serial visual search. Ondansetron at the high dose failed to modify the scopolamine-induced impairments on cognitive, physiological, or behavioral measures. The authors, using a single high dose of ondansetron and a single pretreatment time, emphasized that careful dose-response studies may be required before ruling out possible cholinergic potentiating effects of ondansetron in humans.

In a study of age-associated memory impairment (Crook and Lakin 1991), using a double-blind, placebo-controlled trial and three doses of ondansetron (10, 250, or 1,000 μg po bid), patients were treated for 12 weeks, followed by a 2-week washout period, with assessments being made at the initiation of, during, and at the termination of treatment. Behavioral rating scales and a computerized battery of tests related to learning and memory tasks of daily life were used to assess changes in cognitive performance. Ondansetron caused dose-related effects to enhance acquisition, name-face association—delayed recall, and facial recognition—number recognized before first error, with the intermediate dose being more efficacious than the highest dose. It was concluded that ondansetron merited further study.

Overall, these preliminary studies, although emphasizing the difficulties of dosage selection, offered encouragement to the design of more extensive trials in dementia of the Alzheimer's type. However, a large program of trials has apparently failed to demonstrate a convincing treatment effect on the core cognitive symptoms of dementia or the patient's clinical status (Corn, personal communication). It is hoped that such trials will be published to allow a better understanding of the effect of 5-HT$_3$ receptor antagonists in dementia and to allow a better understanding of the validity of animal models of cognition. Possibly in cognition, as with anxiety, there are subsets of responders in the patient populations examined.

Finally, a study of patients with anxiety and their response to treatment with the benzodiazepines may offer further clues as to the role of serotonin and cognition. The benzodiazepines are known to influence serotonin systems, albeit in a complex manner (see Richards et al. 1991).

Anxiety may be revealing of complex interactions between a primary illness, the degree of cognitive impairment, and the effect of drug treatment. For example, it is well established that patients with anxiety may, as a result of the mood change or benzodiazepine treatment, produce state-dependent alterations in memory (Bower 1981; Eich 1980), an anterograde amnesia occurring as an impairment of acquisition, and, to a lesser extent, retrieval (H. H. Jensen and Poulson 1982). Such studies might yield important information about basic cognitive processing and systems and are important to the patient to assess the degree of clinical significance. Yet studies in subjects with anxiety may have additional benefits. A number of investigations in patients with generalized anxiety disorder have revealed that these patients may process anxiety-related stimuli differently from control subjects (Lister 1991; Lister and Weingartner 1987; Mathews and MacLeod 1986; J. M. G. Williams et al. 1988). Such comparative studies in the future, using the tools of cognitive psychology, selective drug intervention, and brain imaging, may finally allow greatly improved understanding of the brain systems and neurotransmitter mechanisms involved in normal and abnormal cognitive processing.

SUMMARY

In this chapter, we have reviewed the sites and mechanisms of drug action that may modify serotonin function relevant to cognition. A substantial number of animal studies have revealed that an agonist action at the 5-HT$_{1A}$ receptor may impair performance in learning and memory tasks, whereas 5-HT$_3$ receptor antagonists can restore performance in animals that are impaired. The role of the 5-HT$_2$ and the many other serotonin receptor subtypes in cognition remains to be explored. In humans, only the 5-HT$_3$ receptor antagonists have been assessed, and future studies are required to fully establish their potential in age-related memory impairments and dementia. It remains clear that the selective serotonin reuptake inhibitors have a uniquely valuable therapeutic role in patients cognitively disabled with obsessive-compulsive disorder.

The studies provide an exciting foundation for future progress. They have revealed the perennial difficulties of relating the effects of short-term drug administrations in animals with long-term treatments in the clinic that may require weeks or months to show therapeutic benefits; the challenges of designing selective action at the many serotonin receptor subtypes; the presence of distinct serotonin systems and opposing functional roles; and that a combined influence on serotonin and other neurotransmitter systems may be crucially required to demonstrate both profound changes in animal behavior and to secure a therapeutic benefit.

Future progress in serotonin research is dependent on the development of selective ligands for the serotonin receptor subtypes; an appreciation in animal models that more than a serotonin disruption may be required to disrupt learning and memory in a manner relevant to disorders in humans; that therapeutic treatments may require more than a manipulation of a single receptor type; and that instruments used to assess disease impairment and improvement should be adequate to reveal changes in subpopulations of patients from a heterogeneous population. At the most fundamental level, the next generation of animal models should be used to investigate neurotransmitter interactions and, perhaps most exciting, the possibility that serotonin may act as a neuromodulator of cellular changes induced by excitatory amino acids and other neurotransmitter substances. This could complicate and yet transform an understanding of serotonin function and perhaps reveal an additional role for serotonin as important as that which has been afforded by the traditional neurotransmitter hypothesis.

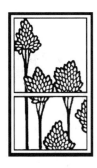

CHAPTER 35

Nicotinic Cholinergic Approaches to Cognitive Enhancement in the Dementias

Paul Newhouse, M.D.

In the not-too-distant past, the presence of central nervous system (CNS) nicotinic receptors was not thought to be a significant part of the cholinergic receptor system of the brain. However, advances in the understanding of the structure, function, and distribution of these receptors have provided the impetus for new studies examining the role(s) that these receptors and associated processes may play in CNS functions. Further motivation has come from the realization that such receptors must be involved in maintenance of cigarette smoking and from clues from studies of degenerative neurological diseases, such as Alzheimer's disease (AD), in which the

This work was supported by National Institute of Mental Health Grant R29-46625 and General Clinical Research Center Grant M01-00109. The author wishes to thank Robert Lenox, Alexandra Potter, Melissa Piasecki, June Corwin, Christina Conrath, Jennifer Geelmuyden, and Judy Kerr for assistance in performing the studies described in this review, as well as Steven Arneric, Michael Decker, and Edward Levin, for many helpful suggestions and permission to summarize extensively from their reviews.

loss of nicotinic receptors has been described (Nordberg 1994). Ongoing investigations of the molecular substructure of CNS nicotinic receptors and their pharmacology have begun to open up new possibilities for novel CNS therapeutics with nicotinic agents (Arneric et al. 1995). Exploiting these possibilities will require understanding of the role(s) that these receptor systems play in human cognitive, behavioral, motor, and sensory functioning. Clues from careful studies of human cognition are beginning to emerge and will provide direction for studies of potentially therapeutic novel nicotinic agents. In this chapter, I review briefly the current understanding of CNS nicotinic receptors, their physiology and pharmacology, and evidence for cognitive effects of nicotine from animal and smoking studies; examine evidence of nicotinic involvement in degenerative neurological diseases; and review studies from our laboratory and others that examine the effects of nicotinic agonists and antagonists on cognitive functioning in AD and Parkinson's disease (PD). Finally, the potential therapeutic role of nicotinic agonists in dementia is discussed.

NICOTINIC RECEPTORS: STRUCTURE AND DISTRIBUTION

Over the past 10 years, extensive studies of the nicotinic receptor have established its basic structure and functional properties (reviewed in Arneric et al. 1995; Changeux et al. 1992). The nicotinic receptor, whether central or peripheral, is a ligand-gated ion channel that transduces (under normal circumstances) sodium ions. The receptor is a pentameric structure composed in the peripheral nervous system of α, β, γ, δ, and ϵ subunits and in the CNS of solely α and β subunits. Neuronal nicotinic receptor genes encode for a variety of molecular subtypes of these constituent units with at least nine α subtypes (α_2–α_9) and at least three β unit subtypes (β_2–β_4). These subunits can assemble into a number of combinations, and many of these combinations have been expressed in oocyte cell preparations (Elgoyen et al. 1994; Luetje and Patrick 1991; Seguela et al. 1993) with varying degrees of similar properties to native receptors. The variety of subunit genes that have been identified suggest the many different combinations that may occur, many of which may have functional properties. Genes for the human α_2–α_5, α_7, β_2, and β_4 subunits have been cloned (Anand and Lindstrom 1990; Chini et al. 1992; Decker et al. 1995; Doucette-Stam et al. 1993).

The particular combination of subunits in a receptor appears to dictate its functional properties, in terms of its physiology and pharmacology. For example, the ability of the receptor to conduct ions is determined by the amino acid composition of the channel portion of the receptor (i.e., the transmembrane domain). This leads to the possibility that certain nicotinic receptors (e.g., $\alpha_4\beta_2$), which generate brief synaptic currents, may have a different functional role than $\alpha_3\beta_4$, which produces prolonged currents (Alkondon and Albuquerque 1993; Decker et al. 1995). However, despite the burgeoning diversity of receptor subunit components and the knowledge of the distribution of their expression within mammalian brain, less is known about the physiological role of these different receptors. The pharmacology of these receptor combinations is also uncertain, but significant progress is being made in establishing specific pharmacological profiles of certain subtype combinations (Arneric et al. 1995).

Thus far, studies of radioligand binding have identified three neuronal nicotinic receptor subtypes: receptors that have a high binding affinity for (−)-nicotine, (−)-cytisine, and methylcarbamylcholine; those that bind α-bungarotoxin (α-BTX); and those that have a selective affinity for neuronal BTX (a different antagonist from α-BTX) (Decker et al. 1995). There appears to be a concordance between the distribution of certain subunit messenger ribonucleic acids (mRNAs) and agonist or antagonist binding. For example, the high-affinity binding of nicotine correlates well with the distribution of the $\alpha_4\beta_2$ subunit mRNAs, and a correlation exists between the distribution of α-BTX binding and the presence of α_7 mRNA (Seguela et al. 1993). In the rat, the greatest concentration of α_7 message is in limbic areas, which may correlate with behavioral/emotional changes seen in neuropsychiatric disease.

Structure-activity relationships for the nicotinic receptor appear complex. For example, antagonists used to map receptors in radioligand binding studies do not appear to bind to the agonist recognition site. The nicotinic agonists nicotine, cytisine, and methylcarbamylcholine all interact with the same acetylcholine binding site (Arneric et al. 1995). By contrast, the nicotinic antagonist mecamylamine does not competitively inhibit nicotine binding and appears to bind inside the ion channel in the transmembrane domain. Other binding sites have been identified such as that identified with radiolabeled physostigmine (B. R. Martin et al. 1993). The nicotinic receptor appears capable of transitioning through several functional states of activity. These distinctive states have different binding characteristics and degrees of ion channel activity (Lena and Changeux 1993). These states are affected by agonist binding through allosteric modulation effects on various subunits. These changes can modify the proportion of receptors that are in various states of sensitization or desensitization to agonists and signal transduction. The transitions between these allosteric states may help explain the effects of certain agonists; for example, certain agonists may convert receptors from a resting state through a low-affinity activated state to a high-affinity desensitized state that is refractory to activation (Arneric et al. 1995). It may be possible to activate nicotinic receptors at sites distinct from the acetylcholine/nicotine recognition site. Certain cholinergic channel activators (Pereira et al. 1993) may increase ion conductance without being subject to the same desensitization mechanisms as the acetylcholine binding site (Arneric et al. 1995). Examples of such compounds include physostigmine and galanthamine, although physostigmine may have other actions, including channel blockade, at nicotinic receptors (Clarke et al. 1994).

Antagonists of nicotinic receptor function similarly can be divided into several types, including noncompetitive and competitive antagonists. Noncompetitive antagonists apparently bind within the ion pore itself and block signal transduction by steric hindrance. Mecamylamine and chlorpromazine are examples of this type of antagonist. Such blockade is enhanced by agonist binding, possibly because a shift in the equilibrium of the receptors toward a channel-open state is produced, allowing entry of the antagonist. Competitive antagonists include dihydro β-erythroidine, which binds to the agonist recognition site. Other compounds, including steroids, calcium channel antagonists (nimodipine), and barbiturates, appear able to modify the properties of the nicotinic receptor through one or more of the mechanisms outlined above.

The particular subunit composition of the receptor appears to have a major impact on the agonist and antagonist sensitivity and the ability of the agonist to produce signal transduction. Both α and β subunit type are important in defining the pharmacological profile of a particular receptor. At this point, only antagonists are useful for defining receptor subtypes, as no agonists exist that have high specificity for a particular $\alpha\beta$ combination (Arneric et al. 1995). For example, α-BTX specifically labels (and blocks) the α_7 homopentamer and has very little effect at other nicotinic acetylcholine receptor subtypes. By contrast, currently available agonists are relatively nonselective and may have a complex pharmacology, including producing agonist activity at some sites and antagonism at others. Whether (–)-cytisine acts as an agonist or antagonist appears determined by the particular β subunits that are present (Arneric et al. 1995). Lobeline, a nicotinic agonist proposed for use in smoking cessation, also acts as a full agonist or antagonist, depending on the experimental system. Newer agonists of interest include several novel compounds. Epibatidine, isolated from the skin of a South American frog

(Badio et al. 1994), is the most potent nicotinic agonist yet isolated, with a K_i of 40 pM at [^{3}H]cytisine sites and is 1,000-fold more potent than nicotine in some assay systems. Anabaseine derivatives, such as 3-(4)-dimethylamino-cinnamylidine anabaseine (DMAC) and 3-(2,4 dimethoxybenzylidene)-anabaseine (DMXB), derived from sea worm toxins (E. M. Meyer et al. 1994), appear to interact with several nicotinic receptor subtypes, including α_7 and $\alpha_4\beta_2$. These compounds may have cytoprotective and long-term potentiation–enhancing effects. ABT-418 is a novel nicotine derivative with good selectivity for the [^{3}H]cytisine site, but is minimally active at the α-BTX receptor in vitro (Arneric et al. 1994). ABT-418 produces some effects similar to those of nicotine itself, but with findings suggestive of greater selectivity for the $\alpha_4\beta_2$ subtype and less selectivity for the α_3 subunit. Overall, the profile suggests that ABT-418 may be a promising selective nicotinic agonist for clinical and research investigations (Arneric et al. 1994).

PHYSIOLOGY

The precise role(s) of CNS nicotinic receptors is unclear. Direct synaptic transmission using nicotinic receptors has been difficult to demonstrate, with the exception of Renshaw cells. Other physiological effects have been documented for nicotinic receptors, particularly involving transmitter release. Evidence suggests that presynaptic nicotinic positive autoreceptors exist on several cell populations in cortical, hippocampal, and cerebellar areas of the rat brain. In vitro studies suggest that nicotinic receptor activation produces release of acetylcholine, dopamine, and other monoamines (Araujo et al. 1988; De Sarno and Giacobini 1989; Rowell and Winkler 1984; Wonnacott et al. 1990). More recently, in vivo studies using microdialysis techniques have verified that nicotinic stimulation produces acetylcholine release under physiological conditions (Quirion et al. 1994). McGehee and colleagues (1995) have shown that nicotine can enhance both glutamatergic and cholinergic fast synaptic transmission in the nanomolar range in an in vitro preparation. This stimulation may occur through nicotinic receptor-induced increases in presynaptic Ca^{2+}. Modifying the excitability of CNS neurons may be one of the primary roles of CNS nicotinic receptors (McGehee et al. 1995); that is, these receptors may act to regulate the gain of excitatory and inhibitory neurotransmission systems rather than being responsible for direct information transfer. It may be that the often contradictory effects of nicotine in cognitive studies may be best understood in this context.

Nicotinic receptors exist on cholinergic cells of the basal forebrain and may have significant effects on overall CNS activity as measured by electroencephalography, cerebral blood flow (CBF) (Linville and Arneric 1991; Linville et al. 1993), and cerebral glucose utilization (London et al. 1990). Generally, it appears that nicotinic stimulation desynchronizes the electroencephalography, increases stimulated CBF, and increases cerebral glucose utilization, effects that are blocked by the antagonist mecamylamine or abolished by cholinergic cell destruction (McCormick 1990).

COGNITIVE EFFECTS OF NICOTINE

Levin (1992) reviewed the extensive animal studies on the cognitive effects of nicotinic agonists and antagonists in rodents and primates. Enhancement on a wide variety of cognitive tasks, including learning, memory, and other performance tasks, has been shown with nicotine. Enhancement with acutely administered nicotine has been described in both short-term (working memory) and long-term (reference) memory. Examples of tasks in which nicotine has been shown to have positive learning and/or memory effects include the Morris water-maze task in rats, in which rats must learn and remember where a submerged platform is located (Decker et al. 1992), and the delayed match-to-sample task in monkeys, in which monkeys must choose a matching probe to a previously viewed target after a variable delay (Buccafusco and Jackson 1991). Not all investigators have found enhancement; some have found that nicotine produces decrements in performance (Dunnett and Martel 1990).

Studies of animals with lesions also reveal that nicotine can restore function to animals with lesion-induced learning deficits, particularly in animals with basal-forebrain cholinergic damage (Ksir and Benson 1983) or lesions of the septohippocampal pathway (Levin 1992). Persisting positive effects of single doses of nicotine have been described (Buccafusco and Jackson 1991), as well as persistence of learning enhancement for several weeks after withdrawal from long-term treatment (Levin and Rose 1990). The mechanism(s) for these effects is unclear, but could include upregulation of receptors, which is seen with long-term nicotine administration (Wonnacott 1990). Experiments with nicotinic antagonists such as mecamylamine have generally showed that antagonists block the positive effects of nicotine on cognitive performance and alone can impair learning and memory at high doses (Levin 1992; Levin et al. 1987; McGurk et al. 1989). Lower doses have not always produced impairment (Clarke and Fibiger 1990).

Studies in humans have spanned several decades and mostly consist of experiments using cigarettes to administer nicotine, usually to smokers deprived of cigarettes for some period of time. Such studies have been extensively reviewed by Levin (1992), Spillich et al. (1992), and critically by Heishman and colleagues (1994). In general, the use of the deprivation model presents problems of interpretation. Although nicotine may "improve" performance in deprived smokers, it appears that this improvement is usually limited to restoring predeprivation performance, which clearly declines during cigarette withdrawal (Snyder and Hennigfield 1989). Whether deprivation-induced impairment of performance returns to predeprivation level and what the time course of recovery to baseline without nicotine replacement is have not been established.

Enhancement of nondeprived smokers and nonsmokers with nicotine has been more difficult to demonstrate. However, several studies with careful experimental designs have found such effects. Provost and Woodward (1991) have shown that nicotine administration to nonsmokers enhances the Stroop effect, suggesting effects on selective attention. (The Stroop effect is the reaction time difference between naming the color of the text of a neutral word and the time taken to name the color of the text of a word when the color conflicts with the text.) Le Houezec and colleagues (1994) have shown that nicotine administration appears to shorten information processing time on harder stimuli in a choice–reaction time (CRT) task and improves reaction time. Rusted and co-workers (1994) have shown that cigarette-administered nicotine to nondeprived smokers enhances recognition memory, especially in light smokers. Wesnes and Revell (1984) have shown that nicotine may act to prevent fatigue-induced deficits in vigilance and long-term performance tasks. However, Newhouse and colleagues (1992b) were able to note only small, short-lived improvements in an attentionally and cognitively demanding vigilance task with intravenous nicotine administration after prolonged total sleep deprivation. It appears that improvement of "normal" performance with nicotine is more likely with tasks that are attentionally and/or cognitively demanding and with tasks that have a large ceiling or when baseline performance is relatively low. However, performance enhancement in cognitively impaired subjects may be more realistic under real-world conditions.

ALZHEIMER'S DISEASE AND NICOTINIC CHOLINERGIC MECHANISMS

Patients with AD have a wide range of cognitive deficits that can be broadly characterized as problems with acquisition, retention, and retrieval of information; access to previously acquired knowledge; decisional processes; and processing capacity. These deficits have been, in part, ascribed to deficits in attentional functioning (Parasuraman and Haxby 1993). The cellular derangements that underlie the development of AD have been the subject of intense investigation over the past decade. Efforts have focused on the role of β-amyloid, its encoding, expression, and processing (Cordell 1994), although the nature of the disease process still eludes investigators. Further, even if the cellular events that lead to disease expression were fully understood, the way in which these derangements lead to cognitive impairment will still need investigation. It will be necessary to understand what neurochemical/cognitive system deficits are produced by cellular derangements in AD if therapeutic strategies are to be intelligently designed. Although treatments aimed at the basic cellular deficits in AD may be helpful to prevent disease progression, it is unlikely that this will eliminate the need for direct treatment of the cognitive failings in AD, which will probably require agents that directly interact with specific neurotransmitter systems. Further, an understanding of how damaged neurotransmitter systems in AD produce impaired cognitive functioning will increase knowledge of how complex cognitive operations take place in the brain.

Although a myriad of neurochemical deficits have been described in AD, explanation of the nature of the cognitive disturbances has been most closely focused on the *cholinergic hypothesis,* which implicates disturbances in central muscarinic cholinergic mechanisms in normal cognitive functioning and disorders of memory function (Bartus et al. 1982; Drachman and Leavitt 1974). Evidence supporting this hypothesis includes significant reductions in choline acetyltransferase (Corkin 1981) and cholinergic cell number in autopsy-confirmed AD (Whitehouse et al. 1982). Antimuscarinic drugs such as scopolamine disrupt some cognitive functions in psychiatrically healthy individuals (Peterson 1977) and have been proposed as a model of the cognitive deficits in AD (Caine et al. 1981; Sitaram et al. 1978).

Studies have examined the cognitive dysfunction brought about by muscarinic cholinergic dysfunction in humans by administering scopolamine to patients with AD, elderly psychiatrically healthy subjects, and elderly patients with depression (Newhouse et al. 1988a; Sunderland et al. 1986). These studies and those of others suggest that scopolamine models some aspects of dementia (e.g., impaired vigilance and discrimination), but not others (e.g., memory acquisition deficit or the high rate of intrusion errors) (Beatty et al. 1986; Grober et al. 1988). It has been argued that muscarinic blockade with scopolamine may produce a deficit in memory retrieval rather than a true acquisition or memory deficit (Callaway et al. 1985; Dunne and Hartley 1985).

The only clinically available cholinergic therapy to date is an anti-cholinesterase (tacrine). Studies have shown short-term improvement in some aspects of memory and a delay in decline in some patients. It has been generally assumed that these effects are solely the result of enhancement of muscarinic mechanisms; however, this assumption may be unwarranted. Direct muscarinic augmentation produces little measurable cognitive improvement and does not generally reproduce the memory-enhancing effects of anticholinesterases (Bruno et al. 1986; Tariot et al. 1988).

Until recently, little attention had been paid to nicotinic mechanisms in explaining either the pathophysiology or treatment of AD. Patients with AD have a marked reduction in cortical nicotinic cholinergic receptor binding compared with that of age-matched control subjects (Aubert et al. 1992; Flynn and Mash 1986; Whitehouse et al. 1986). Psychiatrically healthy elderly subjects show an age-related decline in cortical nicotinic binding (Flynn and Mash 1986).

In animals, nicotine facilitates task acquisition and memory consolidation (Levin 1992). In humans, nicotine is reported to increase arousal and attention as well as decrease reaction time and prevent decline in efficiency over time (Wesnes and Warburton 1983, 1985). In both animals and humans, nicotine improves the subject's ability to withhold responses to inappropriate stimuli (Myrsten et al. 1972; Newhouse et al. 1988b; Wesnes and Warburton 1983). This may be relevant to AD because a cardinal feature of the cognitive disorder of AD and a possible marker of cholinergic dysfunction (Fuld et al. 1982) is the difficulty patients with dementia have in inhibiting inappropriate responses or in responding to inappropriate stimuli. This difficulty in response selection and/or suppression is one explanation of the liberal response bias seen in AD. Nicotine reverses abnormal behavioral effects in the nucleus basalis lesion model of AD (Ksir and Benson 1983). Evidence from studies of CBF also suggests an important nicotinic component to AD. AD is associated with a marked perfusion deficit in parietotemporal cortex in addition to the global decrease in cerebral perfusion. This focal deficit is seen even in early stages of the disease and appears to be specific to AD (Prohovnik et al. 1988). Although the pathophysiology of this deficit is incompletely understood, attempts have been made to model these changes with pharmacological agents. It is of interest that the nicotinic antagonist mecamylamine reliably reproduces this abnormal CBF pattern (in psychiatrically healthy volunteers), whereas the muscarinic antagonist scopolamine does not (Gitelman and Prohovnik 1992). Studies in animals suggest that CBF may be in part controlled by basal forebrain cholinergic neurons (Linville and Arneric 1991), and nicotine reliably augments the enhancement in CBF produced by electrically stimulating this region (Arneric 1989), suggesting an underlying nicotinic mechanism. As the basal forebrain cholinergic neurons are heavily damaged in AD, changes in observed CBF may be secondary to damage to nicotinic systems. Presumably, the inability to autoregulate CBF impairs cognitive functioning. Taken together, these data suggest that 1) the muscarinic (scopolamine) model of dementia does not account for important features of AD and 2) loss of nicotinic receptors may account for other deficits seen in some cortical dementias.

One other aspect of AD suggests a connection to nicotinic mechanisms. Epidemiological studies of AD that assess risk factors show that, as in PD, smokers are at a lower risk for developing AD than nonsmokers, even when other factors are controlled for. P. N. Lee (1994) completed a meta-analysis of these studies and calculated a relative risk of 0.64 for smokers to develop AD. A study by Van Duijn and colleagues (1995) examined the risk of early-onset AD in subjects as a function of their apolipoprotein (APO)-E gene status and family history. The protective effect of smoking was even larger (odds ratio = 7), especially for subjects positive for APO-E4 and with a family history of early-onset disease. Whether the protective effects of smoking are secondary to nicotine is unclear, but in vitro data suggesting a neuroprotective effect of nicotine are consistent with this possibility (Arneric et al. 1995).

PARKINSON'S DEMENTIA AND NICOTINIC MECHANISMS

Changes in CNS cholinergic systems have also been shown to occur in the brains of patients with PD. In particular, a similar loss of cholinergic cells in the basal forebrain nuclei as occurs in AD has been described in PD (Whitehouse et al. 1983). The loss of cholinergic markers in the cortex (E. K. Perry et al. 1985) that may occur in PD may be related to lesions in these nuclei and other cholinergic projections to the cortex (Whitehouse et al. 1988). In patients with PD dementia, the loss of cortical cholinergic markers has been shown to be of greater magnitude and more extensive than that of patients with PD without dementia (E. K. Perry et al. 1985). Studies have shown that, as with AD, a roughly linear relationship exists between the loss of cortical (particularly temporal) cholinergic markers (choline acetyltransferase and acetylcholinesterase) and the degree of cognitive impairment before death (Ruberg et al. 1982). Patients with PD have also been shown to have an exaggerated sensitivity to the cognitive-impairing effects of scopolamine, similar to that seen in AD (Dubois et al. 1987).

Studies have shown a marked reduction in cortical nicotinic receptor binding that parallels the degree of dementia in PD and increasing age (Aubert et al. 1992; Whitehouse et al. 1988). Similarity has been found between the cortical nicotinic binding site loss in PD and AD as well as similar changes in other cholinergic markers. The loss of presynaptic (R. D. Schwartz et al. 1984) cortical nicotinic receptors may reflect degeneration of cortical projections from subcortical structures, notably the nucleus basalis, pedunculopontine, and laterodorsal tegmental nuclei.

Nicotine was examined as a treatment for PD as early as the 1920s (Moll 1926). A number of studies have shown that smokers have a lower than expected incidence of PD, suggesting a protective effect of nicotine (J. A. Baron 1986, 1994; R. J. Baumann et al. 1980). Nicotine has also been shown to counteract the locomotor effects of 1-methyl-4-phenyl-1,2,3,6-tetrahydropyridine (MPTP)-induced lesions in mice, a putative model for PD (Sershen et al. 1987).

Studies of the cognitive deficits seen in PD suggest that cholinergic mechanisms may play a substantial role, particularly in producing so-called subcorticofrontal deficits (Dubois et al. 1990; Reid et al. 1990). Taken together, these results suggest that loss of nicotinic receptors and their associated source and/or target cells may play an important role in the cognitive deficits seen in this disorder.

STUDIES OF NICOTINIC ANTAGONISTS AND AGONISTS IN ALZHEIMER'S DISEASE

One approach to the question of the importance of CNS nicotinic mechanisms for cognitive functioning is to use a nicotinic antagonist to produce a temporary chemical "lesion." Antagonist studies are often more productive in psychiatrically healthy humans than are agonist studies because of the lack of ceiling effects. Newhouse and colleagues (1992a, 1993, 1994) have studied the effects of the centrally active noncompetitive nicotinic antagonist and ganglionic blocker mecamylamine on cognitive functioning. In addition to attempting to establish that nicotinic blockade produced cognitive impairment in humans, these studies also examined whether there might be age- or disease-related changes in sensitivity to nicotinic blockade, which might be indicated by shifts in dose-response curves between groups.

Subjects included healthy young (mean age 23.9) male volunteers and healthy elderly (mean age 62.7) volunteers. Eleven patients with NINCDS-ADRDA diagnoses of AD (mean age 75.2), Global Deterioration Scale (GDS; Reisberg et al. 1982) level 3–5, and 11 patients with early PD (mean age 68.8), Hoehn-Yahr stage 1–2, also participated in the study. Cognitive testing at 2 hours after drug administration consisted of a computer battery, one oral memory test, and behavioral ratings. Tests included the Repeated Acquisition Test (RAT; D. Thompson 1973), which tests a subject's ability to retrieve previously acquired information as well as the ability to learn new information; the High-Low Imagery Test (Corwin et al. 1987), a recognition memory test with high and low imagery words; several reaction-time tasks; and the Selective Reminding Test (Buschke and Fuld 1974). Mecamylamine was administered double-blind in doses of 5, 10, and 20 mg of mecamylamine and placebo.

Mecamylamine administration produced dose-related impairment of the acquisition of new information, with group differences in sensitivity. This was most clearly demonstrated by the RAT, in which subjects learn a button-pushing sequence. The young healthy subjects showed a significant increase in errors after the 20-mg dose. By contrast, the elderly healthy subjects showed significant impairment after the 10- and 20-mg dose, and the subjects with AD showed impairment after all three active doses (5, 10, and 20 mg). In the retrieval condition (old learning), significant dose-related impairments were found in any group.

The selective reminding task, which involves verbal learning, demonstrated a similar pattern. Here, the young healthy subjects showed a small dose-related decline in total recall but no change in recall failure. The elderly healthy subjects showed a significant and substantial increase in recall failure, however, after the 20-mg dose, and the patients with AD showed increased recall failure after the 10- and 20-mg doses. When learning rate (rate of increase in words learned per trial) was calculated, it was found that mecamylamine produced a small dose-related decline in the elderly healthy subjects and no decline across doses in the patients with PD. In the patients with AD, the learning rate actually became negative at 10 and 20 mg of mecamylamine; that is, the patients with AD were actually getting worse with increasing trials. For the High-Low Imagery Test, a test of recognition memory, a dose-related decline was found in discrimination for both healthy groups, with the elderly healthy subjects showing a greater effect than the young. Perhaps more interestingly, in the elderly healthy subjects, mecamylamine produced a dose-related change in response bias, with a significant liberal shift after the 20-mg dose. This did not occur with the young healthy subjects. Regarding psychomotor speed, mecamylamine produced dose-related slowing in a number of tasks that measured reaction time. These included increases in reaction time for the CRT and manikin (spatial rotation) tasks. Elderly subjects tended to show proportionately greater increases in reaction time than the younger subjects did. By contrast, minimal behavioral effects were found.

In summary, the nicotinic antagonist mecamylamine produced impairment of memory acquisition on the RAT, impaired recall on the Selective Reminding Test, slowing of reaction time, and impairment of discrimination and liberalization of response bias on the High-Low Imagery Test. Furthermore, evidence was shown that elderly healthy subjects were proportionately more sensitive to the effects of mecamylamine, and patients with AD were still more responsive, suggesting a continuum of increasing sensitivity with increasing receptor loss. The lack of clinically significant behavioral changes and physical side effects suggests that the cognitive effects were secondary to specific blockade of nicotinic receptors and not the result of nonspecific effects on arousal or overall well-being.

These results suggest that the deficits produced by mecamylamine resemble in several respects those seen in AD and to a lesser extent in PD. Deficits in short- and long-term memory, impaired attention, liberal response bias, and decreases in reaction time are hallmarks of the dementing picture seen in these disorders. The age-related nature of some of the findings suggest that the decline in nicotinic receptors with age produces increased vulnerability to the effects of nicotinic blockade.

NICOTINIC AGONIST STUDIES
IN ALZHEIMER'S DISEASE

Studies by Newhouse and colleagues (1988b, 1993, 1995) have examined the effects of intravenous nicotine on cognitive, behavioral, and physiological functioning in both healthy nonsmokers and patients with AD. The initial study involved 12 patients with AD with moderate dementia (mean GDS score of 4.4) (mean age 66.8) and 11 young healthy nonsmokers (mean age 30.3). Single-blind infusions of saline placebo or nicotine bitartrate were given for 60 minutes at doses of 0.125, 0.25, and 0.5 μg/kg/min of nicotine base in a within-subjects design. Cognitive testing was performed at 0, 30, and 60 minutes and 4, 8, and 24 hours after the start of the infusion. Behavioral ratings were performed and physiological measures were obtained at regular intervals. Blood sampling was used to measure nicotine levels and to assess the effects on certain plasma hormones.

Analysis of the cognitive effects in the group with AD showed no significant effect on immediate correct recall of a word list. However, there was a significant ($P < .05$) dose-related decrease in intrusion errors on this task, with a U-shaped dose-response curve; that is, the middle dose (0.25 µg) produced the biggest decrease in errors. The decline in errors was apparent for words presented at both 30 and 60 minutes after the beginning of the infusion. This decrease in intrusions was not simply the result of suppression of responding, as total word production was not different across doses. Analysis of long-term recall showed that words that were immediately recalled on the 0.25-µg dose were significantly ($P < .05$) more likely to be recalled 8 hours later than words immediately recalled under other doses or placebo. Behavioral measures showed significant dose-related changes. Depressive affect and anxiety self-ratings showed significant increases in both subject groups, particularly after the 0.5-µg dose. The group with AD seemed more sensitive to adverse behavioral effects and showed significant increases in anxiety and depression at the 0.25-µg dose as well. These behavioral effects were closely linked to the drug infusion period and disappeared rapidly after the infusion was terminated.

Neuroendocrine measures (Newhouse et al. 1990) tended to confirm that the doses used were active at CNS nicotinic receptors. Adrenocorticotropic hormone and cortisol showed significant ($P < .01$) dose- and time-related increases in both groups of subjects. The adrenocorticotropic hormone increase was evident by 30 minutes, with the cortisol increase being delayed until 60 minutes, suggesting no direct effect of nicotine on adrenal cortical cells. Reports of physical side effects were generally minimal, although some subjects complained of a mild headache. No consistent report of nausea was found in either group.

Newhouse and co-workers (1995) have reexamined the effects of intravenous nicotine in AD, but with particular attention on tasks that are affected by mecamylamine. Preliminary results suggest that nicotine produces improvements in attentionally driven tasks, with improved reaction time, hits, and false alarms on a continuous performance task. Throughput (speed-accuracy product) was improved as well. Small improvements were seen also in verbal memory tasks, but no improvement was seen in the RAT, which was impaired by mecamylamine.

These findings of the beneficial results of acute nicotinic stimulation in AD have been supported by the studies of Sahakian and colleagues (J. F. Jones 1993; Sahakian and Coull 1994), who have shown that subcutaneous nicotine administration in patients with AD produced improvements in attentional functioning. This group found that nicotine produced a highly significant improvement in accuracy on a sustained visual attention task (which involved the detection of number sequences). Importantly, there was no speed-accuracy tradeoff; that is, patients do not become slower, even though they become more accurate. Further, these researchers showed that the subjects with AD improved in a dose-dependent manner on attentional aspects of a visual short-term memory and attention task. Further support is provided by Parks and colleagues (1994), who have shown that nicotine improves retrieval from long-term semantic memory and increases CBF in AD. More long-term administration of nicotine to AD has also shown promise. A. L. Wilson and colleagues (1995) administered nicotine by patch for 8 days to six patients with AD. Compared with the placebo patch condition, significantly fewer errors were performed on the RAT while subjects were on nicotine. This effect persisted for at least a week after withdrawal.

ATTENTIONAL SYSTEMS IN DEMENTIA: A THERAPEUTIC TARGET FOR NICOTINIC DRUGS

Alzheimer's Disease

In a review of studies of attention in AD, Parasuraman and Haxby (1993) concluded that attentional impairment represents the first cognitive indication of cortical dysfunction. They noted marked deficits in attentional shifting, divided attention, and sustained attentional functioning. Brazzelli and colleagues (1994) have confirmed that patients with AD show significant deficits in vigilance and sustained attention. Deficits in spatial attention shifting in AD appear to correlate with the degree of parietal hypometabolism (Parasuraman et al. 1992), and Parasuraman and colleagues (1992) found that the reduced cholinergic activity seen in AD is associated with an increased cost of incorrect spatial cues (i.e., impaired shifting of attention). Nicotine acts to reduce the cost of invalid cueing (Witte et al. 1997). An attempt to mimic the impairment of spatial attentional shifting seen in AD used the antihistaminic diphenhydramine (Oken et al. 1994), which did not reproduce the impairment, suggesting that the deficit may not involve muscarinic or histaminergic mechanisms. This is consistent with data from Parasuraman et al. (1992), suggesting that this impairment correlates with the decline in parietal blood flow, which may be under nicotinic modulation (Linville and Arneric 1991).

Studies of the deficits seen in early AD also suggest significant deficits in the central executive component of the working memory model of Baddeley (Baddeley et al. 1991). This has been seen in studies that highlight mechanisms involved in allocating attentional resources using dual tasks and requiring divided attention. On dual tasks, patients with AD show a greater degree of impairment than do psychiatrically healthy subjects, even when performance on individual tasks is equivalent (Baddeley et al. 1991). It has been reported that patients with AD show reverse negative priming, that is, facilitation (Szostak et al. 1995), consistent with impairment of inhibitory attentional mechanisms. Baddeley and colleagues (1986) and others (Cossa et al. 1989) have argued that the inability to allocate and direct attention appropriately may be one of the principal deficits observed in AD. Impaired inhibitory mechanisms appear to be an important element of those attentional deficits. Impairment in divided attention in AD appears to be linked to dysfunction of the right frontal lobe (Nestor et al. 1991).

Further, a characteristic change seen in AD on memory tasks is a liberalization of response bias (Snodgrass and Corwin 1988). It has been noted that subjects with AD show high numbers of intrusion errors on recognition memory tasks (Fuld et al. 1982), suggesting a failure of an inhibitory response selection mechanism. This may result from a reduced inhibition of inappropriate information in working memory or as a reduced cholinergic constraint on information processing (Callaway et al. 1992). The nicotinic antagonist mecamylamine appears to reproduce this effect, whereas nicotine antagonizes it.

Parkinson's Disease

Multiple studies of the cognitive deficits in PD have suggested that there is difficulty with selective attentional functioning (R. G. Brown and Marsden 1990; Dalrymple-Alford et al. 1994; Goldenberg et al. 1990; Stam et al. 1993). There appears to be considerable agreement that cognitive impairment in PD may reflect impairment of prefrontal cortex; that is, patients with PD appear "hypofrontal" (Reading 1991; A. E. Taylor et al. 1986). More specifically, the loss of inhibitory attentional processes may be a general mechanism responsible, in part, for the impairment seen early in this disease (Downes et al. 1993). Downes and colleagues (1993) showed that, on a semantic memory search task, subjects with PD were selectively impaired on trials that required them to alternatively switch search strategies and suppress the immediately prior strategy. Subjects with PD were not impaired on trials that did not require this switching. This loss of inhibitory control in PD has also been seen in the Posner covert orienting paradigm (Posner 1980), in which patients with PD do not show the normal reaction-time cost of invalid cueing, although they show the reaction-time benefit of valid cueing (Wright et al. 1990). It appears that patients with PD do not successfully inhibit the noncued direction, as psychiatrically healthy subjects do. Patients with right parietal lobe lesions also have switching difficulties on this task. Further, it has been reported (Downes et al. 1991) that negative priming is impaired in PD. Although R. G. Brown and Marsden (1990, 1991) have proposed that there is an attentional resource deficit problem in PD, a loss of inhibitory control of attention for the contents of working memory may be a more parsimonious explanation of the deficits seen in PD (Downes et al. 1993).

That deficient inhibitory attention may be a primary defect in PD accords with the proposal of Hassler (1978), that the basal ganglia are important for the suppression of extraneous information, and of Robbins and Brown (1990), that the striatum functions to constrain or weight potential responses, as these structures are involved in the pathology of PD. Delong and colleagues (1983) proposed that the basal ganglia are connected to frontal areas through a "complex loop" involving caudate, various nuclei of the thalamus, and prefrontal cortex. These connections, which have significant cholinergic input, may serve as the source of the frontal pathology in PD and may be responsible for deficits in selective attention (the source of the "hypofrontal" effect cited above). Stam and colleagues (1993) have suggested that proper functioning of inhibitory mechanisms in selective attention are dependent on a functioning striatal/thalamic/frontal "loop." In sum, attentional deficits in PD may be secondary to impaired inhibitional functioning of the central executive component of working memory, which may be secondary to damage to the prefrontal and/or parietal cortex and/or known basal ganglia-thalamic-frontal circuits.

Of course differences exist in the attentional impairments of AD and PD. For example, patients with AD show deficits in shifting or disengaging visuospatial attention, suggesting parietal lobe dysfunction, whereas, on the same task, patients with PD show difficulties with sustaining attention (Parasuraman and Haxby 1993). This difference may reflect some of the neurochemical differences between the disorders. Nonetheless, attentional deficits appear to be central to the developing picture of cognitive impairment in AD, particularly deficits involving partitioning attentional resources and/or inhibiting inappropriate processing. Although PD and AD have different underlying cellular and macropathology, a shared loss appears to be nicotinic receptor and cholinergic cell loss. Although the anatomy of the deficits is incompletely understood, especially in AD, this shared damage to cholinergic systems may be responsible for qualitatively similar attentional deficits. This deficiency presents an attractive therapeutic target for nicotinic stimulation.

Other Neuropsychiatric Conditions

Inhibitory attentional deficits linked to nicotinic mechanisms may not be limited to degenerative neuropsychiatric disorders. Several groups (Adler et al. 1982; Braff and Geyer 1990) have shown that patients with schizophrenia (and their first-degree relatives) do not appear to inhibit cortical evoked responses (P50) to repeated sensory stimulation (sensory gating) as psychiatrically healthy subjects do. This appears to be secondary to deficient hippocampal inhibition (C. L. Wilson et al. 1984), probably the result of deficient nicotinic cholinergic input from basal forebrain (Adler et al. 1993). Adler and colleagues (1993) have shown that nicotine can correct this auditory gating impairment in patients with schizophrenia and their first-degree relatives (Adler et al. 1992) and that there is linkage of the P50 auditory gating abnormality to a chromosomal location (15q14) for the α-7 nicotinic receptor gene (R. Freedman et al. 1997).

It has been suggested that abnormalities in attention-deficit/hyperactivity disorder in children and adults may be similar to those seen in early stages of PD (McCracken 1991). Of interest is that nicotinic mechanisms interact closely with dopamine systems (Kirch et al. 1988) and that nicotinic receptors may serve to regulate dopamine release (Clarke and Pert 1985; Rapier et al. 1990) in striatal and mesolimbic pathways. Nicotine is now being tried as an experimental treatment for attention-deficit/hyperactivity disorder in adults (Levin et al. 1995).

NICOTINIC AND MUSCARINIC CONTROL OF ATTENTIONAL MECHANISMS

Studies of animals with central cholinergic lesions produced by either pharmacological inhibition of choline uptake or direct excitotoxic lesions of basal forebrain cholinergic neurons have shown highly specific attentional deficits (Muir et al. 1992; Robbins et al. 1989). These animals showed deficits that might be predicted from studies of humans with AD; that is, they showed increased response latency and increased responsiveness to irrelevant sensory stimuli. Studies by Vidal (1994b) have shown that administration of a nicotinic antagonist into rat prefrontal cortex impairs performance on spatial working memory tasks which normally requires the rat to suppress its preferred alternation strategy. This suggests interference with inhibitory mechanisms by blocking nicotinic receptors, as the animal must inhibit its normal practice of alternating locations to successfully complete the task. Vidal (1994a) has correlated this behavioral result with nicotinic effects on prefrontal glutamatergic synapses. Nicotine appears to increase release of glutamate in rat prefrontal cortex, as measured by in vivo microdialysis, and increase the amplitude of excitatory postsynaptic potentials from the same region. Presynaptic nicotinic receptors may then modulate glutamatergic activity via their presence on thalamocortical afferents (Vidal 1994a).

Studies of the role of central cholinergic systems and attention in humans suggest that these systems appear to help constrain the focus of attention (Callaway et al. 1992). For example, scopolamine appears to not increase stimulus processing time, but rather increases the distraction-time component of reaction time (R. Halliday et al. 1990) that increases behavioral variability and increases the chance for commission errors.

Cholinergic antagonists appear to impair vigilance performance (Wesnes and Revell 1984), which requires the sustained focus of attentional resources and continuous screening out of irrelevant information. Dunne and Hartley (1986) have shown that, in an attentional task, scopolamine decreased the detection of targets in high-probability locations, but increased detection of targets in low-probability locations. This suggests that the cholinergic antagonist impaired the ability to constrain attentional focus to appropriate target areas and decreased the ability to inhibit attention to low-probability areas. Further, they have shown (Dunne and Hartley 1985) that scopolamine impairs detection of target words in a dichotic listening task, but improves detection of distractor words. Muscarinic antagonists have been reported to increase the Stroop effect while not interacting with stimulus processing (Callaway et al. 1992), suggesting an effect on response selection, which in this task involves inhibition of one modality of information over another.

The effects of muscarinic cholinergic agents on memory function have been extensively investigated, and blockade with such agents has been proposed as a possible model for the cognitive failure seen in AD (Sunderland et al. 1988). However, many of the results of such studies can be interpreted as effects on attentional mechanisms or decision processes rather than true memory effects (i.e., effects on encoding, storage, or retrieval) (Beatty et al. 1986).

Wesnes and Warburton (1983) have shown that nicotine improves sustained attention and vigilance performance, particularly over long intervals. Most interestingly, they showed that nicotine appeared to reduce the Stroop effect. This result most strongly argues for an effect on inhibitory mechanisms, as reducing the Stroop effect requires improving the ability to selectively suppress attention to word reading over color naming. This result was confirmed in nonsmokers by Provost and Woodward (1991), who showed a robust effect of nicotine in this paradigm. Parrott and Craig (1992) showed positive effects of nicotine on visual selective attention; rapid information processing showed improvement, and increased speed and accuracy was seen in other tasks, including letter cancellation.

Warburton and Rusted (1993) have summarized the effects of cholinergic, particularly nicotinic, systems on cognition by suggesting that the data support a role for such systems in regulating the functional state of the cortex and the central executive mechanism (or supervisory attentional system). They further conclude that nicotine's most robust memory effects are seen in tasks that have a high attentional requirement, that is, that memory enhancement may be a consequence of improved attentional functioning.

Extensive animal evidence indicates a functional relationship between nicotine and dopamine systems involved in attention and working memory (Levin 1992). Levin and colleagues (1990) have performed an extensive series of studies suggesting complex interactions with several possible anatomical loci for the site(s) of interaction including both limbic and hippocampal areas as well as descending projections to dopamine-containing areas of the mesencephalon via the medial habenula. Nicotinic blockade appears to impair working memory in the rat, an effect reversed by a D_2 agonist or nicotine. The effect is potentiated with a nonselective antagonist (haloperidol) or the D_2 antagonist raclopride, but not with a D_1 antagonist (Levin et al. 1992). The nicotinic blocker mecamylamine decreases dopamine activity in mesolimbic and nigrostriatal systems, suggesting a mechanism for its effect. Nicotinic receptors modulate catecholaminergic transmission, particularly dopaminergic release (Grady et al. 1992), suggesting a tight relationship between the two systems. Full evaluation of this relationship in human attentional functioning will be the subject of future investigations as selective dopamine agents become available for human use.

CONCLUSION

Converging lines of evidence suggest that loss of nicotinic receptors is a marker of the deterioration of brain structure and function in AD and PD. The loss of these receptors and/or their associated processes may be responsible for some of the cognitive changes and blood flow alterations that are seen in these disorders. Nicotinic systems appear important to normal learning and memory, but effects may be, in part, mediated through effects on certain aspects of attentional functioning. Available evidence suggests that nicotinic cholinergic mechanisms may play a critical role in this process. Effects of nicotinic systems may be mediated through catecholaminergic, cholinergic, and/or glutamatergic transmitter mechanisms in widespread projections to prefrontal and/or parietal cortex and basal ganglia-thalamic-prefrontal loops. Stimulation of nicotinic receptors with nicotine and/or novel nicotinic agonists may produce significant improvement in attentional functioning in AD and PD. This could lead to significant therapeutic benefit.

This model, like other models of cholinergic dysfunction, is not intended to explain all the cognitive deficits in AD. Data suggest that nicotinic systems and/or receptors are modulatory of the release of acetylcholine, dopamine, and other neurotransmitters onto their receptors. Therefore, there are probably limits to the actions of this system, and the loss of these receptors may result in the loss of a degree of control of cognitive processes rather than the underlying basic cognitive function itself. Certain cognitive processes affected in AD may not be under nicotinic modulation or influence. For example, relatively little data support that retrieval of long-term memory is influenced positively or negatively by nicotinic agents, although this is disrupted in AD at later stages. Disruptions of language retrieval (dysphasia and aphasia) do not appear to be linked to nicotinic mechanisms (although see Parks et al. 1994). The data supporting nicotinic effects on direct encoding of memories in psychiatrically healthy humans and patients with AD are limited (although better evidence exists in animals). There is little or no evidence linking nicotinic damage to problems of praxis or procedural memory (although this has been little studied). It appears more likely that nicotinic systems act to modulate or control the "front end" of memorial processing, for example, control and partitioning of attentional resources that are critical to appropriate encoding of memories. Further, these mechanisms may help to control the flow of information into and out of working memory, from the outside or from long-term store, inhibiting irrelevant and augmenting salient information. Although stimulation of this system is unlikely to restore full function, it may augment remaining cell connections, increasing information (signal) traffic, and therefore improve cognitive function.

Future directions for research include specific testing of the attentional hypotheses proposed above. Attempting to replicate the attentional impairments of AD and/or PD with the nicotinic antagonist mecamylamine will help establish the relevance of nicotinic mechanisms to these impairments. Studies of functional brain imaging are justified to begin to define the anatomical substrate(s) of the cognitive effects of nicotinic agents. Finally, therapeutic trials of nicotine and novel nicotinic agonists will be performed to assess the realistic likelihood of long-term improvements in functioning. Preliminary evidence suggests that, although attentional effects can be manifested very rapidly with nicotinic agonists, significant learning and memory effects may take longer administration or exposure to nicotinic agonists than can be provided by a single bolus injection. Finally, the evidence that nicotine has cytoprotective effects, coupled with the evidence that smoking is protective against the development of AD and PD, suggests that it may be worthwhile to consider whether chronic nicotine administration may be a useful strategy to try to delay or prevent the clinical onset of the disease. High-risk individuals, identified by either gene status (e.g., APO-E), family history, or cognitive profile, may represent a promising group to test whether chronic nicotinic stimulation can significantly delay the onset of a dementing disorder.

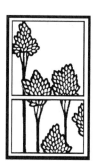

REFERENCES

Abelson JL, Cameron OG: Adrenergic dysfunction in anxiety disorders, in Adrenergic Dysfunction and Psychobiology. Edited by Cameron OG. Washington, DC, American Psychiatric Press, 1995, pp 403–446

Abelson JL, Nesse RM: Cholecystokinin-4 and panic (comment). Arch Gen Psychiatry 47:395, 1990

Abelson JL, Nesse RM: Pentagastrin infusions in patients with panic disorder, I: symptoms and cardiovascular responses. Biol Psychiatry 36:73–83, 1994

Abelson JL, Nesse RM, Vinik AI: Pentagastrin infusions in patients with panic disorder, II: neuroendocrinology. Biol Psychiatry 36:84–96, 1994

Abenhaim L, Moride Y, Brenot F, et al: Appetite-suppressant drugs and the risk of primary pulmonary hypertension. International Primary Pulmonary Hypertension Study Group [see comments]. N Engl J Med 335:609–616, 1996

Abernethy DR, Greenblatt DR, Divoll M, et al: Impairment of diazepam metabolism by low-dose estrogen-containing oral-contraceptive steroids. N Engl J Med 306:791–792, 1982

Abernethy DR, Greenblatt DJ, Ochs HR, et al: Lorazepam and oxazepam kinetics in women on low-dose oral contraceptives. Clin Pharmacol Ther 33:628–632, 1983

Abernethy DR, Greenblatt DJ, Shader RI: Imipramine disposition in users of oral contraceptive steroids. Clin Pharmacol Ther 35:792–797, 1984

Abou-Saleh MT: Lithium and bipolar illness, in Long-Term Treatment of Depression. Edited by Montgomery SA, Rouillon F. Chichester, England, Wiley, 1992, pp 113–138

Abrams R: Electroconvulsive Therapy. New York, Oxford University Press, 1992

Abrams R, Swartz CM, Vedak C: Antidepressant effects of high-dose right unilateral electroconvulsive therapy. Arch Gen Psychiatry 48:746–748, 1991

Adler LE, Pachtman E, Franks RD, et al: Neurophysiological evidence for a defect in neuronal mechanisms involved in sensory gating in schizophrenia. Biol Psychiatry 17:639–654, 1982

Adler LE, Hoffer LD, Griffith J, et al: Normalization of the deficient auditory sensory gating in the relatives of schizophrenics by nicotine. Biol Psychiatry 32:607–616, 1992

Adler LE, Hoffer LD, Wiser A, et al: Normalization of auditory physiology by cigarette smoking in schizophrenic patients. Am J Psychiatry 150:1856–1861, 1993

Adolfsson R, Gottfries CG, Oreland L, et al: Reduced levels of catecholamines in the brain and increased activity of monoamine oxidase in platelets in Alzheimer's disease: therapeutic implications, in Alzheimer's Disease: Senile Dementia and Related Disorders (Ageing, Vol 7). Edited by Katzman R, Terry RD, Bick KL. New York, Raven, 1978, pp 441–451

Agam G, Shapiro J, Bersudsky Y, et al: Effect of high-dose peripheral inositol: brain inositol levels and prevention of behavioral changes due to inositol depletion. Pharmacol Biochem Behav 49:341–343, 1994

Aghajanian GK, Lakoski JM: Hyperpolarization of serotoninergic neurons by serotonin and LSD: studies in brain slices showing increased K^+ conductance. Brain Res 305:181–185, 1984

Aguayo LG: Ethanol potentiates the GABA A activated Cl current in mouse hippocampal and cortical neurons. Eur J Pharmacol 187:127–130, 1990

Ahluwalia P, Singhal RL: Effect of low-dose lithium administration and subsequent withdrawal on biogenic amines in rat brain. Br J Pharmacol 71:601–607, 1980

Ahluwalia P, Singhal RL: Monoamine uptake into synaptosomes from various regions of rat brain following lithium administration and withdrawal. Neuropharmacology 20:483–487, 1981

Ahluwalia P, Singhal RL: Kinetics of the uptake of monoamines into synaptosomes from rat brain: consequences of lithium treatment and withdrawal. Neuropharmacology 24:713–720, 1985

Akindele MO, Evans JI, Oswald I: Monoamine oxidase inhibitors, sleep and mood. Electroencephalogr Clin Neurophysiol 29:47–56, 1970

Akiskal HS: Factors associated with incomplete recovery in primary depressive illness. J Clin Psychiatry 43:266–271, 1982

Akiskal HS: Dysthymic disorder: psychopathology of proposed chronic depressive subtypes. Am J Psychiatry 140:11–20, 1983

Akiskal HS, Rosenthal TL, Haykel RF, et al: Characterological depressions: clinical and sleep EEG findings separating "subaffective dysthymias" from "character spectrum disorders." Arch Gen Psychiatry 37:777–783, 1980

Akiskal HS, Lemmi H, Yerevanian B, et al: The utility of the REM latency test in psychiatric diagnoses: a study of 81 depressed patients. Psychiatry Res 7:101–110, 1982

Alarcon RD, Libb JW, Spittler D: A predictive study of OCD response to CMI. J Clin Psychopharmacol 13:210–213, 1993

Albinsson A, Bjork A, Svartengren J, et al: Preclinical pharmacology of FG5893: a potential anxiolytic drug with high affinity for both 5-HT1A and 5-HT2A receptors. Eur J Pharmacol 22:285–294, 1994

Albus M, Scheibe G: Outcome of panic disorder with or without concomitant depression: a 2-year prospective follow-up study. Am J Psychiatry 150:1878–1880, 1993

Alexander PE: Management of panic disorders. J Psychoactive Drugs 23:329–333, 1991

Alkondon M, Albuquerque EX: Diversity of nicotinic acetylcholine receptors in rat hippocampal neurons, I: pharmacological and functional evidence for distinct structural subtypes. J Pharmacol Exp Ther 265:1455–1473, 1993

Allan AM, Harris RA: Gamma-aminobutyric acid and alcohol actions: neurochemical studies of long sleep and short sleep mice. Life Sci 39:2005–2015, 1986

Allan AM, Harris RA: Both acute and chronic ethanol treatments alter GABA receptor operated chloride channels. Pharmacol Biochem Behav 27:665–670, 1987

Allen L, Tejera C: Treatment of clozapine-induced obsessive-compulsive symptoms with sertraline. Am J Psychiatry 151:1096–1097, 1994

Allikmets LH, Stanley M, Gershon S: The effect of lithium on chronic haloperidol enhanced apomorphine aggression in rats. Life Sci 25:165–170, 1979

Allison JH, Stewart MA: Reduced brain inositol in lithium treated rats. Nature 233:267–268, 1971

Allison K, Paetsch PR, Baker GB, et al: Chronic antidepressant treatment attenuates motor suppressant effects of apomorphine without changing [^{3}H] GBR12935 binding. Eur J Pharmacol 249:125–131, 1993

Altamura C, Maes M, Dai J, et al: Plasma concentrations of excitatory amino acids, serine, glycine, taurine and histidine in major depression. Eur Neuropsychopharmacol 5 (suppl):71–75, 1995

Altemus M, Pigott T, L'Heureux F, et al: CSF somatostatin in obsessive-compulsive disorder. Am J Psychiatry 150:460–464, 1993

Altman HJ, Berman RF: Facilitation of learning and memory following administration of the 5-HT$_3$ receptor antagonists zacopride and dazopride in mice (abstract 16[2]). Paper presented at the 20th annual meeting of the Society for Neuroscience, St. Louis, MO, October 28–November 2, 1990

Altman HJ, Normile HJ: Enhancement of the memory of a previously learned aversive habit following pre-test administration of a variety of serotonergic antagonists in mice. Psychopharmacology 90:24–27, 1986

Altman HJ, Nordy DA, Ogren SO: Role of serotonin in memory facilitation by alaproclate and zimeldine. Psychopharmacology 84:496–502, 1985

Altman HJ, Normile HJ, Galloway MP, et al: Enhanced spatial discrimination learning in rats following 5, 7-DHT-induced serotonergic deafferentation of the hippocampus. Brain Res 518:61–66, 1990

Altshuler LL, Conrad A, Hauser P, et al: Reduction of temporal lobe volume in bipolar disorder: a preliminary report of magnetic resonance imaging. Arch Gen Psychiatry 48:482–483, 1991

Al-Zahrani SS, Ho MY, Al-Ruwaitea AS, et al: Effect of destruction of the 5-hydroxytryptaminergic pathways on the acquisition of temporal discrimination and memory for duration in a delayed conditional discrimination task. Psychopharmacology 123:103–110, 1996

Al-Zahrani SS, Ho MY, Al-Ruwaitea AS, et al: Effect of destruction of the 5-hyroxytryptaminergic pathways on temporal memory: quantitative analysis with a delayed interval bisection task. Psychopharmacology 129:48–55, 1997

American Psychiatric Association: Diagnostic and Statistical Manual: Mental Disorders. Washington, DC, American Psychiatric Association, 1952

American Psychiatric Association: Diagnostic and Statistical Manual of Mental Disorders, 2nd Edition. Washington, DC, American Psychiatric Association, 1968

American Psychiatric Association: Diagnostic and Statistical Manual of Mental Disorders, 3rd Edition. Washington, DC, American Psychiatric Association, 1980

American Psychiatric Association: Diagnostic and Statistical Manual of Mental Disorders, 3rd Edition, Revised. Washington, DC, American Psychiatric Association, 1987

American Psychiatric Association: Practice guideline for major depressive disorder in adults. Am J Psychiatry 150 (suppl):1–26, 1993

American Psychiatric Association: Diagnostic and Statistical Manual of Mental Disorders, 4th Edition. Washington, DC, American Psychiatric Association, 1994

American Psychiatric Association Task Force on Electroconvulsive Therapy: Electroconvulsive Therapy: Report of the Task Force on Electroconvulsive Therapy. Washington, DC, American Psychiatric Press, 1978

American Psychiatric Association Task Force on Electroconvulsive Therapy: The Practice of Electroconvulsive Therapy: Recommendations for Treatment, Training and Privileging. Washington, DC, American Psychiatric Press, 1990

American Sleep Disorders Association: ICSD: The International Classification of Sleep Disorders: Diagnostic and Coding Manual. Rochester, MN, American Sleep Disorders Association, 1990

Amore M, Bellini M, Beradi D, et al: Double-blind comparison of fluvoxamine and imipramine in depressed patients. Current Therapeutic Research 446:815–820, 1989

Amsterdam JD: Use of high dose tranylcypromine in resistant depression, in Refractory Depression. Edited by Amsterdam JD. New York, Raven, 1991, pp 123–130

Amsterdam JD, Berwish N: Treatment of refractory depression with combination reserpine and tricyclic antidepressant therapy. J Clin Psychopharmacol 7:238–242, 1987

Amsterdam JD, Berwish N: High dose tranylcypromine treatment in refractory depression. Pharmacopsychiatry 22:21–25, 1989

Amsterdam JD, Hornig-Rohan M: Treatment algorithms in treatment-resistant depression. Psychiatr Clin North Am 19:371–386, 1996

Amsterdam JD, Mozley PD: Temporal lobe asymmetry with iofetamine (IMP) SPECT imaging in patients with major depression. J Affect Disord 24:43–53, 1992

Amsterdam JD, Brunswick DJ, Mendels J: Reliability of commercially available tricyclic antidepressant levels. J Clin Psychiatry 41:206–207, 1980

Amsterdam JD, Winokur A, Bryant S, et al: The dexamethasone suppression test as a predictor of treatment response. Psychopharmacology 80:43–45, 1983

Amsterdam JD, Maislin G, Droba M, et al: The ACTH stimulation test before and after clinical recovery from depression. Psychiatry Res 20:325–336, 1987a

Amsterdam JD, Marinelli DL, Arger P, et al: Assessment of adrenal gland volume by computed tomography in depressed patients and healthy volunteers: a pilot study. Psychiatry Res 21:189–197, 1987b

Amsterdam JD, Maislin G, Winokur A, et al: Pituitary and adrenocortical responses to ovine corticotropin-releasing hormone stimulation test. Arch Gen Psychiatry 44:775–781, 1987c

Amsterdam JD, Maislin G, Gold PW, et al: The assessment of abnormalities in hormonal responsiveness at multiple levels of the hypothalamic-pituitary-adrenocortical axis in depressive illness. Psychoneuroendocrinology 14:43–62, 1989a

Amsterdam JD, Dunner DL, Fabre LF, et al: Double-blind, placebo-controlled, fixed dose trial of minaprine in patients with major depression. Pharmacopsychiatry 22:137–143, 1989b

Amsterdam JD, Rosenzweig M, Mozley PD: Assessment of adrenocortical activity in refractory depression: steroid suppression with ketoconazole, in Refractory Depression: Current Strategies and Future Directions. Edited by Nolen WA, Zohar J, Roose SP, et al. Chichester, England, Wiley, 1994a, pp 199–210

Amsterdam JD, Maislin G, Potter L: Fluoxetine efficacy in treatment resistant depression. Prog Neuropsychopharmacol Biol Psychiatry 18:243–261, 1994b

Amsterdam JD, Rosenzweig M, Hornig-Rohan M: Clomipramine augmentation in refractory depression. Proceedings of the Third International Conference on Refractory Depression, Napa Valley, CA, October 1995a

Amsterdam JD, Fava M, Rosenbaum J, et al: TRH stimulation test prediction of acute and long-term antidepressant response. Proceedings of the Third International Conference on Refractory Depression, Napa Valley, CA, October 1995b

Amsterdam JD, Mozely PD, Hornig-Rohan M: I-123 Iofetamine (IMP) SPECT brain imaging in depressed patients: normalization of temporal lobe asymmetry during clinical recovery. Depression 3:273–277, 1995/1996

Amsterdam JD, Fawcett J, Quitkin FM, et al: Fluoxetine and norfluoxetine plasma concentrations in major depression: a multicenter study. Am J Psychiatry 154:963–969, 1997

Amsterdam JD, Garcia-Espana F, Fawcett J, et al: Efficacy and safety of fluoxetine in treating bipolar II major depressive episode. J Clin Psychopharmacol 18:435–440, 1998

Anand R, Lindstrom J: Nucleotide sequence of the human nicotinic acetylcholine receptor β2 subunit. Nucleic Acids Res 18:4272–4278, 1990

Ananth J, Solyom L, Bryhtwick S, et al: Clomipramine therapy for obsessive compulsive neurosis. Am J Psychiatry 136:700–720, 1979

Ananth J, Pecknold JC, van den Steen N, et al: Double-blind study of clomipramine and amitriptyline on obsessive neurosis. Prog Neuropsychopharmacol 5:225–262, 1981

Andersen PH: The dopamine uptake inhibitor GBR 12909: selectivity and molecular mechanism of action. Eur J Pharmacol 166:493–504, 1989

Andersen PH, Geisler A: Lithium inhibition of forskolin-stimulated adenylate cyclase. Neuropsychobiology 12:1–3, 1984

Anderson DN, Abou-Saleh MT, Collins J, et al: Pterin metabolism in depression: an extension of the amine hypothesis and possible marker of response to ECT. Psychol Med 22:863–869, 1992

Anderson DN, Wilkinson AM, Abou-Saleh MT, et al: Recovery from depression after electroconvulsive therapy is accompanied by evidence of increased tetra-hydrobiopterin-dependent hydroxylation. Acta Psychiatr Scand 90:10–13, 1994

Anderson IM, Cowen PJ: Effect of pindolol on endocrine and temperature responses to buspirone in healthy volunteers. Psychopharmacology 106:428–432, 1992

Anderson IM, Tomenson BM: Treatment discontinuation with selective serotonin reuptake inhibitors compared with tricyclic antidepressants: a meta-analysis. BMJ 310:1433–1438, 1995

Anderson SMP, Godfrey PP, Grahame-Smith DG: The effects of phorbol esters and lithium on 5-HT release in rat hippocampal slices. Br J Pharmacol 93:96P, 1988

Andrade C, Gangadhar BN, Swaminath G, et al: Predicting the outcome of endogenous depression following electroconvulsive therapy. Convulsive Therapy 4:169–174, 1988

Andreatini R, Leite JR: Evidence against the involvement of ACTH/CRF release or corticosteroid receptors in the anxiolytic effect of corticosterone. Braz J Med Biol Res 27(5):1237–1241, 1994

Angst J: A clinical analysis of the effects of Tofranil in depression. Psychopharmacologia 2:381–407, 1961

Angst J, Wicky W: The epidemiology of frequent and less frequent panic attacks, in Psychopharmacology of Panic (British Association for Psychopharmacology Monograph no 12). Edited by Montgomery AA. New York, Oxford University Press, 1993, pp 7–23

Angst J, Baastrup P, Grof P, et al: The course of monopolar depression and bipolar psychoses. Psychiatria, Neurologia, Neurochirurgia 76:489–500, 1973

Ansseau M, Legros JJ, Mormont C, et al: Intranasal oxytocin in obsessive-compulsive disorder. Psychoneuroendocrinology 12:231–236, 1987

Ansseau M, Olie JP, Von Frencheil R, et al: Controlled comparison of the efficacy and safety of 4 doses of suriclone, diazepam and placebo in generalised anxiety disorder. Psychopharmacology 104:439–443, 1991

Anton RF: Urinary free cortisol in psychotic depression. Biol Psychiatry 2:24–34, 1987

Anton RF Jr, Burch EA Jr: A comparison study of amoxapine versus amitriptyline plus perphenazine in the treatment of psychotic depression. Am J Psychiatry 147:1203–1208, 1990

Anton RF Jr, Burch EA Jr: Response of psychotic depression subtypes to pharmacotherapy. J Affect Disord 28:125–131, 1993

Anton SF, Robinson DS, Roberts DL, et al: Long-term treatment of depression with nefazadone. Psychopharmacol Bull 30:165–169, 1994

Aoba A, Kakita Y, Yamaguchi N, et al: Absence of age effect on plasma haloperidol neuroleptic levels in psychiatric patients. J Gerontol 40:303–308, 1985

Appel SC: Treatment of Alzheimer disease, in Clinical Implications of Neurotrophic Factors. Edited by Appel SC. Philadelphia, PA, Lippincot-Raven, 1997, pp 156–175

Aquilonius SM, Bergstrom K, Eckernas SA, et al: In-vivo evaluation of striatal dopamine reuptake sites using ^{11}C-nomifensin and positron emission tomography. Acta Neurol Scand 76:283–287, 1987

Arai H, Kosaka K, Lizuka R: Changes of biogenic amines and their metabolites in post-mortem brains from patients with Alzheimer-type dementia. J Neurochem 43:388–393, 1984

Arana GW, Baldessarini RJ, Ornsteen M: The dexamethasone suppression test for diagnosis and prognosis in psychiatry. Arch Gen Psychiatry 42:1193–1204, 1985

Arana GW, Santos AB, Laraia EA: Dexamethasone for the treatment of depression: a randomized, placebo-controlled, double-blind trial. Am J Psychiatry 152: 265–267, 1995

Araneda R, Andrade R: 5-Hydroxytryptamine 2 and 5-hydroxytryptamine 1A receptors mediate opposing responses on membrane excitability in rat association cortex. Neuroscience 40:399–412, 1991

Araujo DM, Lapchak PA, Collier B, et al: Characterization of N-[^{3}H]methylcarbamylcholine binding sites and the effect of N-methylcarbamylcholine on acetylcholine release in rat brain. J Neurochem 51:292–299, 1988

Arborelius L, Chergui K, Murase S, et al: The 5-HT$_{1A}$ receptor ligands, (R)-8-OH-DPAT and (S)-UH-301, differentially affect the activity of midbrain dopamine neurons. Naunyn Schmiedebergs Arch Pharmacol 347:353–362, 1995

Archer T, Ogren S-O, Johansson C: The acute effect of p-chloroamphetamine on the retention of fear conditioning in the rat evidence for a role of serotonin in memory consolidation. Neurosci Lett 25:75–82, 1981

Arendrup K, Gregersen G, Hawley J, et al: High-dose dietary myo-inositol supplementation does not alter the ischemia phenomenon in human diabetics. Acta Neurol Scand 80:99–102, 1989

Argentiero V, Tavolato B: Dopamine (DA) and serotonin metabolite levels in the cerebrospinal fluid (CSF) in Alzheimer's presenile dementia under basic conditions and after stimulation with cerebral cortex phospholipids. J Neurol 224:53–58, 1980

Armitage R: Microarchitectural findings in sleep EEG in depression: diagnostic implications. Biol Psychiatry 37:72–84, 1995

Armitage R, Calhon JS, Slegel DE, et al: Interhemispheric EEG coherence in normal controls and unipolar depressed outpatients. Sleep Res 20:356, 1991

Armitage R, Calhoun SJ, Rush J, et al: Comparison of the delta EEG in the first and second non-REM periods in depressed adults and normal controls. Psychiatry Res 41:65–72, 1992a

Armitage R, Roffwarg HP, Rush AJ, et al: Digital period analysis of sleep EEG in depression. Biol Psychiatry 31:52–68, 1992b

Armitage R, Roffwarg HP, Rush AJ: Interhemispheric sleep EEG relationships in depression. Biol Psychiatry 31 (suppl):73A, 1992c

Armitage R, Roffwarg HP, Rush AJ: Digital period analysis of EEG in depression: periodicity, coherence, and interhemispheric relationships during sleep. Prog Neuropsychopharmacol Biol Psychiatry 17:363–372, 1993

Armitage R, Rush AJ, Tivedi M, et al: The effects of nefazodone on sleep architecture in depression. Neuropsychopharmacology 10:123–127, 1994

Arneric SP: Basal forebrain neurons modulate cortical cerebral blood flow: increases by nicotinic cholinergic mechanisms. J Cereb Blood Flow Metab 9 (suppl 1):S502, 1989

Arneric SP, Sullivan JP, Decker MW, et al: ABT-418: a novel cholinergic channel activator (ChCA) for the potential treatment of Alzheimer's disease. Neuropsychopharmacology 10(3S):395S, 1994

Arneric SP, Sullivan JP, Williams M: Neuronal nicotinic receptors: novel targets for central nervous system therapeutics, in Psychopharmacology: The Fourth Generation of Progress. Edited by Bloom FE, Kupfer DJ. New York, Raven, 1995, pp 95–110

Arnsten AFT, Goldman-Rakic PS: Alpha-2-adrenergic mechanisms in prefrontal cortex associated with cognitive decline in aged nonhuman primates. Science 1230:1273–1276, 1985

Arnsten AF, Lin CH, Van Dyck CH, et al: The effects of 5-HT$_3$ receptor antagonists on cognitive performance in aged monkeys. Neurobiol Aging 18:21–28, 1997

Aronson R, Offman JH, Joffe RT, et al: Triiodothyronine augmentation in the treatment of refractory depression: a meta-analysis. Arch Gen Psychiatry 53:842–848, 1996

Arora RC, Meltzer HY: Serotonin 2 (5-HT$_2$) receptor binding in the frontal cortex of schizophrenic patients. J Neural Transm 85:19–29, 1991

Artigas F: 5-HT and antidepressants: new views from microdialysis studies. Trends Pharmacol Sci 14:262, 1993

Artigas F, Perez V, Alvarez E: Pindolol induces a rapid improvement of depressed patients treated with serotonin reuptake inhibitors. Arch Gen Psychiatry 51:248–251, 1994

Åsberg M: Treatment of depression with tricyclic drugs—pharmacokinetic and pharmacodynamic aspects. Pharmakopsychiatrie Neuro-Psychopharmakologie 9(1):18–26, 1976

Åsberg M, Thoren P, Traskman L, et al: "Serotonin depression"—a biochemical subgroup within the affective disorders? Science 191:478–483, 1976

Asher R: Myxoedematous madness. BMJ 2:555–562, 1949

Aston-Jones G, Akoaka H, Charlety P, et al: Serotonin selectively attenuates glutamate-evoked activation of noradrenergic locus coeruleus neurones. J Neurosci 11:760–769, 1991

Atkinson RC, Shiffrin RM: Human memory: a proposed system and its control processes, in The Psychology of Learning and Motivation (Advances in Research and Theory, Vol 2). Edited by Spence KW, Spence TJ. Oxford, England, Oxford University Press, 1968, pp 89–195

Ator NA, Grant KA, Purdy RH, et al: Drug discrimination analysis of endogenous neuroactive steroids in rats. Eur J Pharmacol 241:237–243, 1993

Aubert I, Araujo DM, Cécyre D, et al: Comparative alterations of nicotinic and muscarinic binding sites in Alzheimer's and Parkinson's diseases. J Neurochem 58:529–541, 1992

Aulde J: The use of lithium bromide in combination with solution of potassium citrate. Medical Bulletin (Philadelphia) 9:35–39, 69–72, 228–233, 1887

Austin LS, Lydiard RB, Ballenger JC, et al: Dopamine blocking activity of clomipramine in patients with obsessive-compulsive disorder. Biol Psychiatry 30:225–232, 1991

Austin MP, Dougall N, Ross M, et al: Single photon emission tomography with 99mTc-exametazime in major depression and the pattern of brain activity underlying the psychotic/neurotic continuum. J Affect Disord 26:31–43, 1992

Avery O, Lubrano A: Depression treated with imipramine and ECT: the DeCarolis study reconsidered. Am J Psychiatry 136:559–562, 1979

Avissar S, Schreiber G, Danon A, et al: Lithium inhibits adrenergic and cholinergic increases in GTP binding in rat cortex. Nature 331:440–442, 1988

Axelrod S, Wetzler S: Factors associated with better compliance with psychiatric aftercare. Hospital and Community Psychiatry 40:397–410, 1989

Axelson DA, Doraiswamy PM, Boyko OB, et al: In vivo assessment of pituitary volume with magnetic resonance imaging and systematic stereology: relationship to dexamethasone suppression test results in patients. Psychiatry Res 44:63–70, 1992

Aylward M: Estrogens, plasma tryptophan levels in perimenopausal patients, in The Management of the Menopause and Post-Menopausal Years. Edited by Campbell S. Baltimore, MD, University Park Press, 1976, pp 135–147

Azmitia EC, Dolan K, Whitaker-Azmitia PM: S-100$_\beta$ but not NGF, EGF, insulin or calmodulin functions as a CNS serotonergic growth factor. Brain Res 516:354–356, 1990

Baastrup PC, Poulsen JC, Schou M, et al: Prophylactic lithium: double-blind discontinuation in manic-depressive and recurrent-depressive disorders. Lancet 2:326–330, 1970

Babu GN, Bawari M, Ali MM: Lipid-peroxidation potential, antioxidant status of circumventricular organs of rat brain following neonatal monosodium glutamate. Neurotoxicology 15:773–777, 1994

Bach RO, Gallicchio VS: Lithium and Cell Physiology. New York, Springer-Verlag, 1990

Bacher N: Clonazepam treatment of obsessive compulsive disorder (letter). J Clin Psychiatry 51:168–169, 1990

Baddeley AD: Reading and working memory. Bulletin of the British Psychological Society 35:414–417, 1981

Baddeley AD: Working Memory. Oxford, England, Clarendon, 1986

Baddeley AD: Working memory. Science 255:556–559, 1992

Baddeley A, Logie R, Bressi S, et al: Dementia and working memory. J Exp Psychol 38A:603–618, 1986

Baddeley AD, Bressi S, Sala SD, et al: The decline of working memory in Alzheimer's disease. Brain 114:2521–2542, 1991

Bading H, Ginty DD, Greenberg ME: Regulation of gene expression in hippocampal neurons by distinct calcium signaling pathways. Science 260:181–186, 1993

Badio B, Garraffo HM, Spande TF, Daly JW: Epibatidine: discovery and definition as a potent analgesic and nicotinic agonist. Med Chem Res 4:440, 1994

Baer L, Jenike MA, Black DW, et al: Effect of Axis II diagnoses on treatment outcome with clomipramine in 55 patients with obsessive compulsive disorder. Arch Gen Psychiatry 49:862–866, 1992

Baer L, Rauch SL, Ballantine T, et al: Cingulotomy for intractable obsessive-compulsive disorder. Arch Gen Psychiatry 52:384–392, 1995

Baf MH, Subhash MN, Lakshmana KM, et al: Alterations in monoamine levels in discrete regions of rat brain after chronic administration of carbamazepine. Neurochem Res 19:1139–1143, 1994

Bailey CH, Chen M, Keller F, et al: Serotonin mediated endoxylosis of apCAM an early step of learning-related synaptic growth in aphysia. Science 256:645–649, 1992

Baker GB, Reynolds GP: Biogenic amines and their metabolites in Alzheimer's disease noradrenaline, 5-hydroxytryptamine and 5-hydroxy indole-3-acetic acid depleted in hippocampus but not in substantia innominata. Neurosci Lett 100:335–339, 1989

Baker RW, Chengappa KNR, Baird JW, et al: Emergence of obsessive compulsive symptoms during treatment with clozapine. J Clin Psychiatry 53:439–442, 1992

Bakish D: Fluoxetine potentiation by buspirone: three case histories. Can J Psychiatry 36:749–750, 1991

Bakish D: The use of the reversible monoamine oxidase-A inhibitor brofaromine in social phobia complicated by panic disorder with agoraphobia. J Clin Psychopharmacol 14:74–75, 1994

Bakish D, Saxena BM, Bowen R, et al: Reversible monoamine oxidase-A inhibitors in panic disorder. Clin Neuropharmacol 16 (suppl 2):S77–S82, 1993a

Bakish D, Lapierre Y, Weinstein R, et al: Ritanserin, imipramine and placebo in the treatment of dysthymic disorder. J Clin Psychopharmacol 13:409–414, 1993b

Bakish D, Ravindran A, Hooper C, et al: Psychopharmacological treatment response of patients with a DSM-III diagnosis of dysthymic disorder. Psychopharmacol Bull 30:53–59, 1994

Bakish D, Hooper CL, Filteau MJ, et al: A double-blind placebo-controlled trial comparing fluvoxamine and imipramine in the treatment of panic disorder with or without agoraphobia. Psychopharmacol Bull 32:135–141, 1996

Bakish D, Hooper CL, Thorton MD, et al: Fast onset: an open study of the treatment of major depressive disorder with nefazodone and pindolol combination therapy. Int Clin Psychopharmacol 12:91–97, 1997

Baldwin DS: Depression and sexual function. J Psychopharmacol 10 (suppl 1):30–34, 1996

Ballantine HT, Bouckoms AJ, Thomas EK, et al: Treatment of psychiatric illness by stereotactic cingulotomy. Biol Psychiatry 22:807–819, 1987

Ballenger JC: Medication discontinuation in panic disorder. J Clin Psychiatry 53 (suppl):26–31, 1992

Ballenger JC: Panic disorder: Efficacy of current treatments. Psychopharmacol Bull 29:477–486, 1993

Ballenger JC, Post RM: Therapeutic effects of carbamazepine in affective illness: preliminary report. Communications in Psychopharmacology 2:159–175, 1978

Ballenger JC, Burrows GD, Dupont R, et al: Alprazolam in panic disorder and agoraphobia: results from a multicenter trial, I: efficacy in short term treatment. Arch Gen Psychiatry 45:413–422, 1988

Ballenger JC, McDonald S, Noyes R, et al: The first double blind, placebo controlled trial of a partial benzodiazepine agonist abecarnil (ZK 112-119) in generalized anxiety disorder. Psychopharmacol Bull 27:171–179, 1991

Ballenger JC, Wheadon DE, Steiner M, et al: Double-blind, fixed-dose, placebo-controlled study of paroxetin in the treatment of panic disorder. Am J Psychiatry 155:36–42, 1998

Bammer G: Pharmacological investigation of neurotransmitter involvement, in passive avoidance responding: a review and some new results. Neurosci Biobehav Rev 6:247–296, 1982

Ban TA, Morey L, Aguglia E, et al: Nimodipine in the treatment of old age dementias. Prog Neuropsychopharmacol Biol Psychiatry 14:525–551, 1990

Baptista T, Weiss SRB, Post RM: Carbamazepine attenuates cocaine-induced increases in dopamine in the nucleus accumbens: an in vivo dialysis study. Eur J Pharmacol 236:39–42, 1993

Baraban JM, Worley PF, Snyder SH: Second messenger systems and psychoactive drug focus on the phosphoinositide system and lithium. Am J Psychiatry 146:1251–1260, 1989

Barak Y, Levine J, Belmaker RH: Effects of inositol on lithium induced EEG abnormalities. Eur Neuropsychopharmacol 4:419–420, 1994

Barczak P, Edmunds E, Betts T: Hypomania following complex partial seizures. Br J Psychiatry 152:137–139, 1988

Bardeleben UV, Steiger A, Holsboer F: Effects of fluoxetine upon pharmaco-endocrine and sleep EEG parameters in normal controls. Int Clin Psychopharmacol 4:1–5, 1989

Barden N, Reul JM, Holsboer F: Do antidepressants stabilize mood through actions on the hypothalamic-pituitary-adrenocortical system? Trends Neurosci 18:6–11, 1995

Bark N, Lindenmayer J-P: Ineffectiveness of clomipramine for obsessive-compulsive symptoms in a patient with schizophrenia (letter). Am J Psychiatry 149:136–137, 1992

Barkai IA, Dunner DL, Gross HA, et al: Reduced myo-inositol levels in cerebrospinal fluid from patients with affective disorder. Biol Psychiatry 13:65–72, 1978

Barker AT: An introduction to the basic principles of magnetic nerve stimulation. J Clin Neurophysiol 8:26–37, 1991

Barlow DH: Anxiety and Its Disorders. New York, Guilford, 1988

Barnes JM, Barnes NM, Costall B, et al: 5-HT$_3$ receptors mediate inhibition of acetylcholine release in cortical tissue. Nature 338:762–763, 1989

Barnes JM, Costall B, Coughlan J, et al: The effects of ondansetron, a 5-HT$_3$ receptor antagonist, on cognition in rodents and primates. Pharmacol Biochem Behav 35:955–962, 1990

Barnes NM, Costall B, Naylor RJ, et al: Normal densities of 5-HT$_3$ receptor recognition sites in Alzheimer's disease. Neuroreport 1:253–254, 1990

Barnes R, Veith R, Okimoto J, et al: Efficacy of antipsychotic medications in behaviorally disturbed dementia patients. Am J Psychiatry 139:1170–1174, 1982

Baron BM, Ogden AM, Siegel BW, et al: Rapid down regulation of beta-adrenoceptors by co-administration of desipramine and fluoxetine. Eur J Pharmacol 154:25–134, 1988

Baron JA: Cigarette smoking and Parkinson's disease. Neurology 36:1490–1496, 1986

Baron JA: Epidemiology of smoking and Parkinson's disease, in Effects of Nicotine on Biological Systems II. Edited by Clarke PBS, Quick M, Thuran K, et al. Boston, MA, Birkhäuser, 1994, p S42

Baron M, Gershon ES, Rudy V, et al: Lithium carbonate response in depression. Arch Gen Psychiatry 32:1107–1111, 1975

Barr LC, Goodman WK, Price LH, et al: The serotonin hypothesis of OCD: implications of pharmacologic challenge studies. J Clin Psychiatry 4:17–28s, 1992

Barr LC, Goodman WK, Price LH: The serotonin hypothesis of obsessive compulsive disorder. Int Clin Psychopharmacol 8 (suppl 2):79–82, 1993

Barr LC, Goodman WK, McDougle CJ, et al: Tryptophan depletion in patients with OCD who respond to serotonin reuptake inhibitors. Arch Gen Psychiatry 51:309–17, 1994

Barrett RP, Rowan MJ: Low dose interaction of the 5-HT$_{1A}$ ligand gepirone with atropine on spatial learning in the rat (abstract). Br J Pharmacol 101:516P, 1990

Barrett RP, Rowan MJ: The effects of the 5-HT$_{1A}$ ligand MDL73005EF on the spatial learning impairment produced by either gepirone or atropine (abstract). Br J Pharmacol 107:4P, 1992

Barton BM, Gitlin MJ: Verapamil in treatment-resistant mania: an open trial. J Clin Psychopharmacol 7:101–103, 1987

Bartus RT: Cholinergic drug effects on memory and cognition in animals, in Aging in the 1980s: Psychological Issues. Edited by Poon LW. Washington, DC, American Psychological Association, 1980, pp 168–184

Bartus RT: Age-related memory loss and cholinergic dysfunction: possible directions based on animal models, in Strategies for the Development of an Effective Treatment for Senile Dementia. Edited by Crook T, Gershon S. New Canaan, CT, Mark Powley Associates, 1981, pp 71–90

Bartus R, Dean R, Beer B, et al: The cholinergic hypothesis of geriatric memory dysfunction. Science 217:408–417, 1982

Bartus RT, Dean RL, Pontecorvo MJ, et al: The cholinergic hypothesis: a historical overview, current perspectives, and future directions. Ann N Y Acad Sci 444:332–358, 1985

Bass EW, Means A, McMillen B: Buspirone impairs performance of a three-choice working memory escape task in rats. Brain Res Bull 28:455–461, 1992

Bastani B, Arora RC, Meltzer HY: Serotonin uptake and imipramine binding in the blood platelets of OCD patients. Biol Psychiatry 30:131–139, 1991

Bauer MS, Whybrow PC: Rapid cycling bipolar affective disorder, II: treatment of refractory rapid cycling with high-dose levothyroxine: a preliminary study. Arch Gen Psychiatry 47:435–440, 1990

Bauer MS, Whybrow PC, Winokur A: Rapid cycling bipolar affective disorder, I: association with grade I hypothyroidism. Arch Gen Psychiatry 47:427–432, 1990

Baulieu EE: Steroid hormones in the brain: several mechanisms? in Steroid Hormone Regulation of the Brain (Wenner-Gren Center International Symposium Series, Vol 34). Edited by Fuxe K, Gustafsson JA, Wetterberg L. Oxford, England, Pergamon, 1981, pp 3–14

Baulieu EE, Robel P: Neurosteroids: a new brain function? J Steroid Biochem Mol Biol 37:395–403, 1990

Baumann P: Clinical pharmacokinetics of citalopram and other selective serotonergic reuptake inhibitors (SSRIs). Int Clin Psychopharmacol 6 (suppl 5):13–20, 1992

Baumann RJ, Jameson HD, McKean HD, et al: Cigarette smoking and Parkinson's disease, I: comparison of cases with matched neighbors. Neurology 30:839–843, 1980

Baxter BL, Gluckman MI: Iprindole: an antidepressant which does not block REM sleep. Nature 223:750–752, 1969

Baxter LR, Phelps ME, Mazziotti JC, et al: Cerebral metabolic rates for glucose in mood disorders. Arch Gen Psychiatry 42:441–447, 1985

Baxter LR Jr, Thompson JM, Schwartz JM, et al. Trazodone treatment response in obsessive-compulsive disorder—correlated with shifts in glucose metabolism in the caudate nuclei. Psychopathology 20 (suppl 1):114–122, 1987

Beale MD, Kellner CH, Pritchett JT, et al: Stimulus dose-titration in ECT: a 2-year clinical experience. Convulsive Therapy 10:171–176, 1994

Beale MD, Kellner CH, Pritchett JT, et al: ECT for OCD. J Clin Psychiatry 56:81–82, 1995

Beani L, Tanganelli S, Antonelli T, et al: Noradrenergic modulation of cortical acetylcholine release is both direct and gamma-aminobutyric acid-mediated. J Pharmacol Exp Ther 236:230–236, 1986

Beatty WW, Butters N, Janowsky D: Patterns of memory failure after scopolamine treatment: implications for the cholinergic hypothesis of dementia. Behavioral and Neural Biology 45:196–211, 1986

Bech P: A review of the antidepressant properties of serotonin reuptake inhibitors. Advances in Biological Psychiatry 17:58–69, 1988

Bech P: Clinical properties of citalopram in comparison with other antidepressants: a quantitative meta-analysis, in Citalopram: The New Antidepressant from Lundbeck Research. Proceedings of a Symposium 11 August 1988. Edited by Montgomery SA. New York, Excerpta Medica, 1989, pp 56–68

Bech P, Bolwig TG, Kramp P, et al: The Bech-Rafaelsen Mania Scale and the Hamilton Depression Scale. Acta Psychiatr Scand 59:420–430, 1979

Beck AT, Ward CH, Mendelson M, et al: An inventory for measuring depression. Arch Gen Psychiatry 4:561–571, 1961

Beck AT, Rush AJ, Shaw BF, et al: Cognitive Therapy of Depression. New York, Guilford, 1979

Beckmann H, St-Laurent J, Goodwin FK: The effect of lithium on urinary MHPG in unipolar and bipolar depressed patients. Psychopharmacologia 42:277–282, 1975

Beersma DGM, van den Hoofdakker RH: Can non-REM sleep be depressogenic? J Affect Disord 24:101–108, 1992

Beigel A, Murphy DL: Assessing clinical characteristics of the manic state. Am J Psychiatry 128:688–694, 1971

Beiko J, Candusso L, Cain DP: The effect of nonspatial water maze pretraining in rats subjected to serotonin depletion and muscarinic receptor antagonism: a detailed behavioural assessment of spatial performance. Behav Brain Res 88:201–211, 1997

Bel N, Artigas F: Fluvoxamine preferentially increases extracellular 5-hydroxy-tryptamine in the raphe nuclei: an in vivo microdialysis study. Eur J Pharmacol 229:101–103, 1992

Belcheva I, Belcheva S, Petkov, et al: Asymmetry in behavioral responses to cholecystokinin microinjected into rat nucleus accumbens and amygdala. Neuropharmacology 33:995–1002, 1994

Belelli D, Lan N, Gee KW: Anticonvulsant steroids and the GABA/benzodiazepine receptor-chloride ionophore complex. Neurosci Biobehav Rev 14:315–322, 1990

Bellaire W, Demisch K, Stoll K-D: Carbamazepine vs. lithium. Application in the prophylaxis of recurrent affective and schizoaffective psychoses. Muenchener Medizinische Wochenschrift 132:S82–S86, 1990

Belmaker RH: Receptors, adenylate cyclase, depression, and lithium. Biol Psychiatry 16:333–350, 1981

Belmaker RH, Kon M, Epstein RP, et al: Partial inhibition by lithium of the epinephrine-stimulated rise in plasma cyclic GMP in humans. Biol Psychiatry 15:3–8, 1980

Belmaker RH, Revasov A, Bersudsky, et al: Inositol passes the blood brain barrier sufficiently to reverse lithium effects on behavior in rats. Clin Neuropharmacol 15 (suppl 1):606–607, 1992

Benca RM, Obermeyer WH, Thisted RA, et al: Sleep and psychiatric disorders: a metaanalysis. Arch Gen Psychiatry 49:651–668, 1992

Benfield P, Ward A: Fluvoxamine: a review of its pharmacodynamic and pharmacokinetic properties and therapeutic efficacy in depressive illness. Drugs 32:313–334, 1986

Benjamin J, Levine J, Fux M, et al: Inositol treatment for panic disorder: a double-blind placebo-controlled crossover trial. Am J Psychiatry 152:1084–1086, 1995

Benkelfat C, Bradwejn J, Meyer E, et al: Neuroanatomical correlates of CCK-4-induced-panic in normals. Am J Psychiatry 152:1180–1184, 1995

Benkert O, Gründer G, Wetzel H: Dopamine autoreceptor agonists in the treatment of schizophrenia and major depression. Pharmacopsychiatry 25:254–260, 1992

Benkert O, Grunder G, Wetzel H, et al: A randomized, double-blind comparison of a rapidly escalating dose of venlafaxine and imipramine in inpatients with major depression and melancholia. J Psychiatr Res 30:441–452, 1996

Berelowitz M, Firestone SL, Frohman LA: Effects of growth hormone excess and deficiency on hypothalamic somatostatin content and release and on tissue somatostatin distribution. Endocrinology 109:714–719, 1981

Beresford IJ, Hall MD, Clark CR, et al: Cholecystokinin modulation of [3H]noradrenaline release from superfused hypothalamic slices. Neurosci Lett 88:227–232, 1988

Berger M, Riemann D: REM sleep in depression—an overview. J Sleep Res 2:211–223, 1993

Berger M, Emrich HM, Lund R, et al: Sleep-EEG variables as course criteria and predictors of antidepressant therapy with fluvoxamine/oxaprotiline. Advances in Pharmacotherapy 2:110–120, 1986

Berger M, Riemann D, Höchli D, et al: The cholinergic rapid eye movement sleep induction test with RS-86. Arch Gen Psychiatry 46:421–428, 1989

Berger PA, Tinklenberg JR: Neuropeptides and senile dementia, in Strategies for the Development of an Effective Treatment for Senile Dementia. Edited by Crook T, Gershon S. New Canaan, CT, Mark Powley Associates, 1981, pp 155–171

Berggren U: Effects of short-term lithium administration on tryptophan levels and 5-hydroxytryptamine synthesis in whole brain and brain regions in rats. J Neural Transm 69:115–121, 1987

Bergiannaki JD, Soldatos CR, Sakkas PN, et al: Longitudinal studies of biologic markers for depression in male anorectics. Psychoneuroendocrinology 12:237–239, 1987

Berk M, Bodemer W, Van Oudenhove T, et al: Dopamine increases platelet intracellular calcium in bipolar affective disorder and controls. Int Clin Psychopharmacol 9:291–293, 1994

Berk M, Kirchmann NH, Butkow N: Lithium blocks $45Ca^{2+}$ uptake into platelets in bipolar affective disorder and controls. Clin Neuropharmacol 19:48–51, 1996

Berman RM, Darnel AM, Anand A, et al: Effect of pindolol in hastening response to fluoxetine in the treatment of major depression: a double-blind placebo-controlled trial. Am J Psychiatry 154:37–43, 1997

Bernardi M, Vergoni AV, Sandrini M, et al: Influence of ovariectomy, estradiol and progesterone on the behavior of mice in an experimental model of depression. Physiol Behav 45:1067–1068, 1989

Bernasconi R: The GABA hypothesis of affective illness: influence of clinically effective antimanic drugs on GABA turnover, in Basic Mechanisms in the Action of Lithium. Edited by Emrich HM, Adenhoff JB, Lux HM. Amsterdam, Excerpta Medica, 1982, pp 183–192

Bernstein GA, Borchardt CM: Anxiety disorders of childhood and adolescence: a critical review. J Am Acad Child Adolesc Psychiatry 30:519–532, 1991

Bernstein I, Williams L, Ramsay M: The expression of aggression in old world monkeys. International Journal of Primatology 4:113–124, 1983

Berrettini WH, Nurnberger JI Jr, Hare T, et al: Plasma and CSF GABA in affective illness. Br J Psychiatry 141:483–487, 1982

Berrettini WH, Nurnberger JI Jr, Hare TA, et al: Reduced plasma and CSF gamma-aminobutyric acid in affective illness. Biol Psychiatry 18:185–194, 1983

Berrettini WH, Nurnberger JI, Scheinin M, et al: Cerebrospinal fluid and plasma monoamines and their metabolites in euthymic bipolar patients. Biol Psychiatry 20:257–269, 1985a

Berrettini WH, Nurnberger JI Jr, Chan JS, et al: Pro-opiomelanocortin-related peptides in cerebrospinal fluid: a study of manic-depressive disorder. Psychiatry Res 16:287–302, 1985b

Berrettini WH, Nurnberger JI Jr, Hare TA, et al: CSF GABA in euthymic manic-depressive patients and controls. Biol Psychiatry 21:844–846, 1986

Berrettini WH, Nurnberger JI Jr, Zerbe RL, et al: CSF neuropeptides in euthymic bipolar patients and controls. Br J Psychiatry 150:208–212, 1987

Berridge MJ: Inositol trisphosphate, calcium, lithium, and cell signaling. JAMA 262:1834–1841, 1989

Berridge MJ, Downes CP, Hanley MR: Lithium amplifies agonist-dependent phosphatidyl-inositol responses in brain and salivary glands. Biochem J 206:587–595, 1982

Berridge MJ, Downes CP, Hanley MR: Neural and developmental actions of lithium: a unifying hypothesis. Cell 59:411–419, 1989

Berrios GE: Conceptual problems in diagnosing schizophrenic disorders, in Advances in the Neurobiology of Schizophrenia. Edited by Den Boer JA, Westenberg HGM, Van Praag HM. New York, Wiley, 1995

Bersudsky Y, Vinnitsky I, Grisaru N, et al: The effect of inositol on lithium-induced polyuria-polydipsia in rats and humans. Human Psychopharmacology 7:403–407, 1992

Bersudsky Y, Vinnitsky I, Ghelber D, et al: Mechanism of lithium lethality in rats. J Psychiatr Res 4:415–422, 1993a

Bersudsky Y, Vinnitsky I, Grisaru N, et al: Dose-response and time-curve of inositol prevention of Li-pilocarpine seizures. Eur Neuropsychopharmacol 2:428–429, 1993b

Bhattacharya SK, Glover V, Sandler M, et al: Raised endogenous monoamine oxidase inhibitor output in post withdrawal alcoholics: effects of L-dopa and ethanol. Biol Psychiatry 17:687–694, 1982

Bianchi C, Siniscalchi A, Beani L: 5-HT$_{1A}$ agonists increase and 5-HT$_3$ agonists decrease acetylcholine efflux from the cerebral cortex of freely moving guinea-pigs. Br J Pharmacol 101:448–452, 1990

Bianchi G, Caccia S, Della Vedove F, et al: The alpha-2-adrenoceptor antagonist activity of ipsapirone and gepirone is mediated by their common metabolite 1-(2-pyrimidinyl)-piperazine (PMP). Eur J Pharmacol 151:365–371, 1988

Biederman J, Rosenbaum JF, Chaloff J, et al: Behavioral inhibition as a risk factor, in Anxiety Disorders in Children and Adolescents. Edited by March JS. New York, Guilford, 1995

Biegon A, Reches A, Snyder L, etal: Serotonergic and noradrenergic receptors in the rat brain: modulation by chronic exposure to ovarian hormones. Life Sci 32:2015–2021, 1983

Bijak M: Prolonged treatment with antidepressant drugs increases the excitatory effect of quinpirole in hippocampal slices. Pol J Pharmacol 45:381–390, 1993

Bing O, Moller C, Engel JA, et al: Anxiolytic-like action of centrally administered galanin. Neurosci Lett 164:17, 1993

Birbaumer N, Schmidt RF: Biologische Psychologie, 2nd Edition. Berlin, Germany, Springer-Verlag, 1991

Biro E, Sarnyai Z, Penke B, et al: Role of endogenous corticotropin-releasing factor in mediation of neuroendocrine and behavioral responses to cholecystokinin octapeptide sulfate ester in rats. Neuroendocrinology 57:340–345, 1993

Bitran D, Hilvers RJ, Kellogg CK: Anxiolytic effects of 3a-hydroxy-5a-pregnan-20-one, endogenous metabolite of progesterone that are active at the GABA receptor. Brain Res 561:157–161, 1991

Bitran D, Purdy RH, Kellogg CK: Anxiolytic effect of progesterone is associated with increases in cortical allopregnanolone and GABAa receptor Function. Pharmacol Biochem Behav 45:423–428, 1993

Bitran JA, Potter WZ, Manji HK, et al: Chronic Li^+ attenuates agonist- and phorbol ester-mediated Na^+/Ha^+ antiporter activity in HL-60 cells. Eur J Pharmacol 188:193–202, 1990

Bixler EO, Kales A, Santen R, et al: Effects of flurazepam (Dalmane) on anterior pituitary secretion. Research Communications in Chemical Pathology and Pharmacology 14(3):421–429, 1976

Bixler EO, Kales A, Soldatos CR, et al: Prevalence of sleep disorders in the Los Angeles metropolitan area. Am J Psychiatry 136:1257–1262, 1979

Bjork K: The efficacy of zimelidine in preventing depressive episodes in recurrent major depressive disorders—a double-blind placebo-controlled study. Acta Psychiatr Scand Suppl 308:182–189, 1983

Black B, Uhde TW, Taneer ME: Fluoxetine for the treatment of social phobia (letter). J Clin Psychopharmacol 12:293–295, 1992

Black DW, Winokur G, Nasrallah A: The treatment of depression: electroconvulsive therapy versus antidepressants—a naturalistic evaluation of 1,495 patients. Compr Psychiatry 28:169–182, 1987

Black DW, Bell S, Hulbert J, et al: The importance of Axis II in patients with major depression: a controlled study. J Affect Disord 14:115–122, 1988a

Black DW, Winokur G, Hulbert J, et al: Predictors of immediate response in the treatment of mania: the importance of comorbidity. Biol Psychiatry 24:191–198, 1988b

Black DW, Wesner R, Bowers W, et al: A comparison of fluvoxamine, cognitive therapy and placebo in the treatment of panic disorder. Arch Gen Psychiatry 50:44–50, 1993

Blackburn IM, Eunson KM, Bishop S: A two-year naturalistic follow-up of depressed patients treated with cognitive therapy, pharmacotherapy and a combination of both. Affect Disord 10:67–75, 1986

Blackshear PJ: The MARCKS family of cellular protein kinase C substrates. J Biol Chem 268:1501–1504, 1993

Blancquaert JP, Lefebvre RA, Willems JL: Antiaversive properties of opioids in the conditioned taste aversion test in the rat. Pharmacol Biochem Behav 27:437–441, 1987

Blazer DG: Epidemiology of depression: prevalence and incidence, in Principles and Practice of Geriatric Psychiatry. Edited by Copelan JRM, Abou-Saleh MT, Blazer DG. Chichester, England, Wiley, 1994

Blessed G, Tomlinson BE, Roth M: The association between quantitative measures of dementia and senile change in the cerebral grey matter of elderly subjects. Br J Psychiatry 144:797–811, 1968

Blier P, Bergeron R: Effectiveness of pindolol with selected antidepressant drugs in the treatment of major depression. J Clin Psychopharmacol 15:217–222, 1995

Blier P, de Montigny C: Short-term lithium administration enhances serotonergic neurotransmission: electrophysiological evidence in the rat CNS. Psychopharmacology 113:69–77, 1985

Blier P, de Montigny C: Lack of efficacy of lithium augmentation in obsessive-compulsive disorder: the perspective of different regional effects of lithium on serotonin release in the central nervous system. J Clin Psychopharmacol 12:65–66, 1992

Blier P, de Montigny C: Current advances and trends in the treatment of depression. Trends Pharmacol Sci 15:220–226, 1994

Blier P, de Montigny C, Tardif D: Short-term lithium treatment enhances responsiveness of postsynaptic 5-HT1A receptors without altering 5-HT autoreceptor sensitivity: an electrophysiological study in the rat brain. Synapse 1:225–232, 1987

Blier P, Bergeron R, Hebert C: Differential effectiveness of pindolol addition in treatment-resistant obsessive-compulsive disorder and depression. Poster No. 7, New Clinical Drug Evaluation Unit (NCDEU) Program, 35th Annual Meeting, Orlando, FL, May 31–June 3, 1995

Blin J, Baron JC, Dubois B, et al: Loss of brain 5-HT$_2$ receptors in Alzheimer's disease: in vivo assessment with positron emission tomography and fluorine-18 setoperone. Brain 116:497–510, 1993

Blois R, Gaillard JM: Effects of moclobemide on sleep in healthy human subjects. Acta Psychiatr Scand Suppl 360:63–75, 1990

Bloom FE, Baetge G, Deyo S, et al: Chemical and physiological aspects of the actions of lithium and antidepressant drugs. Neuropharmacology 22:359–365, 1983

Bobon DP, Gottfries CG (eds): Clinical Physiognomy of Thioxanthenes (special issue). Acta Psychiatrica Belgica 74:441–568, 1974

Bockaert J: Serotonin receptors: from genes to pathology, in Critical Issues in the Treatment of Affective Disorders. Edited by Langer SZ, Brunello N, Racagni G, et al. Basel, Switzerland, Karger, 1994, pp 1–8

Boden PR, Woodruff GN, Pinnock RD: Pharmacology of a cholecystokinin receptor on 5-hydroxytryptamine neurons in dorsal raphe of the rat. Br J Pharmacol 102:635–638, 1991

Bodkin JA, White K: Clonazepam in the treatment of obsessive compulsive disorder associated with panic disorder in one patient. J Clin Psychiatry 50:265–266, 1989

Bodrick NC, DeLong AF, Bonate PL, et al: Xanomeline, a specific M1 agonist: early clinical trials, in Alzheimer Disease: Therapeutic Strategies. Edited by Giacobini E, Becker R. Boston, MA, Birkhäuser, 1994, pp 234–238

Böhm C, Placchi M, Stallone G, et al: A double-blind comparison of buspirone, clobazam, and placebo in patients with anxiety treated in a general practice setting. J Clin Psychopharmacol 10:38s–42s, 1990

Bohmann D: Transcription factor phosphorylation: a link between signal transduction and the regulation of gene expression. Cancer Cells 2:337–343, 1990

Bolden-Watson C, Richelson E: Blockade by newly developed antidepressants of biogenic amine uptake into rat brain synaptosomes. Life Sci 52:1023–1029, 1993

Bolla KI, McCann UD, Ricaurte GA: Memory impairment in abstinent MDMA ("Ecstasy") users. Neurology 51:1532–1537, 1998

Bolwig TG: The influence of electrically induced seizures on deep brain structures, in ECT: Basic Mechanisms. Edited by Lerer B, Weiner RD, Belmaker RH. London, John Libbey, 1984, pp 132–138

Bolwig TG: Regional cerebral blood flow in affective disorder. Acta Psychiatr Scand 371:48–53, 1993

Bond PA, Jenner JA, Sampson DA: Daily variation of the urine content of 3-methoxy 4-hydroxyphenylglycol in two manic-depressive patients. Psychol Med 2:81–85, 1972

Bond PA, Brooks BA, Judd A: The distribution of lithium, sodium and magnesium in rat brain and plasma after various periods of administration of lithium in the diet. Br J Pharmacol 53:235–239, 1975

Bonner TI, Buckley NJ, Young AC, et al: Identification of a family of muscarinic acetylcholine receptor genes. Science 237:527–532, 1987

Booth M, Hunt JN, Miles JM, et al: Comparison of gastric emptying and secretion in men and women with reference to prevalence of duodenal ulcer in each sex. Lancet 1:657–659, 1957

Borbely AA: A two-process model of sleep regulation. Human Neurobiology 1:195–204, 1982

Borbely AA: The S-deficiency hypothesis of depression and the two-process model of sleep regulation. Pharmacopsychiatry 20:23–29, 1987

Borbely AA, Wirz-Justice A: Sleep, sleep deprivation and depression. Human Neurobiology 1:205–210, 1982

Borbely AA, Tobler I, Loepfe M, et al: All-night spectral analysis of the sleep EEG in untreated depressives and normal controls. Psychiatry Res 12:27–33, 1984

Borcherding BG, Keysor CS, Rapoport JL, et al: Motor/vocal tics and compulsive behaviors on stimulant drugs: is there a common vulnerability? Psychiatry Res 33:83–94, 1990

Borison RL, Albrecht JW, Diamond BI: Efficacy and safety of a putative anxiolytic agent: ipsapirone. Psychopharmacol Bull 26:219–222, 1990

Born GVR, Grignani G, Martin K: Long-term effect of lithium on the uptake of 5-hydroxytryptamine by human platelets. Br J Clin Pharmacol 9:321–325, 1980

Borsini F, Meli A: Is the forced swimming test a suitable model for revealing antidepressant activity? Psychopharmacology 94:147–160, 1988

Borsini F, Lecci A, Mancinelli A, et al: Stimulation of dopamine D_2 but not D_1 receptors reduces immobility time of rats in the forced swimming test: implication for antidepressant activity. Eur J Pharmacol 148:301–307, 1988

Bouchard JM, Delaunay J, Delisle J-P, et al: Citalopram versus maprotiline: a controlled clinical multicenter trial in depressed patients. Acta Psychiatr Scand 76:583–592, 1987

Bouckoms AJ: The role of stereotactic cingulotomy in the treatment of intractable depression, in Refractory Depression (Advances in Neuropsychiatry and Psychopharmacology Series, Vol 2). Edited by Amsterdam JD. New York, Raven, 1991, pp 233–242

Bouckoms A, Mangini L: Pergolide: an antidepressant adjuvant for mood disorders? Psychopharmacol Bull 29:207–211, 1993

Boulenger JP, Jolicoeur F, Cadieux A, et al (eds): Are peripheral mechanisms involved in CCK-4-induced panic attacks? Paper presented at the 19th CINP Congress, Washington DC, June 1994, pp 117–174

Bouthillier A, de Montigny C: Long term benzodiazepine treatment reduces neuronal responsiveness to cholecystokinin: an electrophysiological study in the rat. Eur J Pharmacol 115:135–138, 1988

Bouwer C, Stein DJ: Buspirone is an effective augmenting agent of SSRIs in severe treatment-refractory depression. S Afr Med J 87 (suppl 4):534–537, 540, 1997

Bowden CL: Predictors of response to divalproex and lithium. J Clin Psychiatry 56 (suppl):25–30, 1995

Bowden CL, Huang LG, Javors MA, et al: Calcium function in affective disorders and healthy controls. Biol Psychiatry 23:367–376, 1988

Bowden C, Cheetham SC, Crompton MR, et al: Dopamine and its metabolites in depressed suicide victims (abstract). Can J Physiol Pharmacol 72 (suppl 1):386, 1994a

Bowden CL, Brugger AM, Swann AC, et al: Efficacy of divalproex vs lithium and placebo in the treatment of mania. JAMA 271:918–924, 1994b

Bowen DM, Davison AN: Biochemical studies of nerve cells and energy metabolism in Alzheimer's disease. Br Med Bull 42:75–80, 1986

Bowen DM, Smith CB, White P: Accelerated ageing or selective neuronal loss as an important cause of dementia? Lancet 1:11–14, 1979

Bowen DM, Smith CB, White P, et al: Biochemical assessment of serotonergic and cholinergic dysfunction and cerebral atrophy in Alzheimer's disease. J Neurochem 41:266–272, 1983

Bowen DM, Francis PT, Procter AW, Young AB: Treatment of Alzheimer's disease. J Neurol Neurosurg Psychiatry 55:328–336, 1992

Bower GH: Mood and memory. Am Psychol 36:129–148, 1981

Bowers MB, Heninger GR: Lithium: clinical effects and cerebrospinal fluid acid monoamine metabolites. Communications in Psychopharmacology 1:135–145, 1977

Bowlby MR: Pregnenolone sulfate potentiation of N-methyl-D-aspartate receptor channels in hippocampal neurons. Mol Pharmacol 43:813–819, 1993

Boyer W: Serotonin uptake inhibitors are superior to omopramine and alprazolam in alleviating panic attacks: a meta-analysis. Int Clin Psychopharmacol 10:45–49, 1995

Boyer WF, Blumhardt CL: The safety profile of paroxetine. J Clin Psychiatry 53 (suppl 2):61–66, 1992

Boyer WF, Feighner JP: A placebo-controlled double-blind multicenter trial of two doses of ipsapirone versus diazepam in generalized anxiety disorder. Int Clin Psychopharmacol 8:173–176, 1993

Boyle WJ, Smeal T, Defize LH, et al: Activation of protein kinase C decreases phosphorylation of c-Jun at sites that negatively regulate its DNA-binding activity. Cell 64:573–584, 1991

Brabbins CJ, Dewey ME, Copeland JRM, et al: Insomnia in the elderly: prevalence, gender differences and relationships with morbidity and mortality. Int J Geriatr Psychiatry 8:473–480, 1993

Bradford LD: Preclinical pharmacology of fluvoxamine (Floxyrol). Proceedings of the International Symposium on Fluvoxamine in Depressive Disorder, Amsterdam, September 8–9, 1984, pp 13–17

Bradford LD, Stevens G: Double-blind placebo controlled fixed dose studies of flesonoxan in generalized anxiety disorders. Abstract 167, American College of Neuropsychopharmacology Annual Meeting, San Juan, Puerto Rico, December 1994

Bradwejn J, de Montigny C: Benzodiazepines antagonize cholecystokinin-induced activation of rat hippocampal neurons. Nature 312:363–364, 1984

Bradwejn J, Koszycki D: Comparison of CO2-induced panic attacks with cholecystokinin-induced panic attacks in PD. Prog Neuropsychopharmacol Biol Psychiatry 15:237–239, 1991

Bradwejn J, Koszycki D: CCK-4 and panic attacks in man, in Multiple Cholecystokinin Receptors in Man. Edited by Iversen S, Dourish C, Cooper F. Oxford, England, Oxford University Press, 1992, pp 121–131

Bradwejn J, Koszycki D: The cholecystokinin hypothesis of anxiety and panic disorders. Ann N Y Acad Sci 713:273–282, 1994a

Bradwejn J, Koszycki D: Imipramine antagonizes the panicogenic effects of CCK-4 in panic disorder patients. Am J Psychiatry 151:261–263, 1994b

Bradwejn J, Koszycki D, Meterissian G: Cholecystokinin-tetrapeptide induced panic attacks in patients with panic disorder. Can J Psychiatry 35:83–85, 1990

Bradwejn J, Koszycki D, Bourin M: Dose ranging study of the effect of CCK-4 in healthy volunteers. J Psychiatry Neurosci 16:260–264, 1991a

Bradwejn J, Koszycki D, Shroqui C: Enhanced sensitivity to cholecystokinin tetrapeptide in panic disorder. Arch Gen Psychiatry 48:603–610, 1991b

Bradwejn J, Koszycki D, Couetoux du Tertre A, et al: The cholecystokinin hypothesis of panic and anxiety disorders: a review. J Psychopharmacol 6:345, 1992a

Bradwejn J, Koszycki D, Annable L: A dose-ranging study of the behavioral and cardiovascular effects of CCK-tetrapeptide in PD. Biol Psychiatry 32:903–912, 1992b

Bradwejn J, Koszycki D, Payeur R: Study of the replication of action of cholecystokinin in panic disorders. Am J Psychiatry 149:962–964, 1992c

Bradwejn J, Koszycki D, Couetoux-Dutertre AC, et al: L-365,260, a CCK-B receptor antagonist, blocks CCK-4 panic (oral presentation). Presented at the annual meeting of the Anxiety Disorders Association of America (NR 235), Charleston, SC, March 20, 1993

Bradwejn J, Koszycki D, Couetoux du Tertre A, et al: Effects of flumazenil on cholecystokinin-tetrapeptide-induced panic symptoms in healthy volunteers. Psychopharmacology 114:257–261, 1994a

Bradwejn J, Koszycki D, Couetoux-Dutertre A: L-365,260: a CCK-B antagonist blocks CCK-4-panic in panic disorder. Arch Gen Psychiatry 51:486–493, 1994b

Bradwejn J, Koszycki D, Annable L, et al: The panicogenic effects of cholecystokinin tetrapeptide are anatgonized by L-365,260, a central cholecystokinin receptor antagonist in patients with panic disorder. Arch Gen Psychiatry 51:486–493, 1994c

Bradwejn J, Koszycki D, Paradis M, et al: Effect of CI-988 on cholecystokinin tetrapeptide-induced panic symptoms in healthy volunteers. Biol Psychiatry 38:742–746, 1995

Brady KT, Sonne SC, Anton R, Ballenger JC: Valproate in the treatment of acute bipolar affective episodes complicated by substance abuse: a pilot study. J Clin Psychiatry 56:118–121, 1995

Braff DL, Geyer MA: Sensorimotor gating and schizophrenia: human and animal model studies. Arch Gen Psychiatry 47:181–188, 1990

Bramanti P, Bianchi L, Benedetto M, et al: Study of the hypnic effect of amineptine evaluation by polygraphy and tests. Prog Neuropsychopharmacol Biol Psychiatry 9:157–165, 1985

Brambilla F, Bellodi L, Perna G: Lymphocyte cholecystokinin concentrations in panic disorder. Am J Psychiatry 150:1111–1113, 1993

Brambilla F, Perna G, Barberi A, et al: Alpha-2-adrenergic receptor sensitivity in panic disorder, I: GH response to GHRH and clonidine stimulation in panic disorder. Psychoneuroendocrinology 1:1–9, 1995

Brami BA, Leli U, Hauser G: Influence of lithium on second messenger accumulation in NG108-15 cells. Biochem Biophys Res Commun 174:606–612, 1991a

Brami BA, Leli U, Hauser G: Origin of the diacylglycerol produced in excess of inositol phosphates by lithium in NG108-15 cells. J Neurochem 57 (suppl):S9, 1991b

Brandt L, Saveland H, Ljunggren B, et al: Control of epilepsy partialis continuans with intravenous nimodipine: report of two cases. J Neurosurg 69:949–950, 1988

Brantigan CO, Brantigan TA, Joseph N: Effect of beta-blockade and beta-stimulation on stage fright. Am J Med 72:88–94, 1982

Braughler JM, Hall ED, Jacobsen EJ, et al: The 21 aminosteroids: potent inhibitors of lipid peroxidation for the treatment of central nervous system trauma and ischemia. Drug Future 14:143–152, 1989

Brazzelli M, Cocchini G, Della Sala S, et al: Alzheimer patients show a sensitivity decrement over time on a tonic alertness task. J Clin Exp Neuropsychol 16:851–860, 1994

Breier A: Serotonin, schizophrenia and antipsychotic drug action. Schizophr Res 14:187–202, 1995

Brennan MJW, Sandyk R, Barsook D: Use of sodium valproate in the management of affective disorders: basic and clinical aspects, in Anticonvulsants in Affective Disorders. Edited by Emrich HM, Okuma T, Müller AA. Amsterdam, Excerpta Medica, 1984, pp 56–65

Briley M, Chopin P, Moret C: New concepts in Alzheimer's disease. Neurobiol Aging 7:57–62, 1986

Briley M, Chopin P, Moret C: The role of serotonin in anxiety: behavioral approaches, in New Concepts in Anxiety. Edited by Briley M, File SE. London, Macmillan, 1991, pp 56–73

Brinton RD: The neurosteroid 3a-hydroxy-5a-pregnan-20-one induces cytoarchitectural regression in cultured fetal hippocampal neurons. J Neurosci 14:2763–2774, 1994

Britton KT, Morgan J, Rivier J, et al: Chlordiazepoxide attenuates response suppression induced by corticotropin-releasing factor in the conflict test. Psychopharmacology 86:170–174, 1985

Britton KT, Lee G, Vale W, et al: Corticotropin releasing factor (CRF) receptor antagonist blocks activating and "anxiogenic" actions of CRF in the rat. Brain Res 369:303–306, 1986

Britton KT, Page M, Baldwin H, et al: Anxiolytic activity of steroid anesthetic alphaxalone. J Exp Pharmacol Ther 258:124–129, 1991

Britton KT, McLeod S, Koob GF, et al: Pregnane steroid alphaxolane attenuates anxiogenic behavioral effects of corticotropin releasing factor and stress. Pharmacol Biochem Behav 41:399–403, 1992

Broekkamp CL, Garrigon D, Lloyd KG: Serotonin mimetic and antidepressant drugs on passive avoidance learning by olfactory bulbectomized rats. Pharmacol Biochem Behav 13:643–646, 1980

Broocks A, Pigott TA, Canter S, et al: Acute administration of ondansetron and M-CPP in patients with obsessive-compulsive disorder (OCD) and controls: behavioural and biological results. Biol Psychiatry 31:174A, 1992

Brotman AW, Farhadi AM, Gelenberg AJ: Verapamil treatment of acute mania. J Clin Psychiatry 47:136–138, 1986

Brown AS, Gershon S: Dopamine and depression. J Neural Transm 91:75–109, 1993

Brown D, Silverstone T, Cookson J: Carbamazepine compared to haloperidol in acute mania. Int Clin Psychopharmacol 4:229–238, 1989

Brown GM: Endocrine aspects of psychosocial dwarfism, in Hormones, Behavior, and Psychopathology. Edited by Sachar E. New York, Raven, 1975

Brown GR, Rundell JR: A prospective study of psychiatric aspects of early HIV disease in women. Gen Hosp Psychiatry 15:139–147, 1993

Brown GW, Harris TO: Aetiology of anxiety and depressive disorders in an inner-city population, 1: early adversity. Psychol Med 23:143–154, 1993

Brown GW, Harris T, Copeland JR: Depression and loss. Br J Psychiatry 130:1–18, 1977

Brown RG, Marsden CD: Cognitive function in Parkinson's disease: from description to theory. Trends Neurosci 13:21–29, 1990

Brown RG, Marsden CD: Dual task performance and processing resources in normal subjects and patients with Parkinson's disease. Brain 114:215–231, 1991

Brown RP, Frances A, Kocsis JH, et al: Psychotic vs. nonpsychotic depression: comparison of treatment response. J Nerv Ment Dis 170:635–637, 1982

Brown SA, Irwin M, Schuckit MA: Changes in anxiety among abstinent male alcoholics. J Stud Alcohol 52:55–61, 1991

Browne M, Horn E, Jones TT: The benefits of clomipramine-fluoxetine combination in obsessive compulsive disorder. Can J Psychiatry 38(4):242–243, 1993

Bruguerolle B, Toumi M, Faraj F, et al: Influence of menstrual cycle on theophylline pharmacokinetics in asthmatics. Eur J Clin Pharmacol 39:59–61, 1990

Brun A: An overview of light and electron microscopic changes, in Alzheimer's Disease. Edited by Reisberg B. New York, Free Press, 1983, pp 37–47

Brunet G, Cerlich B, Robert P, et al: Open trial of a calcium antagonist, nimodipine in acute mania. Clin Neuropharmacol 13:224–228, 1990

Bruno G, Mohr E, Gillespie M, et al: Muscarinic agonist therapy of Alzheimer's disease. Arch Neurol 43:659–661, 1986

Buccafusco JJ, Jackson WJ: Beneficial effects of nicotine administered prior to a delayed matching-to-sample task in the young and aged monkeys. Neurobiol Aging 12:233–238, 1991

Buchan H, Johnstone E, McPherson K, et al: Who benefits from electroconvulsive therapy? Combined results of the Leicester and Northwick Park trials. Br J Psychiatry 160:355–359, 1992

Buchanan CM, Eccles JS, Becker JB: Are adolescents the victims of raging hormones? Evidence for activational effects of hormones on moods and behavior at adolescence. Psychol Bull 111:62–107, 1992

Buchsbaum MS, Wu J, DeLisi LE, et al: Frontal cortex and basal ganglia metabolic rates assessed by positron emission tomography with [18F]2-deoxyglucose in affective illness. J Affect Disord 10:137–152, 1986

Buhot MC, Patra SK, Naili S: Spatial memory deficits following stimulation of hippocampal 5-HT$_{1B}$ receptors in the rat. Eur J Pharmacol 285:221–228, 1995

Buijs RM, De Vries GJ, Van Leeuwen FW: The distribution and synaptic release of oxytocin in the central nervous system, in Oxytocin: Clinical and Laboratory Studies. Edited by Amico JA, Robinson AG. Amsterdam, Elsevier, 1985, pp 77–86

Buck KJ, Harris RA: Benzodiazepine agonist and inverse agonist actions on GabaA receptor-operated chloride channels, II: chronic effects of ethanol. J Pharmacol Exp Ther 253:713–719, 1990

Bunce K, Tyers M, Beranek P: Clinical evaluation of 5-HT$_3$ receptor antagonists as anti-emetics. Trends Pharmacol Sci 12:46–48, 1991

Bunney WE: Neuronal receptor function in psychiatry: strategy and theory, in Neuroreceptors: Basic and Clinical Aspects. Edited by Usdin E, Bunney WE Jr, Davis JM. New York, Wiley, 1981

Bunney WE Jr, Davis JM: Norepinephrine in depressive reactions: a review. Arch Gen Psychiatry 13:483–494, 1965

Bunney WE, Garland BL: Lithium and its possible modes of action, in Neurobiology of Mood Disorders. Edited by Post RM, Ballenger J. Baltimore, MD, Williams & Wilkins, 1984, pp 731–743

Bunney WE, Garland-Bunney BL: Mechanism of action of lithium in affective illness: basic and clinical implications, in Psychopharmacology: The Third Generation of Progress. Edited by Meltzer HY. New York, Raven, 1987, pp 553–565

Bunney WE Jr, Hamburg DA: Methods for reliable longitudinal observation of behavior. Arch Gen Psychiatry 9:280–294, 1963

Burke WJ, Roccaforte WH, Wengel SP, et al: L-Deprenyl in the treatment of mild dementia of the Alzheimer type: results of a 15-month trial. J Am Geriatr Soc 41:1219–1225, 1993

Burke WJ, Dewan V, Wengel SP, et al: The use of selective serotonin reuptake inhibitors for depression and psychosis complicating dementia. Int J Geriatr Psychiatry 12:519–525, 1997

Burns G, Herz A, Nikolarakis KE: Stimulation of hypothalamic opioid peptide release by lithium is mediated by opioid autoreceptors: evidence from a combined in vitro, ex vivo study. Neuroscience 36:691–697, 1990

Burt DR, Kamatchi GL: GABA A receptor subtypes: from pharmacology to molecular biology. FASEB J 5:2916–2923, 1991

Buschke H, Fuld P: Evaluating storage retention, and retrieval in disordered memory and learning. Neurology 24:1019–1025, 1974

Butcher SP, Liptropt J, Arbuthnott GW: Characterisation of methylphenidate and nomifensin-induced dopamine release in rat striatum using in vivo brain microdialysis. Neurosci Lett 122:245–248, 1991

Butelman ER: The effect of NMDA antagonists in the radial arm maze with interposed delay. Pharmacol Biochem Behav 35:533–536, 1990

Butler PD, Weiss JM, Stout JC, et al: Corticotropin-releasing factor produces fear-enhancing and behavioral activating effects following infusion into the locus coeruleus. J Neurosci 10:176–183, 1990

Buxbaum JD, Gandy SE, Cicchetti P: Processing of Alzheimer beta/A4 amyloid precursor protein: modulation by agents that regulate protein phosphorylation. Proc Natl Acad Sci U S A 87:6003–6006, 1990

Bylund DB: Subtypes of alpha 1- and alpha 2-adrenergic receptors. FASEB J 6(3):832–839, 1992

Cabrera JF, Muhlbauer HD, Schley J, et al: Long-term randomized clinical trial on oxcarbazepine vs lithium in bipolar and schizoaffective disorders: preliminary results. Pharmacopsychiatry 19:282–283, 1986

Cade JFJ: Lithium salts in the treatment of psychotic excitement. Med J Aust 36:349–352, 1949

Caillard V: Treatment of mania using a calcium antagonist—preliminary trial. Neuropsychobiology 14:23–26, 1985

Caine ED, Polinsky RJ: Haloperidol induced dysphoria in patients with Tourette syndrome. Am J Psychiatry 236:1216–1217, 1979

Caine ED, Weingartner H, Ludlow EA, et al: Qualitative analysis of scopolamine-induced amnesia. Psychopharmacology 74:74–80, 1981

Calabrese JR, Delucchi GA: Spectrum of efficacy of valproate in 55 rapid-cycling manic depressives. Am J Psychiatry 147:431–434, 1990

Calabrese JR, Markowitz PJ, Kimmel SE, et al: Spectrum of efficacy of valproate in 78 rapid-cycling bipolar patients. J Clin Psychopharmacol 12 (suppl):53–56, 1992

Calabrese JR, Woyshville MJ, Kimmerl SE, et al: Predictors of valproate response in bipolar rapid cycling. J Clin Psychopharmacol 13:280–283, 1993a

Calabrese JR, Rapport DJ, Kimmel SE, et al: Rapid cycling bipolar disorder and its treatment with valproate. Can J Psychiatry 38 (suppl 2):S57–S61, 1993b

Caldwell BM, Watson RI: Evaluation of psychologic effects of sex hormone administration in aged women: results of therapy after 6 months. J Gerontol 7:228–244, 1952

Calev A, Fink M, Petrides G, et al: Caffeine pretreatment enhances clinical efficacy and reduces cognitive effects of electroconvulsive therapy. Convulsive Therapy 9:95–100, 1993

Callaway E, Halliday R, Naylor H, et al: Effects of oral scopolamine on human stimulus evaluation. Psychopharmacology 85:133–138, 1985

Callaway E, Halliday R, Naylor H: Cholinergic activity and constraints on information processing. Biol Psychol 33:1–21, 1992

Calvocoressi L, Lewis B, Harris M, et al: Family accommodation in obsessive compulsive disorder. Am J Psychiatry 152:441–443, 1995

Cameron DL, Williams JT: Dopamine D_1 receptors facilitate transmitter release. Nature 366:344–347, 1993

Cameron OG, Smith CB: Comparison of acute and chronic lithium treatment on 3H-norepinephrine uptake by rat brain slices. Psychopharmacology 67:81–85, 1980

Cantello R, Gianell M, Civardi C, et al: Magnetic brain stimulation: the silent period after the motor evoked potential. Neurology 42:1951–1959, 1992

Canton T, Doble A: Evidence for different binding domains on the GABAa benzo-diazepine receptor for benzodiazepines and cyclopyrrolones. Clin Neuro-pharmacol 15 (suppl 1 pt B):125, 1992

Cantor P, Rehfeld JF: Cholecystokinin in pig plasma: release of components devoid of a bioactive COOH-terminus. Am J Physiol 256:53–61, 1989

Caplan LR, Ahmed I: Depression and neurological disease: their distinction and asso-ciation. Gen Hosp Psychiatry 14:177–185, 1992

Carey GJ, Costall B, Domeney AM: Behavioral effects of anxiogenic agents in the common marmoset. Pharmacol Biochem Behav 42:143–153, 1992

Carlberg C, Wiesenberg I: The orphan receptor family RZR/ROR, melatonin, and lipooxygenase: an unexpected relationship. J Pineal Res 18:171–178, 1995

Carli M, Samanin R: 8-hydroxy-2-di-n-propylaminotetralin impairs spatial learning in a water maze role of postsynaptic 5-HT$_{1A}$ receptors. Br J Pharmacol 105: 720–726, 1992

Carli M, Tranchina S, Samanin R: 8-Hydroxy-2-(di-n-propylamino)tetralin, a 5-HT$_{1A}$ receptor agonist, impairs performance in a passive avoidance task. Eur J Pharmacol 211:227–234, 1992

Carli M, Luschi R, Garofalo P: 8-OH-DPAT impairs spatial but not visual learning in a water maze by stimulating 5-HT$_{1A}$ receptors in the hippocampus. Behav Brain Res 67:67–74, 1995a

Carli M, Luschi R, Samanin R: (S)-WAY100135, a 5-HT$_{1A}$ receptor antagonist, pre-vents the impairment of spatial learning caused by intra-hippocampal scopol-amine. Eur J Pharmacol 283:133–139, 1995b

Carli M, Luschi R, Samanin R: Dose-related impairment of spatial learning by intrahippocampal scopolamine : antagonism by ondansetron, a 5-HT$_3$ receptor an-tagonist. Behav Brain Res 82:185–194, 1997

Carlsson A: Aging and brain neurotransmitters, in Strategies for the Development of an Effective Treatment for Senile Dementia. Edited by Crook T, Gershon S. New Canaan, CT, Mark Powley Associates, 1981, pp 93–104

Carman JS, Wyatt ES, Smith W, et al: Calcium and calcitonin in bipolar illness, in Neurobiology of Mood Disorders. Edited by Post RM, Ballenger JC. Baltimore, MD, Williams & Wilkins, 1984, pp 340–355

Carmiliet EE: Influence of lithium ions on the transmembrane potential and cation content of cardiac cells. J Gen Physiol 47:501–530, 1964

Carney MWP, Roth M, Garside RF: The diagnosis of depressive syndromes and the prediction of ECT response. Br J Psychiatry 111:659–674, 1965

Carroll BJ, Martin FI, Davis B: Pituitary-adrenal function in depression. Lancet 556:1373–1374, 1968

Carroll BJ, Curtis GC, Mendels J: Cerebrospinal fluid and plasma free cortisol con-centration in depression. Psychol Med 6:235–244, 1976a

Carroll BJ, Curtis GC, Mendels J: Neuroendocrine regulation in depression. I: limbic system—adrenocortical dysfunction. Arch Gen Psychiatry 33:1039–1044, 1976b

Carroll BJ, Curtis GC, Mendels J: Neuroendocrine regulation in depression, II: discrimination of depressed from nondepressed patients. Arch Gen Psychiatry 33:1051–1058, 1976c

Carroll BJ, Greden JF, Feinberg M, et al: Neuroendocrine dysfunction in genetic subtypes of primary unipolar depression. Psychiatry Res 2:251–258, 1980

Carta A, Calvani M: Acetyl-L-carnitine: a drug able to slow the progress of Alzheimer's disease? Ann N Y Acad Sci 640:228–232, 1991

Carter MM, Hollon SD, Carson R, Shelton RC: Effects of a safe person on induced distress following a biological challenge in panic disorder with agoraphobia. J Abnorm Psychol 194:156–161, 1995

Cartwright RD: Rapid eye movement sleep characteristics during and after mood disturbing events. Arch Gen Psychiatry 40:197–201, 1983

Casas M, Alvarez E, Duro P, et al: Antiandrogenic treatment of obsessive-compulsive neurosis. Acta Psychiatr Scand 73:221–222, 1986

Casebolt TL, Jope RS: Long-term lithium treatment selectively reduces receptor-coupled inositol phospholipid hydrolysis in rat brain. Biol Psychiatry 25:329–340, 1989

Casebolt TL, Jope RS: Effects of chronic lithium treatment of protein kinase C and cyclic AMP-dependent protein phosphorylation. Biol Psychiatry 29:233–243, 1991

Casey DA, Davis MH: Obsessive-compulsive disorder responsive to electroconvulsive therapy in an elderly woman. South Med J 87:862–864, 1994

Casey ML, McDonald PC, Simpson ER: Endocrinological changes in pregnancy, in Williams Textbook of Endocrinology, 7th Edition. Edited by Wilson JD, Doster DW. Philadelphia, PA, WB Saunders, 1985, pp 442–447

Casper JL: Bigraphic d'une idee fixe. Traduction de Lalaune G. Archiv de Neurologic 1:270–287, 1902

Caspers H, Speckmann EJ: Cerebral PO2, PCO2 and pH: changes during convulsion activity and their significance for spontaneous arrest of seizures. Epilepsia 13:669–725, 1972

Cassady SL, Taker GK: Addition of fluoxetine to clozapine (letter). Am J Psychiatry 149:1274, 1992

Cassano GB, Petracca A, Parugi G, et al: Clomipramine for panic disorder, I: the first 10 weeks of a long-term comparison with imipramine. J Affect Disord 14:123–127, 1988

Cassidy WL, Flanagan NB, Spellman M, et al: Clinical observations in manic depressive disease. JAMA 164:1535–1546, 1957

Catalano M, Bellodi L, Lucca A, et al: Lithium and alpha-2-adrenergic receptors: effects of lithium ion on clonidine-induced growth hormone release. Neuroendocrinology Letters 6:61–66, 1984

Cataldo AM, Paskevich PA, Kominami E, et al: Lysosomal hydrolases of different classes are abnormally distributed in brains of patients with Alzheimer's disease. Proc Natl Acad Sci U S A 88:10998–11002, 1991

Catapano F, Monteleone P, Maj M, et al: Dexamethasone suppression test and response to serotonergic drugs in OCD. European Psychiatry 6:273–274, 1991

Ceccherini-Nelli A, Guazzelli M: Treatment of refractory OCD with the dopamine agonist bromocriptine. J Clin Psychiatry 55:415–416, 1994

Celotti F, Melcangi RC, Martini L: The 5a-reductase in the brain: molecular aspects and relation to brain function. Frontiers in Neuroendocrinology 13:163–215, 1992

Cerletti U, Bini L: Un nuovo metodo di shock-terapie "L'electroshock." Boll Acad Med Roma 64:136–138, 1938

Cervo L, Rossi C, Samanin R: The role of serotonin and dopamine in brain in the antidepressant-like effect of clonidine in the forced swimming test. Neuropharmacology 31:331–335, 1992

Ceulemans DLS, Hoppenbrouwers MLJA, Gelders YG, et al: The influence of ritanserin, a serotonergic antagonist, in anxiety disorders: a double-blind placebo-controlled study versus lorazepam. Pharmacopsychiatry 8:303–305, 1985

Chagraoui A, Vasse M, Protais P: Effects of chronic treatments with amineptine and desipramine on motor responses involving dopaminergic systems. Psychopharmacology 102:201–206, 1990

Chalmers DT, Lopez JF, Vazquez DM, et al: Regulation of hippocampal 5-HT1A receptor gene expression by dexamethasone. Neuropsychopharmacology 10:215–222, 1994

Chamba G, Lemoine P, Flachaire E, et al: Increased serotonin platelet uptake after tianeptine administration in depressed patients. Biol Psychiatry 30:609–617, 1991

Chambers CA, Bain J, Rosbottom R, et al: Carbamazepine in senile dementia and overactivity—a placebo controlled double blind trial. IRCS Med Sci 10:505–506, 1982

Chan CH, Janicak PG, Davis JM, et al: Response of psychotic and nonpsychotic depressed patients to tricyclic antidepressants. J Clin Psychiatry 48:197–200, 1987

Chan-Palay V, Asan E: Alterations in catecholamine neurons of the locus coeruleus in senile dementia of the Alzheimer type and in Parkinson's disease with and without dementia and depression. J Comp Neurol 287:373–392, 1989

Chan-Palay V, Hochli M, Jentsch L, et al: Raphe serotonin neurons in the human brain stem in normal controls and patients with senile dementia of the Alzheimer type and Parkinsons disease: relationship to monoamine oxidase enzyme localization. Dementia 3:253–269, 1992

Changeux JP, Galzi JL, Devilliers-Thiery A, et al: The functional architecture of the acetylcholine nicotinic receptor explored by affinity labeling and site-directed mutagenesis. Q Rev Biophys 25:395–432, 1992

Chao HM, Spencer RL, Frankfurt M, et al: The effects of hormone manipulation on amyloid precursor protein APP695 mRNA expression in the rat hippocampus. J Neuroendocrinol 6:517–521, 1994

Chao MV: Neurotrophic receptors: a window into neuronal differentiation. Neuron 9:583–593, 1992

Charney DS, Nelson JC: Delusional and nondelusional unipolar depression: further evidence for distinct subtypes. Am J Psychiatry 138:328–333, 1981

Charney DS, Menekes DB, Heninger GR: Receptor sensitivity and the mechanism of action of antidepressant treatment. Arch Gen Psychiatry 38:1160–1180, 1981

Charney DS, Price LH, Heninger GR: Desipramine-yohimbine combination treatment for refractory depression. Arch Gen Psychiatry 43:1155–1161, 1986

Charney DS, Goodman WK, Price LH, et al: Serotonin function in OCD: a comparison of the effects of tryptophan and mCPP in patients and healthy subjects. Arch Gen Psychiatry 45:177–185, 1988

Charney DS, Woods SW, Nagy LM, et al: Noradrenergic function in panic disorder. J Clin Psychiatry 51:5–11, 1990

Charney DS, Deutch AY, Krystal JH, et al: Psychobiologic mechanisms of posttraumatic stress disorder. Arch Gen Psychiatry 50:294–305, 1993

Chassen JB: Intensive design: statistics and the single case, in Research Designs and Methods in Psychiatry. Edited by Fava M, Rosenbaum JF. Amsterdam, Elsevier, 1992, pp 173–183

Chatellier G, Lacomblez L: Tacrine (tetrahydroamino-acridine; THA) and lecithin in senile dementia of the Alzheimer type: a multicentre trial. BMJ 300:495–499, 1990

Chen C: Sleep, depression and antidepressants. Br J Psychiatry 135:385–402, 1979

Chen C, Harris P, Crisp AH: Sleep, mood and maprotiline—a preliminary report, in Depression: The Biochemical and Physiological Role of Ludiomil. Edited by Jukes A. England, CIBA, 1977, pp 103–114

Chen G, Yuan P, Hawver D, et al: Increase in AP-1 transcription factor DNA binding activity by valproic acid. Neuropsychopharmacology 16:238–245, 1997

Chen G, Yuan PX, Jiang Y, et al: Valproate robustly enhances AP-1 mediated gene expression. Mol Brain Res 64:52–58, 1999

Chen J, Rasenick MM: Chronic treatment of C6 glioma cells with antidepressant drugs increases functional coupling between G protein (G_s) and adenylyl cyclase. J Neurochem 64:724–732, 1995

Cheng B, McMahon DG, Mattson MP: Modulation of calcium current, intracellular calcium levels and cell survival by glucose deprivation and growth factors in hippocampal neurons. Brain Res 607:275–285, 1993

Cheng CHK, Costall B, Kelly ME, et al: Actions of 5-hydroxytryptophan to inhibit and disinhibit mouse behaviour in the light dark test. Eur J Pharmacol 255:39–49, 1994

Chevalier JF, Mendlewicz J, Coupez R, et al: Safety and efficacy of alpidem, in Imidazopyridines in Anxiety Disorders: A Novel Experimental and Therapeutic Approach. Edited by Bartholini G, Garreau M, Morselli PL. New York, Raven, 1993, pp 193–199

Chini B, Clementi F, Hukovic N, Sher E: Neuronal type α-bungarotoxin receptors and the α5-nicotinic receptor subunit gene are expressed in neuronal and nonneuronal human cell lines. Proc Natl Acad Sci U S A 89:1572–1576, 1992

Choi DW, Hartley DM: Calcium and glutamate-induced cortical neuronal death, in Molecular and Cellular Approaches to the Treatment of Neurological Disease. Edited by Waxman SG. New York, Raven, 1993, pp 23–34

Chouinard G, Goodman W, Greist J, et al: Results of a double-blind placebo controlled trial of a new serotonin uptake inhibitor, sertraline, in the treatment of OCD. Psychopharmacol Bull 26:279–284, 1990

Chouinard G, Jones B, Remington G, et al: A Canadian multicenter placebo-controlled study of fixed doses of risperidone and haloperidol in the treatment of chronic schizophrenic patients. J Clin Psychopharmacol 13:25–40, 1993

Chouinard G, Belanger M-C, Sultan S, et al: Potentiation of fluoxetine by aminoglutethimide steroid suppression in OCD: a case report (NR397), in 1995 New Research Program and Abstracts, American Psychiatric Association 148th Annual Meeting, Miami, FL, May 20–25, 1995. Washington, DC, American Psychiatric Association, 1995

Christie BR, Kerr DS, Abraham WC: Flip side of synaptic plasticity: long-term depression mechanisms in the hippocampus. Hippocampus 4:127–135, 1994

Christie JE, Shering PM, Ferguson J, et al: Physostigmine and arecoline: effects of intravenous infusion in Alzheimer presenile dementia. Br J Psychiatry 138:46–50, 1981

Christodoulou GN, Malliaras DE, Lykouras EP, et al: Possible prophylactic effect of sleep deprivation. Am J Psychiatry 135:375–376, 1978

Chrousos GP, Gold PW: The concept of stress and stress system disorders: overview of physical and behavioral homeostasis [published erratum appears in JAMA 268:200, 1992]. JAMA 267:1244–1252, 1992

Chuang DM: Neurotransmitter receptors and phophonositide turnover. Annu Rev Pharmacol Toxicol 29:71–110, 1989

Chuang DM, Gao X-M, Paul SM: N-methyl-D-aspartate exposure blocks glutamate toxicity in cultured cerebellar granule cells. Mol Pharmacol 42:210–216, 1992

Chugh Y, Saha N, Sankaranarayanan A, et al: Enhancement of memory retrieval and attenuation of scopolamine-induced amnesia following administration of 5-HT$_3$ antagonist ICS 205–930. Pharmacol Toxicol 69:105–106, 1991

Ciraulo DA, Jaffe JH: Tricyclic antidepressants in the treatment of depression associated with alcoholism. Clin Psychopharmacol 1:146, 1981

Ciraulo DA, Barnhill JG, Jaffe JH: Clinical pharmacokinetics of imipramine and desipramine in alcoholics and normal volunteers. Pharmacol Ther 43:539–548, 1988

Claassen V: Review of the pharmacology and pharmacokinetics of fluvoxamine. Br J Pharmacol 15 (suppl 3):349S–355S, 1983

Claghorn JL, Lesem MD: A double-blind placebo-controlled study of Org 3770 in depressed outpatients. J Affect Disord 34:165–171, 1995

Clark C, Rosenblatt S: A multicentre study of sertraline in the treatment of diabetic obesity. Paper presented at Progress in the Treatment of Simple and Complicated Obesity, Lisbon, 19 September, 1989

Clark CP, Alexopoulos GS, Kaplan J: Prolactin and clinical response to electroconvulsive therapy in depressed geriatric inpatients: a preliminary report. Convulsive Therapy 11:24–31, 1995

Clark DM: Cognitive mediation of panic attacks induced by biological challenge tests. Adv Behav Res Ther 15:75–84, 1993

Clark M, Massenburg GS, Weiss SRB, et al: Analysis of the hippocampal $GABA_A$ receptor system in kindled rats by autoradiographic and in situ hybridization techniques: contingent tolerance to carbamazepine. Brain Res Mol Brain Res 26:309–319, 1994

Clarke PBS, Fibiger HC: Reinforced alternation performance is impaired by muscarinic but not by nicotinic receptor blockade in rats. Behav Brain Res 36:203–207, 1990

Clarke PBS, Pert A: Autoradiographic evidence for nicotine receptors on nigrostriatal and mesolimbic dopaminergic neurons. Brain Res 348:355–358, 1985

Clarke PB, Reuben M, el-Bizri H: Blockade of nicotinic receptors by physostigmine, tacrine, and other cholinesterase inhibitors in rat striatum. Br J Pharmacol 111:695–702, 1994

Clary C, Schweizer E: Treatment of MAOI hypertensive crisis with sublingual nifedipine. J Clin Psychiatry 48:249–250, 1987

Clary C, Mandos LA, Schweizer E: Results of a brief survey on the prescribing practices for monoamine oxidase inhibitor antidepressants. J Clin Psychiatry 51:226–231, 1990

Clerc GE, Ruimy P, Verdeau Pailles J: A double-blind comparison of venlafaxine and fluoxetine in patients hospitalized for major depression and melancholia: the Venlafaxine French Inpatient Study Group. Int Clin Psychopharmacol 9:139–143, 1994

Clineschmidt BV, Zacchei AG, Totaro JA, et al: Fenfluramine and brain serotonin. Ann N Y Acad Sci 305:222–241, 1978

Clinical Research Centre, Division of Psychiatry: The Northwick Park ECT trial: predictors of response to real and simulated ECT. Br J Psychiatry 144:227–237, 1984

CMI Collaborative Study Group: CMI in the treatment of patients with OCD. Arch Gen Psychiatry 48:730–738, 1991

Coccaro EF, Zembishlany Z, Thorne A, et al: Pharmacologic treatment of noncognitive behavioral disturbances in elderly demented patients. Am J Psychiatry 147:1640–1645, 1990a

Coccaro E, Gabriel S, Siever L: Buspirone challenge: preliminary evidence for a role for central 5-HT1A receptor function in impulsive aggressive behavior in humans. Psychopharmacol Bull 26:393–405, 1990b

Coffey CE, Figiel GS, Weiner RD, et al: Caffeine augmentation of ECT. Am J Psychiatry 147:579–585, 1990

Coffey CE, Lucke J, Weiner RD, et al: Seizure threshold in electroconvulsive therapy, I: initial seizure threshold. Biol Psychiatry 37:713–720, 1995a

Coffey CE, Lucke J, Weiner RD, et al: Seizure threshold in electroconvulsive therapy (ECT), II: the anticonvulsant effect of ECT. Biol Psychiatry 37:777–788, 1995b

Cohen MR, Niska RW: Localized right hemisphere dysfunction and recurrent mania. Am J Psychiatry 137:847–848, 1980

Cohen RM, Pickar D, Garnett D, et al: REM sleep suppression induced by selective monoamine oxidase inhibitors. Psychopharmacology 78:137–140, 1982

Coleman BS, Block AB: Fluvoxamine maleate, a serotonergic antidepressant: a comparison with chlorimipramine. Prog Neuropsychopharmacol Biol Psychiatry 6:475–478, 1982

Colin SF, Chang HC, Mollner S, et al: Chronic lithium regulates the expression of adenylate cyclase and Gi-protein alpha subunit in rat cerebral cortex. Proc Natl Acad Sci U S A 88:10634–10637, 1991

Collard KJ: Lithium effects on brain 5-HT metabolism, in Lithium in Medical Practice. Edited by Johnson FN, Johnson S. Lancaster, United Kingdom, MTP Press, 1978, pp 123–133

Collard KJ, Roberts MHT: Effects of lithium on the elevation of forebrain 5-hydroxyindoles by tryptophan. Neuropharmacology 16:671–673, 1977

Consolo S, Bertorelli R, Russi G, et al: Serotonergic facilitation of acetylcholine release in vivo from rat dorsal hippocampus via serotonin 5-HT$_3$ receptors. J Neurochem 62:2254–2261, 1994

Constantopoulos A, Papadaki-Papandreou U, Papaconstantinou E: Increased beta-endorphin but not Leu-enkephalin in plasma due to preoperative stress. Experientia 51(1):16–18, 1995

Cook EH, Rowlett R, Jaselskis C, et al: Fluoxetine treatment of children and adults with autistic disorder and mental retardation. J Am Acad Child Adolesc Psychiatry 31:739–745, 1992

Coope J: Is oestrogen therapy effective in the treatment of menopausal depression. Journal of the Royal College of General Practitioners 31:134–40, 1981

Coope J, Thomson J, Poller L: Effects of "natural estrogen" replacement therapy on menopausal symptoms and blood clotting. BMJ 4:139–143, 1975

Cooper GL: The safety of fluoxetine—an update. Br J Psychiatry 153 (suppl 3):77–86, 1988

Cooper J: On the publication of the Diagnostic and Statistical Manual of Mental Disorders: Fourth Edition (DSM-IV). Br J Psychiatry 166:4–8, 1995

Cooper JR, Bloom FE, Roth RH: The Biochemical Basis of Neuropharmacology, 6th Edition. New York, Oxford University Press, 1991, p 261

Cooper TB, Simpson GM: The 24-hour serum lithium level as a prognosticator of dosage requirements: a 2-year follow-up study. Am J Psychiatry 133:440–443, 1976

Cooper TB, Bergner PE, Simpson GM: The 24-hour serum lithium level as a prognosticator of dosage requirements. Am J Psychiatry 130:601–603, 1973

Coplan JD, Rosenblum LA, Friedman S, et al: Effects of oral yohimbine administration in differentially reared nonhuman primates. Neuropsychopharmacology 6:31–37, 1992a

Coplan J, Sharma T, Rosenblum LA: Effects of sodium lactate infusion on cisternal lactate and carbon dioxide levels in nonhuman primates. Am J Psychiatry 149:1369–1373, 1992b

Coplan JD, Gorman JM, Klein DF: Serotonin-related function in panic disorder: a critical overview. Neuropsychopharmacology 6(3):189–200, 1992c

Coplan JD, Rosenblum LA, Andrews M, et al: Persistent elevations of CSF CRF, somatostatin, HVA and 5-HIAA in grown nonhuman primates exposed to early life stressors. Paper presented at the annual meeting of the American College of Neuropsychopharmacology, San Juan, Puerto Rico, December 1994

Coplan JD, Papp LA, Pine DS, et al: Clinical improvement with fluoxetine therapy normalizes noradrenergic function in panic disorder. Paper presented at the annual meeting of the American College of Neuropsychopharmacology, San Juan, Puerto Rico, December 1995a

Coplan JD, Pine D, Papp LA, et al: Noradrenergic/HPA axis uncoupling in panic disorder. Neuropsychopharmacology 13:65–73, 1995b

Coplan JD, Papp LA, Martinez J, et al: Persistence of blunted human growth hormone response to clonidine in panic disorder following fluoxetine treatment. Am J Psychiatry 152:619–622, 1995c

Coplan JD, Andrews MW, Rosenblum LA, et al: Persistent elevations of cerebrospinal fluid concentrations of corticotropin-releasing factor in adult nonhuman primates exposed to early-life stressors: implications for the pathophysiology of mood and anxiety disorders. Proc Natl Acad Sci U S A 93:1619–1623, 1996

Coppen A: Depressive states and indolealkylamines, in Advances in Pharmacology, Vol 6. Edited by Garattini S, Shore PA. New York, Academic Press, 1968, pp 283–291

Coppen A, Shaw DM: Mineral metabolism in melancholia. BMJ 2:1439–1444, 1963

Coppen A, Shaw DM, Malleson A, et al: Mineral metabolism in mania. BMJ 1:71–75, 1966

Coppen A, Noguera R, Bailey J, et al: Prophylactic lithium in affective disorders: controlled trial. Lancet 2:275–279, 1971

Coppen A, Peet M, Bailey J, et al: Double-blind and open prospective studies of lithium prophylaxis in affective disorders. Psychiatria, Neurologia, Neurochirurgia 76:500–510, 1973

Coppen A, Ghose K, Montgomery S, et al: Continuation therapy with amitriptyline in depression. Br J Psychiatry 133:28–33, 1978

Coppen A, Swade C, Wood K: Lithium restores abnormal platelet 5-HT transport in patients with affective disorders. Br J Psychiatry 136:235–238, 1980

Coppen A, Swade C, Jones SA, et al: Depression and tetrahydrobiopterin: the folate connection. J Affect Disord 16:103–107, 1989

Cordell B: β-Amyloid formation as a potential therapeutic target for Alzheimer's disease. Annu Rev Pharmacol Toxicol 34:69–89, 1994

Corkin S: Acetylcholine, aging, and Alzheimer's disease: implications of treatment. Trends Neurosci 4:287–290, 1981

Corn THE: New antidepressants—a look to the future, in Psychopharmacology of Depression. Edited by Montgomery SA, Corn THE. Oxford, England, Oxford University Press, 1994, p 14

Corona GL, Cucchi ML, Santagostino G, et al: Blood noradrenaline and 5-HT levels in depressed women during amitriptyline or lithium treatment. Psychopharmacology 77:236–241, 1982

Corpéchot C, Robel P, Axelson M, et al: Characterization and measurement of dehydroepiandrosterone sulphate in the rat brain. Proc Natl Acad Sci U S A 78:4704–4707, 1981

Corpéchot C, Young J, Calvel M, et al: 3a-hydroxy-5a-pregnan-20-one and its precursors in the brain, plasma, and steroidogenic glands of male and female rats. Endocrinology 133:1003–1009, 1993

Corwin J, Peselow E, Fieve R, et al: Memory in untreated depression: severity and task requirement effects. Paper presented at the annual meeting of the American College of Neuropsychopharmacology, San Juan, Puerto Rico, December 1987

Coryell W, Winokur G: Course and outcome, in Handbook of Affective Disorders. Edited by Paykel ES. New York, Guilford, 1982, pp 93–108

Coryell W, Zimmerman M: Outcome following ECT for primary unipolar depression: a test of newly proposed response predictors. Am J Psychiatry 141:862–867, 1984

Coryell W, Gaffney G, Burkhardt PE: The dexamethasone suppression test and familial subtypes of depression: a naturalistic replication. Biol Psychiatry 17:33–40, 1982

Coryell W, Pfohl B, Zimmerman M: The clinical and neuroendocrine features of psychotic depression. J Nerv Ment Dis 172:521–528, 1984

Coryell W, Endicott J, Andreasen NC, et al: Depression and panic attacks: the significance of overlap as reflected in follow up and family study data. Am J Psychiatry 145:293–300, 1988

Cossa FM, Della Sala S, Spinnler H: Selective visual attention in Alzheimer's and Parkinson's patients: memory- and data-driven control. Neuropsychologia 27:887–892, 1989

Costa E, Guidotti A: Diazepam binding inhibitor (DBI): a peptide with multiple biological actions. Life Sci 49:325–344, 1991

Costa E, Auta J, Guidotti A, et al: The pharmacology of neurosteroidogenesis. J Steroid Biochem Mol Biol 49:385–389, 1994

Costa LG: Signal-transduction mechanisms in developmental neurotoxicity: the phosphoinositide pathway. Neurotoxicology 15:19–27, 1994

Costall B, Naylor RJ: Astra award lecture: the psychopharmacology of 5-HT3 receptors. Pharmacol Toxicol 71:401, 1992a

Costall B, Naylor RJ: 5-HT receptors and antipsychotic drugs, in Central Serotonin Receptors and Psychotropic Drugs. Edited by Marsden CA, Heal DJ. London, Blackwell Scientific, 1992b, pp 198–221

Costello EJ, Angold A: Epidemiology, in Anxiety Disorders in Children and Adolescents. Edited by March JS. New York, Guilford, 1995

Cotman CW, Pike CJ: Beta-amyloid and its contribution to neurodegeneration in Alzheimer disease, in Alzheimer Disease. Edited by Terry RD, Katzman R, Bick K. New York, Raven, 1994, pp 305–316

Cottraux J: Behavioral psychotherapy for OCD. International Review of Psychiatry 1(3):227–34, 1989

Cottraux J, Mollard E, Bouvard M, et al: A controlled study of fluvoxamine and exposure in obsessive-compulsive disorder. Int Clin Psychopharmacol 5(1):17–30, 1989

Coulter DM, Edwards IR: Mianserin and agranulocytosis in New Zealand. Lancet 336:785–787, 1990

Court JA, Perry EK: CNS nicotinic receptors. Possible therapeutic targets in neurodegenerative disorders. CNS Drugs 2(3):216–233, 1994

Covi L, Lipman RS, Derogatis LR, et al: Drugs and group psychotherapy in neurotic depression. Am J Psychiatry 131:191–198, 1974

Cowen PJ: Neuroendocrine measures of 5-HT receptor subtype function in depression, in Serotonin, CNS Receptors and Brain Function (Advances in the Biosciences, Vol 85). Edited by Bradley PB, Handley SL, Cooper SJ, et al. Oxford, England, Pergamon, 1992, pp 287–296

Cowen PJ, McCance SL, Cohen PR, et al: Lithium increases 5-HT-mediated neuroendocrine responses in tricyclic resistant depression. Psychopharmacology (Berl) 99:230–232, 1989

Cowley DS, Arana GW: The diagnostic utility of lactate sensitivity in panic disorder. Arch Gen Psychiatry 47:277–284, 1990

Cox BJ, Swinson RP, Morrison B, Lee PS: Clomipramine, fluoxetine and behavior therapy in the treatment of obsessive-compulsive disorder: a meta-analysis. J Behav Ther Exp Psychiatry 24:2, 149–153, 1993a

Cox BJ, Hasey G, Swinson RP, et al. The symptom structure of panic attacks in depressed and anxious patients. Can J Psychiatry 38:181–184, 1993b

Cox RF, Meller E, Waszczak BL: Electrophysiological evidence for a large receptor reserve for inhibition of dorsal raphe cell firing by 5-HT1A agonists. Synapse 14:297–304, 1993

Coxhead N, Silverstone T, Cookson J: Carbamazepine versus lithium in the prophylaxis of bipolar affective disorder. Acta Psychiatr Scand 85:114–118, 1992

Coyle JT, Price DL, DeLong MR: Alzheimer's disease: a disorder of cortical cholinergic innervation. Science 219:1184–1190, 1983

Crawley JN: Subtype-selective cholecystokinin receptor antagonists block cholecystokinin modulation of dopamine-mediated behaviors in the rat mesolimbic pathway. J Neurosci 12:3380–3391, 1992

Crawley JN, Glowa JR, Majewska MD, et al: Anxiolytic activity of an endogenous adrenal steroid. Brain Res 398:382–385, 1986

Crawley J, Ninan P, Pickar D: Neuropharmacological antagonism of the B-carboline-induced "anxiety" response in rhesus monkeys. J Neurosci 5:455–485, 1995

Crews FT, Paul SM, Goodwin FK: Acceleration of β-receptor desensitization in combined administration of antidepressants and phenoxybenzapine. Nature 290:787–789, 1981

Criswell HE, Simpson PE, Knapp DJ, et al: Effect of zolpidem on GABA aminobutyric acid-induced inhibition predicts the interaction of ethanol with GABA on individual neurons in several rat brain regions. J Pharmacol Exp Ther 273:526–538, 1995

Crook TH, Lakin M: Effects of ondansetron image-associated memory impairment, in Biological Psychiatry: Proceedings of the 5th World Congress of Biological Psychiatry, Florence, 9–14 June 1991. Edited by Racagni G, Brunello N, Fukuda T. New York, Excerpta Medica, 1991, pp 1–4

Crook T, Bartus RT, Ferris St. H, et al: Age-associated memory impairment: proposed diagnostic criteria and measures of clinical change—report of a National Institute of Health Work Group. Developmental Neuropsychology 2(4):261–276, 1986

Cross AJ, Crow TJ, Johnson JA: Monoamine metabolism in senile dementia of Alzheimer type. J Neurol Sci 60:383–393, 1983

Cross AJ, Crow TJ, Johnson JA: Studies on neurotransmitter receptor systems in cortex and hippocampus in senile dementia of the Alzheimer type. J Neurol Sci 64:109–117, 1984

Cross AJ, Slater P, Perry EK, et al: An autoradiographic analysis of serotonin receptors in human temporal cortex changes in Alzheimer-type dementia. Neurochem Int 13:89–96, 1988

Crow TJ, Grove-White IG: Analysis of the learning deficit following hyoscine administration to man. Br J Pharmacology 49:322–327, 1973

Csonka E, Fekete M, Nagy G, et al: Anxiogenic effect of cholecystokinin in rats, in Peptides. Edited by Penke B, Török A. New York, Walter de Gruyter, 1988, pp 249–252

Cummings JL: Depression and Parkinson's disease: a review. Am J Psychiatry 149:443–454, 1992

Cummings JL: Depression in neurologic diseases. Psychiatric Annals 24:525–531, 1994

Cummings JL, Cunningham K: Obsessive-compulsive disorder in Huntington's disease. Biol Psychiatry 31:263–270, 1992

Cummings JL, Mendez MF: Secondary mania with focal cerebrovascular lesions. Am J Psychiatry 141:1084–1087, 1984

Cummings JL, Miller B, Hill MA, et al: Neuropsychiatric aspects of multi-infarct dementia and dementia of the Alzheimer type. Arch Neurol 44:389–393, 1987

Cundall RL, Brooks PW, Murray LG: A controlled evaluation of lithium prophylaxis in affective disorders. Psychol Med 2:308–311, 1972

Cutler NR, Haxy J, Kay AD, et al: Evaluation of zimeldine in Alzheimer's disease: cognitive and biochemical measures. Arch Neurol 42:744–748, 1985

Czyrak A: The effect of chronic nifedipine and ECS in the forced swimming test in rats. Pol J Pharmacol 45:191–195, 1993

Czyrak A, Mogilnicka E, Maj J: Dihydropyridine calcium channel antagonists as antidepressant drugs in mice and rats. Neuropharmacology 28:229–233, 1989

Daan S, Beersma DGM, Borbely AA: Timing of human sleep: recovery process gated by a circadian pacemaker. Am J Physiol 246:R161–R178, 1984

Dager SR, Rainey JM, Kenny MA: Central nervous system effects of lactate infusion in primates. Biol Psychiatry 27:193–204, 1990

Dahlström A, Fuxe K: Evidence for the existence of monoamine containing neurons in the central nervous system: I. Demonstration of monoamines in the cell bodies of brainstem neurons. Acta Physiol Scand 62:1–55, 1964

Dalrymple-Alford JC, Kalders AS, Jones RD, et al: A central executive deficit in patients with Parkinson's disease. J Neurol Neurosurg Psychiatry 57:360–367, 1994

Daly E, Gray A, Barlow D, et al: Measuring the impact of menopausal symptoms on quality of life. BMJ 307:836–840, 1993

Dampney RAL, Czachurski J, Dembowsky K, et al: Afferent connections and spinal projections of the pressor region in the rostral ventrolateral medulla of the cat. J Auton Nerv Syst 20:73–86, 1977

Dampney RAL, Goodchild AK, Robertson LG, et al: Role of ventrolateral medulla in vasomotor regulation: a correlative anatomical and physiological study. Brain Res 249:223–235, 1982

Danion J: A placebo controlled study with GBR 12909, a dopamine uptake inhibitor (abstract). Biol Psychiatry 29:635, 1991

Danish University Antidepressant Group: Citalopram: clinical effect profile in comparison with clomipramine: a controlled multicenter study. Psychopharmacology 90:131–138, 1986

Danish University Antidepressant Group: Paroxetine: a selective serotonin reuptake inhibitor showing better tolerance but weaker antidepressant effect profile in comparison with clomipramine: a controlled multicentre study. J Affect Disord 18:289–299, 1990

D'Aquila PS, Sias A, Gessa GL, et al: The NMDA receptor antagonist MK-801 prevents imipramine-induced supersensitivity to quinpirole. Eur J Pharmacol 224:199–302, 1992

D'Aquila PS, Collu M, Pani L, et al: Antidepressant-like effect of selective dopamine D_1 receptor agonists in the behavioural despair animal model of depression. Eur J Pharmacol 262:107–111, 1994

Dassa D, Kaladjian A, Azorin JM, et al: Clozapine in the treatment of psychotic refractory depression. Br J Psychiatry 163:822–824, 1993

Daugé V, Steimes P, Derrien M, et al: CCK8 effects on motivational and emotional states of rats involve CCKA receptors of the postero-median part of the nucleus accumbens. Pharmacol Biochem Behav 34:157–163, 1989

Davidson J: Seizures and bupropion: a review. J Clin Psychiatry 50:256–261, 1989

Davidson J, Pelton S: Forms of atypical depression and their response to antidepressant drugs. Psychiatry Res 17:87–95, 1986

Davidson JR, Miller R, Turnbull CD, et al: Atypical depression. Arch Gen Psychiatry 39:527–534, 1982

Davidson JRT, Potts NLS, Richichi EA, et al: The Brief Social Phobia Scale. J Clin Psychiatry 52 (suppl):48–51, 1991a

Davidson JRT, Ford SM, Smith RD, et al: Long-term treatment of social phobia with clonazepam. J Clin Psychiatry 52 (suppl):16–20, 1991b

Davidson JRT, Potts N, Richichi E, et al: Treatment of social phobia with clonazepam and placebo. J Clin Psychopharmacol 13:423–428, 1993

Davies P: Theoretical treatment possibilities for dementia of the Alzheimer type: the cholinergic hypothesis, in Strategies for the Development of an Effective Treatment for Senile Dementia. Edited by Crook T, Gershon S. New Canaan, CT, Mark Powley Associates, 1981, pp 19–32

Davies P, Maloney AJF: Selective loss of central cholinergic neurons in Alzheimer's disease. Lancet 2:1403, 1976

Davis KL, Powchik P: Tacrine. Lancet 345:625–630, 1995

Davis KL, Hollister LE, Overall J, et al: Physostigmine: effects on cognition and affect in normal subjects. Psychopharmacologia 51:23–27, 1976

Davis KL, Mohs RC, Tinklenberg JR, et al: Physostigmine: improvement of long-term memory processes in normal humans. Science 201:272–274, 1978

Davis KL, Mohs RC, Davis BM, et al: Cholinomimetic agents and human memory: clinical studies in Alzheimer's disease and scopolamine dementia, in Strategies for the Development of an Effective Treatment for Senile Dementia. Edited by Crook T, Gershon S. New Canaan, CT, Mark Powley Associates, 1981, pp 53–69

Davis KL, Thal LJ, Gamzu ER, et al. and the Tacrine Collaborative Study Group: A double-blind placebo-controlled multicenter study of tacrine for Alzheimer's disease. N Engl J Med 327:1253–1259, 1992

De Bellis MD, Gold PW, Geracioti TD Jr, et al: Association of fluoxetine treatment with reductions in CSF concentrations of corticotropin-releasing hormone and arginine vasopressin in patients with major depression. Am J Psychiatry 150:656–657, 1993

de Beurs E, van Balkom AJLM, Lange A, et al: Treatment of panic disorder with agoraphobia: comparison of fluvoxamine, placebo, and psychological panic management combined with exposure and of exposure in vivo alone. Am J Psychiatry 152:683–691, 1995

de Boer T, Ruigt SF: The selective α_2-adrenoceptor antagonist mirtazapine (Org 3770) enhances noradrenergic and 5-HT$_{1A}$-mediated serotonergic neurotransmission. CNS Drugs 4(1):29–38, 1995

de Boer TH, Maura G, Raiteri M, et al: Neurochemical and autonomic pharmacological profiles of the 6-aza-analogue of mianserin, org 3770 and its enantiomers. Neuropharmacology 27:399–408, 1988

de Falco FA, Bartiromo U, Majello L, et al: Calcium antagonist nimodipine in intractable epilepsy. Epilepsia 33:343–345, 1992

de Jonge M, Freidl A, de Vry J: CNS pharmacology of nimodipine: antidepressants effects, drug discrimination and Ca^{2+} imaging, in Drugs in Development, Vol 2: Ca^{2+} Antagonists in the CNS. Edited by Scriabine A, Janis RA, Triggle DJ. Branford, CT, Neva Press, 1993, pp 165–174

de Montigny C: Cholecystokinin tetrapeptide induces panic-like attacks in healthy volunteers. Arch Gen Psychiatry 46:511–517, 1989

de Montigny C: Lithium addition in refractory depression, in Refractory Depression: Current Strategies and Future Directions. Edited by Nolen WA, Zohar J, Roose SP, et al. Chichester, England, Wiley, 1994, pp 47–57

de Montigny C, Grunberg F, Mayer A, et al: Lithium induces rapid relief of depression in tricyclic antidepressant drug non-responders. Br J Psychiatry 138:252–256, 1981

de Montigny C, Cournoyer G, Morissette R, et al: Lithium carbonate addition in tricyclic antidepressant-resistant unipolar depression: correlations with the neurobiologic actions of tricyclic antidepressant drugs and lithium ion on the serotonin system. Arch Gen Psychiatry 40:1327–1334, 1983

De Montis GM, Devoto P, Gessa GL, et al: Central dopaminergic transmission is selectively increased in the limbic system of rats chronically exposed to antidepressants. Eur J Pharmacol 180:31–35, 1990

De Montis MG, Gambarana C, Meloni D, et al: Long-term imipramine effects are prevented by NMDA receptor blockade. Brain Res 606:63–67, 1993

De Sarno P, Giacobini E: Modulation of acetylcholine release by nicotinic receptors in the rat brain. J Neurosci Res 22:194–200, 1989

De Vos H, Vauquelin G, De Keyser J, et al: Regional distribution of alpha$_{2A}$ and alpha$_{2B}$-adrenoceptor subtypes in post mortem human brain. J Neurochem 58:1555–1560, 1992

De Vos H, Bricca G, De Keyser J, et al: Imidazoline receptors, non-adrenergic idazoxan binding sites and a_2-adrenoceptors in the human central nervous system. Neuroscience 59:589–598, 1994

Debonnel G, Gronier B, Bergeron R, et al: Neuropeptides, neurosteroids and sigma ligands: interactions in the modulation of the NMDA response of hippocampal neurons (abstract). Paper presented at the annual meeting of the American College of Neuropsychopharmacology, San Juan, Puerto Rico, December 1994

DeBree H, Van der Schoot JB, et al: Fluvoaxmine maleate: disposition in man. Eur J Drug Metab Pharmacokinet 8:175–179, 1983

Decker MW, Majchrzak MJ, Anderson DJ: Effects of nicotine on spatial memory deficits in rats with septal lesions. Brain Res 572:281–285, 1992

Decker MW, Brioni JD, Bannon AW, et al: Diversity of neuronal nicotinic acetylcholine receptors: lessons from behavior and implications for CNS therapeutics. Life Sci 56:545–570, 1995

Deckner ML, Frisen J, Verge VMK, et al: Localization of neurotrophin receptors in olfactory epithelium and bulb. Neuroreport 5:301–304, 1993

Dehlin O, Hedenrud B, Jansson P, et al: A double blind comparison of alaproclate and placebo in the treatment of patients with senile dementia. Acta Psychiatr Scand 71:190–196, 1985

Deicken RF: Verapamil treatment of bipolar depression (letter). J Clin Psychopharmacol 10:148–149, 1990

DeKloet ER, Reul JMHM: Tonic influence and feedback action of corticosteroids: a concept arising from heterogeneity of brain receptor system. Psychoneuroendocrinology 12:83–105, 1987

DeKloet ER, Kovacs GL, Szabo G, et al: Decreased serotonin turnover in the dorsal hippocampus of rat brain shortly after adrenalectomy: selective normalization after corticosterone substitution. Brain Res 239:659–663, 1982

Del Zompo M, Bernadi F, Burrai C, et al: A double-blind study of minaprine versus amitriptyline in major depression. Neuropsychobiology 24:79–83, 1991

Delespaul PhAEG: Schizophrenics in Daily Life. Maastricht, Universiteitspers Maastricht, 1995

Delgado PL, Goodman WK, Price LH, et al: Fluvoxamine/pimozide treatment of concurrent Tourette's and obsessive compulsive disorder. Br J Psychiatry 157:762–765, 1990a

Delgado PL, Charney DS, Price LH, et al: Serotonin function and the mechanism of antidepressant action: reversal of antidepressant-induced remission by rapid depletion of plasma tryptophan. Arch Gen Psychiatry 47:411–418, 1990b

Delgado PL, Price LH, Miller HL, et al: Rapid serotonin depletion as a provocative challenge test for patients with major depression: relevance to antidepressant action and the neurobiology of depression. Psychopharmacol Bull 27:321–330, 1991

Della-Fera MA, Baile CA: Cholecystokinin octapeptide: continuous picomole injections into the cerebral ventricles of sheep suppress feeding. Science 206:471–473, 1979

Delong MR, Georgopoulos AP, Crutcher MD: Cortico-basal ganglia relations and coding of motor performance. Exp Brain Res 49 (suppl 7):30–40, 1983

Deltito JA: Valproate pretreatment for difficult-to-treat patients with OCD. J Clin Psychiatry 55:500, 1994

Delvenne V, Delecluse F, Hubain P, et al: Regional cerebral blood flow in patients with affective disorders. Br J Psychiatry 157:359–365, 1990

Demirgoren S, Majewska MD, Spivak CE, London ED: Receptor binding and electrophysiological effects of dehydroepiandrosterone sulfate, an antagonist of the GABAa receptor. Neuroscience 45:127–135, 1991

Den Boer JA, Westenberg HGM: Effect of a serotonin and noradrenalin uptake inhibitor in panic disorder, a double-blind comparative study with fluvoxamine and maprotiline. Int Clin Psychopharmacol 3:59–74, 1988

Den Boer JA, Westenberg HGM: Serotonin function in panic disorder: a double-blind placebo-controlled study with fluvoxamine and ritanserin. Psychopharmacology 102:85–94, 1990

Den Boer JA, Westenberg HGM: No evidence for anticompulsive action of oxytocin. Clin Neuropharmacol 15(1):307B, 1992a

Den Boer JA, Westenberg HGM: Oxytocin in obsessive compulsive disorder. Peptides 13(6):1083–1085, 1992b

Den Boer JA, Westenberg HGM, Kamerbeek WDJ, et al: Effect of serotonin uptake inhibitors in anxiety disorders: a double-blind comparison of clomipramine and fluvoxamine. Int Clin Psychopharmacol 2:21–32, 1987

Den Boer JA, Westenberg HGM, De Vries H: The MSH/ACTH analog ORG 2766 in anxiety disorders. Peptides 13:109–112, 1992

Den Boer JA, Van Vliet IM, Westenberg HG: Recent advances in the psychopharmacology of social phobia. Prog Neuropsychophamacol Biol Psychiatry 18:625–645, 1994

Denavit-Saubié M, Hurlé MA, Morin-Surun MP, et al: The effects of cholecystokinin-8 in the nucleus tractus solitarius, in Neuronal Cholecystokinin. Edited by Vanderhaeghen JJ, Crawley JN. New York, New York Academy of Sciences, 1985, pp 375–384

Denicoff KD, Smith-Jackson E, Disney E, et al: Comparative prophylactic efficacy of lithium, carbamazepine, and the combination in the treatment of bipolar affective illness. J Clin Psychiatry 58:470–478, 1997

DeNinno MP, Schrenleber R, Mackenzie R, et al: A68930: a potent agonist selective for the dopamine D_1 receptor. Eur J Pharmacol 199:209–219, 1991

Dennerstein L, Spencer-Gardner C, Gotts G, et al: Progesterone and the premenstrual syndrome: a double-blind cross-over trial. BMJ 290:1617–1621, 1985

Denoble VJ, Schrack LM, Reigel AL, et al: Visual recognition in squirrel monkeys effects of serotonin antagonists on baseline and hypoxia induced performance deficits. Pharmacol Biochem Behav 39:991–996, 1991

Depue RA, Karuss SP, Spoont MR: A two-dimensional threshold model of seasonal bipolar affective disorder, in Psychopathology: An Interactional Perspective. Edited by Magnusson D, Ohman A. Orlando, FL, Academic Press, 1987, pp 95–123

Depue RA, Arbisi P, Spoont MR, et al: Dopamine functioning in the behavioural facilitation system and seasonal variation in behaviour: normal populations and clinical studies, in Seasonal Affective Disorders and Phototherapy. Edited by Rosenthal NE, Blehar MC. New York, Guilford, 1989, pp 230–259

Derkach V, Surprenant A, North RA: 5-HT3 receptors are membrane ion channels. Nature 339:706–709, 1989

Derrien M, McCort-Tranchepain I, Ducos B, et al: Heterogeneity of CCK-B receptors involved in animal models of anxiety. Pharmacol Biochem Behav 49:133, 1994

Desai NG, Gangadhar BN, Channabasavanna SM, et al: Carbamazepine hastens therapeutic action of lithium in mania (abstract). Proceedings of the International Conference on New Directions in Affective Disorders, 1987, p 97

Deschenes RJ, Lorenz LJ, Haun RS, et al: Cloning and sequence analysis of a cDNA encoding rat preprocholecystokinin. Proc Natl Acad Sci U S A 81:726–730, 1984

Deschodt-Lanckman M, Bui ND, Noyer M, et al: Degradation of cholecystokinin-like peptides by a crude rat brain synaptosomal fraction: a study by high-pressure-liquid chromatography. Regul Pept 2:15–30, 1981

Detre T, Himmelhock J, Swartzburg M, et al: Hypersomnia and manic-depressive disease. Am J Psychiatry 128:1303–1305, 1972

Deutch AY, Roth RH: The determinants of stress-induced activation of the prefrontal cortical dopamine system, in Progress in Brain Research, Vol 85. Edited by Uylings HBM, van Eden CG, De Bruin JPC, et al. Amsterdam, Elsevier, 1990, pp 357–393

Deutsch JA: The cholinergic synapse and the site of memory. Science 174:788–794, 1971

Deutsch SI, Mastropaolo J: Discriminative stimulus properties of midazolam are shared by a GABA-receptor positive neurosteroid. Pharmacol Biochem Behav 46:963–965, 1993

Deutsch SI, Mastropaolo J, Hitri A: GABA-active steroids: endogenous modulators of GABA-gated chloride ion conductance. Clin Neuropharmacol 15:352–364, 1992

Devanand DP, Decina P, Sackeim HA, et al: Status epilepticus during ECT in a patient receiving theophylline. J Clin Psychopharmacol 8:153, 1988

Devanand DP, Sackeim HA, Brown RP, et al: A pilot study of haloperidol treatment of psychosis and behavioral disturbance in Alzheimer's disease. Arch Neurol 46:854–857, 1989

Devanand DP, Cooper T, Sackeim HA, et al: Low dose oral haloperidol and blood levels in Alzheimer's disease: a preliminary study. Psychopharmacol Bull 28:169–173, 1992

Devanand DP, Shapira B, Petty F, et al: Effects of electroconvulsive therapy on plasma GABA. Convulsive Therapy 11:3–13, 1995

DeVane CL: Pharmacokinetics of the newer antidepressants: clinical relevance. Am J Med 97 (suppl 6A):13S–23S, 1994

DeVeaugh-Geiss J, Bell J: Multicenter trial of a 5HT3 antagonist, ondansetron, in social phobia. Poster presented at the annual meeting of the American College of Neuropsychopharmacology, San Juan, Puerto Rico, December 1994

DeVeaugh-Geiss J, Katz R, Landau P, et al: Clinical predictors of treatment response in OCD: exploratory analyses from multicenter trials of CMI. Psychopharmacol Bull 26:54–59, 1990

Devous MD, Rush AJ, Schlesser MA, et al: Single-photon tomographic determination of regional cerebral blood flow in psychiatric disorders. J Nucl Med 25:P57, 1984

DeVries MH, Raghoebar M, Mathlener IS, et al: Single and multiple oral dose fluvoxamine in young and elderly subjects. Ther Drug Monit 14:493–498, 1992

Dewan MJ, Haldipur CV, Lane EE, et al: Bipolar affective disorder, I: comprehensive quantitative computed tomography. Acta Psychiatr Scand 77:670–676, 1988

DeWied D, Jolles J: Neuropeptides derived from pro-opiocortin: behavioral, physiological, and neurochemical effects. Physiol Rev 62(3):976–1059, 1992

deWitte PH, Heideberg C, Roques PB: Kelatorphan, a potent enkephalinase inhibitor, and opioid receptor agonist DAGO and DTLET, differentially modulate self-stimulation behavior depending on the site of administration. Neuropharmacology 28:667–676, 1989

D'haenen HA, Bossuyt A: Dopamine D_2 receptors in depression measured with single photon emission computed tomography. Biol Psychiatry 35:128–132, 1994

Di Costanzo E, Schifano F: Lithium alone or in combination with carbamazepine for the treatment of rapid-cycling bipolar affective disorder. Acta Psychiatr Scand 83:456–459, 1991

Di Perri R, Mailland F, Bramanti P: The effects of amineptine on the mood and nocturnal sleep of depressed patients. Prog Neuropsychopharmacol Biol Psychiatry 11:65–70, 1987

Dick DAT, Naylor GJ, Dick EG: Effect of lithium on sodium transport across membranes, in Lithium in Medical Practice. Edited by Johnson FN, Johnson S. Lancaster, England, MTP Press, 1978, pp 183–192

Dick P, Ferrero E: A double-blind comparison study of the clinical efficacy of fluvoxamine and chlorimipramine. Br J Clin Pharmacol 15 (suppl 3):419S–425S, 1983

Diehl DJ, Gershon S: The role of dopamine in mood disorders. Compr Psychiatry 33:115–120, 1992

Dillier N: Worldwide clinical experience with Ludiomil. Activitas nervosa superior. 24:40–52, 1982

Dilsaver SC, Coffman JA: Cholinergic hypothesis of depression: a reappraisal. J Clin Psychopharmacol 9:173–179, 1989

Dilsaver SC, Hariharan M: Amitriptyline-induced supersensitivity of a central muscarinic mechanism: lithium blocks amitriptyline-induced supersensitivity. Psychiatry Res 25:181–186, 1988

Dilsaver SC, Hariharan M: Chronic treatment with lithium produces supersensitivity to nicotine. Biol Psychiatry 25:792–795, 1989

Divish MM, Sheftel G, Boyle A, et al: Differential effect of lithium on fos protooncogene expression mediated by receptor and postreceptor activators of protein kinase C and cyclic adenosine monophosphate: model for its antimanic action. J Neurosci Res 28:40–48, 1991

Division of Neuropharmacological Drug Products, U.S. Food and Drug Administration: Tacrine as a treatment for Alzheimer's disease: an interim report from the FDA. N Engl J Med 324:349–352, 1991

Divoll M, Greenblatt DJ, Harmatz JS, et al: Effect of age and gender on disposition of temazepam. J Pharm Sci 70:1104–1107, 1981

Dixon JF, Lee CH, Los GV, et al: Lithium enhances accumulation of [^{3}H] inositol radioactivity and mass of second messenger inositol 1,4,5-triphosphate in monkey cerebral cortex slices. J Neurochem 59:2332–2335, 1992

Dixon JF, Los GV, Hokin LE: Lithium stimulates glutamate "release" and inositol 1,4,5-triphosphate accumulation via activation of the N-methyl-D-aspartate receptor in monkey and mouse cerebral cortex slices. Proc Natl Acad Sci U S A 91:8358–8362, 1994

Doble A, Canton T, Piot O, et al: The pharmacology of cyclopyrrolone derivatives acting at the GABA a benzodiazepine receptor. Adv Biochem Psychopharmacol 47:407–418, 1992

Dockray GJ, Gregory RA, Hutchison JB, et al: Isolation, structure and biological activity of two cholecystokinin octapeptides from sheep brain. Nature 274:711–713, 1978

Dodd J, Kelly JS: The actions of cholecystokinin and related peptides on pyramidal neurones of the mammalian hippocampus. Brain Res 205:337–350, 1981

Dodd PR, Edwardson JA, Dockray GJ: The depolarization-induced release of cholecystokinin C-terminal octapeptide (CCK-8) from rat synaptosomes and brain slices. Regul Pept 1:17–19, 1980

Doerr P, Berger M: Physostigmine-induced escape from dexamethasone in normal adults. Biol Psychiatry 18:261–268, 1983

Donnell CD, McNally RJ: Anxiety sensitivity and panic attacks in a nonclinical population. Behav Res Ther 28:83–85, 1990

Donnelly EF, Goodwin FK, Waldman IN, et al: Prediction of antidepressant responses to lithium. Am J Psychiatry 135:552–556, 1978

Donoghue JM, Tylee A: The treatment of depression: prescribing patterns of antidepressants in primary care in the UK. Br J Psychiatry 168:164–168, 1996

Doogan DP: Toleration and safety of sertraline: experience world-wide. Int Clin Psychopharmacol 6 (suppl 2):47–56, 1991

Doogan DP, Caillard V: Sertraline in the prevention of depression. Br J Psychiatry 160:217–222, 1992

Dose M, Emrich HM, Cording-Tommel C, et al: Use of calcium antagonists in mania. Psychoneuroendocrinology 11:241–243, 1986

Dostert P, Benedetti MS, Pogessi I: Review of the pharmacokinetics and metabolism of reboxetine, a selective noradrenaline reuptake inhibitor. Eur Neuropsychopharmacol 7 (suppl 1): S23–S35, 1997

Doucette-Stamm L, Monteggia L, Donnelly Roberts D, et al: Cloning and sequence of the human a7 nicotinic acetylcholine receptor. Drug Dev Res 30:252–256, 1993

Dourish CT, Hutson PH, Ahlenius S (eds): Brain 5-HT1A Receptors. Horwood, NJ, Chichester Press, 1987

Dousa TP: Interaction of lithium with vasopressin-sensitive cyclic AMP system of human renal medulla. Endocrinology 95:1359–1366, 1974

Dousa T, Hechter O: The effect of NaCl and LiCl on vasopressin-sensitive adenyl cyclase. Life Sci 9:765–770, 1970a

Dousa T, Hechter O: Lithium and brain adenyl cyclase. Lancet 1:834–835, 1970b

Downes JJ, Sharp HM, Sagar HJ: The time course of negative priming in Parkinson's disease. J Clin Exp Neuropsychol 13:75, 1991

Downes JJ, Sharp HM, Costall BM, et al: Alternating fluency in Parkinson's disease. An evaluation of the attentional control theory of cognitive impairment. Brain 116:887–902, 1993

Drachman DA, Glosser G: Pharmacologic strategies in aging and dementia, in Strategies in the Development of an Effective Treatment for Senile Dementia. Edited by Crook T, Gershon S. New Canaan, CT, Mark Powley Associates, 1981, pp 35–51

Drachman D, Leavitt J: Human memory and the cholinergic system. Arch Neurol 30:113–121, 1974

Drake ME: Episodic depression and hypomania with temporal lobe EEG paroxysms. Psychosomatics 29:354–357, 1988

Drevets WC, Rubin EH: Psychotic symptoms and the longitudinal course of senile dementia of the Alzheimer type. Biol Psychiatry 25:39–48, 1989

Drugan RC, Philip HV: Central and peripheral benzodiazepine receptors: involvement in an organism's response to physical and psychological stress. Neurosci Behav Rev 15:277, 1991

Drummond AH, Raeburn CA: The interaction of lithium with thyrotropin releasing hormone-stimulated lipid metabolism in GH3 pituitary tumor cells. Biochem J 224:129–136, 1984

Dryman A, Eaton WW: Affective symptoms associated with the onset of major depression in the community: findings from the US National Institute of Mental Health Epidemiologic Catchment Area Program. Acta Psychiatr Scand 84:1–5, 1991

Dubois B, Danze F, Pillon B, et al: Cholinergic-dependent cognitive deficits in Parkinson's disease. Ann Neurol 22:26–30, 1987

Dubois B, Pillon R, Lhermitte F, et al: Cholinergic deficiency and frontal dysfunction in Parkinson's disease. Ann Neurol 28:117–121, 1990

Dubovsky SL: Beyond the serotonin reuptake inhibitors: rationales for the development of new serotonergic agents. J Clin Psychiatry 55 (suppl 2): 34–44, 1994

Dubovsky SL: Calcium channel antagonists as novel agents for manic-depressive disorder, in Textbook of Psychopharmacology. Edited by Schatzberg AF, Nemeroff CB. Washington DC, American Psychiatric Press, 1995, pp 377–88

Dubovsky SL, Franks RD: Intracellular calcium in affective disorders: a review and an hypothesis. Biol Psychiatry 18:781–797, 1983

Dubovsky SL, Franks RD: Verapamil: a new antimanic drug with potential interactions with lithium. J Clin Psychiatry 48:371–372, 1987

Dubovsky SL, Franks RD, Lifschitz M, et al: Effectiveness of verapamil in the treatment of a manic patient. Am J Psychiatry 139:502–504, 1982

Dubovsky S, Franks R, Schrier D: Phenelzine-induced hypomania: effect of verapamil. Biol Psychiatry 20:1009–1014, 1985

Dubovsky SL, Franks RD, Allen S: Calcium antagonists in mania: a double-blind study of verapamil. Psychiatry Res 18:309–320, 1986

Dubovsky SL, Christiano J, Daniell LC, et al: Increased platelet intracellular calcium concentration in patients with bipolar affective disorders. Arch Gen Psychiatry 46:632–638, 1989

Dubovsky SL, Lee C, Christiano J, et al: Elevated platelet intracellular calcium concentration in bipolar depression. Biol Psychiatry 29:441–450, 1991a

Dubovsky SL, Lee C, Christiano J, et al: Lithium lowers platelet intracellular ion concentration in bipolar patients. Lithium 2:167–174, 1991b

Dubovsky SL, Murphy J, Thomas M, et al: Abnormal intracellular calcium ion concentration in platelets and lymphocytes of bipolar patients. Am J Psychiatry 149:118–120, 1992a

Dubovsky SL, Murphy J, Christiano J, et al: The calcium second messenger system in bipolar disorders: data supporting new research directions. J Neuropsychiatry Clin Neurosci 4:3–14, 1992b

Dubovsky SL, Thomas M, Hijazi A, et al: Intracellular calcium signalling in peripheral cells of patients with bipolar affective disorder. Eur Arch Psychiatry Clin Neurosci 243:229–234, 1994

Duman RS, Heninger GR, Nestler EJ: Adaptations of receptor-coupled signal transduction pathways underlying stress- and drug-induced neural plasticity. J Nerv Ment Dis 182:692–700, 1994

Dunbar GC, Fuell DL: The anti-anxiety and anti-agitation effects of paroxetine in depressed patients. Int Clin Psychopharmacol 6 (suppl 4):81–90, 1992

Dunleavy DLF, Oswald I: Phenelzine, mood response and sleep. Arch Gen Psychiatry 28:353–356, 1973

Dunleavy DLF, Brezinova V, Oswald I, et al: Changes during weeks in effects of tricyclic drugs on the human sleeping brain. Br J Psychiatry 120:663–672, 1972

Dunn AJ, Berridge CW: Physiological and behavioral responses to corticotropin-releasing factor administration: is CRF a mediator of anxiety or stress responses? Brain Res 15:71, 1990

Dunn CG, Quinlan D: Indicators of ECT response and non-response in the treatment of depression. J Clin Psychiatry 39:620–622, 1978

Dunne MP, Hartley LR: The effects of scopolamine upon verbal memory: evidence for an attentional hypothesis. Acta Psychologica 58:205–217, 1985

Dunne MP, Hartley LR: Scopolamine and the control of attention in humans. Psychopharmacology 89:94–97, 1986

Dunner DL, Dunbar GC: Optimal dose regimen for paroxetine. J Clin Psychiatry 53 (suppl 2):21–26, 1992

Dunner DL, Fieve RR: Clinical factors in lithium carbonate prophylaxis failure. Arch Gen Psychiatry 30:229–233, 1974

Dunner DL, Stallone FL, Fieve RR: Lithium carbonate and affective disorders, V: a double-blind study of prophylaxis of depression in bipolar illness. Arch Gen Psychiatry 33:117–120, 1976

Dunner DL, Ishiki D, Avery DH, et al: Effectiveness of alprazolam and diazepam in patients with panic disorder: a controlled study. J Clin Psychiatry 47:458–460, 1986

Dunnett SB, Martel FL: Proactive interference effects on short-term memory in rats, I: basic parameters and drug effects. Behav Neurosci 104:655–665, 1990

Dunnett SB, Wareham AT, Torres EM: Cholinergic blockade in prefrontal cortex and hippocampus disrupts short-term memory in rats. Neuroreport 1:61–64, 1990

Durlach-Misteli C, Van Ree JM: Dopamine and melatonin in the nucleus accumbens may be implicated in the mode of action of antidepressant drugs. Eur J Pharmacol 217:15–21, 1992

Dursun SM, Reveley MA: Obsessive-compulsive symptoms and clozapine (letter). Br J Psychiatry 165:267–268, 1994

Duterte-Boucher D, Leclère J-F, Panissand C, et al: Acute effects of direct dopamine agonists in the mouse behavioural despair test. Eur J Pharmacol 154:185–190, 1988

Dwoskin LP, Jewell AL, Cassis LA: DuP 753, a non-peptide angiotensin II-1 receptor antagonist, alters dopaminergic function in rat striatum. Arch Pharmacol 345:153–159, 1992

Dysken MW, Mendels J, LeWitt P: Milacemide: a placebo-controlled study in senile dementia of the Alzheimer type. J Am Geriatr Soc 40:503–506, 1992

Dysken MW, Johnson SB, Holden L, et al: Haloperidol concentrations in patients with Alzheimer's Disease. Am J Geriatr Psychiatry 2:124–133, 1994

Eagger SA, Levy R, Sahakian BJ: Tacrine in Alzheimer's disease. Lancet 337:989–929, 1991

Eales MG, Layeni AO: Exacerbation of obsessive-compulsive symptoms associated with clozapine. Br J Psychiatry 164:687–688, 1994

Eaton SA, Salt TE: Modulatory effects of serotonin on excitatory amino acid responses and sensory synaptic transmission in the ventrobasal thalamus. Neuroscience 33:285–292, 1989

Eaton WW, Kessler RC, Wittchen HU, et al: Panic disorder and panic in the United States. Am J Psychiatry 151:413–420, 1994

Ebadi MS, Simmons VJ, Hendrickson MJ, et al: Pharmacokinetics of lithium and its regional distribution in rat brain. Eur J Pharmacol 27:324–329, 1974

Ebert D, Feistel H, Kaschka W, et al: Single photon emission computerised tomography assessment of cerebral dopamine D_2 receptor blockade in depression before and after sleep deprivation—preliminary results. Biol Psychiatry 35:880–885, 1994

Ebstein R, Belmaker R, Grunhaus L, et al: Lithium inhibition of adrenaline-stimulated adenylate cyclase in humans. Nature 259:411–413, 1976

Ebstein RP, Hermoni M, Belmaker RH: The effect of lithium on noradrenaline-induced cyclic AMP accumulation in rat brain: inhibition after chronic treatment and absence of supersensitivity. J Pharmacol Exp Ther 213:161–167, 1980

Ebstein RP, Lerer B, Shlaufman M, et al: The effect of repeated electroconvulsive shock treatment and chronic lithium feeding on the release of norepinephrine from rat cortical vesicular preparations. Cell Mol Neurobiol 3:191–201, 1983

Ebstein RP, Moscovich D, Zeevi S, et al: Effect of lithium in vitro and after chronic treatment on human platelet adenylate cyclase activity: prosreceptor modification or second messenger signal amplification. Psychiatry Res 21:221–228, 1987

Eccleston D, Cole AJ: Calcium-channel blockade and depressive illness. Br J Psychiatry 156:889–891, 1990

Eckmann VF: Double-blind clinical study with the calcium antagonist flunarizine in cerebral circulatory disturbances. Arzneimittel-Forschung 35:1276–1279, 1985

Edelbroek PM, Linnsen CG, Zitman FG, et al: Analgesic and antidepressive effects of low-dose amitriptyline in relation to its metabolism in patients with chronic pain. Clin Pharmacol Ther 39:156–162, 1986

Edelfors S: Distribution of sodium, potassium and lithium in the brain of lithium-treated rats. Acta Pharmacol Toxicol 37:387–392, 1975

Efron R: Post-epileptic paralysis: theoretical critique and report of a case. Brain 84:381–394, 1961

Ehlers CL, Reed TK, Henriksen SJ: Effects of corticotropin-releasing factor and growth hormone-releasing factor on sleep and activity in rats. Neuroendocrinology 42:467–474, 1986

Ehrensing RH, Kastin AJ: Dose-related biphasic effect of prolyl-leucylglycinamide (MIF-1) in depression. Am J Psychiatry 135:562–566, 1978

Ehrlich BE, Diamond JM, Fry V, et al: Lithium's inhibition of erythrocyte cation countertransport involves a slow process in the erythrocyte. J Membr Biol 75:233–240, 1983

Eich JE: The cue-dependent nature of state-dependent retrieval. Mem Cognit 8:157–173, 1980

Eimerl S, Schramm N: The quantity of calcium that appears to induce neuronal death. J Neurochem 62:1223–1226, 1994

Eisenberg J, Asnis G: Lithium as an adjunct treatment in obsessive-compulsive disorder. Am J Psychiatry 142:663, 1985

Eison A, Eison M: Serotonergic mechanisms in anxiety. Prog Neuropsychopharmacol Biol Psychiatry 18:47–62, 1994

Eison MS: The new generation of serotonergic anxiolytics: possible clinical roles. Psychopathology 22 (suppl 1):13–20, 1989

Elgoyen AB, Johnson D, Boulter J, et al: Cloning and functional expression of $\alpha 9$: a novel acetylcholine-gated ion channel, in International Symposium on Nicotine: The Effects of Nicotine on Biological Systems II. Edited by Clarke PBS, Quick M, Thuran K, et al. Basel, Switzerland, Birkhäuser Verlag, 1994, p P7

Elkin I, Shea T, Watkins JT, et al: National Institute of Mental Health Treatment of Depression Collaborative Research Program: general effectiveness of treatments. Arch Gen Psychiatry 46:971–982, 1989

Elliott HL, Jones CR, Vincent J, et al: The alpha adrenoceptor antagonist properties of idazoxan in normal subjects. Clin Pharmacol Ther 36:190–196, 1984

Ellis J, Lenox RH: Chronic lithium treatment prevents atropine-induced supersensitivity of the muscarinic phosphoinositide response in rat hippocampus. Biol Psychiatry 28:609–619, 1990

Ellis J, Lenox RH: Receptor coupling to G proteins: interactions not affected by lithium. Lithium 2:141–147, 1991

El-Mallakh RS: The ionic mechanism of lithium action. Lithium 1:87–92, 1990

Elphick M: Clinical issues in the use of carbamazepine in psychiatry: a review. Psychol Med 19:591–604, 1989a

Elphick M: Effects of carbamazepine on dopamine function in rodents. Psychopharmacology 99:532–536, 1989b

Elphick M, Lyons F, Cowen PJ: Low tolerability of carbamazepine in psychiatric patients may restrict its clinical usefulness. J Psychopharmacol 2:1–4, 1988

Emamghoreishi M, Schlichter L, Li PP, et al: High intracellular calcium concentrations in transformed lymphoblasts from subjects with bipolar I disorder. Am J Psychiatry 154:976–982, 1997

Emmanuel NP, Lydiard RB, Ballenger J: Treatment of social phobia with bupropion. J Clin Psychopharmacol 11:276–277, 1991

Emptage NJ, Marcus EA, Stark LL, et al: Differential modulatory actions of serotonin in aphysia sensory neurons: implications for development and learning. Semin Neurosci 6:21–33, 1994

Emrich HM: Studies with oxcarbazepine (Trileptal) in acute mania, in Carbamazepine and Oxcarbazepine in Psychiatry. Edited by Emrich H, Schiwy W, Silverstone T. London, CNS Publishers, 1990, pp 83–88

Emrich HM, von Zerssen D, Kissling W, et al: Effect of sodium valproate on mania: the GABA hypothesis of affective disorders. Archiv fur Psychiatrie und Nervenkrankheiten 229:1–16, 1980

Emrich HM, von Zerssen D, Kissling W, et al: On a possible role of GABA in mania: therapeutic efficacy of sodium valproate, in GABA and Benzodiazepine Receptors. Edited by Costa E, Dicharia G, Gessa GL. New York, Raven, 1981, pp 287–296

Emrich HM, Dose M, Von Zerssen D: The use of sodium valproate, carbamazepine and oxcarbazepine in patients with affective disorders. J Affect Disord 8:243–250, 1985

Emson PC, Lee CM, Rehfeld JF: Cholecystokinin peptides: vesicular localization and calcium dependent release from rat brain in vitro. Life Sci 26:2157–2162, 1980

Endicott J, Spitzer RL: A diagnostic interview: the Schedule for Affective Disorders and Schizophrenia. Arch Gen Psychiatry 35:837–844, 1978

Endicott J, Spitzer RL, Fleiss JL: The Global Assessment Scale: a procedure for measuring overall severity of psychiatric disturbance. Arch Gen Psychiatry 33:766–771, 1976

Eng J, Shiina Y, Pan Y-CE, et al: Pig brain contains cholecystokinin octapeptide and several cholecystokinin desoctapeptides. Proc Natl Acad Sci U S A 80:6381–6385, 1983

Engel J, Berggren U: Effects of lithium on behaviour and central monoamines. Acta Psychiatr Scand Suppl 280:133–143, 1980

Engel J Jr, Ackermann RF, Caldecott-Hazard S, et al: Epileptic activation of antagonistic systems may explain paradoxical features of experimental and human epilepsy, a review and hypothesis, in Kindling 2. Edited by Wada JA. New York, Raven, 1981, pp 193–217

Enns M, Karvelas L: Electrical dose titration for electroconvulsive therapy: a comparison with dose prediction methods. Convulsive Therapy 11:86–93, 1995

Enz A, Gray JA, Spiegel R: Muscarinic agonists for senile dementia: past experience and future trends, in Cholinergic Basis for Alzheimer Therapy. Edited by Becker R, Giacobini E. Boston, MA, Birkhäuser, 1991, pp 370–376

Eraker SA, Kirscht JP, Becker MH: Understanding and improving patient compliance. Ann Intern Med 100:258, 1984

Eric L: A prospective double-blind comparative multicentre study of paroxetine and placebo in preventing recurrent major depressive episodes. Biol Psychiatry 29:25–45, 1991

Eriksson E: Brain neurotransmission in panic disorder. Acta Psychiatr Scand Suppl 335:31–37, 1987

Ernsberger P, Giuliano R, Willette RN, et al: Role of imidazole receptors in the vasodepressor response to clonidine analogs in the rostral ventrolateral medulla. J Pharmacol Exp Ther 253:408–418, 1990

Eroglu L, Hizal A, Koyuncuoglu H: The effect of long-term concurrent administration of chlorpromazine and lithium on the striatal and frontal cortical dopamine metabolism in rats. Psychopharmacology 73:84–86, 1981

Erzegovesi S, Ronchi P, Smeraldi E: 5-HT-2 receptor and fluvoxamine effect in obsessive-compulsive disorder. Hum Psychopharmacol 7:287–289, 1992

Essig CF, Flanary G: The importance of the convulsion in occurrence and rate of development of electroconvulsive threshold elevation. Exp Neurol 14:448–452, 1966

Estes WK, Skinner BF: Some quantitative properties of anxiety. J Exp Psychol 29:390–400, 1941

Eugster HP, Probst M, Wurgler FE, Sengstag C: Caffeine, estradiol, and progesterone interact with human CYP1A1 and CYP1A2. Evidence from cDNA-directed expression in Saccharomyces cerevisiae. Drug Metab Dispos 21(1):43–49, 1993

Evans L, Moore G, Cox J: Zimeldine—a serotonin uptake blocker—in the treatment of phobic anxiety. Prog Neuropsychopharmacol Biol Psychiatry 4:75–79, 1980

Evans L, Kenardy P, Hoey H: Effect of a selective serotonin uptake inhibitor in agoraphobia with panic attacks. Acta Psychiatr Scand 73:40–53, 1986

Evans MS, Zorumski CF, Clifford DB: Lithium enhances neuronal muscarinic excitation by presynaptic facilitation. Neuroscience 38:457–468, 1990

Eysenck HJ: The Biological Basis of Personality. Springfield, IL, Charles C Thomas, 1967

Eysenck MW: A Handbook of Cognitive Psychology. Hillsdale, NJ, Lawrence Erlbaum Associates, 1984

Eysselein V, Eberlein G, Ho FJ, et al: An amino-terminal fragment of cholecystokinin-58 is present in the gut: evidence for a similar processing site of procholecystokinin in canine gut and brain. Reg Peptides 22:205–215, 1988

Fabre L, Vettraine J, Birkhimmer L, et al: Fluvoxamine in the treatment of depression: a double-blind comparison with imipramine and placebo in outpatients with major depression. Paper presented at the 18th CINP Congress, Nice, France, 1992

Faedda GL, Baldessarini RJ, Tohen M, et al: Episode sequence in bipolar disorder and response to lithium treatment. Am J Psychiatry 148:1237–1239, 1991

Falkenburg T, Mohammed AK, Henriksson B, et al: Increased expression of brain-derived neurotrophic factor mRNA in rat hippocampus is associated with improved spatial memory and enriched environment. Neurosci Lett 138: 153–156, 1992

Fallon BA, Campeas R, Schneier FR, et al: Open trial of intravenous clomipramine in five treatment-refractory patients with obsessive-compulsive disorder. J Neuropsychiatry Clin Neurosci 4:70–75, 1992

Fallon BA, Liebowitz MR, Campeas R, et al: Intravenous clomipramine for clomipramine-refractory OCD (Abstract NR448). Paper presented at the 148th annual meeting of the American Psychiatric Association, Miami, FL, May 20–25, 1995

Falloon IR, Lloyd GG, Harpin RE: The treatment of social phobia: real-life rehearsal with nonprofessional therapists. J Nerv Ment Dis 169:180–184, 1981

Farlow M, Gracon SI, Hershey LA, et al: A controlled trial of tacrine in Alzheimer's disease. JAMA 268:2523–2529, 1992

Fava GA, Molnar G, Block B, et al: The lithium loading dose method in a clinical setting. Am J Psychiatry 141:812–813, 1984

Fava M: High-dose fluoxetine in the treatment of depressed patients not responsive to a standard dose of fluoxetine. J Affect Disord 25:229–234, 1992

Fava M, Davidson KG: Definition and epiemiology of treatment-resistant depression. Psychiatr Clin North Am 19:179–200, 1996

Fava M, Rosenbaum JF, McGrath PJ, et al: Lithium and tricyclic augmentation of fluoxetine treatment for resistant major depression: a double-blind, controlled study. Am J Psychiatry 151:1372–1374, 1994

Fawcett J: Suicide risk factors in depressive disorders and panic disorder. J Clin Psychiatry 53 (suppl 3):9–13, 1992

Fawcett J: Progress in treatment resistant depression: we have a long way to go. Psychiatric Annals 24:214–216, 1994

Fawcett J, Kravitz HM: Treatment refractory depression, in Common Treatment Problems in Depression. Edited by Schatzberg AF. Washington, DC, American Psychiatric Press, 1985, pp 2–27

Fawcett J, Kravitz HM: Anxiety syndromes and their relationship to depressive illness. J Clin Psychiatry 44:8–11, 1988

Fedele E, Andrioli GC, Ruelle A, et al: Release-regulating dopamine autoreceptors in human cerebral cortex. Br J Pharmacol 110:20–22, 1993

Feder R: Lithium augmentation of clomipramine. J Clin Psychiatry 49:458, 1988

Feighner JP: Busporine in the long-term treatment of generalised anxiety disorder. J Clin Psychiatry 48 (suppl):3–6, 1987

Feighner JP, Cohen JB: Analysis of individual symptoms in generalized anxiety disorder: a pooled, multi-study, double evaluation of buspirone. Neuropsychobiology 21:124–130, 1989

Feighner JP, Herbstein J, Damlouju N: Combined MAOI, TCA and direct stimulant therapy of treatment resistant depression. J Clin Psychiatry 6:206–209, 1985

Feighner JP, Pambakian R, Fowler RC, et al: A comparison of nefazadone, imipramine and placebo in patients with moderate to severe depression. Psychopharmacol Bull 25:219–221, 1989a

Feighner JP, Boyer WF, Meredith CF, et al: A double-blind comparison of fluoxetine, imipramine and placebo in outpatients with major depression. Int Clin Psychopharmacol 4:127–134, 1989b

Feinberg I, Fein G, Floyd TC: Period and amplitude analysis of NREM EEG in sleep: repeatability of results in young adults. Electroencephalogr Clin Neurophysiol 48:212–221, 1980

Fekete M, Varszegi M, Kadar T, et al: Effect of cholecystokinin octapeptide sulphate ester on brain monoamines in the rat. Acta Physiol Acad Sci Hung 57:37–46, 1981a

Fekete M, Kadar T, Penke B, et al: Influence of cholecystokinin octapeptide sulfate ester on brain monoamine metabolism in rats. J Neural Transm 50:81–88, 1981b

Feldman JD, Noshirvani H, Chu C: Improvement in female patients with severe obsessions and/or compulsions treated with cyproterone acetate (letter). Acta Psychiatr Scand 78:254, 1988

Feldman M, Walker P, Goldschmiedt M, et al: Role of affect and personality in gastric acid secretion and serum gastrin concentration: comparative studies in normal men and in male duodenal ulcer patients. Gastroenterology 102:175–180, 1992

Fensbo C, Montgomery SA, Andersen J, et al: GBR 12909. A dose response relationship of the selective dopamine reuptake inhibitor in major depression (abstract). Abstracts of the 17th CINP Congress, Kyoto, Japan, September 10–14 1990, p 83

Fenton WS, McGlashan TH: The prognostic significance of obsessive-compulsive symptoms in schizophrenia. Am J Psychiatry 143:437–441, 1986

Ferbert A, Priori A, Rothwel JC, et al: Interhemispheric inhibition of the human motor cortex. J Physiol Lond 453:525–546, 1992

Fergusson DM, Horwood AJ, Lynskey MT: Maternal depressive symptoms and depressive symptoms in adolescence. J Child Psychol Psychiatry 36:1161–1178, 1995

Fernandez-Cordoba E, López-Ibor AJ: La monoclorimiprimina en enfermos psiquiatricos resistantes a otros tratamientos. Actas Lusco Espanolas de Neurologia Y Psiquatria 26:119–147, 1967

Fernandez-Guasti A, Picazo O: The actions of diazepam and serotonergic anxiolytics vary according to the gender and the estrous cycle phase. Pharmacol Biochem Behav 37:77–81, 1990

Feuillade P, Pringuey D, Belugou JL, et al: Trimipramine: acute and lasting effects on sleep in healthy and major depressive subjects. J Affect Disord 24:135–146, 1992

Fibiger HC, Vincent SR: Anatomy of central cholinergic neurons, in Psychopharmacology: The Third Generation of Progress. Edited by Meltzer HY. New York, Raven, 1987, pp 211–218

Fibiger HC, Lepiane FG, Phillips AG: Disruption of memory produced by stimulation of the dorsal raphe nucleus: mediation by serotonin. Brain Res 155:380–386, 1978

Fieve RR, Platman SR, Plutchik RR: The use of lithium in affective disorders, I: acute endogenous depression. Am J Psychiatry 125:79–83, 1968

Fieve RR, Kumbaraci T, Dunner DL: Lithium prophylaxis of depression in bipolar I, bipolar II, and unipolar patients. Am J Psychiatry 133:925–930, 1976

File SE: Rapid development of tolerance to the sedative effects of lorazepam and triazolam in rats. Psychopharmacology 73:240–245, 1981

File SE: Animal models of different anxiety states. Adv Biochem Psychopharmacol 48:93–113, 1995

Fink G, Sarkar DK, Dow RC, et al: Sex difference in response to alphaxolone may be estrogen dependent. Nature 298:270–272, 1982

Fink M: ECT: A last resort treatment for resistant depression, in Treating Resistant Depression. Edited by Zohar J, Belmaker RH. Great Neck, NY, PMA, 1987

Fink M: A trial of ECT is essential before a diagnosis of refractory depression is made, in Refractory Depression (Advances in Neuropsychiatry and Psychopharmacology, Vol 2). Edited by Amsterdam JD. New York, Raven, 1991, pp 87–92

Finn DA, Gee KW: The influence of estrous cycle on neurosteroid potency at the g-aminobutyric acid A receptor complex. J Pharmacol Exp Ther 265:1374–1379, 1993

Fisher A, Barak D: Progress and perspectives in new muscarinic agonists. Drug News and Perspective 7(8):453–464, 1994

Fisher A, Heldman E Gurwitz D, et al: Selective signaling via novel muscarinic agonists: implications for Alzheimer's disease treatment and clinical update, in Alzheimer Disease: Therapeutic Strategies. Edited by Giacobini E, Becker R. Boston, MA, Birkhäuser, 1994, pp 219–223

Fisher SK, Heacock AM, Agranoff BW: Inositol lipids and signal transduction in the nervous system: an update. J Neurochem 58:18–38, 1992

Fisone G, Wu CF, Consolo S, et al: Galanin inhibits acetylcholine release in the ventral hippocampus of the rat: histochemical, autoradiographic, in vivo, and in vitro studies. Proc Natl Acad Sci U S A 84:7339–7343, 1987

Flament MF, Rapoport JL, Berg CJ, et al: CMI treatment of childhood OCD: a double-blind study. Arch Gen Psychiatry 42:977, 1985

Fleischmann A, Steppel J, Leon A, et al: The effect of transcranial magnetic stimulation compared with electroconvulsive shock on rat apomorphine-induced stereotypy. Eur Neuropsychopharmacol 4:449–450, 1994

Fleischmann A, Prolov K, Abarbanel J, et al: The effect of transcranial magnetic stimulation of the rat brain on behavioral models of depression. Brain Res 699(1):130–132, 1995

Fletcher A, Bill DJ, Bill SJ, et al: WAY100135: a novel, selective antagonist of presynaptic and postsynaptic 5-HT$_{1A}$ receptors. Eur J Pharmacol 237:283–291, 1993

Fletcher A, Forster EA, Bill DJ, et al: Electrophysiological, biochemical, neurohormonal and behavioural studies with WAY-100635, a potent, selective and silent 5-HT$_{1A}$ receptor antagonist. Behav Brain Res 73:337–353, 1996

Fletcher PJ, Higgins GA: Differential effects of ondansetron and alpha-flupenthixol on responding for conditioned reward. Psychopharmacology 134: 64–72, 1997

Flood JF, Smith GE, Roberts E: Dehydroepiandrosterone and its sulfate enhance memory retention in mice. Brain Res 447:269–277, 1988

Flood JF, Baker ML, Davis JL: Modulation of memory processing by glutamic receptor agonists and antagonists. Brain Res 521:197–202, 1990

Flood JF, Morley JE, Roberts E: Memory-enhancing effects in male mice of pregnenolone and steroids metabolically derived from it. Proc Natl Acad Sci U S A 89:1567–1571, 1992

Flood JF, Farr SA, Uezo K, et al: The pharmacology of post-trial memory processing in septum. Eur. J Pharmacol 350:31–38, 1998

Flor-Henry P: Psychosis and temporal lobe epilepsy: a controlled investigation. Epilepsia 10:363–395, 1969

Flynn D, Mash D: Characterization of l-[^{3}H]nicotine binding in human cerebral cortex: comparison between Alzheimer's disease and the normal. J Neurochem 47:1948–1954, 1986

Folstein MF, Folstein SE, McHugh PR: Mini-Mental State: a practical method for grading the cognitive state of patients for the clinician. J Psychiatr Res 12:189–198, 1975

Fontaine E: Novel serotonergic mechanisms and clinical experience with nefazadone. Clin Neuropsychopharmacol 16 (suppl 3):S45–S51, 1994

Fontaine R, Chouinard G: Antiobsessive effect of fluoxetine. Am J Psychiatry 142:989, 1985

Fontaine R, Ontiveros A, Elie R, et al: A double-blind comparison of nefazadone, imipramine and placebo in major depression. J Clin Psychiatry 55:234–241, 1994

Fontana DJ, Daniels SE, Henderson C, et al: Ondansetron improves cognitive performance in the Morris water maze spatial navigation task. Psychopharmacology 120:409–417, 1995

Foote SL, Freedman R, Oliver AP: Effects of putative neurotransmitters on neuronal activity in monkey auditory cortex. Brain Res 86:229–242, 1975

Ford DE, Kamerow DB: Epidemiologic study of sleep disturbances and psychiatric disorders: an opportunity for prevention? JAMA 262:1479–1484, 1985

Foreman MM, Gehlert DR, Schaus JM: Quinelorane, a potent and selective dopamine agonist for the "D_2-like" receptor family. Neurotransmissions 11:1–5, 1995

Forn J, Valdecasas FG: Effects of lithium on brain adenyl cyclase activity. Biochem Pharmacol 20:2773–2779, 1971

Forrest DV: Bipolar illness after right hemispherectomy: a response to lithium carbonate and carbamazepine. Arch Gen Psychiatry 39:817–819, 1982

Förstner U, Bohus M, Gebicke-Harter PJ, et al: Decreased agonist-stimulated Ca^{2+} response in neutrophils from patients under chronic lithium therapy. Eur Arch Psychiatry Clin Neurosci 243:240–243, 1994

Fozard JR: Neuronal 5-HT receptors in the periphery. Neuropharmacology 23:1473–1486, 1984

Fozard JR: Pharmacological relevance of 5HT-3 receptors, in Serotonin Receptor Subtypes: Pharmacological Significance and Clinical Implications. Edited by Langer SZ, Brunello N, Racagni G, et al. International Academy for Biomedical and Drug Research. Basel, Switzerland, Karger, 1992, pp 44–55

Franc JE, Duncan GF, Farmen RH, et al: High performance liquid chromatographic method for the determination of nefazodone and its metabolites in human plasma using laboratory robotics. J Chromatogr B Biomed Sci Appl 570:129–138, 1991

Frances A, Hall W: Work in progress on the DSM-IV mood disorders, in Diagnosis of Depression. Edited by Feighner JP, Boyer WF. Chichester, England, Wiley, 1991, pp 49–78

Frances A, Brown RP, Kocsis JH, et al: Psychotic depression: a separate entity? Am J Psychiatry 138:831–833, 1981

Francis PT, Pangalos MM, Bowen DM: Animal and drug modelling for Alzheimer synaptic pathology. Prog Neurobiol 39:517–545, 1992

Frank E, Kupfer DJ, Perel JM, et al: Three-year outcomes for maintenance therapies in recurrent depression. Arch Gen Psychiatry 47:1093–1099, 1990

Frank E, Prien R, Jarrett RB, et al: Conceptualization and rationale for consensus definitions of terms in major depressive disorder. Arch Gen Psychiatry 48:851–855, 1991

Frank E, Kupfer DJ, Perel JM, et al: Comparison of full-dose versus half-dose pharmacotherapy in the maintenance treatment of recurrent depression. J Affect Disord 27:139–145, 1993

Frankland PW, Josselyn SA, Bradwejn J, et al: Activation of amygdala cholecystokinin B receptors potentiates the acoustic startle response in the rat. J Neurosci 17:1838–1847, 1997

Fraser RM, Glass IB: Unilateral and bilateral ECT in elderly patients: a comparative study. Acta Psychiatr Scand 62:13–31, 1980

Frederick DL, Ali SF, Slikker W, et al: Behavioural and neurochemical effects of chronic methylenedioxymethamphetamine (MDMA) treatment in rhesus monkeys. Neurotoxicol Teratol 17:531–543, 1995

Frederick DL, Ali SF, Gillam MP, et al: Acute effects of dexfenfluramine (d-Fen) and methylenedioxymethamphetamine (MDMA) before and after short-course, high dose treatment. Ann N Y Acad Sci 844:183–190, 1998

Fredericson Overø K, Toft B, Christophersen L, et al: Kinetics of citalopram in elderly patients. Psychopharmacology 86:253–257, 1985

Freedman DD, Waters DD: "Second generation" dihydropyridine calcium antagonists: greater vascular selectivity and some unique applications. Drugs 34:578–598, 1987

Freedman R, Coon H, Myles-Worsley M, et al: Linkage of a neurophysiological deficit in schizophrenia to a chromosome 15 locus. Proc Natl Acad Sci U S A 94:587–592, 1997

Freeman CPL, Trimble MR, Deatin JFW, et al: Fluvoxamine vs CMI in the treatment of OCD: a multicenter, randomized, double-blind, parallel-group comparison. J Clin Psychiatry 55:301–305, 1994

Freeman EW, Purdy RH, Coutifaris C, et al: Anxiolytic metabolites of progesterone: correlation with mood and performance measures following oral progesterone administration to healthy female volunteers. Neuroendocrinology 58:478–484, 1993

Freeman TW, Clothier JL, Pazzaglia P, et al: A double-blind comparison of valproate and lithium in the treatment of acute mania. Am J Psychiatry 149:108–111, 1992

Frenchman IB, Prince T: Clinical experience with risperidone, haloperidol, and thioridazine for dementia-associated behavioral disturbances. Int Psychogeriatr 9:431–435, 1997

Frey WH, Liu J, Thorne RG, et al: Intranasal delivery of 125 I-labeled nerve growth factor to the brain via the olfactory route, in Research Advances in Alzheimer's Disease and Related Disorders. Edited by Iqbal K, Mortimer JA, Winblad B, et al. Chichester, England, Wiley, 1995, pp 329–335

Friedman E, Gershon S: Effect of lithium on brain dopamine. Nature 243:520–521, 1973

Friedman E, Wang H-Y: Effect of chronic lithium treatment on 5-hyroxytryptamine autoreceptors and release of 5-[3H]hydroxytryptamine from rat brain cortical, hippocampal, and hypothalamic slices. J Neurochem 50:195–201, 1988

Friedman E, Dallob A, Levine G: The effect of long-term lithium treatment on reserpine-induced supersensitivity in dopaminergic and serotonergic transmission. Life Sci 25:1263–1266, 1979

Friedman L, Ecker J, Sullivan J, et al: A comparative study of the abuse potential of nefazodone, amphetamines, diazepam and placebo in normal volunteers. Paper presented at the meeting of the New Clinical Drugs Evaluation Unit, Boca Raton, FL, May 26–29, 1992

Friedman S, Sunderland GS, Rosenblum LA: A non-human model for panic disorder. Psychiatry Res 23:65–75, 1987

Friess E, Trachsel L, Guldner J, et al: DHEA administration increases rapid eye movement sleep and EEG power in the sigma frequency range. Am J Physiol 268:E107–E113, 1995

Frisoni GB, De Leo D, Rozzini R, et al: Psychic correlates of sleep symptoms in the elderly. Int J Geriatr Psychiatry 7:891–898, 1992

Fritschy J, Benke D, Mertens S, et al: 5 types of type A GABA receptors identified in neurons by double and triple immunofluorescence staining with subunit specific antibodies. Proc Natl Acad Sci U S A 89:6726–6730, 1992

Frye CA, Duncan JE: Progesterone metabolites effective at the GABAa receptor complex attenuate pain sensitivity in rats. Brain Res 643:194–203, 1994

Frye CA, Cuevas CA, Crystal S, et al: Diet and estrous cycle influence pain sensitivity in rats. Pharmacol Biochem Behav 45:255–260, 1993

Frye PE, Arnold LE: Persistent amphetamine-induced compulsive rituals: response to pyridoxine (B6). Biol Psychiatry 16:583–587, 1981

Fukunaga K, Soderling TR: Activation of Ca^{2+}/calmodulin-dependent protein kinase II in cerebellar granule cells by N-methyl-D-aspartate receptor activation. Mol Cell Neurosci 1:133–138, 1990

Fuld P, Katzman R, Davies P, et al: Intrusions as a sign of Alzheimer dementia: chemical and pathological verification. Ann Neurol 11:155–159, 1982

Fuller RW, Hemrick-Luecke SK: Antagonism by tomoxetine of the depletion of norepinephrine and epinephrine in rat brain by αmethyl-*m*-tyrosine. Res Commun Chem Pathol Pharmacol 41:169–172, 1983

Fuster JM: The Prefrontal Cortex: Anatomy, Physiology and Neuropsychology of the Frontal Lobe. New York, Raven, 1989

Fyro B, Petterson U, Sedvall G: The effect of lithium treatment on manic symptoms and levels of monoamine metabolites in cerebrospinal fluid of manic depressive patients. Psychopharmacologia 44:99–103, 1975

Gabriel SM, Harsutunian V: Alterations in galanin peptide in Alzheimer's disease (AD) contrast with acute, experimentally induced lesions in adult rats (abstract). Paper presented at the annual meeting of the American College of Neuropsychopharmacology, San Juan, Puerto Rico, December 1994

Gadde KM, Krishnan KRR: Endocrine factors in depression. Psychiatric Annals 24: 521–524, 1994

Gaillard JM, Blois R, Couto L, et al: Modifications of paradoxical sleep by desipramine in elderly depressed patients. Advances in Biological Psychiatry 13:224–228, 1983

Galeotti N, Ghelardini C, Bartolini A: Role of 5-HT_4 receptors in the mouse passive avoidance test. J Pharmacol Exp Ther 286:1115–1121, 1998

Gallager DW, Pert A, Bunney WE Jr: Haloperidol-induced presynaptic dopamine supersensitivity is blocked by chronic lithium. Nature 273:309–312, 1978

Ganguli R, Reynolds CF III, Kupfer DJ: Electroencephalographic sleep in young never-medicated schizophrenics. Arch Gen Psychiatry 44:36–44, 1987

Gao XM, Fukamauchi F, Chuang DM: Long-term biphasic effects of lithium treatment on phospholipase C-coupled M3-muscarinic acetylcholine receptors in cultured cerebellar granule cells. Neurochem Int 22:395–403, 1993

Gao XM, Margolis RL, Leeds P, et al: Carbamazepine induction of apoptosis in cultured cerebellar neurons: effects of N-methyl-D-aspartate, aurintricarboxylic acid and cycloheximide. Brain Res 703: 63–71, 1995

Garattini S: Pharmacology of amineptine, an antidepressant agent acting on the dopaminergic system: a review. Int Clin Psychopharmacol 12 (suppl 3):S15–S19, 1997

Garattini S, Mennini T: Pharmacology of amineptine: synthesis and updating. Clin Neuropharmacol 12 (suppl):S13–S18, 1989

Garcia-Sainz JA, Gutierrez VG: Activation of protein kinase C alters the interaction of alpha2 adrenoceptors and the inhibitory G protein (Gi) in human platelets. FEBS Lett 257:427–430, 1989

Garcia-Sevilla JA, Guimon J, Garcia-Vallejo P, et al: Biochemical and functional evidence of supersensitive platelet alpha-2-adrenoceptors in major affective disorder: effect of long-term lithium carbonate treatment. Arch Gen Psychiatry 43:51–57, 1986

Gardette R, Krupa M, Crepel F: Differential effects of serotonin on the spontaneous discharge and on the excitatory amino acid-induced responses of deep cerebellar nuclei neurones in rat cerebellar slices. Neuroscience 23:491–500, 1987

Garrod AB: The Nature and Treatment of Gout and Rheumatic Gout. London, Walton and Maberly, 1859

Garvey MJ, Mungas D, Tollefson GD: Hypersomnia in major depressive disorders. J Affect Disord 6:283–286, 1984

Garza-Trevino ES: Verapamil versus lithium in acute mania (NR27), in 1990 New Research Program and Abstracts, American Psychiatric Association 143rd Annual Meeting, New York, NY, May 12–17, 1990. Washington, DC, American Psychiatric Association, 1990

Garza-Trevino ES, Overall JE, Hollister LE: Verapamil versus lithium in acute mania. Am J Psychiatry 149:121–122, 1992

Gauss CJ: Geburten im künstlichen Dämmerschlaf. Archives of Gynecology 78:579–631, 1906

Gauthier S, Bouchard R, Lamontagne A, et al: Tetrahydro-aminoacridine-lecithin combination treatment in patients with intermediate stage Alzheimer's disease: results of a Canadian double-blind, cross-over, multicentre study. N Engl J Med 322:1272–1276, 1990

Ge X, Lorenz FO, Conger RD, et al: Trajectories of stressful life events and depressive symptoms during adolescence. Dev Psychol 30:467–483, 1994

Gee KW: Steroid modulation of the GABA/benzodiazepine receptor-linked chloride ionophore. Mol Neurobiol 2:291–317, 1988

Gee KW, Bolger MB, Brinton RE, et al: Steroid modulation of the chloride ionophore in rat brain: structure-activity requirements, regional dependence and mechanism of action. J Pharmacol Exp Ther 246:803–812, 1988

Gehlert DR: Subtypes of receptors for neuropeptide Y: implications for the targeting of therapeutics. Life Sci 55(8):551–562, 1994

Geisler A, Klysner R, Andersen PH: Influence of lithium in vitro and in vivo on the catecholamine-sensitive cerebral adenylate cyclase systems. Acta Pharmacologica et Toxicologica 56:80–97, 1985

Geizer M, Ancill RJ: Combination of risperidone and donepezil in Lewy body dementia. Can J Psychiatry 43:421–422, 1998

Gelenberg AJ, Wojcik JD, Falk WE, et al: Tyrosine for depression: a double-blind study. J Affect Disord 19:125–132, 1990

Gelernter CS, Uhde TW, Cimbolic P, et al: Cognitive-behavioral and pharmacological treatments of social phobia: a controlled study. Arch Gen Psychiatry 48:938–945, 1991

Gelfand EW, Dosch HM, Hastings B, et al: Lithium: a modulator of cyclic AMP-dependent events in lymphocytes. Science 203:365–367, 1979

Geller I, Seifter J: The effects of meprobamate, d-amphetamine and promazine on experimentally induced conflict in the rat. Psychopharmacologia 1:482–492, 1967

Gengo F, Timko J, D'Antonio J, et al: Prediction of dosage of lithium carbonate: use of a standard predictive method. J Clin Psychiatry 41:319–321, 1980

Geoffroy M, Mogilnicka E, Nielsen M, et al: Effect of nifedipine on the shuttlebox escape deficit induced by inescapable shock in the rat. Eur J Pharmacol 154:277–283, 1988

George DT, Nutt DJ, Dwyer BA, et al: Alcoholism and panic disorders: is the co-morbidity more than coincidence? Acta Psychiatr Scand 81:97–107, 1988

George MS, Guidotti A, Rubinow D, et al: CSF neuroactive steroids in affective disorders: pregnenolone, progesterone, and DBI. Biol Psychiatry 35:775–780, 1994

George MS, Wassermann, EM, Williams WA: Daily repetitive transcranial magnetic stimulation (rTMS) improves mood in depression. Neuroreport 6(14):1853–1856, 1995

Georgotas A, Stokes P, McCue RE, et al: The usefulness of DST in predicting response to antidepressants: a placebo-controlled study. J Affect Disord 11:21–28, 1986

Georgotas A, McCue RE, Cooper TB: A placebo-controlled comparison of nortriptyline and phenelzine in maintenance therapy of elderly depressed patients. Arch Gen Psychiatry 46:783–786, 1989

Gerken A, Maier W, Holsboer F: Weekly monitoring of dexamethasone suppression response in depression: its relationship to change of body weight and psychopathology. Psychoneuroendocrinology 10:261–271, 1985

Geula C, Mesulam MM: Cholinergic systems and related neuropathological predilection patterns in Alzheimer disease, in Alzheimer Disease. Edited by Terry RD, Katzman R, Bick K. New York, Raven, 1994, pp 263–291

Gex-Fabry M, Balant-Georgia A, Balant LP, et al: Clomipramine metabolism: model based analysis of variability factors from drug monitoring data. Clin Pharmacokinet 19:241–255, 1990

Ghadirian AM, Engelsman F, Dhar V, et al: The psychotropic effects of inhibitors of steroid biosynthesis in depressed patients refractory to treatment. Biol Psychiatry 37:369–375, 1995

Giacobini E, Becker R: Current Research in Alzheimer Therapy: Cholinesterase Inhibitors. New York, Taylor & Francis, 1988

Giacobini E, Becker R (eds): Alzheimer Disease: Therapeutic Strategies. Boston, MA, Birkhäuser, 1994

Giannini AJ, Houser WL, Loiselle RH, et al: Antimanic effects of verapamil. Am J Psychiatry 141:1602–1603, 1984

Giannini AJ, Taraszewsky R, Loiselle RH: Verapamil and lithium in maintenance therapy of manic patients. J Clin Pharmacol 27:980–982, 1987

Giannini AJ, Sullivan BS, Folts DJ: Comparison of lithium carbonate, valproic acid and verapamil in the treatment of manic symptoms (abstract). J Clin Pharmacol 29:832, 1989

Giannini AJ, Melemis SM, Martin DM, et al: Symptoms of premenstrual syndrome as a function of beta-endorphin: two subtypes. Prog Neuropsychopharmacol Biol Psychiatry 18:321–327, 1994

Gibbs DM: Vasopressin and oxytocin: hypothalamic modulators of the stress response: a review. Psychoneuroendocrinology 22:131–140, 1986

Gierz M, Campbell SS, Gillin JC: Sleep disturbances in various nonaffective psychiatric disorders. Psychiatr Clin North Am 4:565–581, 1987

Gifford RW: Management of hypertensive crises. JAMA 266:829–835, 1991

Giles DE, Roffwarg HP, Rush AJ: REM latency concordance in depressed family members. Biol Psychiatry 22:910–914, 1987

Giles DE, Biggs MM, Rush AJ, et al: Risk factors in families of unipolar depression, I: psychiatric illness and reduced REM latency. J Affect Disord 14:51–59, 1988

Giles HG, Sellers EM, Naranho A, et al: Dispisition of intravenous diazepam in young men and women. Eur J Clin Pharmacol 20:207–213, 1981

Gillett G, Ammor S, Fillion G: Serotonin inhibits acetylcholine release from rat striatum slices: evidence for a presynaptic-mediated effect. J Neurochem 45:1687–1691, 1985

Gillig P, Sackellares S, Greenberg HS: Right hemisphere partial complex seizures: mania, hallucinations, and speech disturbances during ictal events. Epilepsia 29:26–29, 1988

Gillin JC: Sleep studies in affective illness: diagnostic, therapeutic and pathophysiological implications. Psychiatr Ann 13:367–384, 1983a

Gillin JC: The sleep therapies of depression. Prog Neuropsychopharmacol Biol Psychiatry 7:351–364, 1983b

Gillin JC, Shiromani Y: Cholinergic mechanisms in sleep: basic and clinical applications, in Sleep and Biological Rhythms. Edited by Montplaisir J, Godbout R. New York, Oxford University Press, 1990, pp 186–208

Gillin JC, Lipper S, Sitaram N, et al: The effects of clorgyline and paragyline on the sleep of depressed patients. Sleep Res 7:109–111, 1976

Gillin JC, Wyatt RJ, Fram D, et al: The relationship between changes in REM sleep and clinical improvement in depressed patients treated with amitriptyline. Psychopharmacology 59:267–272, 1978

Gillin JC, Duncan WB, Murphy DL, et al: Age-related changes in sleep in depressed and normal subjects. Psychiatry Res 4:73–78, 1981

Gillin JC, Sitaram N, Wehr T, et al: Sleep and affective illness, in Neurobiology of Mood Disorders. Edited by Post RM, Ballenger JC. Baltimore, MD, Williams & Wilkins, 1984, pp 157–189

Gillin JC, Sutton L, Ruiz C: The cholinergic rapid eye movement induction test with arecoline in depression. Arch Gen Psychiatry 48:264–270, 1991

Gintzler JH, Bohan M: Pain thresholds are elevated during pseudopregnancy. Brain Res 507:312–316, 1990

Giros B, Caron MG: Molecular characterisation of the dopamine transporter. Trends Pharmacol Sci 14:43–49, 1993

Giros B, Wang Y-M, Suter S, et al: Delineation of discrete domains for substrate, cocaine, and tricyclic antidepressant interactions using chimeric dopamine-norepinephrine transporters. J Biol Chem 269:15985–15988, 1994

Giros B, Jaber M, Jones SR, et al: Hyperlocomotion and indifference to cocaine and amphetamine in mice lacking the dopamine transporter. Nature 379:606–612, 1996

Gitelman DR, Prohovnik I: Muscarinic and nicotinic contributions to cognitive function and cortical blood flow. Neurobiol Aging 13:313–318, 1992

Gitlin MJ, Weiss J: Verapamil as maintenance treatment in bipolar illness: a case report. J Clin Psychopharmacol 4:341–343, 1984

Gittelman-Klein R, Klein DF: Controlled imipramine treatment in school phobia. Arch Gen Psychiatry 25:204–207, 1971

Gjessing R, Jenner F (eds): Somatology of Periodic Catatonia. Oxford, England, Pergamon, 1976

Glassman AH, Roose SP: Delusional depression: a distinct clinical entity? Arch Gen Psychiatry 38:424–427, 1981

Glassman AH, Kantor SJ, Shostak M: Depression, delusions, and drug response. Am J Psychiatry 132:716–719, 1975

Glassman AH, Perel JM, Shostak M, et al: Clinical implications of imipramine plasma levels for depressive illness. Arch Gen Psychiatry 34:197–204, 1977

Gleason RP, Schneider LS: Carbamazepine treatment of agitation in Alzheimer's outpatients refractory to neuroleptics. J Clin Psychiatry 51:115–118, 1990

Glen AIM, Johnson AL, Shepherd M: Continuation therapy with lithium and amitriptyline in unipolar depressive illness: a randomized double-blind controlled trial. Psychol Med 14:37–50, 1984

Glue P, Nutt D: Clonidine challenge testing of alpha-2-adrenoceptor function in man: the effects of mental illness and psychotropic medication. J Psychopharmacol (Oxf) 2:119–137, 1988

Glue PW, Cowen PJ, Nutt DJ, et al: The effect of lithium on 5-HT mediated neuroendocrine response and platelet 5-HT receptors. Psychopharmacology 90:398–402, 1986

Glue P, Wilson S, Lawson C, et al: Acute and chronic idazoxan in normal volunteers: biochemical, physiological and psychological effects. J Psychopharmacol (Oxf) 5:394–401, 1991

Goa KL, Ward A: Buspirone: a preliminary review of its pharmacological properties and therapeutic efficacy as an anxiolytic. Drugs 32:114–129, 1986

Godfrey PP: Potentiation by lithium of CMP-phosphatidate formation in carbachol-stimulated rat cerebral-cortical slices and its reversal by myo-inositol. Biochem J 258:621–624, 1989

Godfrey PP, McClue SJ, White AM, et al: Subacute and chronic in vivo lithium treatment inhibits agonist- and sodium fluoride-stimulated inositol phosphate production in rat cortex. J Neurochem 52:498–506, 1989

Goetz RR, Klein DF, Gully R, et al: Panic attacks during placebo procedures in the laboratory: physiology and symptomatology. Arch Gen Psychiatry 50:280–285, 1993

Gold BI, Bowers MB, Roth RH, et al: GABA levels in CSF of patients with psychiatric disorders. Am J Psychiatry 137:362–364, 1980

Gold LH, Balster RL: Evaluation of nefazadone self-administration in rhesus monkeys. Drug Alcohol Depend 28:241–247, 1991

Gold MS, Pottash ALC, Extein I: Hypothyroidism in depression: evidence from complete thyroid function evaluation. JAMA 245:1919–1922, 1981

Gold MS, Pottash AC, Sweeney D, et al: Antimanic, antidepressant, and antipanic effects of opiates: clinical, neuroanatomical, and biochemical evidence. Ann N Y Acad Sci 398:140–150, 1982a

Gold MS, Pottash AC, Extein I: Symptomless autoimmune thyroiditis in depression. Psychiatry Res 6:261–269, 1982b

Gold MS, Miller NS, Hoffman NG: Depression in drug dependency. Paper presented at the annual meeting of the American Psychiatric Association, Philadelphia, PA, May 25, 1994

Gold PW, Loriaux DL, Roy A, et al: Responses to corticotropin releasing hormone in the hypercortisolism of depression and Cushing's disease: pathophysiologic and diagnosis implications. N Engl J Med 314:1329–1335, 1986

Gold PW, Goodwin FK, Chrousos GP: Clinical and biochemical manifestations of depression: relation to the neurobiology of stress. Part I. N Engl J Med 319:348–353, 1988a

Gold PW, Goodwin FK, Chrousos GP: Clinical and biochemical manifestations of depression: relation to the neurobiology of stress. Part II. N Engl J Med 319:413–420, 1988b

Goldberg H, Clayman P, Skorecki K: Mechanism of Li inhibition on vasopressin-sensitive adenylate cyclase in cultured renal epithelial cells. Am J Physiol 24:F995–F1002, 1988

Golden RN, Morris JE, Sack DA: Combined lithium-tricyclic treatment of obsessive-compulsive disorder. Biol Psychiatry 23:181–185, 1988

Goldenberg G, Lang W, Podreka I, et al: Are cognitive deficits in Parkinson's disease caused by frontal lobe dysfunction? Journal of Psychophysiology 4:137–144, 1990

Goldgaber D, Harris HW, Hla T: Interleukin-1 regulates synthesis of amyloid beta-protein precursor mRNA in human endothelial cells. Proc Natl Acad Sci U S A 86:7606–7610, 1989

Goldman-Rakic PS: Cortical localization of working memory, in Brain Organization and Memory: Cells, Systems, and Circuits. Edited by Gaugh JL, Weinberger NM, Lynch G. New York, Oxford University Press, 1990

Goldstein S: Treatment of social phobia with clonidine. Biol Psychiatry 22:369–372, 1987

Goltermann NR, Rehfeld JF, Røigaard-Petersen H: In vivo biosynthesis of cholecystokinin in rat cerebral cortex. J Biol Chem 255:6181–6185, 1980

Goncalves N, Stoll KD: Carbamazepine in manic syndromes: a controlled double-blind study. Nervenarzt 56:43–47, 1985

Gonella G, Baignoli G, Ecari U: Fluvoxamine and imipramine in the treatment of depressive patients: a double-blind placebo-controlled study. Curr Med Res Opin 12:177–184, 1990

Goodlet I, Mireylees SE, Sugrue MF: Effects of mianserin, a new antidepressant, on the in vitro and in vivo uptake of monoamines. Br J Pharmacol 61:307–313, 1977

Goodman LS, Gilman A (eds): Goodman and Gilman's The Pharmacological Basis of Therapeutics, 7th Edition. New York, Macmillan, 1985

Goodman WK, Price LH, Rasmussen SA, et al: Efficacy of fluroxamine in obsessive-compulsive disorder: a double-blind comparison with placebo. Arch Gen Psychiatry 46:36–44, 1989a

Goodman WK, Price LH, Rasmussen SA, et al: The Yale-Brown Obsessive Compulsive Scale (Y-BOCS), part I: development, use, and reliability. Arch Gen Psychiatry 46:1006–1011, 1989b

Goodman WK, Price LH, Rasmussen SA, et al: The Yale-Brown Obsessive Compulsive Scale (Y-BOCS), part II: validity. Arch Gen Psychiatry 46:1012–1016, 1989c

Goodman WK, McDougle CJ, Price LH, et al: Beyond the serotonin hypothesis: a role for dopamine in some forms of obsessive compulsive disorder? J Clin Psychiatry 51 (suppl):36–43, 1990a

Goodman WK, Price LH, Delgado PL, et al: Specificity of serotonin reuptake inhibitors in the treatment of obsessive compulsive disorder: comparison of fluvoxamine and desipramine. Arch Gen Psychiatry 47:577–585, 1990b

Goodman WK, Rasmussen SA, Foa EB, et al: Obsessive compulsive disorder, in Clinical Evaluation of Psychotropic Drugs: Principles and Guidance. Edited by Prien RF, Robinson DS. New York, Raven, 1994, pp 431–466

Goodnick P: Effects of lithium on indices of 5HT and catecholamines in the clinical content: a review. Lithium 1:65–73, 1990

Goodnick PF, Fieve RR, Schlegel A, et al: Predictors of interepisode symptoms and relapse in affective disorder patients treated with lithium carbonate. Am J Psychiatry 144:367–369, 1987

Goodnick PJ: Nimodipine treatment of rapid cycling bipolar disorder (letter). J Clin Psychiatry 56:330, 1995

Goodnick PJ, Gershon ES: Lithium, in Handbook of Neurochemistry. Edited by Lajtha A. New York, Plenum, 1985, pp 103–149

Goodnick PJ, Meltzer HY: Neurochemical changes during discontinuation of lithium prophylaxis, I: increases in clonidine-induced hypotension. Biol Psychiatry 19:883–889, 1984

Goodwin FK: The biology of recurrence: new directions for the pharmacologic bridge. J Clin Psychiatry 50 (suppl):40–44, 1989

Goodwin FK: Clinical Psychiatric News 11, 1994

Goodwin FK, Jamison KR: Course and outcome, in Manic-Depressive Illness. New York, Oxford University Press, 1990a, pp 127–156

Goodwin FK, Jamison KR: Manic-Depressive Illness. New York, Oxford University Press, 1990b

Goodwin FK, Roy-Byrne P: Treatment of bipolar disorders, in Psychiatry Update: The American Psychiatric Association Annual Review, Vol 6. Edited by Hales RE, Francis AJ. Washington, DC, American Psychiatric Press, 1987, p 89

Goodwin FK, Murphy DL, Bunney WE: Lithium-carbonate treatment in depression and mania: a longitudinal double-blind study. Arch Gen Psychiatry 21:486–496, 1969

Goodwin FK, Murphy DL, Dunner DL, et al: Lithium response in unipolar versus bipolar depression. Am J Psychiatry 129:76–79, 1972

Goodwin GM, DeSouza RJ, Wood AJ, et al: The enhancement by lithium of the 5-HT1A mediated serotonin syndrome produced by 8-OH-DPAT in the rat: evidence for a post-synaptic mechanism. Psychopharmacology 90:488–493, 1986a

Goodwin GM, DeSouza RJ, Wood AJ, et al: Lithium decreases 5-HT1A and 5-HT2 receptor and alpha-2 adrenoceptor mediated function in mice. Psychopharmacology 90:482–487, 1986b

Goodwin GM, Austin M-P, Ross M, et al: State changes in brain activity shown by the uptake of ^{99m}Tc exametazime with single photon emission tomography in major depression before and after treatment. J Affect Disord 29:243–253, 1993

Goodyear IM, Wright C, Altham P: Maternal adversity and recent stressful life events in anxious and depressed children. J Child Psychol Psychiatry 29:651–667, 1988

Gordon CT, Rapoport JL, Hamburger SD, et al: Differential response of seven subjects with autistic disorder to clomipramine and desipramine. Am J Psychiatry 149:363–366, 1992

Gorman JM, Hatterer JA: The role of thyroid hormone in refractory depression, in Refractory Depression: Current Strategies and Future Directions. Edited by Nolen WA, Zohar J, Roose SP, et al. Chichester, England, Wiley, 1994, pp 121–128

Gorman JM, Kent JM: SSRIs and SNRIs: broad spectrum of efficacy beyond major depression. J Clin Psychiatry 60 (suppl 4):33–38, 1999

Gorman JM, Papp LA: Respiratory physiology and panic, in Neurobiology of Panic Disorder. Edited by Ballenger JC. New York, Alan R Liss, 1990

Gorman JM, Liebowitz MR, Fyer AJ, et al: Treatment of social phobia with atenolol. J Clin Psychopharmacol 5:298–301, 1985

Gorman JM, Fyer MR, Liebowitz MR: Pharmacologic provocation of panic attacks, in Psychopharmacology: A Third Generation of Progress. Edited by Meltzer HY. New York, Raven, 1987, pp 980–983

Gorman JM, Liebowitz MR, Fyer AJ, et al: An open trial of fluoxetine in the treatment of panic attacks [published erratum appears in J Clin Psychopharmacol 8:13, 1988]. J Clin Psychopharmacol 7:329–332, 1988

Gorman JM, Liebowitz MR, Fyer AJ, et al: Neuro-anatomical hypothesis for panic disorder. Am J Psychiatry 146:148–161, 1989

Göthert M: Presynaptic effects of 5-HT, in Aspects of Synaptic Transmission: LTP, Galanin, Opioids, Autonomic and 5-HT. Edited by Stone TW. New York, Taylor & Francis, 1991, pp 314–329

Gottesfeld Z, Ebstein BS, Samuel D: Effect of lithium on concentrations of glutamate and GABA levels in amygdala and hypothalamus of rat. Nature 234:124–125, 1971

Gottfries CG: Review of treatment strategies. Acta Neurol Scand Suppl 139:63–68, 1992

Gottfries CG, Nyth AL: Effect of citalopram—a selective 5-HT reuptake blocker in emotionally disturbed patients with dementia. Ann N Y Acad Sci 640:276–279, 1991

Gottfries CG, Roos BE: Monoamine metabolites in cerebrospinal fluid (CSF) in patients with organic presenile and senile dementia. Aktuelle Gerontologie 6:37–42, 1976

Gottfries CG, Kjallquist K, Ponten U, et al: Cerebrospinal fluid pH and monoamine and glucolytic metabolites in Alzheimer's disease. Br J Psychiatry 124:280–287, 1974

Gourch A, Orosco M, Rodriguez M, et al: Effects of a new cholecystokinin analogue (JMV 236) on food intake and brain monoamines in the rat. Neuropeptides 15(1):37–41, 1990

Gowers WR: Epilepsy and Other Convulsive Diseases (1881). New York, Dover Publications, 1964, pp 77–86

Grady TA, Pigott TA, L'Heureux F, et al: Seizure associated with fluoxetine and adjuvant buspirone therapy (letter). J Clin Psychopharmacol 12:70–71, 1992

Grady TA, Pigott TA, L'Heureux FL, et al: Double-blind study of adjuvant buspirone for fluoxetine-treated patients with obsessive-compulsive disorder. Am J Psychiatry 150:819–821, 1993

Grahame-Smith DG, Green AR: The role of brain 5-hydroxytryptamine in the hyperactivity produced in rats by lithium and monoamine oxidase inhibition. Br J Pharmacol 52:19–26, 1974

Grahame-Smith DG, Green AR, Costain DW: Mechanism of the antidepressant action of electroconvulsive therapy. Lancet 1:254–256, 1978

Gram LF, Christiansen J: First-pass metabolism of imipramine in man. Clin Pharmacol Ther 17:555–563, 1975

Granon S, Poucet B, Thinus-Blanc C, et al: Nicotine and muscarinic receptors in the rat prefrontal cortex: differential roles in working memory, response selection and effortful processing. Psychopharmacology 119:139–144, 1995

Gravem A, Amthor KF, Astrup C, et al: A double-blind comparison of citalopram (Lu 10–171) and amitriptyline in depression. Acta Psychiatr Scand 75:478–486, 1987

Gray JA: The Neuropsychology of Anxiety: An Enquiry Into the Functions of the Septo-Hippocampal System. Oxford, England, Oxford University Press, 1982

Greden JF: Antidepressant maintenance medications: when to discontinue and how to stop. J Clin Psychiatry 54 (suppl 8):39–45, 1993

Greden JF, Gardner R, King D, et al: Dexamethasone suppression test in antidepressant treatment of melancholia. Arch Gen Psychiatry 40:493–505, 1983

Green AI, Austin CP: Psychopathology of pancreatic cancer: a psychobiologic probe. Psychosomatics 34:208–221, 1993

Green AR: Alterations in monoamine mediated behaviours and biochemical changes after repeated ECS: studies in their possible association, in ECT Basic Mechanisms. Edited by Lerer B, Weiner RD, Belmaker RH. London, John Libbey, 1984, pp 5–17

Green AR, Butt D, Cowen P: Increased seizure threshold following convulsion, in Psychopharmacology of Convulsants. Edited by Sandler M. Oxford, England, Oxford University Press, 1982, pp 16–26

Greenberg PE, Stiglin LE, Finkelstein SN, et al: The economic burden of depression in 1990. J Clin Psychiatry 54 (suppl 11):405–418, 1993a

Greenberg PE, Stiglin LE, Finkelstein SN, et al: Depression: a neglected major illness. J Clin Psychiatry 54:419–424, 1993b

Greenblatt DJ, Shader RI, Franke K, et al: Kinetics of intravenous chlordiazepoxide: sex differences in drug distribution. Clin Pharmacol Ther 22:893–903, 1977

Greenblatt DJ, Divoll M, Harmatz JS, et al: Oxazepam kinetics: effects of age and sex. J Pharmacol Exp Ther 215:86–91, 1980

Greenblatt DJ, Friedman H, Burstein ES, et al: Trazodone kinetics: effects of age, gender, and obesity. Clin Pharmacol Ther 42:193–200, 1987

Greenblatt M, Grosser GH, Wechsler H: Differential response to hospitalized depressed patients to somatic therapy. Am J Psychiatry 120:935–943, 1964

Greenhouse JB, Kupfer DJ, Frank E, et al: Analysis of time to stabilization in the treatment of depression: biological and clinical correlates. J Affect Disord 13:259–266, 1987

Greenhouse JB, Stangl D, Kupfer DJ, et al: Methodologic issues in maintenance therapy clinical trials. Arch Gen Psychiatry 48:313–318, 1991

Greenspan K, Schildkraut JJ, Gordon EK, et al: Catecholamine metabolism in affective disorders, 3: MHPG and other catecholamine metabolites in patients treated with lithium carbonate. J Psychiatr Res 7:171–183, 1970

Greil WW, Ludwig-Mayerhofer, et al: Lithium vs carbamazepine in the maintenance treatment of schizoaffective disorder: a randomised study. European Archives of Psychiatry and Clinical Neuroscience 247(1):42–50, 1997a

Greil WW, Ludwig-Mayerhofer, et al: Lithium versus carbamazepine in the maintenance treatment of bipolar disorders: a randomised study. J Affect Disord 43(2):151–161, 1997b

Greist JH: Fluvoxamine treatment of OCD, in Biological Psychiatry: Proceedings of the 5th World Congress of Biological Psychiatry, Florence, 9–14 June 1991. Edited by Racagni G, Brunello N, Fukuda T. New York, Excerpta Medica, 1991

Greist JH: An integrated approach to treatment of obsessive compulsive disorder. J Clin Psychiatry 53 (suppl):38–41, 1992

Greist JH, Chouinard G, DuBoff E, et al: Double-blind comparison of three doses of sertraline and placebo in the treatment of outpatients with OCD. 9th World Congress of Psychiatry, Rio de Janeiro, Brazil, June 1993a

Greist JH, Chouinard G, DuBoff E, et al: Long-term sertraline treatment of OCD. 9th World Congress of Psychiatry, Rio de Janeiro, Brazil, June 1993b

Greist JH, Chouinard G, DuBoff E, et al: Double-blind parallel comparison of three dosages of sertraline and placebo in outpatients with obsessive-compulsive disorder. Arch Gen Psychiatry 52:289–295, 1995a

Greist JH, Jefferson JW, Kobak KA, et al: Efficacy and tolerability of serotonin transport inhibitors in obsessive-compulsive disorder: a meta-analysis. Arch Gen Psychiatry 52:53–60, 1995b

Greist JH, Jenike MA, Robinson DS, et al: Efficacy of fluvoxamine in obsessive-compulsive disorder: results of a multicentre, double-blind, placebo-controlled trial. European Journal of Clinical Research 7:195–204, 1995c

Griffin WST, Stanley LC, Ling C, et al: Brain interleukin 1 and S-100 immunoreactivity are elevated in Down syndrome and Alzheimer disease. Proc Natl Acad Sci U S A 86:7611–7615, 1989

Grisaru N, Yaroslavsky U, Abarbanel J, et al: Transcranial magnetic stimulation in depression and schizophrenia. Eur Neuropsychopharmacol 4:287–288, 1994

Grober E, Buschke H, Crystal H, et al: Screening for dementia by memory testing. Neurology 38:900–903, 1988

Grobin AC, Roth RH, Deutch AY: Regulation of the prefrontal cortical dopamine system by the neuroactive steroid 3a-21-dihydroxy-5a-pregnane-20-one. Brain Res 578:351–356, 1992

Grof E, Brown GM, Grof P, et al: Effects of lithium administration on plasma catecholamines. Psychiatry Res 19:87–92, 1986

Grof P, Angst J, Haines T: The clinical course of depression: practical issues, in Classification and Prediction of Outcome of Depression. Edited by Angst J. New York, F. K. Schattauer Verlag, 1973, pp 141–155

Grof P, Alda M, Grof E, et al: The challenge of predicting response to stabilizing lithium treatment. Br J Psychiatry 163 (suppl):16–19, 1993

Gross G, Hanft G, Mehdorn HM: Demonstration of α_{1A} and α_{1B}-adrenoceptor binding sites in human brain tissue. Eur J Pharmacol 169:325–328, 1989

Grossi E, Sacchetti E, Vita A, et al: Carbamazepine vs. chlorpromazine in mania: a double-blind trial, in Anticonvulsants in Affective Disorders. Edited by Emrich HM, Okuma T, Muller AA. Amsterdam, Excerpta Medica, 1984, pp 177–187

Grossman E, Rea RF, Hoffman A, et al: Yohimbine increases sympathetic nerve activity and norepinephrine spillover in normal volunteers. Am J Physiol 2601 (1 pt 2):R142–R147, 1991

Grunhaus L: Clinical and psychobiological characteristics of simultaneous panic disorder and major depression. Am J Psychiatry 145:1214–1221, 1988

Grunze H, Walden J, Wolf R, et al: Combined treatment with lithium and nimodipine in a bipolar I manic syndrome. Prog Neuropsychopharmacol Biol Psychiatry 20:419–426, 1996

Guarneri P, Papadoupoulas V, Pan B, et al: Regulation of pregnenolone synthesis in C6-2B glioma cells by 4' -chlorodiazepam. Proc Natl Acad Sci U S A 89):5118–5122, 1992

Guelfi JD, Pichot P, Dreyfus JF: Efficacy of tianeptine in anxious depressed patients: results of a multi-center trial versus amitriptyline. Neuropsychobiology 22:41–48, 1989

Guelfi JD, White AG, Hackett D, et al: Effectiveness of venlafaxine in hospitalized patients with major depression and melancholia. J Clin Psychiatry 56:450–458, 1995

Guerciolini R, Szumlanski C, Weinshilboum RM: Human liver xanthine oxidase: nature and extent of individual variation. Clin Pharmacol Ther 50:663–672, 1991

Guisti P, Ducic I, Puia G, et al: Imidazenil: a new partial positive allosteric modulator of gamma-amniobutyric acid (GABA) action of GABAa receptors. J Pharmacol Exp Ther 266:1018–1028, 1993

Gulley LR, Nemeroff CB: The neurobiological basis of mixed depression-anxiety states. J Clin Psychiatry 54 (suppl):16–19, 1993

Gur RC, Gur RE, Obrist WD, et al: Sex and handedness differences in cerebral blood flow during rest and cognitive activity. Science 217:659–661, 1982

Guttmacher LB, Murphy DL, Insel TR: Pharmacologic models of anxiety. Compr Psychiatry 24:312–326, 1993

Guy W: Clinical Global Impressions, in ECDEU Assessment Manual for Psychopharmacology. Publication ADM 76-338. Washington, DC, U.S. Department of Health, Education and Welfare, 1976, pp 217–222

Gwirtsman HE, Szuba MP, Toren L, et al: The antidepressant response to tricyclics in major depressives is accelerated with adjunctive use of methylphenidate. Psychopharmacol Bull 30:157–164, 1994

Gyermek L, Soyka LF: Steroid anesthetics. Anesthesiology 42:331–344, 1975

Haas S, Vincent K, Holt J, et al: Divalproex: a possible treatment alternative for demented, elderly aggressive patients. Ann Clin Psychiatry 9:145–147, 1997

Hablitz JJ, Langmoen IA: Excitation of hippocampal pyramidal cells by glutamate in the guinea pig and rat. J Physiol 325:317–331, 1982

Haddjeri N, Blier P, De Montigny C: Noradrenergic modulation of central serotonergic neurotransmission: acute and long-term actions of mirtazapine. Int Clin Psychopharmacol 10 (suppl 4):11–18, 1995

Hafizi S, Palij P, Stamford JA: Activity of two primary human metabolites of nomifensin on stimulated efflux and uptake of dopamine in the striatum: in vivo voltammetric data in slices of rat brain. Neuropharmacology 31:817–824, 1992

Haggerty JG, Stern RA, Mason G, et al: Subclinical hypothyroidism: a modifiable risk factor for depression? Am J Psychiatry 150:508–510, 1993

Halbreich U: Treatment of premenstrual syndromes with progesterone antagonists (e.g., RU-486): political and methodological issues. Psychiatry 53:407–409, 1990

Halbreich U: Menstrually related disorders: what we do know, what we do not know, what we only believe that we know and what we know we do not know. Crit Rev Neurobiol 9:163–175, 1995

Halbreich U: Premenstrual syndromes, in Psychiatric Issues in Women (Bailliere's International Clinical Psychiatry), Vol 2. Edited by Halbreich U. London, Tindall, 1996, pp 667–686

Halbreich U: Role of estrogen in postmenopausal depression. Neurology 48 (5 suppl 7):S16–S19, 1997

Halbreich U, Wamback SJ: Clinical psychotropic effects of gonadal hormones in women, in Psychoneuroendocrinology for the Clinician. Edited by Wolkowitz O, Rothschild A. Washington, DC, American Psychiatric Press (in press)

Halbreich U, Asnis G, Ross D, et al: Amphetamine-induced dysphoria in postmenopausal women. Br J Psychiatry 138:470–473, 1981

Halbreich U, Asnis GM, Shindledecker R, et al: Cortisol secretion in endogenous depression, I: basal plasma levels. Arch Gen Psychiatry 42:904–908, 1985a

Halbreich U, Asnis GM, Shindledecker R, et al: Cortisol secretion in endogenous depression, II: time-related functions. Arch Gen Psychiatry 42:909–914, 1985b

Halbreich U, Yonkers K, Kahn L: Gender differences in dysthymia, in Mood Disorders in Women. Edited by Steiner M, Yonkers K, Eriksson E. London, Dunitz Publication (in press)

Halenda SP, Volpi M, Zavoico GB, et al: Effects of thrombin, phorbol myristate acetate, and prostaglandin D2 on 40–41 kDa protein that is ADP ribosylated by pertussis toxin in platelets. FEBS Lett 204:341–346, 1986

Hall RC, Gardner ER, Popkin MK, et al: Unrecognized physical illness prompting psychiatric admission: a prospective study. Am J Psychiatry 138:629–635, 1981

Hallcher LM, Sherman WR: The effects of lithium ion and other agents on the activity of myo-inositol-1-phosphatase from bovine brain. J Biol Chem 255: 10896–10901, 1980

Halle MT, Dilsaver SC: Comorbid panic disorder in patients with winter depression. Am J Psychiatry 150:1108–1110, 1993

Hallett M, Cohen LG: Magnetism: a new method for stimulation of nerve and brain. JAMA 262:538–541, 1989

Halliday GM, McCann HL, Pamphlett R, et al: Brain stem synthesising neurones in Alzheimer's disease: a clinicopathological correlation. Acta Neuropathol 84:638–650, 1992

Halliday R, Gregory K, Naylor H, et al: Beyond drug effects and dependent variables: the use of the Poisson-Erlang model to assess the effects of d-amphetamine on information processing. Acta Psychologica 73:35–54, 1990

Hallman M, Bry K, Hoppu K, et al: Inositol supplementation in premature infants with respiratory distress syndrome. N Engl J Med 326:1233–1239, 1992

Hamik A, Peroutka S: MCPP interaction with neurotransmitter receptors in human brain. Biol Psychiatry 25:569–575, 1989

Hamilton JA, Grant M: Sex differences in metabolism and pharmacokinetics: Effects on agent choice and dosing. NIMH Conference, Bethesda, MD, November 4, 1993

Hamilton J, Parry B: Sex-related differences in clinical drug response: implications for women's health. J Am Med Womens Assoc 38(5):126–131, 1983

Hamilton JA, Yonkers KA: Sex differences in pharmacokinetics of psychotropic medications, part 1: physiological basis for effects, in Psychopharmacology of Women: Sex, Gender and Hormonal Considerations, Vol 1. Edited by Jensvold MJ, Halbreich U, Hamilton JA. Washington, DC, American Psychiatric Press, 1996

Hamilton JA, Lloyd C, Alagna SW, et al: Gender, depressive subtypes, and gender-age effects on antidepressant response: hormonal hypotheses. Psychopharmacol Bull 20:475–480, 1984

Hamilton M: The assessment of anxiety states by rating. Br J Med Psychol 32:50–55, 1959

Hamilton M: A rating scale for depression. J Neurol Neurosurg Psychiatry 12:56–62, 1960

Hamilton M: Drug resistant depressions: response to ECT. Pharmacopsychiatry 7:205–206, 1974

Hamilton M, White J: Factors related to the outcome of depression treated with ECT. Journal of Mental Science 106:1031–1041, 1960

Hammarback S, Backstrom T: Induced anovulation as treatment of premenstrual tension syndrome: a double-blind crossover study with GnRH-agonist versus placebo. Acta Obstet Gynecol Scand 67:159–166, 1988

Hamon M: Neuropharmacology of anxiety-perspectives and prospects. Trends Pharmacol Sci 15(2):36–39, 1994

Hamon M, Bourgoin S, Gozlan H: Effet de la tianeptine sur la liberation in vitro de 3H-5-HT et sur les divers types de recepteurs serotonergiques dans le systeme nerveux central chez le rat. J Psychiatr Biol Ther March:32–35, 1988

Handley SL, McBlane JW: 5HT drugs in animal models of anxiety. Psychopharmacology 112:13–20, 1993

Hansen S, Ferreira A, Selart ME: Behavioral similarities between mother rats and benzodiazepine-treated non-maternal animals. Psychopharmacol 86:344–347, 1985

Hantz P, Caradoc-Davies G, Caradoc-Davies T: Depression in Parkinson's disease. Am J Psychiatry 151:1010–1014, 1994

Haresh H, Aizenberg D, Munitz H: Trazodone in clomipramine-resistant obsessive-compulsive disorder. Clin Neuropharmacol 13:322–328, 1990

Harrington MA, Zhong P, Garlow SJ, et al: Molecular biology of serotonin receptors. J Clin Psychiatry 53 (suppl 10):8–27, 1992

Harris B, Szulecka TK, Anstee JA: Fluvoxamine versus amitriptyline in depressed hospital outpatients: a multicentre double-blind comparison trial. British Journal of Clinical Research 2:81–88, 1991

Harrison NL, Majewska MD, Harrington JW, et al: Structure-activity relationships for steroid interaction with the g-aminobutyric acid A receptor complex. J Pharmacol Exp Ther 241:346–353, 1987

Harrison-Read PE: Evidence from behavioural reactions to fenfluramine, 5-hydroxyptryptophan, and 5-methoxy-N,N-dimethyltryptamine for differential effects of short-term and long-term lithium on indoleaminergic mechanisms in rats. Br J Pharmacol 66:144–145, 1979

Harro J, Vasar E: Cholecystokinin-induced anxiety: how is it reflected in studies on exploratory behaviour? Neurosci Biobehav Rev 15:473–477, 1991a

Harro J, Vasar E: Evidence that CCK-B receptors mediate the regulation of exploratory behaviour in the rat. Eur J Pharmacol 193:379–381, 1991b

Harro J, Pold M, Vasar E: Anxiogenic-like action of caerulein, a CCK-8 receptor agonist, in the mouse: influence of acute and subchronic diazepam treatment. Naunyn Schmiedebergs Arch Pharmacol 341:62–67, 1990a

Harro J, Lang A, Vasar E: Long-term diazepam treatment produces changes in cholecystokinin receptor binding in rat brain. Eur J Pharmacol 10:77–83, 1990b

Harro J, Kiivet RA, Lang A, et al: Rats with anxious or non-anxious type of exploratory behaviour differ in their brain CCK-8 and benzodiazepine receptor characteristics. Behav Brain Res 39:63–71, 1990c

Harro J, Oopik T, Vasar E: CCK receptor agonists and antagonists in the rodent models of anxiety and drug abuse. Eur Neuropsychopharmacol 2(3):192–193, 1992a

Harro J, Jossan SS, Oreland L, et al: Changes in cholecystokinin receptor binding in rat brain after selective dopaminemage of locus coeruleus projections by DSP-4 treatment. Naunyn Schmiedebergs Arch Pharmacol 346:425–431, 1992b

Harro J, Löfberg C, Rehfeld J, et al: Brain cholecystokinin levels and receptor binding in anxiety states. Eur Neuropsychopharmacol 4:352, 1994

Harro J, Vasar E, Oreland L, et al: Animal studies on CCK and anxiety, in Cholecystokinin and Anxiety: From Neuron to Behavior. Edited by Bradwejn J, Vasar E. Austin, TX, RG Landes, 1995, pp 57–72

Hartmann E, Cravens J: The effects of long term administration of psychotropic drugs on human sleep, III: the effects of amitriptyline. Psychopharmacologia 33:185–202, 1973

Harto N, Branconnier RJ: Clinical profile of gepirone, a nonbenzodiazepine anxiolytic. Psychopharmacol Bull 24:154–160, 1988

Hassan AHS, von Rosenstiel P, Patchev VK, et al: Exacerbation of apoptosis in the dentate gyrus of the aged rat by dexamethasone and the protective role of corticosterone. Exp Neurol 140(1):43–52, 1996

Hassler R: Striatal control of locomotion, intentional actions and of integrating and perceptive activity. J Neurol Sci 36:187–224, 1978

Hathaway SR, McKinley JC: The Minnesota Multiphasic Personality Inventory Manual. New York, Psychological Corporation, 1983

Hayes SG: Long-term use of valproate in primary psychiatric disorders. J Clin Psychiatry (suppl 3):35S–39S, 1989

Hayward C: Psychiatric illness and cardiovascular disease risk. Epidemiol Rev 17:129–138, 1995

Healy D, O'Halloran A, Carney PA, et al: Platelet 5-HT uptake in delusional and nondelusional depressions. J Affect Disord 10:233–239, 1986

Hedgepeth CM, Conrad LJ, Zhang J, et al: Activation of the Wnt signaling pathway: a molecular mechanism for lithium action. Dev Biol 185:82–91, 1997

Hefti F: Growth factors and neurodegeneration, in Neurodegenerative Diseases. Edited by Calne D. Philadelphia, PA, WB Saunders, 1994, pp 177–194

Hefti F, Hartikka J, Knusel B: Function of neurotrophic factors in the adult and aging brain and their possible use in the treatment of neurodegenerative diseases. Neurobiol Aging 10:515–533, 1989

Hefti F, Vernero JL, Widmer HR, et al: Nerve growth factor therapy for Alzheimer's disease: comparison with brain-derived neurotrophic factor, in Research Advances in Alzheimer's Disease and Related Disorders. Edited by Iqbal K, Mortimer JA, Winblad B, et al. Chichester, England, Wiley, 1995, pp 321–328

Hefti I: Nerve growth factor (NGF) promotes survival of septal cholinergic neurons after fimbrial transection. J Neurosci 6:2155–2162, 1986

Heilig M, McLeod S, Brot M, et al: Anxiolytic-like action of neuropeptide Y: mediation by Y1 receptors in amygdala, and dissociation from food intake effects. Neuropsychopharmacology 8(4):357–363, 1993

Heimann H: Therapy resistant depressions: symptoms and syndromes. Pharmakopsychiatrie Neuro-Psychopharmakologie 7:156–163, 1974

Heinrichs SC, Pich EM, Miczek KA, et al: Corticotropin-releasing factor antagonist reduces emotionality in socially defeated rats via direct neurotropic action. Brain Res 581:190–197, 1992

Heinrichs SC, Menzaghi F, Pich EM, et al: Anti-stress action of a corticotropin-releasing factor antagonist on behavioral reactivity to stressors of varying type and intensity. Neuropsychopharmacology 11(3):179–186, 1994

Heishman SJ, Taylor RC, Henningfield JE: Nicotine and smoking: a review of effects on human performance. Exp Clin Psychopharmacol 2:345–395, 1994

Henderson VW, Roberts E, Wimer C, et al: Multicenter trial of naloxone in Alzheimer's disease. Ann Neurol 25:404–406, 1989

Hendrie CA, Dourish CT: Effects of cholecystokinin tetrapeptide and the CCK-B antagonist LY 288513 in a putative model of panic in the mouse, in Ethology and Psychopharmacology. Edited by Cooper SJ, Hendrie CA. Chichester, England, Wiley, 1994, pp 110–132

Heninger GR, Charney DS, Sternberg DE: Lithium carbonate augmentation of antidepressant treatment: an effective prescription for treatment-refractory depression. Arch Gen Psychiatry 40:1335–1342, 1983

Henry JA: Overdose and safety with fluvoxamine. Int Clin Psychopharmacol 6 (suppl 3):41–47, 1991

Henry JA: The safety of antidepressants. Br J Psychiatry 160:439–441, 1992

Henry JA, Alexander CA, Sener EK: Relative mortality from overdose of antidepressants. BMJ 310:221–224, 1995

Herberg LJ, Watkins PJ: Epileptiform seizures induced by hypothalamic stimulation in the rat, resistance to fits following fits. Nature 209:515–516, 1966

Herberg LJ, Tress KH, Blundell JE: Raising the threshold in experimental epilepsy by hypothalamic and septal stimulation and by audiogenic seizures. Brain 92:313–328, 1969

Herman JB, Rosenbaum JF, Brotman AW: The alprazolam to clonazepam switch for the treatment of panic disorder. J Clin Psychophamacol 7:175–178, 1987

Herrmann N: Valproic acid treatment of agitation in dementia. Can J Psychiatry 43:69–72, 1998

Hermann N, Eryavec G: Buspirone in the management of agitation and aggression associated with dementia. Am J Geriatr Psychiatry 1:249–253, 1993

Hermann N, Rivard MF, Flynn M, et al: Risperidone for the treatment of behavioral disturbances in dementia: a case series. J Neuropsychiatry Clin Neurosci 10:220–223, 1998

Hermann RC, Dorwart RA, Hoover CW, et al: Variation in ECT use in the United States. Am J Psychiatry 152:869–875, 1995

Hermesh H, Aizenberg D, Munitz H: Trazodone treatment of CMI resistant OCD. Clin Neuropharmacol 13:322–328, 1990

Hermoni M, Lerer B, Ebstein RP, et al: Chronic lithium prevents reserpine-induced supersensitivity of adenylate cyclase. J Pharm Pharmacol 32:510–511, 1980

Hertzman PA, Blevins WL, Mayer J, et al: Association of the eosinophilia-myalgia syndrome with the ingestion of tryptophan [see comments]. N Engl J Med 322:869–873, 1990

Herz LR, Volicer L, Ross V, et al: Pharmacotherapy of agitation in dementia. Am J Psychiatry 149:1757–1758, 1992

Herzog DB, Keller MB, Lavori PW, et al: Short term prospective study of recovery in bulimia. Psychiatry Res 23:45–55, 1988

Hesketh JE, Nicolaou NM, Arbuthnott GW, et al: The effect of chronic lithium administration on dopamine metabolism in rat striatum. Psychopharmacology 56:163–166, 1978

Heurteaux C, Baumann N, Lachapelle F, et al: Lithium distribution in the brain of normal mice and of "quacking" dysmyelinating mutants. J Neurochem 46:1317–1321, 1986

Heuser IJE, Yassouridis A, Holsboer F: The combined dexamethasone/CRH test: a refined laboratory test for psychiatric disorders. J Psychiatr Res 28:341–356, 1994

Heuser IJE, Schweiger U, Gotthardt U, et al: Pituitary-adrenal-system regulation and psychopathology during amitriptyline treatment in elderly depressed patients and in normal comparison subjects. Am J Psychiatry 153:93–99, 1996

Hewlett WA, Vinogradov S, Agras WS: Clonazepam treatment of obsessions and compulsions. J Clin Psychiatry 51:158–161, 1990

Hewlett WA, Vinogradov S, Agras WS: Clomipramine, clonazepam, and clonidine treatment of obsessive-compulsive disorder. J Clin Psychopharmacol 12: 420–430, 1992a

Hewlett WA, Vinogradov S, Martin K, et al: Fenfluramine stimulation of prolactin in OCD. Psychiatry Res 42:81–92, 1992b

Hiatt JF, Floyd TC, Katz PH, et al: Further evidence of abnormal non-rapid-eye-movement sleep in schizophrenia. Arch Gen Psychiatry 42:797–802, 1985

Hicks TP, Krupa M, Crepel F: Selective effects of serotonin upon excitatory amino acid-induced depolarisations of Purkinje cells in cerebellar slices from young rats. Brain Res 492:371–376, 1989

Higley JD, Suomi SJ: Temperamental reactivity in nonhuman primates, in Temperament in Childhood. Edited by Kohnstamm D, Bates JE, Rothbart MK. Chichester, England, Wiley, 1989, pp 153–167

Higuchi T, Yamazaki O, Takazawa A, et al: Effects of carbamazepine and valproic acid on brain immunoreactive somatostatin and gamma-aminobutyric acid in amygdaloid-kindled rats. Eur J Pharmacol 125:169–175, 1986

Hilger PA: Applied anatomy and physiology of the nose, in Boie's Fundamentals of Otolaryngology, 6th Edition. Edited by Adams GL, Boies LR, Hilger PA. Philadelphia, PA, WB Saunders, 1989, pp 177–195

Hill DR, Woodruff GN: Differentiation of central cholecystokinin receptor binding sites using the non-peptide antagonists MK-329 and L-365,260. Brain Res 526:276–283, 1990

Hill DR, Campbell NJ, Shaw TM, et al: Autoradiographic localization and biochemical characterization of peripheral type CCK receptors in rat CNS using highly selective nonpeptide CCK antagonists. J Neurosci 7:2967–2976, 1987

Hill DR, Singh L, Boden P, et al: Detection of CCK receptor subtypes in mammalian brain using highly selective non-peptide antagonists, in Multiple Cholecystokinin Receptors in the CNS. Edited by Cooper ST, Dourish CD, Iversen SD, et al. New York, Oxford University Press, 1992, pp 57–76

Hill DR, Woodruff GN, Hughes J: Cholecystokinin receptor subtypes and their potential involvement in anxiety, in Abstracts of Panels and Posters of the 32nd Annual Meeting of American College of Neuropsychopharmacology, Honolulu, HI, American College of Neuropsychopharmacology, 1993, p 58

Himmelhoch JM: Major mood disorders related to epileptic changes, in Psychiatric Aspects of Epilepsy. Edited by Blumer D. Washington, DC, American Psychiatric Press, 1984, pp 271–294

Himmelhoch JM, Mulla D, Neil JF, et al: Incidence and significance of mixed affective states in a bipolar population. Arch Gen Psychiatry 33:1062–1066, 1976

Himmelhoch JM, Thase ME, Mallinger AC, et al: Tranylcypromine versus imipramine in anergic bipolar depression. Am J Psychiatry 148:910–916, 1991

Hirvonen MR, Paljarri L, Naukkarinen A, et al: Potentiation of malaoxon-induced convulsions by lithium: early neuronal injury, phosphoinositide signaling and calcium. Toxicol Appl Pharmacol 104:276–289, 1990

Hitzemann R, Mark C, Hirschowitz J, et al: RBC lithium transport in the psychoses. Biol Psychiatry 25:296–304, 1989

Hjorth S: Functional differences between ascending 5-HT systems, in Serotonin, CNS Receptors and Brain Function (Advances in the Biosciences, Vol 85). Edited by Bradley PB, Handley SL, Cooper SJ, et al. Oxford, England, Pergamon, 1992, pp 203–218

Ho AKS, Tsai CS: Lithium and ethanol preference. J Pharm Pharmacol 27:58–60, 1975

Ho AKS, Loh HH, Craves F, et al: The effect of prolonged lithium treatment on the synthesis rate and turnover of monoamines in brain regions of rats. Eur J Pharmacol 10:72–78, 1970

Hobson JA, McCarley RW, Wyzinski PW: Sleep cycle oscillation: reciprocal discharge by two brainstem neuronal groups. Science 189:55–58, 1975

Hobson JA, Lydic R, Baghdoyan HA: Evolving concepts of sleep cycle generation: from brain centers to neuronal populations. Behav Brain Sci 9:371–448, 1986

Hobson RF: Prognostic factors in ECT. J Neurol Neurosurg Psychiatry 16:275–281, 1953

Hodges H, Sowinski P, Sinden JD, et al: The selective 5-HT$_3$ receptor antagonist, WAY100289, enhances spatial memory in rats with ibotenate lesions of the forebrain cholinergic projection system. Psychopharmacology 117:318–332, 1995

Hodges H, Sowinski P, Turner JJ, et al: Comparison of the effects of the 5-HT$_3$ receptor antagonists WAY-100579 and ondansetron on spatial learning in the water maze in rats with excitotoxic lesions of the forebrain cholinergic system. Psychopharmacology 125:146–161, 1996

Hoehn-Saric R, Fawcett J, Munjack DJ, et al: A multicentre, double-blind, placebo-controlled study of fluvoxamine in the treatment of panic disorder. Neuropsychopharmacology 10:102S, 1994

Hofer M, Pagliusi SR, Hohn A, et al: Regional distribution of brain-derived neurotrophic factor mRNA in the adult mouse brain. EMBO J 9:2458–2464, 1990

Hoflich G, Kasper S, Hufnagel A, et al: Application of transcranial magnetic stimulation in treatment of drug-resistant major depression—a report of two cases. Human Psychopharmacology 8:361–365, 1993

Hokfelt T, Xu Z, Ji RR, et al: Plasticity and expression of galanin in peripheral and central neurons (abstract). Paper presented at the 33rd annual meeting of the American College of Neuropsychopharmacology, San Juan, Puerto Rico, December 1994

Hokin-Neaverson M, Jefferson JW: Deficient erythrocyte Na,K-ATPase activity in different affective states in bipolar affective states in bipolar affective disorder and normalization by lithium therapy. Neuropsychobiology 22:18–25, 1989a

Hokin-Neaverson M, Jefferson JW: Erythrocyte sodium pump activity in bipolar affective disorder and other psychiatric disorders. Neuropsychobiology 22:1–7, 1989b

Hokin-Neaverson M, Burckhardt WA, Jefferson JW: Increased erythrocyte Na$^+$ pump and Na-K-ATPase activity during lithium therapy. Research Communications in Chemical Pathology and Pharmacology 14:117–126, 1976

Holazo AA, Winkler MB, Patel IH: Effects of age, gender and oral contraceptives on intramuscular midazolam pharmacokinetics. J Clin Pharmacol 28:1040–1045, 1988

Holland RL: Fluvoxamine in panic disorder: after discontinuation? Neuropsychopharmacology 10:102S, 1994

Holland RL, Fawcett J, Hoehn-Saric R, et al: Long-term treatment of panic disorder with fluvoxamine in outpatients who had completed double-blind studies. Neuropsychopharmacology 10:102S, 1994

Hollander E, Fay M, Liebowitz MR: Clonidine and clomipramine in obsessive-compulsive disorder. Am J Psychiatry 145:388–389, 1988a

Hollander E, Fay M, Cohen B, et al: Serotonergic and noradrenergic sensitivity in obsessive-compulsive disorder: behavioral findings. Am J Psychiatry 145:1015–1017, 1988b

Hollander E, DeCaria CM, Schneier FR, et al: Fenfluramine augmentation of serotonin reuptake blockade antiobsessional treatment. J Clin Psychiatry 51:119–123, 1990a

Hollander E, Schiffman E, Cohen B, et al: Signs of central nervous system dysfunction in obsessive-compulsive disorder. Arch Gen Psychiatry 47:27–32, 1990b

Hollander E, Mullen L, DeCaria CM, et al: Obsessive compulsive disorder, depression, and fluoxetine. J Clin Psychiatry 52:418–422, 1991

Hollander E, De Caria CM, Nitescu A, et al: Serotonergic function in OCD. Arch Gen Psychiatry 49:21–28, 1992

Hollander E, Stein DJ, De Caria E, et al: A pilot study of biological predictors of treatment outcome in OCD. Biol Psychiatry 33:747–749, 1993

Hollister LE: Monitoring tricyclic antidepressant plasma concentrations. JAMA 241:2530–2533, 1979

Holloway W, McNally RJ: Effects of anxiety sensitivity on the response to hyperventilation. J Abnorm Psychol 96:330–334, 1987

Holmberg G: Effect on electrically induced convulsions of the number of previous treatments in a series. Arch Neurol Psychiatry 71:619–623, 1954

Holsboer F: Neuroendocrinology of affective disorder, in Psychopharmacology: The Fourth Generation of Progress. Edited by Bloom FE, Kupfer DJ. New York, Raven, 1995, pp 263–291

Holsboer F, Barden N: Antidepressants and hypothalamic-pituitary-adrenocortical regulation. Endocr Rev 17(2):187–205, 1996

Holsboer F, Liebl R, Hofschuster E: Repeated dexamethasone suppression test during depressive illness: normalization of test result compared with clinical improvement. J Affect Disord 4:93–101, 1982

Holsboer F, von Bardeleben U, Gerken A, et al: Blunted corticotropin and normal cortisol response to human corticotropin-releasing factor in depression. N Engl J Med 311:1127, 1984

Holsboer F, Gerken A, von Bardeleben U, et al: Human corticotropin-releasing hormone in depression. Biol Psychiatry 21:609–611, 1986

Holsboer F, von Bardeleben U, Wiedemann K, et al: Serial assessment of corticotropin-releasing hormone response after dexamethasone in depression—implications for pathophysiology of DST nonsuppression. Biol Psychiatry 22:228–234, 1987

Holsboer F, von Bardeleben U, Steiger A: Effects of intravenous corticotropin-releasing hormone upon sleep-related growth hormone surge and sleep EEG in man. Neuroendocrinology 48:32–38, 1988

Holsboer F, Spengler D, Heuser I: The role of corticotropin-releasing hormone in the pathogenesis of Cushing's disease, anorexia nervosa, alcoholism, affective disorders and dementia, in Progress in Brain Research, Vol 93. Edited by Swaab DF, Hofmann MA, Mermiran M, et al. Amsterdam, Elsevier, 1992, pp 385–417

Holsboer F, Lauer CJ, Schreiber W, et al: Altered hypothalamic-pituitary-adrenocortical regulation in healthy subjects at high familial risk for affective disorders. Neuroendocrinology 62:340–347, 1995

Holsboer-Trachsler E, Stohler R, Hatzinger M: Repeated administration of the combined dexamethasone/human corticotropin releasing hormone stimulation test during treatment of depression. Psychiatry Res 38:163–171, 1991

Holsboer-Trachsler E, Hemmeter U, Hatzinger M, et al: Sleep deprivation and bright light as potential augmenters of antidepressant drug treatment—neurobiological and psychometric assessment of course. J Psychiatr Res 28:381–399, 1994

Holttum JR, Gershon S: The cholinergic model of dementia, Alzheimer type: progression from the unitary transmitter concept. Dementia 3:174–185, 1992

Honchar MP, Olney JW, Sherman WR: Systemic cholinergic agents induce seizures and brain damage in lithium-treated rats. Science 220:323–325, 1983

Honchar MP, Ackermann KE, Sherman WR: Chronically administered lithium alters neither myo-inositol monophosphatase nor phosphoinositide levels in rat brain. J Neurochem 53:590–594, 1989

Hong E, Meneses A: Systemic injection of p-chloramphetamine eliminates the effect of the 5-HT$_3$ compounds on learning. Pharmacol Biochem Behav 53:765–769, 1996

Hong J-S, Tilson HA, Yoshikawa K: Effects of lithium and haloperidol administration on the rat brain levels of Substance P. J Pharmacol Exp Ther 224:590–597, 1983

Honig A, Bartlett JR, Bouras N, et al: Amino acid levels in depression: a preliminary investigation. J Psychiatr Res 22:159–164, 1989

Honjo H, Ogino Y, Natitoh K, et al: In vivo effects by estrone sulphate on the central nervous system on senile dementia (Alzheimer's type). Journal of Steroid Biochemistry 34:521–525, 1989

Hoover TM: CI-979/RU 35926: a novel muscarinic agonist for the treatment of Alzheimer's disease, in Alzheimer Disease: Therapeutic Strategies. Edited by Giacobini E, Becker R. Boston, MA, Birkhäuser, 1994, pp 239–243

Hordern A, Holt NF, Burt CG, et al: Amitriptyline in depressive states: phenomenology and prognostic considerations. Br J Psychiatry 10:815–825, 1963

Horn JL: The theory of fluid and crystallized intelligence in relation to concepts of cognitive psychology and aging in adulthood, in Aging and Cognitive Processes, Vol 8. Edited by Craik FIM, Trehub S. New York, Plenum, 1982, pp 237–278

Hornig M, Mozely PD, Amsterdam JD: HMPAO SPECT brain imaging in treatment-resistant depression. Prog Neuropsychopharmacol Biol Psychiatry 21:1097–1114, 1997

Hornig-Rohan M, Amsterdam JD: Clinical and biological correlates of treatment-resistant depression: an overview. J Clin Psychiatry 24:220–227, 1994

Horowski R, Wachtel L, Turski L, et al: Glutamate excitotoxicity as a possible pathogenetic mechanism in chronic neurodegeneration, in Neurodegenerative Diseases. Edited by Calne DB. Philadelphia, PA, WB Saunders, 1994, pp 163–174

Hoschl C: Verapamil for depression? Am J Psychiatry 140:1100, 1983

Hoschl C, Kozeny J: Verapamil in affective disorders: a controlled, double-blind study. Biol Psychiatry 25:128–140, 1989

Hoschl C, Vackova J, Janda B: Mood stabilizing effect of verapamil. Abstracts of the 17th CINP Congress, Kyoto, Japan, September 10–14, 1990, Vol 1, abstract no P-11-4-15, 1990, p 95

Hoschl C, Vackova J, Janda B: Mood stabilizing effect of verapamil. Bratisl Lek Listy 93:208–209, 1992

Hotta I, Yamawaki S: Possible involvement of presynaptic 5-HT autoreceptors in effect of lithium on 5-HT release in hippocampus of rat. Neuropharmacology 27:987–992, 1988

Hough CJ, Irwin RP, Gao X-M, et al: Carbamazepine inhibition of N-methyl-D-aspartate-evoked calcium influx in rat cerebellar granule cells. J Pharmacol Exp Ther 276:143–149, 1996

Houslay MD: "Crosstalk": a pivotal role for protein kinase C in modulating relationships between signal transduction pathways. Eur J Biochem 195:9–27, 1991

Howland RH: Thyroid dysfunction in refractory depression: implications for pathophysiology and treatment. J Clin Psychiatry 54:47–54, 1993

Hoyer D: Functional correlates of serotonin 5-HT1 recognition sites. J Recept Res 8:59–81, 1988

Hoyer D, Clarke DE, Fozard JR, et al: VII International Union of Pharmacology classification of receptors for 5-hydroxtryptamine. Pharmacol Rev 46:157–203, 1994

Hsiao JK, Manji HK, Chen GA, et al: Lithium administration modulates platelet Gi in humans. Life Sci 50:227–233, 1992

Hsiao JK, Colison J, Bartko JJ, et al: Monoamine neurotransmitter interactions in drug-free and neuroleptic-treated schizophrenics. Arch Gen Psychiatry 50:606–614, 1993

Hu ZY, Bourreau E, Jung-Testas I, et al: Neurosteroids: oligodendrocyte mitochondria convert cholesterol to pregnenolone: Proc Natl Acad Sci U S A 84:8215–8219, 1987

Huang KP: The mechanism of protein kinase C activation. Trends Neurosci 12:425–432, 1989

Huang S, Fortune KP, Wank SA, et al: Multiple affinity states of different cholecystokinin receptors. J Biol Chem 269:26121–26126, 1994

Hudson JL, Pope HG, Jonas JM, et al: Phenomenologic relationship of eating disorders to major affective disorder. Psychiatry Res 9:345–354, 1983

Huey LY, Janowshy, DS, Judd LL, et al: Effects of lithium carbonate on methylphenidate-induced mood, behavior, and cognitive processes. Psychopharmacology 73:161–164, 1981

Huff FJ, Mickel SF, Corkin S, et al: Cognitive functions affected by scopolamine in Alzheimer's disease and normal aging. Drug Development Research 12:271–278, 1988

Huganir RL, Greengard P: Regulation of neurotransmitter receptor desensitization by protein phosphorylation. Neuron 5:555–567, 1990

Hughes J, Boden P, Costall B, et al: Development of a class of selective cholecystokinin type B receptor antagonists having potent anxiolytic activity. Proc Natl Acad Sci U S A 87:6728–6732, 1990

Hulme EC, Birdsall NJM, Buckley NJ: Muscarinic receptor subtypes. Annu Rev Pharmacol Toxicol 30:633–637, 1990

Hunt CM, Westerkam WR, Stave GM: Effect of age and gender on the activity of human hepatic CYP3A. Biochem Pharmacol 44:275–283, 1992

Hunter T, Karin M: The regulation of transcription by phosphorylation. Cell 70:377–387, 1992

Husain MM, Lewis SF, Thornton WL: Maintenance ECT for refractory obsessive-compulsive disorder (letter). Am J Psychiatry 150:1899–1900, 1993

Hwang EC, Van Woert MH: Antimyoclonic action of clonazepam: the role of serotonin. Eur J Pharmacol 60:31–40, 1979

Hyttel J: Citalopram: pharmacological profile of a specific serotonin reuptake inhibitor with antidepressant activity. Prog Neuropsychopharmacol Biol Psychiatry 6:277–295, 1982

Hyttel J: Pharmacological characterization of selective serotonin reuptake inhibitors (SSRIs). Int Clin Psychopharmacol 9 (suppl 1):19–26, 1994

Hytell J, Larsen J-J: Serotonin-selective antidepressants. Acta Pharmacol Toxicol 56 (suppl 1):146–153, 1985

Imperato A, Cabib S, Puglisi-Allegra S: Repeated stressful experiences differently affect the time-dependent responses of the mesolimbic dopamine system to the stressor. Brain Res 601:333–336, 1993

Imperato A, Obinu MC, Cabib S, et al: Effects of subchronic minaprine on dopamine release in the ventral striatum and on immobility in the forced swimming test. Neurosci Lett 166:69–72, 1994

Inghilleri M, Berardelli A, Cruccu G, et al: Silent period evoked by transcranial stimulation of the human cortex and cervicomedullary junction. J Physiol (Lond) 466:521–34, 1993

Insel TR: Oxytocin—a neuropeptide for affiliation: evidence from behavioral, receptor autoradiographic, and comparative studies. Psychoneuroendocrinology 17:3–35, 1992

Insel TR, Alterman I, Murphy DL: Antiobsessional and anti-depressant effects of CMI in the treatment of OCD. Psychol Bull 18:115–117, 1982a

Insel TR, Gillin JC, Moore A, et al: The sleep of patients with obsessive-compulsive disorder. Arch Gen Psychiatry 39:1372–1377, 1982b

Insel TR, Hamilton JA, Guttmacher LB, et al: D-amphetamine in obsessive-compulsive disorder. Psychopharmacology 80:231–235, 1983a

Insel TR, Murphy DL, Cohen RM, et al: OCD: a double-blind trial of CMI and clorgyline. Arch Gen Psychiatry 40:605–612, 1983b

Insel TR, Mueler EA, Alterman I, et al: OCD and serotonin: is there a connection? Biol Psychiatry 20:1174–1188, 1985

Insel TR, Scanlan J, Champoux M, et al: Rearing paradigm in a nonhuman primate affects response to b-CCE challenge. Psychopharmacology 96:81–86, 1988

Invernizzi G, Aguglia E, Bertolino A, et al: The efficacy and safety of tianeptine in the treatment of depressive disorder: results of a controlled double-blind multicentre study vs. amitriptyline. Neuropsychobiology 30(2–3):85–93, 1994

Invernizzi R, Belli S, Samanin R: Citalopram's ability to increase the extracellular concentrations of serotonin in the dorsal raphe prevents the drug's effect in the frontal cortex. Brain Res 584:322–324, 1992a

Invernizzi R, Pozzi L, Vallebuona F, et al: Effect of amineptine on regional extracellular concentrations of dopamine and noradrenaline in the rat brain. J Pharmacol Exp Ther 262:769–774, 1992b

Irwin RP, Magarakis NJ, Rogawski MA, et al: Pregnenolone sulfate augments NMDA receptor mediated increases in intracellular Ca^{2+} in cultured rat hippocampal neurons. Neurosci Lett 141:30–34, 1992

Ishibashi S, Oomura Y, Okajima T, et al: Cholecystokinin, motilin and secretin effects on the central nervous system. Physiol Behav 23:401–403, 1979

Ishii T: Distribution of Alzheimer's neurofibrillary changes in the brain stem and hypothalamus of senile dementia. Acta Neuropathol 6:181–187, 1966

Itil TM, Itil KZ: The significance of pharmacodynamic measurements of bioavailability and bioequivalence of psychotropic drugs using CEEG and dynamic brain mapping. J Clin Psychiatry 47:20–27, 1986

Itoh S, Takashima A, Katsuura G: Effect of cholecystokinin tetrapeptide amide on the metabolism of 5-hydroxytryptamine in the rat brain. Neuropharmacology 27:427–431, 1988

Iversen SD: 5-HT and anxiety. Neuropharmacology 23:156–164, 1984

Iwamori M, Moser HW, Kishimoto Y: Steroid sulfatase in brain: comparison of sulfohydrolase activities for various steroid sulfates in normal and pathological brains, including various forms of metachromatic leukodystrophy. J Neurochem 27:1389–1395, 1976

Jackson D, Stachowiak MK, Bruno JP, et al: Inhibition of striatal acetylcholine release by endogenous serotonin. Brain Res 457:259–266, 1988

Jacobs S, Hansen F, Kasl S, et al: Anxiety disorders during acute bereavement: risk and risk factors. J Clin Psychiatry 51:269–274, 1990

Jacobsen FM: Possible augmentation of antidepressant response by buspirone. J Clin Psychiatry 52:217–220, 1991

Jacobsen FM: Fluoxetine-induced sexual dysfunction and an open trial of yohimbine. J Clin Psychiatry 53:119–122, 1992

Jacobsen FM: Risperidone in the treatment of severe affective illness and refractory OCD (NR275), in 1995 New Research Program and Abstracts, American Psychiatric Association 148th Annual Meeting, Miami, FL, May 20–25, 1995. Washington, DC, American Psychiatric Association, 1995, p 129

Jacobson AF, Dominguez RA, Goldstein BJ, et al: Comparison of buspirone and diazepam in generalised anxiety disorder. Pharmacotherapy 5:290–296, 1985

Jacobson NS, Dobson K, Fruzzetti AE, et al: Marital therapy as a treatment for depression. J Consult Clin Psychol 59:547–557, 1991

Jacobson SJ, Jones K, Johnson K, et al: Prospective multicentre study of pregnancy outcome after lithium exposure during first trimester. Lancet 339:530–533, 1992

Jain VK: A psychiatric study of hypothyroidism. Psychiatr Clin North Am 5:121–130, 1972

Jakala P, Sirvio J, Riekkinen P, et al: Effects of p-chlorophenylalanine and methysergide on the performance of a working memory test. Pharmacol Biochem Behav 44:411–418, 1993

Jakovljevic M, Mewett S: Comparison between paroxetine, imipramine and placebo in preventing recurrent major depressive episodes. Eur Neuropsychopharmacol 1:440, 1991

James SP, Potter L, Berwish N, et al: Polysomnography in refractory depression, in Refractory Depression (Advances in Neuropsychiatry and Psychopharmacology, Vol 2). Edited by Amsterdam JD. New York, Raven, 1991

Janicak PG, Lipinski J, Davis JM, et al: Parenteral S-adenosyl-methionine (SAMe) in depression: literature review and preliminary data. Psychopharmacol Bull 25:238–242, 1989

Janicak PG, Sharma RP, Pandey G, et al: Verapamil for the treatment of acute mania: a double-blind, placebo-controlled trial. Am J Psychiatry 155:972–973, 1998

Janis RA, Triggle DJ: Drugs acting on calcium channels, in Calcium Channels: Their Properties, Functions, Regulation, and Clinical Relevance. Edited by Hurwitz L, Partridge LD, Leach JK. Boca Raton, FL, CRC, 1991, pp 195–249

Janowski DS, El-Yousef MK, Davis JM, et al: A cholinergic adrenergic hypothesis of mania and depression. Lancet 2:632–635, 1972

Jarrett DB, Miewald JM, Kupfer DJ: Acute changes in sleep-related hormone secretion of depressed patients following oral imipramine. Biol Psychiatry 24:541–554, 1988

Jarvik LF: Calcium channel blocker nimodipine for primary degenerative dementia. Biol Psychiatry 30:1171–1172, 1991

Jeanblanc W, Davis YB: Risperidone for treating dementia associated aggression. Am J Psychiatry 152:1239, 1995

Jenden DJ: Chemistry and biochemical pharmacology of cholinergic neurons, in Psychopharmacology: The Third Generation of Progress. Edited by Meltzer HY. New York, Raven, 1987, pp 233–239

Jenike MA: Drug treatment of obsessive-compulsive disorder, in Obsessive Compulsive Disorders: Theory and Management, 2nd Edition. Edited by Jenike MJ, Baer L, Minichiello WE. Littleton, MA, PSG Publishing, 1990, pp 249–282

Jenike MA, Baer L: An open trial of buspirone in OCD. Am J Psychiatry 145:1285–1286, 1988

Jenike MA, Brotman AW: The EEG in obsessive compulsive disorder. J Clin Psychiatry 45:122–124, 1984

Jenike MA, Surman OS, Cassem NH, et al: Monoamine oxidase inhibitors in obsessive-compulsive disorder. J Clin Psychiatry 144:131–132, 1983

Jenike MA, Baer L, Minichiello WE, et al: Concomitant obsessive-compulsive disorder and schizotypal personality disorder. Am J Psychiatry 143:530–533, 1986

Jenike MA, Hyman S, Baer L, et al: A controlled trial of fluvoxamine in OCD. Am J Psychiatry 147:1209–1215, 1990

Jenike MA, Baer L, Buttolph L: Buspirone augmentation of fluoxetine in patients with obsessive compulsive disorder. J Clin Psychiatry 52:13–14, 1991a

Jenike MA, Baer L, Ballantine HT, et al: Cingulotomy for refractory obsessive-compulsive disorder: a long-term follow-up of 33 patients. Arch Gen Psychiatry 48:548–555, 1991b

Jenike MA, Rauch SL, Cummings JL, et al: Recent developments in neurobiology of obsessive-compulsive disorder. J Clin Psychiatry 57:492–503, 1996

Jenner PN: Paroxetine: an overview of dosage, tolerability, and safety. Int Clin Psychopharmacol 6 (suppl 4):69–80, 1992

Jensen HH, Poulson JC: Amnesic effects of diazepam: 'drug dependence' explained by state dependent learning. Scand J Psychol 23:107–111, 1982

Jensen HH, Hutchings B, Poulsen JC: Conditioned emotional responding under diazepam: a psychophysiological study of state-dependent learning. Psychopharmacology 98:392–397, 1989

Jensen S, Plaetke R, Holik J, et al: Linkage analysis of the D_1 dopamine receptor gene and manic depression in six families. Hum Hered 42:269–275, 1992

Jeste DV, Eastham JH, Lacro JP, et al: Management of late-life psychosis. J Clin Psychiatry 57 (suppl 3):39–45, 1996

Jeste DV, Eastham JH, Lohr JB, et al: Treatment of disordered behavior and psychosis, in Clinical Geriatric Psychopharmacology, 3rd Edition. Edited by Salzman C. Baltimore, MD, Williams & Wilkins, 1998, pp 107–149

Jimerson DC, Post RM, Carman JS, et al: CSF calcium: clinical correlates in affective illness and schizophrenia. Biol Psychiatry 14:37–51, 1979

Joffe RT, Levitt AJ: Major depression and subclinical (Grade 2) hypothyroidism. Psychoneuroendocrinology 17:215–221, 1992

Joffe RT, Levitt AJ: The thyroid and depression, in The Thyroid Axis and Psychiatric Illness. Edited by Joffe RT, Levitt AJ. Washington, DC, American Psychiatric Press, 1993, pp 195–253

Joffe RT, Schuller DR: An open study of buspirone augmentation of serotonin reuptake inhibitors in refractory depression. J Clin Psychiatry 54:269–271, 1993

Joffe RT, Singer W: A comparison of triiodothyronine and thyroxine in the potentiation of tricyclic antidepressants. Psychiatry Res 32:241–251, 1990

Joffe RT, Swinson RP: Carbamazepine in obsessive-compulsive disorder. Biol Psychiatry 22:1169–1171, 1987

Joffe RT, Swinson RP: Total sleep deprivation in patients with obsessive-compulsive disorder. Acta Psychiatr Scand 77:483–487, 1988

Joffe RT, Swinson RP, Levitt AJ: Acute psychostimulant challenge in primary obsessive-compulsive disorder. J Clin Psychopharmacol 11:237–241, 1991

Johns CA, Greenwald BS, Mohs RC, et al: The cholinergic treatment strategy in aging and senile dementia. Pharmacological Bulletin 19:185–197, 1983

Johnson BB, Naylor GJ, Dick EG, et al: Prediction of clinical course of bipolar manic depressive illness treated with lithium. Psychol Med 10:329–334, 1980

Johnson G, Gershon S, Burdock E, et al: Comparative effects of lithium and chlorpromazine in the treatment of manic states. Br J Psychiatry 119:267–276, 1971

Johnson J, Weissman MM, Klerman GL: Panic disorder, comorbidity, and suicide attempts. Arch Gen Psychiatry 47:805–808, 1990

Johnson MR, Lydiard RB, Ballenger JC: Panic disorder. Pathophysiology and drug treatment. Drugs 49:328–344, 1995

Johnson RD, Minneman KP: α_1-Adrenergic receptors and stimulation of [3H]inositol metabolism in rat brain: regional distribution and parallel inactivation. Brain Res 341:7–15, 1985

Johnson RM, Inouye GT, Eglen RM: 5-HT$_3$ receptor ligands lack modulatory influence on acetylcholine release in rat entorhinal cortex. Naunyn Schmiedebergs Arch Pharmacol 347:241–247, 1993

Johnson RW, Reisine T, Spotnitz S, et al: Effect of desipramine and yohimbine on alpha-2- and beta-adrenoreceptor sensitivity. Eur J Pharmacol 67:123–127, 1980

Johnston DG, Troyer IE, Whitsett SF: Clomipramine in the treatment of agoraphobic women. Biol Psychiatry 25:101–104, 1988

Johnston JA, Lineberry CG, Ascher JA, et al: A 102-center prospective study of seizure in association with bupropion. J Clin Psychiatry 52 (suppl 11):450–456, 1991

Johnstone EC, Owens DGC, Crow TJ, et al: Hypothyroidism as a correlate of lateral ventricular enlargement in manic-depressive and neurotic illness. Br J Psychiatry 148:317–321, 1986

Jolas T, Schreiber R, Laporte AM, et al: Are postsynaptic 5-HT1A receptors involved in the anxiolytic effects of 5-HT1A receptor agonists and in their inhibitory effects on the firing of serotonergic neurons in the rat? J Pharmacol Exp Ther 272:920–929, 1995

Jolles J: Vasopressin-like peptides and the treatment of memory disorders in man. Prog Brain Res 60:169–182, 1983

Jones FD, Maas JW, Dekirmenjian H, et al: Urinary catecholamine metabolites during behavioral changes in a patient with manic-depressive cycles. Science 179:300–302, 1973

Jones JF: Viral etiology of chronic fatigue syndrome, in Chronic Fatigue and Related Immune Deficiency Syndromes. Edited by Goodnick PJ, Klimas NG. Washington, DC, American Psychiatric Press, 1993, pp 23–43

Jonsson B, Bebbington PE: What price depression?, The cost of depression and the cost-effectiveness of pharmacological treatment. Br J Psychiatry 164:665–673, 1994

Jope RS: Effects of lithium treatment in vitro and in vivo on acetylcholine metabolism in rat brain. J Neurochem 33:487–495, 1979

Jope RS: Anti-bipolar therapy: mechanism of action of lithium. Mol Psychiatry (in press)

Jope RS, Williams MB: Lithium and brain signal transduction systems. Biochem Pharmacol 47:429–441, 1994

Jope RS, Jenden DJ, Ehrlich BE, et al: Choline accumulates in erythrocytes during lithium therapy. N Engl J Med 299:833–834, 1978

Jope RS, Jenden DJ, Ehrlich BE, et al: Erythrocyte choline concentrations are elevated in manic patients. Proc Natl Acad Sci U S A 77:6144–6146, 1980

Jope RS, Morrisett RA, Snead OC: Characterization of lithium potentiation of pilocarpine induced status epilepticus in rats. Exp Neurol 91:471–480, 1986

Jordan D, Spyer KM: Brainstem integration of cardiovascular and pulmonary afferent activity. Prog Brain Res 67:295–314, 1986

Jorge RE, Robinson RG, Starkstein SE, et al: Secondary mania following traumatic brain injury. Am J Psychiatry 150:916–921, 1993

Jovanovic UJ: Studies with maprotiline on waking states and on sleep patterns in healthy subjects and in depressed patients, in Depression: The Biochemical and Physiological Role of Ludiomil. Edited by Jukes A. England, CIBA, 1977, pp 85–101

Joyce D, Hurwitz HMB: Avoidance behaviour in the rat after 5-hydroxytryptophan (5-HTP) administration. Psychopharmacologia 5:424–430, 1964

Joyce EM: The neurochemistry of Korsakoff's syndrome, in Cognitive Neurochemistry. Edited by Stahl SM, Iversen SD, Goodman EC. Oxford, England, Oxford Science Publications, 1987, pp 327–345

Judd FK, Chua P, Lynch C, et al: Fenfluramine augmentation of clomipramine treatment of obsessive compulsive disorder. Aust N Z J Psychiatry 25:412–414, 1991

Judge R, Steiner M: The long-term efficacy and safety of paroxetine in panic disorder. Eur J Neuropsychopharmacol 6 (suppl 3):207, 1996

Julius D, McDermott AB, Axel R, et al: Molecular characterization of a functional cDNA encoding the serotonin 1C receptor. Science 241:558–564, 1988

Jung-Testas I, Hu ZY, Beaulieu EE, et al: Neurosteroids: biosynthesis of pregnenolone and progesterone in primary cultures of rat glial cells. Endocrinology 125:2083–2091, 1989

Kabakov AY, Karkanias NB, Lenox RH, et al: Synapse-specific accumulation of lithium in intracellular microdomains: a model for uncoupling coincidence detection in the brain. Synapse 28:271–279, 1998

Kafka M, Wirz-Justice A, Naber D, et al: Effect of lithium on circadian neurotransmitter receptor rhythms. Neuropsychobiology 8:41–50, 1982

Kagan J, Reznick JS, Snidman N: The physiology and psychology of behavioral inhibition. Child Dev 58:1459–1473, 1987

Kagan J, Reznick JS, Snidman N: Biological bases of childhood shyness. Science 240:167–171, 1990

Kahn RS, Moore C: Serotonin in the pathogenesis of anxiety, in Biology of Anxiety Disorders. Edited by Hoehn-Saric R, McLoad R. Washington, DC, American Psychiatric Press, 1993

Kahn RS, Westenberg HGM: L-5-Hydroxytryptophan in the treatment of anxiety disorders. J Affect Disord 8:197–200, 1985

Kahn RS, Westenberg HGM, Verhoeven WMA, et al: Effects of a serotonin precursor and uptake inhibitor in anxiety disorders: a double-blind comparison of 5-hydroxytryptophan, clomipramine and placebo. Int J Clin Psychopharmacol 2:33–45, 1987

Kahn RS, van Praag HM, Wetzler S, et al: Serotonin and anxiety revisited. Biol Psychiatry 23:189–208, 1988

Kakigi T, Tanimoto K, Maeda K: The effect of various antidepressants on the concentration of somatostatin in the rat brain. Jpn J Psychiatry Neurol 44:145, 1990

Kalasapudi VD, Sheftel G, Divish MM, et al: Lithium augments fos protoonocogene expression in PC12 pheochromocytoma cells: implications for therapeutic action of lithium. Brain Res 521:47–54, 1990

Kales A: Pharmacology of Sleep. Handbook of Experimental Pharmacology. Berlin, Springer-Verlag, 1995

Kalin NH, Shelton SJ: Defensive behaviors in infant rhesus monkeys: environmental cues and neurochemical regulation. Science 243:1718–1721, 1989

Kalinowsky LB, Kennedy F: Observations in electric shock therapy applied to problems of epilepsy. J Nerv Ment Dis 98:56–67, 1943

Kampen D, Sherwin B: Estrogen use and verbal memory in healthy postmenopausal women. Obstet Gynecol 83:979–983, 1994

Kane JM, Quitkin FM, Rifkin A, et al: Lithium carbonate and imipramine in the prophylaxis of unipolar and bipolar II illness: a prospective placebo-controlled comparison. Arch Gen Psychiatry 39:1065–1069, 1982

Kaneno S, Komatsu H, Fukamauchi F, et al: Biochemical basis of antidepressant-effect of low dose of sulpiride. Japanese Journal of Psychiatry and Neurology 45:131–132, 1991

Kaneyuki T, Morimasa T, Shohmori T: Action of peripherally administered cholecystokinin on monoaminergic and GABAergic neurons in the rat brain. Acta Med Okayama 43:153–159, 1989

Kantor SJ, Glassman AH: Delusional depression: natural history and response to treatment. Br J Psychiatry 131:351–360, 1977

Kao KR, Elinson RP: Dorsalization of mesoderm induction by lithium. Dev Biol 132:81–90, 1989

Kao KR, Elinson RP: The legacy of lithium effects on development. Biol Cell 90:585–589, 1998

Kapur S, Mann JJ: Role of the dopaminergic system in depression. Biol Psychiatry 32:1–17, 1992

Karajgi B, Rifkin A, Doddi S, et al: The prevalence of anxiety disorders in patients with chronic obstructive pulmonary disease. Am J Psychiatry 147:200–201, 1990

Karazman R, Konig G, Langer G, et al: Narcotherapy in resistant depressive patients, in Refractory Depression (Advances in Neuropsychiatry and Psychopharmacology, Vol 2). Edited by Amsterdam JD. New York, Raven, 1991, pp 223–231

Katada T, Gillman AG, Watanabe Y, et al: Protein C phosphorylates the inhibitory guanine-nucleotide-binding regulatory component and apparently suppresses its function in hormonal inhibition of adenylate cyclase. Eur J Biochem 151:431–437, 1985

Kato G, Weitsch AF: Neurochemical profile tianeptine, a new antidepressant. Clin Neuropharmacol 11 (suppl 2):S43–S50, 1988

Katon W, Sullivan M: Depression and chronic medical illness. J Clin Psychiatry 51 (6 suppl):3, 1990

Katon W, Von Korff M, Lin E, et al: Adequacy and duration of antidepressant treatment in primary care. Med Care 30:67–76, 1992

Katona CL, Hunter BN, Bray J: A double-blind comparison of the efficacy and safety of paroxetine and imipramine in the treatment of depression with dementia. Int J Geriatr Psychiatry 13:100–108, 1998

Katschnig H, Merz WA, Berger P, et al: Attack related treatment of panic disorder with bretazenil: a randomised placebo controlled clinical trial, in Biological Psychiatry: Proceedings of the 5th World Congress of Biological Psychiatry, Florence, Italy, June 9–14, 1991. Edited by Racagni G, Brunello N, Fukuda T. New York, Excerpta Medica, 1991, pp 709–712

Katterndahl DA, Realini JP: Lifetime prevalence of panic states. Am J Psychiatry 150:246–249, 1993

Katz IR, Jeste DV, Mintzer JE, et al: Comparison of risperidone and placebo for psychosis and behavioral disturbances associated with dementia: a randomized, double-blind trial: Risperidone Study Group. J Clin Psychiatry 60:107–115, 1999

Katz JL, Kuperberg A, Pollack CP, et al: Is there a relationship between eating disorder and affective disorder? New evidence from sleep recordings. Am J Psychiatry 141:753–759, 1984

Katz RJ, DeVeaugh-Geiss J: The antiobsessional effects of clomipramine do not require concomitant affective disorder. Psychiatry Res 31:121–129, 1990

Katzelnick DJ, Jefferson JW, Greist JH, et al: Sertraline in social phobia: a double-blind, placebo-controlled crossover pilot study. Poster presentation at the annual meeting of the New Clinical Drug Evaluation Unit, Marco Island, FL, June 1994

Katzelnick DJ, Kobak KA, Greist JH: Sertraline in social phobia: a double blind, placebo-controlled crossover study. Am J Psychiatry 152:1368–1371, 1995

Kaufman I, Rosenblum LA: A behavioral taxonomy for M nemestrina and M radiata: based on longitudinal observations of family groups in the laboratory. Primates 7:205, 1966

Kavaliers M, Wiebe JP: Analgesic effects of the progesterone metabolite, 3a-hydroxy-5a-pregnan-20-one, and possible modes of action. Brain Res 415:393–398, 1987

Kawachi I, Sparrow D, Vokonas PS, et al: Decreased heart rate variability in men with phobic anxiety: data from the Normative Aging Study. Am J Cardiol 75:882–885, 1995

Kawashima K, Araki H, Uchiymya Y, et al: Amygdaloid catecholaminergic mechanisms involved in suppressive effects of electroconvulsive shock on duration of immobility in rats forced to swim. Eur J Pharmacol 141:1–6, 1987

Keck PE Jr, McElroy SL: New uses for antidepressants: social phobia. J Clin Psychiatry 58 (suppl 14):32–36, 1997

Keck PE Jr, McElroy SL, Nemeroff CB: Anticonvulsants in the treatment of bipolar disorder. J Neuropsychiatry 4:395–405, 1992a

Keck PE Jr, McElroy SL, Vuckovic A, et al: Combined valproate and carbamazepine treatment of bipolar disorder. J Neuropsychiatry Clin Neurosci 4:319–322, 1992b

Keck PE Jr, McElroy SL, Tugrul KC, et al: Valproate oral loading in the treatment of acute mania. J Clin Psychiatry 54:305–308, 1993

Keck PE Jr, McElroy SL, Strakowski SM, et al: Pharmacologic treatment of schizoaffective disorder. Psychopharmacology 114:529–538, 1994

Keller MB: Chronic and recurrent affective disorders: Incidence, course, and influencing factors, in Chronic Treatments in Neuropsychiatry. Edited by Kemali D, Recagni G. New York, Raven, 1985

Keller MB, Baker MA: The clinical course of panic disorder and depression. J Clin Psychiatry 53 (suppl 3):5–8, 1992

Keller MB, Hanks DL: Course and outcome in panic disorder and depression. J Clin Psychopharmacol Biol Psychiatry 17:551–570, 1993

Keller MB, Shapiro RW: "Double depression": superimposition of acute depressive episodes on chronic depressive disorders. Am J Psychiatry 139:438–442, 1982

Keller MB, Shapiro RW, Lavori PW, et al: Recovery in major depressive disorder: analysis with the life table and regression models. Arch Gen Psychiatry 39:905–910, 1982a

Keller MB, Shapiro RW, Lavori PW, et al: Relapse in major depressive disorder: analysis with the life table. Arch Gen Psychiatry 39:911–915, 1982b

Keller MB, Klerman GL, Lavori PW, et al: Treatment received by depressed patients. JAMA 248:1848–1855, 1982c

Keller MB, Lavori PW, Klerman GL, et al: Low levels and lack of predictors of somatotherapy and psychotherapy received by depressed patients. Arch Gen Psychiatry 43:458–466, 1986

Keller MB, Labori PW, Mueller TI, et al: Time to recovery, chronicity, and levels of psychopathology in major depression. Arch Gen Psychiatry 49:809–816, 1992

Kellner CH, Nixon DW, Bernstein HJ: ECT—drug interactions: a review. Psychopharmacol Bull 27:595–609, 1991

Kellner CH, Beale MD, Pritchett JT, et al: Electroconvulsive therapy and Parkinson's disease: the case for further study. Psychopharmacol Bull 30:495–500, 1994

Kellner M, Wiedemann K, Krieg J-C, et al: Effects of the dopamine autoreceptor agonist roxindole in patients with depression and panic disorder (abstract). Neuropsychopharmacology 10:101S, 1994

Kelly GR, Scott JE, Mamon J: Medication compliance and health education among outpatients with chronic mental disorders. Med Care 28:1181–1197, 1990

Kendall DA, Nahorski SR: Acute and chronic lithium treatments influence agonist- and depolarization-stimulated inositol phospholipid hydrolysis in rat cerebral cortex. J Pharmacol Exp Ther 241:1023–1027, 1987

Kendall DA, Stancel GM, Enna SJ: The influence of sex hormones on antidepressant-induced alterations in neurotransmitter receptor binding. J Neurosci 2:354–360, 1981

Kendell RE: Schizophrenia: clinical features, in Psychiatry, Vol 1. Edited by Michels R, Chvenar JO, Keith H, et al. New York, Basic Books, 1987

Kendler KS, Heath AC, Martin NG, et al: Symptoms of anxiety and depression: same genes, different environments? Arch Gen Psychiatry 44:451–457, 1987

Kendler KS, Kessler RC, Neale MC, et al: The prediction of major depression in women: toward an integrated etiologic model. Am J Psychiatry 150: 1139–1148, 1993

Kendler KS, Walters EE, Neale MC, et al: The structure of the genetic and environmental risk factors for six major psychiatric disorders in women. Arch Gen Psychiatry 52:374–383, 1995

Kennedy ED, Challiss RJ, Nahorski SR: Lithium reduces the accumulation of inositol polyphosphate second messengers following cholinergic stimulation of cerebral cortex slices. J Neurochem 53:1652–1655, 1989

Kennedy ED, Challiss RAJ, Ragan CI, et al: Reduced inositol polyphosphate accumulation and inositol supply induced by lithium in stimulated cerebral cortex slices. Biochem J 267:781–786, 1990

Kennett GA, Whitton P, Shah K, et al: Anxiogenic-like effects of mCPP and TFMPP in animal models are opposed by 5-HT$_{1C}$ receptor antagonists. Eur J Pharmacol 164:445–454, 1989

Kennett GA, Pittaway K, Blackburn TP: Evidence that 5-HT2C receptor antagonists are anxiolytic in the rat Geller-Seifter model of anxiety. Psychopharmacology 114:90–96, 1994

Keppel Hesselink JM: Promising anxiolytics? A new class of drugs: the azapirones, in Serotonin 1A Receptors in Depression and Anxiety. Edited by Stahl SM, Gastpar M, Keppel Hesselink JM, et al. New York, Raven, 1992, p 171

Kerkhofs M, Rielaert C, de Maertelaer V, et al: Fluoxetine in major depression: efficacy, safety and effects on sleep polygraphic variables. Int Clin Psychopharmacol 5:253–260, 1990

Kessler R, McGonagle K, Zhao S, et al: Lifetime and 12-month prevalence of DSM-III-R psychiatric disorders in the United States. Arch Gen Psychiatry 51:8–19, 1994

Ketter TA, Pazzaglia PJ, Post RM: Synergy of carbamazepine and valproic acid in affective illness: case report and review of literature. J Clin Psychopharmacol 12:276–281, 1992

Ketter TA, Flockhart DA, Post RM, et al: The emerging role of cytochrome P450 3A in psychopharmacology. J Clin Psychopharmacol 15:387–398, 1995

Ketter TA, Kimbrell TA, George MS, et al: Baseline hypermetabolism may predict carbamazepine response, and hypometabolism nimodipine response in mood disorders (abstract). Paper presented at the 20th CINP Congress, Melbourne, Australia, June 1996

Keynes RS, Swan RC: The permeability of frog muscle fibers to lithium ions. J Physiol 147:626–638, 1959

Khanna S: Carbamazepine in obsessive-compulsive disorder. Clin Neuropharmacol 11:478–481, 1988

Khanna S, Gangadhar BN, Sinha V, et al: Electroconvulsive therapy in obsessive-compulsive disorder. Convulsive Therapy 4:314–320, 1988

Kim CK, Pinel JP, Hudda MM, et al: Tolerance to the anticonvulsant effects of phenobarbital, trimethadione, and clonazepam in kindled rats: cross tolerance to carbamazepine. Pharmacol Biochem Behav 41:115–120, 1992

Kim MH, Neubig RR: Membrane reconstitution of high affinity alpha-2-adrenergic agonist binding with guanine nucleotide regulatory proteins. Biochemistry 26:3664–3672, 1987

Kim SW: Trazodone in the treatment of obsessive-compulsive disorder: a case report. J Clin Psychopharmacol 7:278–279, 1987

Kim SW, Dysken MW, Pandey GN, et al: Platelet 3H-imipramine binding sites in OC behavior. Biol Psychiatry 30:467–474, 1991

Kindler S, Shapira B, Hadjez J, et al: Factors influencing response to bilateral electroconvulsive therapy in major depression. Convulsive Therapy 7:245–254, 1991

Kirch DG, Alho AM, Wyatt RJ: Hypothesis: a nicotine-dopamine interaction linking smoking with Parkinson's disease and tardive dyskinesia. Cell Mol Neurobiol 8:285–291, 1988

Kirkegaard C: The thyrotropin response to thyrotropin-releasing hormone in endogenous depression. Psychoneuroendocrinology 6:189–212, 1981

Kirkwood C, Moore A, Hayes P, et al: Influence of the menstrual cycle and gender on alprazolam pharmacokinetics. Clin Pharmacol Ther 50:404–409, 1991

Kishimoto A, Okuma T: Antimanic and prophylactic effects of carbamazepine in affective disorders, in Biological Psychiatry 1985. Edited by Shagass C, Josiassen RC, Bridger WH, et al. New York, Elsevier, 1986, pp 883–885

Kishimoto H, Takazu O, Ohno S, et al: ^{11}C-glucose metabolism in manic and depressed patients. Psychiatry Res 22:81–88, 1987

Kislauskis E, Dobner PR: Mutually dependent response elements in the cis-regulatory region of the neurotensin/neuromedin N gene integrate environmental stimuli in PC12 cells. Neuron 4:783–795, 1990

Kiwit JC, Hertel A, Matuschek AE: Reversal of chemoresistance in malignant gliomas by calcium antagonists: correlation with the expression of multidrug-resistant p-glycoprotein. J Neurosurg 81:587–594, 1994

Klaiber EL, Broverman DM, Vogel W, et al: Estrogen therapy for persistant depression in women. Arch Gen Psychiatry 36:550–554, 1979

Klawans HL, Weiner WJ, Nausieda PA: The effect of lithium on an animal model of tardive dyskinesia. Prog Neuropsychopharmacol 1:53–60, 1976

Klein DF: Delineation of two drug-responsive anxiety syndromes. Psychopharmacologia 5:397–408, 1964

Klein DF: Anxiety reconceptualized. Compr Psychiatry 21:411–427, 1980

Klein DF: False suffocation alarms, spontaneous panics, and related conditions: an integrative hypothesis. Arch Gen Psychiatry 50:306–317, 1993

Klein DF, Fink M: Psychiatric reaction patterns to imipramine. Am J Psychiatry 119:432–438, 1962

Klein E, Bental E, Lerer B, et al: Carbamazepine and haloperidol vs. placebo and haloperidol in excited psychoses. Arch Gen Psychiatry 41:165–170, 1984a

Klein E, Hefez A, Lavie P: Effects of clomipramine infusion on sleep in depressed patients. Neuropsychobiology 1:85–88, 1984b

Klein E, Lavie P, Meiraz R, et al: Increased motor activity and recurrent manic episodes: risk factors that predict rapid relapse in remitted bipolar disorder patients after lithium discontinuation—a double blind study. Biol Psychiatry 31:279–284, 1992

Klein PS, Melton DA: A molecular mechanism for the effect of lithium on development. Proc Natl Acad Sci U S A 93:8455–8459, 1996

Klein RG: Is panic disorder associated with childhood separation anxiety disorder? Clin Neuropharmacol 18 (suppl 2):S7–S14, 1995

Klemfuss H, Kripke DF: Effects of lithium on circadian rhythms, in Chronopharmacology, Cellular and Biochemical Interactions. Edited by Lemmer B. New York, Marcel Dekker, 1989, pp 281–297

Klepner CA, Lippa AS, Benson DI, et al: Resolution of two biochemically and pharmacologically distinct benzodiazepine receptors. Pharmacol Biochem Behav 11:457–462, 1979

Klerman GL: Treatments for panic disorder. J Clin Psychiatry 53 (suppl):14–19, 1992

Klerman GL, Weissman MM: The course, morbidity, and costs of depression. Arch Gen Psychiatry 49:831–834, 1992

Klerman GL, DiMascio A, Weissman MM, et al: Treatment of depression by drugs and psychotherapy. Am J Psychiatry 131:186–191, 1984

Kleven MS, Seiden LS: D-, L- and DL-fenfluramine cause long-lasting depletions of serotonin in rat brain. Brain Res 505:351–353, 1989

Kligman D, Marshak D: Purification and characterization of a neurite extension factor from bovine brain. Proc Natl Acad Sci U S A 82:7136–7139, 1985

Klimek V, Maj J: Repeated administration of antidepressants enhances agonist affinity for mesolimbic D_2 receptors. J Pharm Pharmacol 41:555–558, 1989

Klinkhamer P, Szelies B, Heiss WD: Effect of phosphatidylserine on cerebral glucose metabolism in Alzheimer's disease. Dementia 1:197–201, 1990

Knapp MJ, Knoppman DS, Solomon PR, et al: A 30-week randomized controlled trial of high-dose tacrine in patients with Alzheimer's disease. JAMA 271:985–991, 1994

Knesevich JW: Successful treatment of obsessive-compulsive disorder with clonidine hydrochloride. Am J Psychiatry 139:364–365, 1982

Knowles JB, Cairns J, McLean AW, et al: The sleep of remitted bipolar depressives: comparison with sex and age-matched controls. Can J Psychiatry 31:295–298, 1986

Knusel B, Beck KD, Winslow JW, et al: Brain-derived neurotrophic factor administration protects basal forebrain cholinergic but not nigral dopaminergic neurons from degenerative changes after axotomy in the adult rat brain. J Neurosci 12:4391–4402, 1992

Knutti R, Rothweiler H, Schlatter C: Effect of pregnancy on the pharmacokinetics of caffeine. Eur J Clin Pharmacol 21:121–126, 1981

Kocsis JH, Francis AJ: A critical discussion of DSM-III dysthymia disorder. Am J Psychiatry 144:1534–1542, 1987

Kocsis JH, Croughan JL, Katz MM, et al: Response to treatment with antidepressants of patients with severe or moderate nonpsychotic depression and of patients with psychotic depression. Am J Psychiatry 147:621–4, 1990

Koczkas S, Weissman A: A pilot study of the effect of the 5-HT-uptake inhibitor, zimeldine, on phobic anxiety. Acta Psychiatr Scand 290:328–341, 1981

Koenig JI, Meltzer HY, Gudelsky GA: Alterations of hormonal responses following lithium treatment in the rat. Proceedings of the 8th International Congress of Endocrinology, 1984, p 1037

Koenigsberg HW, Pollak CP, Fine J, et al: Cardiac and respiratory activity in panic disorder: effects of sleep and sleep lactate infusions. Am J Psychiatry 151:1148–1152, 1994

Kofman O, Belmaker RH: Intracerebroventricular myo-inositol antagonizes lithium-induced suppression of rearing behaviour in rats. Brain Research 534:345–347, 1990

Kofman O, Belmaker RH: Biochemical, behavioral and clinical studies of the role of inositol in lithium treatment and depression. Biol Psychiatry 34:839–852, 1993

Kofman O, Belmaker RH, Grisaru N, et al: Myo-inositol attenuates two specific behavioral effects of accute lithium in rats. Psychopharmacol Bull 27:185–190, 1991

Kofman O, Sherman WR, Katz V, et al: Restoration of brain myo-inositol levels in rats increases latency to lithium-pilocarpine seizures. Psychopharmacology 10:229–234, 1993

Koizumi HM: Obsessive-compulsive symptoms following stimulants. Biol Psychiatry 20:1332–1333, 1985

Kokate TG, Svensson BE, Rogawski MA: Anticonvulsant activity of neurosteroids: correlation with g-aminobutyric acid-evoked chloride current potentiation. J Pharmacol Exp Ther 270:1223–1229, 1994

Kokka N, Sapp DW, Witte U, et al: Sex difference in sensitivity to pentylenetetrazol but not GABAa receptor binding. Pharmacol Biochem Behav 43:441–447, 1992

Kolbinger HM, Hoflich G, Hufnagel A, et al: Transcranial magnetic stimulation (TMS) in the treatment of major depression—a pilot study. Human Psychopharmacology 10:305–310, 1995

Kook KA, Stimmel GL, Wilkins JN, et al: Accuracy and safety of a priori lithium loading. J Clin Psychiatry 46:49–51, 1985

Kopala L, Honer WG: Risperidone, serotonergic mechanisms, and obsessive-compulsive symptoms in schizophrenia (letter). Am J Psychiatry 151: 1714–1715, 1994

Kopelman MD: The cholinergic neurotransmitter system in human memory and dementia: a review. Q J Exp Psychol A 38:535–573, 1986

Kopelman MD, Corn TH: Cholinergic 'blockade' as a model for cholinergic depletion: a comparison of the memory deficits with those of Alzheimer-type dementia and the alcoholic Korsakoff syndrome. Brain 111:1079–1110, 1988

Kordower JH, Le HK, Mufson EJ: Galanin immunoreactivity in the primate central nervous system. J Comp Neurol 319:479–500, 1992

Kornstein SG, Yonkers KA, Schatzberg A, et al: Premenstrual exacerbation of depression. Poster presentation at the 35th annual meeting of the NCDEU, Orlando, FL, 1995

Korte M, Carroll P, Wolf E, et al: Hippocampal long-term potentiation is impaired in mice lacking brain-derived neurotrophic factor. Proc Natl Acad Sci U S A 92:8856–8860, 1995

Kosofsky BE, Molliver ME: The serotonergic innervation of cerebral cortex: different classes of axon terminals arise from dorsal and median raphe nuclei. Synapse 1:153–168, 1987

Koszycki D, Bradwejn J, Bourin M: Comparison of the effects of cholecystokinin and carbon dioxide in healthy volunteers. Eur Neuropharmacology 1:137–141, 1991

Koszycki D, Cox BJ, Bradwejn J: Anxiety sensitivity and response to CCK-4 in healthy volunteers. Am J Psychiatry 150:1881–1883, 1993

Koszycki D, Zacharko R, Le Melledo J-M, et al: Effect of acute tryptophan depletion on behavioral, cardiovascular and hormonal sensitivity to cholecystokinin-tetrapeptide challenge in healthy volunteers. Biol Psychiatry 40:648–655, 1996a

Koszycki D, Zacharko R, Bradwejn J: Personality correlates of behavioral response to CCK-4 in patients with panic disorder. Psychiatry Res 62:131–138, 1996b

Koszycki D, Zacharko RM, Le Melledo JM, et al: Behavioral, cardiovascular, and neuroendocrine profiles following CCK-4 challenge in healthy volunteers: a comparison of panickers and nonpanickers. Depress Anxiety 8:1–7, 1998

Kovacs GL: Oxytocin and behavior, in Neurobiology of Oxytocin. Edited by Ganten D, Pfaff D. Heidelberg, Springer-Verlag, 1986, pp 91–120

Kraepelin E: Manic-depressive illness. Edinburgh, Livingstone, 1921

Kral VA: Senescent forgetfulness: benign and malignant. Journal of the Canadian Medical Association 86:257–260, 1962

Kramer MS, Cutler NR, Ballenger JC, et al: A placebo-controlled trial of L-365,260, a CCKB antagonist, in panic disorder. Biol Psychiatry 37:462–466, 1995

Krauss GL, Fisher RS: Cerebellar and thalamic stimulation for epilepsy, in Electrical and Magnetic Stimulation of the Brain and Spinal Cord. Edited by Devinsky O, Beric A. New York, Raven, 1993, pp 231–245

Krell RD, Goldberg AM: Effect of acute and chronic administration of lithium on steady-state levels of mouse brain choline and acetylcholine. Biochem Pharmacol 22:3289–3291, 1973

Krieger C, Jones K, Kim SU, et al: The role of intracellular free calcium in motor-neuron disease. J Neurol Sci 124:27–32, 1994

Kroboth PD, Smith RB, Stoehr GP, et al: Pharmacodynamic evaluation of the benzodiazepine—oral contraceptive interaction. Clin Pharmacol Ther 38:525–532, 1985

Kroessler D: Relative efficacy rates for therapies of delusional depression. Convulsive Therapy 1:173–182, 1985

Krog-Meyer I, Kirkegaard C, Kinje B, et al: Effects of amitriptyline on the thyrotropin response to TRH in endogenous depression. Psychiatry Res 15:145–151, 1985

Krueger RB, Sackeim HA: Electroconvulsive therapy and schizophrenia, in Schizophrenia. Edited by Hirsch SR, Weinberger D. New York, Blackwell, 1995, pp 503–545

Krueger RB, Sackeim HA, Gamzu ER: Pharmacological treatment of the cognitive side effects of ECT: a review. Psychopharmacol Bull 28:409–424, 1992

Krueger RB, Fama JM, Devanand DP, et al: Does ECT permanently alter seizure threshold? Biol Psychiatry 33:272–276, 1993

Krystal AD, Weiner RD, McCall WV, et al: The effects of ECT stimulus dose and electrode placement on the ictal electroencephalogram: an intraindividual crossover study. Biol Psychiatry 34:759–767, 1993

Krystal AD, Weiner RD, Coffey CE: The ictal EEG as a marker of adequate stimulus intensity with unilateral ECT. J Neuropsychiatry Clin Neurosci 7:295–303, 1995

Ksir C, Benson D: Enhanced behavioral response to nicotine in an animal model of Alzheimer's disease. Psychopharmacology 81:272–273, 1983

Ktonas PY: Period amplitude EEG analysis. Sleep 10:505–507, 1987

Kuhar MJ: Recent progress in dopamine transporter research (abstract). Eur Neuropsychopharmacol 4:248–249, 1994

Kumar KB, Nalini K, Karanth KS: Effects of p-chlorophenylalamine induced depletion of brain serotonin on retrieval of appetitive and aversive memories. Indian J Exp Biol 33:837–840, 1995

Kunik ME, Puryear L, Orengo CA, et al: The efficacy and tolerability of divalproex sodium in elderly demented patients with behavioral disturbances. Int J Geriatr Psychiatry 13:29–34, 1998

Kunovac JL, Stahl SM: Biochemical pharmacology of serotonin receptor subtypes: hypothesis for clinical applications of selective serotonin ligands. International Review of Psychiatry 7:55–67, 1995

Kupfer DJ: REM latency: a psychobiologic marker for primary depressive disease. Biol Psychiatry 1:159–174, 1976

Kupfer DJ: Neurophysiological "markers"—EEG sleep measures. J Psychiatry Res 18:467–475, 1984

Kupfer DJ: Long-term treatment of depression. J Clin Psychiatry 52 (suppl 5):28–34, 1991

Kupfer DJ: Maintenance treatment in recurrent depression: current and future directions: the first William Sargant Lecture. Br J Psychiatry 161:309–316, 1992

Kupfer DJ, Bowers MB: REM sleep and central monoamine oxidase inhibition. Psychopharmacologia 27:183–190, 1972

Kupfer DJ, Foster FG: EEG sleep and depression, in Sleep Disorders: Diagnosis and Treatment. Edited by Williams RL, Karacan I. New York, Wiley, 1978, pp 163–204

Kupfer DJ, Himmelhoch JM, Schwartzberg M, et al: Hypersomnia in manic-depressive disease. Diseases of the Nervous System 33:720–724, 1972

Kupfer DJ, Spiker DG, Coble P, et al: Amitriptyline and EEG sleep in depressed patients, I: drug effects. Sleep 1:149–159, 1978

Kupfer DJ, Coble P, Kane J, et al: Imipramine and EEG sleep in children with depressive symptoms. Psychopharmacology 60:117–123, 1979

Kupfer DJ, Broudy D, Coble PA, et al: EEG sleep and affective psychosis. J Affect Disord 2:17–25, 1980

Kupfer DJ, Spiker DG, Rossi A, et al: Nortriptyline and EEG sleep in depressed patients. Biol Psychiatry 17:535–546, 1982a

Kupfer DJ, Spiker DG, Rossi A, et al: Recent diagnostic and treatment advances in REM sleep and depression, in Treatment of Depression: Old Controversies and New Approaches. Edited by Clayton P, Barrett J. New York, Raven, 1982b, pp 31–35

Kupfer DJ, Ulrich RF, Coble PA, et al: Application of automated REM and slow wave sleep analysis, I: normal and depressed subjects. Psychiatry Res 13:325–334, 1984

Kupfer DJ, Grochocinski VJ, McEachran AB: Relationship of awakening and delta sleep in depression. Psychiatry Res 19:297–304, 1986

Kupfer DJ, Ehlers CJ, Pollock BG, et al: Clomipramine and EEG sleep in depression. Psychiatry Res 30:165–180, 1989a

Kupfer DJ, Reynolds CF III, Ehlers CL: Comparison of EEG sleep measures among depressive subtypes and controls in older individuals. Psychiatry Res 27:13–21, 1989b

Kupfer DJ, Frank E, Ehlers CL: EEG sleep in young depressives: first and second night effects. Biol Psychiatry 25:87–97, 1989c

Kupfer DJ, Frank E, McEachran AB, et al: Delta sleep ratio. Arch Gen Psychiatry 47:1100–1105, 1990

Kupfer DJ, Perel JM, Pollock BG, et al: Fluvoxamine versus desipramine: comparative polysomnographic effects. Biol Psychiatry 29:23–40, 1991

Kupfer DJ, Frank E, Perel JM, et al: Five-year outcome for maintenance therapies in recurrent depression. Arch Gen Psychiatry 49:769–773, 1992

Kupfer DJ, Ehlers CL, Frank E, et al: Persistent effects of antidepressants: EEG sleep studies in depressed patients during maintenance treatment. Biol Psychiatry 35:781–793, 1994

Kusumi I, Koyama T, Yamashita I: Thrombin-induced platelet calcium mobilization is enhanced in bipolar disorders. Biol Psychiatry 32:731–734, 1992

Kutsuwada T, Kashiwabuchi N, Mori X, et al: Molecular diversity of the NMDA receptor channel. Nature 358:36–41, 1992

Laakso ML, Oja SS: Transport of tryptophan and tyrosine in rat brain slices in the presence of lithium. Neurochem Res 4:411–423, 1979

Lacroix C, Fiet J, Benais JP, et al: Simultaneous radioimmunoassay of progesterone, androst-4-ene-dione, pregnenolone, dehydroepiandrosterone and 17-hydroxyprogesterone in specific regions of human brain. J Steroid Biochem 28:317–325, 1987

Ladd CO, Owens MJ, Nemeroff CB: Persistent changes in corticotropin-releasing factor neuronal system induced by maternal deprivation. Endocrinology 137:1–7, 1996

Lader M: Ondansetron in the treatment of anxiety, in Biological Psychiatry: Proceedings of the 5th World Congress of Biological Psychiatry, Florence, Italy, June 9–14, 1991. Edited by Racagni G, Brunello N, Fukuda T. New York, Excerpta Medica, 1991

Lagarde D, Laurent J, Milhaud C, et al: Behavioral effects induced by beta CCE in free or restrained rhesus monkeys (Macaca mulatta). Pharmacol Biochem Behav 35:713–719, 1990

Lalonde R, Vikis-Freibergs V: Manipulations of 5-hydroxytryptamine activity and memory in the rat. Pharmacol Biochem Behav 22:377–382, 1985

Lam HR, Christensen S: Regional and subcellular localization of Li^+ and other cations in the rat brain following long-term lithium administration. J Neurochem 59:1372–1380, 1992

Lambert PA: Acute and prophylactic therapies of patients with affective disorders using valpromide (dipropylacetamide), in Anticonvulsants in Affective Disorders. Edited by Emrich HM, Okuma T, Müller AA. Amsterdam, Excerpta Medica, 1984, pp 56–65

Lambert PA, Cavaz G, Borselli S, et al: Action neuropsychotrop d'un nouvel anti-epileptique: Le Dépamide. Ann Med Psychol (Paris) 1:707–710, 1966

Lan NC, Gee KW, Bolger MB, et al: Differential responses to expressed recombinant human g-aminobutyric acid A receptors to neurosteroids. J Neurochem 57:1818–1821, 1991

Landgraf R, Gerstberger R, Montkowski A, et al: V1 vasopressin receptor antisense oligo-deoxynucleotide into septum reduces vasopressin binding, social discrimination abilities, and anxiety-related behavior in rats. J Neurosci 15:4250–4258, 1995

Lange C: Om Periodiske Depressionstilstande og deres Patogenese. Copenhagen, Jacob Lunds Forlag, 1886

Langer G, Konig G, Hatzinger R, et al: Response of thyrotropin to TRH as a predictor of treatment outcome: prediction of recovery and relapse in treatment with antidepressants. Arch Gen Psychiatry 43:861–868, 1986

Langer SZ: Presynaptic regulation of the release of catecholamines. Biochem Pharmacol 23:1793–1800, 1974

Langer SZ, Arbilla S, Benavides J, et al: Zolpidem and alpidem: two imidazopyridines with selectivity for omega-1 and omega-3 receptor subtypes, in GABA and Benzodiazepine Receptor Subtypes. Edited by Biggio G, Costa E. New York, Raven, 1990, p 61

Lanthier A, Patwardhan VV: Sex steroids and 5-en-3β-hydroxysteroids in specific regions of human brain and plasma. J Steroid Biochem 25:445–449, 1986

Lapierre YD: Pharmacological therapy of dysthymia. Acta Psychiatr Scand Suppl 383:42–48, 1994

Lapierre YD, Browne M, Horn E, et al: Treatment of major affective disorder with fluvoxamine. J Clin Psychiatry 48:65–68, 1987

Lapierre YD, Ravindran AV, Bakish D: Dysthymia and serotonin. Int Clin Psychopharmacol 8 (suppl 2):87–90, 1993

Lapin I, Oxenkrug G: Intensification of the central serotonergic process as a possible determinant of thymoleptic effect. Lancet 1:132–136, 1969

Larkin JG, McKee PJ, Blacklaw J, et al: Nimodipine in refractory epilepsy: a placebo-controlled, add-on study. Epilepsy Res 9:71–77, 1991

Larsson LI, Rehfeld JF: Localization and molecular heterogeneity of cholecystokinin in the central and peripheral nervous system. Brain Res 165:201–218, 1979

Laruelle M, Abi-Dargham A, Casanova M, et al: Selective abnormality of prefrontal serotonergic receptors in schizophrenia: a post mortem study. Arch Gen Psychiatry 50:810–818, 1993

Lauer CJ, Schreiber W, Holsboer F, et al: In quest of identifying vulnerability markers for psychiatric disorders by all-night polysomnography. Arch Gen Psychiatry 52:145–153, 1995

Lavretsky H, Sultzer D: A structured trial of risperidone for the treatment of agitation in dementia. Am J Geriatr Psychiatry 6:127–135, 1998

Lawlor BA, Sunderland T, Mellow AM, et al: Hyper responsivity to the serotonin agonist m-chlorophenylpiperazine in Alzheimer's disease: a controlled study. Arch Gen Psychiatry 46:542–549, 1989a

Lawlor BA, Sunderland T, Mellow AM, et al: A preliminary study of the effects of intravenous m-chlorophenylpiperazine, a serotonin agonist, in elderly subjects. Biol Psychiatry 25:679–686, 1989b

Lawton BP, Brody EM: Assessment of older people. Self-maintaining and instrumental activities of daily living. Gerontology 9:176–186, 1969

Le Goascogne C, Robel P, Gouezou M, et al: Neurosteroids: cytochrome P450scc in rat brain. Science 237:1212–1214, 1987

Le Houezec J, Halliday R, Benowitz NL, et al: A low dose of nicotine improves information processing in non-smokers. Psychopharmacology 114:628–634, 1994

Leber P: Guidelines for the Clinical Examination of Antidementia Drugs. Washington, DC, Food and Drug Administration, 1991

Leckman JF, Weissman MM, Prusoff BA, et al: Subtypes of depression: family study perspective. Arch Gen Psychiatry 41:833–838, 1984

Leckman JF, Hardin MT, Riddle MA, et al: Clonidine treatment of Gilles de la Tourette syndrome. Arch Gen Psychiatry 48:324–328, 1991

Leckman JF, Goodman WK, North WG, et al: The role of central oxytocin in obsessive compulsive disorder and related normal behavior. Psychoneuroendocrinology 19(8):723–749, 1994

Leckman JF, Pauls DL, Cohen DJ: Tic disorders, in Psychopharmacology: The Fourth Generation of Progress. Edited by Bloom FE, Kupfer DJ. New York, Raven, 1995, pp 1665–1674

Lecrubier Y, Judge R: Long-term evaluation of paroxetine, clomipramine and placebo in panic disorder. Acta Psychiatr Scand 95:153–160, 1997

Lecrubier Y, Puech AJ, Azcona A, et al: A randomized double-blind placebo-controlled study of tropisetron in the treatment of outpatients with generalized anxiety disorder. Psychopharmacology 112:129, 1993

Lecrubier Y, Pletan Y, Selles A, et al: Clinical efficacy of milnacipran: placebo-controlled trials. Int Clin Psychopharmacol 11 (suppl 4):29–34, 1996

Lecrubier Y, Bakker A, Dunbar G, et al: A comparison of paroxetine, clomipramine and placebo in the treatment of panic disorder. Acta Psychiatr Scand 95:145–152, 1997

LeDoux JE: Brain mechanisms of emotion and emotional learning. Curr Opin Neurobiol 2:191–197, 1992

Lee G, Lingsch C, Lyle PT, et al: Lithium treatment strongly inhibits choline transport in human erythrocytes. Br J Clin Pharmacol 1:365–370, 1974

Lee KF, Li E, Huber J, et al: Targeted mutation of the gene encoding the low affinity NGF receptor p75 leads to deficits in the peripheral nervous system. Cell 69:737–749, 1992

Lee M, Strahlendorf JC, Strahlendorf HK: Modulatory action of serotonin on glutamate induced excitation of cerebellar Purkinje cells. Brain Res 361:107–113, 1986

Lee PN: Smoking and Alzheimer's disease: a review of the epidemiologic evidence. Neuroepidemiology 13:131–144, 1994

Lee YM, Beinborn M, McBride EW, et al: The human brain cholecystokinin-B/gastrin receptor: cloning and characterization. J Biol Chem 268:8164–8169, 1993

Legris P, George Y, Boval P, et al: A comparative study of alpidem versus buspirone, in Imidazopyridines in Anxiety Disorders: A Novel Experimental and Therapeutic Approach. Edited by Bartholini G, Garreau M, Morselli PL. New York, Raven, 1993, pp 183–192

Leis AA, Kofler M, Stokic DS, et al: Effect of the inhibitory phenomenon following magnetic stimulation of cortex on brainstem motor neuron excitability and on the cortical control of brainstem reflexes. Muscle Nerve 16:1351–1358, 1993

Lemke MR: Effect of carbamazepine on agitation in Alzheimer's inpatients refractory to neuroleptics. J Clin Psychiatry 56:354–357, 1995

Lemus CZ, Robinson DG, Kronig M, et al: Behavioral responses to a dopaminergic challenge in obsessive-compulsive disorder. J Anxiety Disord 5:369–373, 1991

Lena C, Changeux JP: Allosteric modulations of the nicotinic acetylcholine receptor. Trends Neurosci 16:181–186, 1993

Lenox RH, Manji HK: Lithium, in The American Psychiatric Press Textbook of Psychopharmacology. Edited by Nemeroff C, Schatzberg A. Washington, DC, American Psychiatric Press, 1995, pp 303–349

Lenox RH, Watson DG: Lithium and the brain: a psychopharmacological strategy to a molecular basis for manic-depressive illness. Clin Chem 40(2):309–314, 1994

Lenox RH, Watson DG, Patel J, et al: Chronic lithium administration alters a prominent PKC substrate in rat hippocampus. Brain Res 570:333–340, 1992

Lenzi A, Lazzerini F, Grossi E, et al: Use of carbamazepine in acute psychosis: a controlled study. J Int Med Res 14:78–84, 1986

Leonard BE: Commentary on the mode of action of benzodiazepines. J Psychiatr Res 27 (suppl 1):193, 1993

Leonard BE, Song C: The effects of the central administration of neuropeptide Y on behaviour, neurotransmitter and immune functions in the olfactory bulbectomized rat model of depression (abstract). Paper presented at the 33rd annual meeting of the American College of Neuropsychopharmacology, San Juan, Puerto Rico, December 1994

Leonard HL, Swedo SE, Koby E, et al: Treatment of OCD with CMI and desmethylimipramine in children and adolescents. Arch Gen Psychiatry 46:1088–1092, 1989

Leonard HL, Swedo SE, Lenane MC, et al: A double-blind desipramine substitution during long-term CMI treatment in children adolescents with OCD. Arch Gen Psychiatry 48:922–927, 1991

Leonard HL, Topol D, Bukstein O, et al: Clonazepam as an augmenting agent in the treatment of childhood-onset obsessive-compulsive disorder. J Am Acad Child Adolesc Psychiatry 33:792–794, 1994

Lepine J, Gastpar M, Mendlewiez J, et al: Depression in the community: the first pan-European study DEPRES (Depression Research in European Society). Int Clin Psychopharmacol 12(1):19–29, 1997

Lerer B: Neurochemical and other neurobiological consequences of ECT: implications for the pathogenesis and treatment of affective disorders, in Psychopharmacology, The Third Generation of Progress. Edited by Meltzer HY. New York, Raven, 1987, pp 577–588

Lerer B, Stanley M: Effect of chronic lithium on cholinergically mediated responses and [3H]QNB binding in rat brain. Brain Res 344:211–219, 1985

Lerer B, Weiner RD, Belmaker RH: Introduction, in ECT: Basic Mechanisms. Edited by Lerer B, Weiner RD, Belmaker RH. London, John Libbey, 1984, pp 1–4

Lerer B, Moore N, Meyendorff E, et al: Carbamazepine versus lithium in mania: a double-blind study. J Clin Psychiatry 48:89–93, 1987

Lerer B, Shapira B, Calev A, et al: Antidepressant and cognitive effects of twice- versus three-times-weekly ECT. Am J Psychiatry 152:564–570, 1995

Lesch KP, Manji HK: Signal-transducing G proteins and antidepressant drugs: evidence for modulation of alpha subunit gene expression in rat brain. Biol Psychiatry 32:549–579, 1992

Letemendia FJJ, Delva NJ, Rodenburg M, et al: Therapeutic advantage of bifrontal electrode placement in ECT. Psychol Med 23:349–360, 1993

Letty S, Child R, Dumis A, et al: 5-HT$_4$ receptors improve social olfactory memory in the rat. Neuropharmacology 36:681–687, 1997

Levin E: Nicotinic systems and cognitive function. Psychopharmacology 108:417–431, 1992

Levin E, Rose JE: Anticholinergic sensitivity following chronic nicotine administration as measured by radial-arm maze performance in rats. Behav Pharmacol 1:511–520, 1990

Levin E, Castonguay M, Ellison GD: Effects of the nicotinic receptor blocker mecamylamine on radial arm maze performance in rats. Behavioral and Neural Biology 48:206–212, 1987

Levin E, McGurk SR, Rose JE, et al: Cholinergic-dopaminergic interactions in cognitive performance. Behavioral and Neural Biology 54:271–299, 1990

Levin E, McGurk SR, Rose JE, et al: Reversal of a mecamylamine-induced cognitive deficit with the D$_2$ agonist, LY 171555. Pharmacol Biochem Behav 33:919–922, 1992

Levin E, Connors CK, Sparrow E, et al: Nicotine effects in attention deficit hyperactivity disorder. Paper presented at 1st annual meeting, Society for Research on Nicotine and Tobacco, San Diego, March 24–25, 1995

Levine J, Rapaport A, Lev L, et al: Inositol treatment raises CSF inositol levels. Brain Res 627:168–170, 1993

Levine J, Pomerantz T, Belmaker RH: The effect of inositol on cognitive processes and mood states in normal volunteers. Eur Neuropsychopharmacol 4:418–419, 1994

Levine J, Barak Y, Gonsalves M, et al: A double-blind controlled trial of inositol treatment of depression. Am J Psychiatry 152:792–794, 1995a

Levine J, Pomerantz T, Stier S, et al: Lack of effect of 6 g inositol treatment on post-ECT cognitive function in humans. J Psychiatr Res 29:487–489, 1995b

Levy A, Zohar J, Belmaker RH: The effect of chronic lithium pretreatment on rat brain muscarinic receptor regulation. Neuropharmacology 21:1199–1201, 1983

Levy AB, Dixon KN, Schmidt H: Sleep architecture in anorexia nervosa and bulimia. Biol Psychiatry 23:99–101, 1988

Lewis PR, Shute CCD: The cholinergic limbic system. Brain 90:521–540, 1967

Lewy AJ, Nurnberger JI, Wehr TA: Supersensitivity to light: possible trait marker for manic-depressive illness. Am J Psychiatry 142:725–727, 1985

Lewy AJ, Hughes RJ, Bauer VK, et al: Melatonin modulation of brain and behavior: clinical aspects, in Hormonal Modulation of Brain and Behavior. Edited by Halbreich U. Washington, DC, American Psychiatric Press (in press)

Leysen D, Pinder RM: Toward third generation antidepressants. Annual Report in Medicinal Chemistry 29:1–12, 1994

Leysen JE: 5HT2-Receptors: location, pharmacological, pathological and physiological role, in Serotonin Receptor Subtypes: Pharmacological Significance and Clinical Implications. Edited by Langer SZ, Brunello N, Racagni G, et al. International Academy for Biomedical and Drug Research. Basel, Switzerland, Karger, 1992, pp 31–43

Li PP, Tam YK, Young LT, et al: Lithium decreases Gs, Gi-1 and Gi-2 alpha-subunit mRNA levels in rat cortex. Eur J Pharmacol 206:165–166, 1991

Lieblich I, Yirmiya R: Naltrexone reverses a long term depressive effect of a toxic lithium injection on saccharin preference. Physiol Behav 39:547–550, 1987

Liebowitz MR: Social phobia. Mod Probl Pharmacopsychiatry 22:141–173, 1987

Liebowitz MR, Quitkin FM, Stewart JW, et al: Phenelzine vs. imipramine in atypical depression: a preliminary report. Arch Gen Psychiatry 41:669–677, 1984

Liebowitz MR, Quitkin FM, Stewart JW, et al: Antidepressant specificity in atypical depression. Arch Gen Psychiatry 45:129–137, 1988

Liebowitz MR, Schneier F, Campeas R, et al: Phenelzine vs atenolol in social phobia. Arch Gen Psychiatry 49:290–300, 1992

Liebowitz MR, Coplan JD, Martinez J, et al: Effects of intravenous diazepam pretreatment on lactate-induced panic. Psychiatry Res 58:127–138, 1995

Liebsch G, Landgraf R, Gerstberger R, et al: Chronic infusion of a CRH_1 receptor antisense oligodeoxynucleotide into the central nucleus of the amygdala reduced anxiety-related behavior in socially defeated rats. Regul Pept 59:229–239, 1995

Liljenberg B, Almwvist M, Hetta J, et al: Affective disturbance and insomnia: a population study. Eur J Psychiatry 3(2):91–98, 1989

Limouzin-Lamothe M, Mairon N, LeGal J, et al: Quality of life after the menopause: influence of hormonal replacement therapy. Am J Obstet Gynecol 170:618–624, 1994

Lin A, Smeal T, Binetruy B, et al: Control of AP-1 activity by signal transduction cascades. Adv Second Messenger Phosphoprotein Res 28:255–260, 1993

Lindefors N, Linden A, Brene S, et al: CCK peptides and mRNA in the human brain. Prog Neurobiol 40:671–690, 1993

Lindelius R, Nilsson CG: Flunarizine as maintenance treatment of a patient with bipolar disorder. Am J Psychiatry 149:139, 1992

Lindenmayer J-P, Bernstein-Hyman R, Grochowski S: Five-factor model of schizophrenia. J Nerv Ment Disord 182:631–638, 1994

Lingsch C, Martin K: An irreversible effect of lithium administration to patients. Br J Pharmacol 57:323–327, 1976

Linnoila M, Karoum F, Rosenthal N, et al: Electroconvulsive treatment and lithium carbonate. Arch Gen Psychiatry 40:677–680, 1983

Linnoila M, Miller TL, Barko J, et al: Five antidepressant treatments in depressed patients. Arch Gen Psychiatry 41:688–692, 1984

Linville DG, Arneric SP: Cortical cerebral blood flow governed by the basal forebrain: age related impairments. Neurobiol Aging 12:503–510, 1991

Linville DG, Williams S, Arneric SP: Basal forebrain control of cortical cerebral blood flow is independent of local cortical neurons. Brain Res 622:26–34, 1993

Lipsedge MS, Prothero W: Clonidine and clomipramine in obsessive-compulsive disorder. Am J Psychiatry 144:965–966, 1987

Lisanby SH, Devanand DP, Prudic J, et al: Prolactin response to electroconvulsive therapy: effects of electrode placement and stimulus dosage. Biol Psychiatry 43:146–155, 1998

Lishman WA: Intracranial infections, in Organic Psychiatry: The Psychological Consequences of Cerebral Disorder, 2nd Edition. Edited by Lishman WA. London, Blackwell Scientific, 1987a, pp 289–313

Lishman WA: The senile dementias, presenile dementias and pseudodementias, in Organic Psychiatry: The Psychological Consequences of Cerebral Disorder, 2nd Edition. Edited by Lishman WA. London, Blackwell Scientific, 1987b, pp 370–427

Lishman WA (ed): Organic Psychiatry: The Psychological Consequences of Cerebral Disorder, 3rd Edition. London, Blackwell Scientific, 1998

Lister RG: Anxiety and cognition, in New Concepts in Anxiety. Edited by Briley M, File SE. Basingstoke, England, Macmillan, 1991, pp 64–79

Lister RG, Karanian JW: RO15–4513 induces seizures in DBA/2 mice undergoing alcohol withdrawal. Alcohol 4:409–411, 1987

Lister RG, Weingartner H: Neuropharmacological strategies for understanding psychobiological determinants of cognition. Hum Neurobiol 6:119–127, 1987

Litman RE, Hong WW, Weissman EM, et al: Idazoxan, an alpha-$_2$ antagonist, augments fluphenazine in schizophrenic patients: a pilot study. J Clin Psychopharmacol 13:264–267, 1993

Litman RE, Su TP, Potter WZ, et al: Idazoxan and response to typical neuroleptics in treatment-resistant schizophrenia: comparison with the atypical neuroleptic, clozapine. Br J Psychiatry 168:571–579, 1996

Little A, Levy R, Chuaqui-Kidd P, et al: A double-blind placebo-controlled trial of high-dose lecithin in Alzheimer's disease. J Neurol Neurosurg Psychiatry 12:110–118, 1985

Little JT, Broocks A, Martin A, et al: Serotonergic modulation of anticholinergic effects on cognition and behaviour in elderly humans. Psychopharmacology 120:280–288, 1995

Livingston G, Hawkins A, Graham N, et al: The Gospel Oak study: prevalence rates of dementia, depression and activity limitation among elderly residents in Inner London. Psychol Med 20:137–146, 1990

Livingston-Van Noppen B, Rasmussen SA, Eisen J, et al: Family function and treatment of obsessive-compulsive disorder, in Obsessive-Compulsive Disorders: Theory and Management, 2nd Edition. Edited by Jenike MA, Baer L, Minichiello WE. Littleton, MA, Year Book, 1990, pp 325–340

Lloyd KG, Morselli PL, Bartholini G: GABA and affective disorders. Med Biol 65:159–165, 1987

Lo DC: Neurotrophic factors and synaptic plasticity. Neuron 15:979–981, 1995

Loewenstein RJ, Weingartner H, Gillin JC, et al: Disturbance of sleep and cognitive functioning in patients with dementia. Neurobiol Aging 3:371–377, 1982

Lombroso PJ, Scahill L, King RA, et al: Risperidone treatment of children and adolescents with chronic tic disorders: a preliminary report [see comments] [published erratum appears in J Am Acad Child Adolesc Psychiatry 35:394, 1996]. J Am Acad Child Adolesc Psychiatry 34:1147–1152, 1995

Lonati-Galligani M, Emrich HM, Raptis C, et al: Effect of in vivo lithium treatment on (-) isoproterenol-stimulated cAMP accumulation in lymphocytes of healthy subjects and patients with affective psychoses. Pharmacopsychiatry 22:241–245, 1989

Londborg PD, Wolkow R, Smith WT, et al: Sertraline in the treatment of panic disorder—a multi-site, double-blind, placebo-controlled, fixed-dose investigation. Br J Psychiatry 173:54–60, 1998

London E, Fanelli RJ, Kimes A, et al: Effects of chronic nicotine on cerebral glucose utilization in the rat. Brain Res 520:208–214, 1990

Lonnqvist J, Sihvo S, Syvälahti E, et al: Moclobemide and fluoxetine in atypical depression: a double-blind trial. J Affect Disord 32:169–177, 1994

Loo H, Malka R, Defance R, et al: Tianeptine and amitriptyline: controlled double-blind trial in depressed alcoholic patients. Neuropsychobiology 19:79–85, 1988

López-Ibor JJ Jr: Serotonin and psychiatric disorders. Int Clin Psychopharmacol 7 (suppl 2):5–11, 1992

López-Ibor JJ, Gueli JD, Pletan Y, et al: Milnacipran and selective serotonin reuptake inhibitors in major depression. Int Clin Psychopharmacol 11 (suppl 4):41–46, 1996

Lorr M, Klett CJ, McNair DM, et al: Inpatient Multidimensional Psychiatric Scale. Palo Alto, CA, Consulting Psychologists Press, 1962

Louilot A, Mocaer E, Simon H, et al: Difference in the effects of the antidepressant tianeptine on dopaminergic metabolism in the prefrontal cortex and nucleus accumbens of the rat: a voltametric study. Life Sci 47:1083–1089, 1990

Lovenberg TW, Liaw CW, Grigoriadis DE, et al: Cloning and characterization of a functionally distinct corticotropin-releasing factor receptor subtype from rat brain. Proc Natl Acad Sci U S A 92:836–840, 1995

Lucey JV, Butcher G, Clare AW, et al: The ant pituitary responds normally to protirelin in OCD. Acta Psychiatr Scand 145:1089–1093, 1993

Lucki I, Rickels K, Giesecke MA, et al: Differential effects of the anxiolytic drugs, diazepam and buspirone, on memory function. Br J Clin Pharmacol 23:207–211, 1987

Luetje CW, Patrick J: Both α and β-subunits contribute to the agonist sensitivity of neuronal nicotinic receptors. J Neurosci 11:837–845, 1991

Luine VN, Khylchevskaya RJ, McEwen BS: Effect of gonadal steroids on activities of monoamine oxidase and choline acetylase in rat brain. Brain Res 86:293–306, 1975

Lundberg JM, Terenius L, Hokfelt T, et al: Neuropeptide Y (NPY)-like immunoreactivity in peripheral noradrenergic neurons and effects of NPY on sympathetic function. Acta Physiol Scand 116:477–480, 1982

Lupu-Meiri M, Lipinsky D, Ozaki S, et al: Independent external calcium entry and cellular calcium mobilization in Xenopus oocytes. Cell Calcium 16:20–28, 1994

Lusznat RM, Murphy DP, Nunn CM: Carbamazepine vs lithium in the treatment and prophylaxis of mania. Br J Psychiatry 153:198–204, 1988

Lydiard RB: Obsessive-compulsive disorder successfully treated with trazodone. Psychosomatics 27:858–859, 1986

Lydiard RB: Desipramine in agoraphobia with panic attacks: an open, fixed-dose study. J Clin Psychopharmacol 7:258–260, 1987

Lydiard RB, Laraia MT, Howell EF, et al: Alprazolam in the treatment of social phobia. J Clin Psychiatry 49:17–19, 1988

Lydiard RB, Ballenger JC, Elinwood E, et al: CSF monoamine metabolites in OCD. Paper presented at 143rd annual meeting of the American Psychiatric Association, New York, May 12–17, 1990

Lydiard RB, Ballenger J, Laraia M, et al: CSF cholecystokinin concentrations in patients with panic disorder and normal comparisons subjects. Am J Psychiatry 149:691–693, 1992

Lydiard RB, Brewerton TD, Fossey MD, et al: CSF cholecystokinin octapeptide in patients with bulimia nervosa and in normal comparison subjects. Am J Psychiatry 150:1099–1101, 1993

Lykouras E, Malliaras O, Christodoulou GN, et al: Delusional depression: phenomenology and response to treatment: a prospective study. Acta Psychiatr Scand 73:324–329, 1986

MacDonald PC, Dombroski RA, Casey ML: Recurrent secretion of progesterone in large amounts: an endocrine/metabolic disorder unique to young women? Endocr Rev 12(4):372–401, 1991

MacEwan WG, Remick RA: Treatment resistant depression: a clinical perspective. Can J Psychiatry 33:788–792, 1988

Macher JP, Siechel JP, Serre C, et al: Double-blind placebo-controlled study of milnacipran in hospitalized patients with major depressive disorders. Neuropsychobiology 22:77–82, 1989

Maddock RJ, Carter CS, Blacker KH, et al: Relationship of past depressive episodes to symptom severity and treatment response in panic disorder with agoraphobia. J Clin Psychiatry 54:88–95, 1993

Maeda Y, Hayashi T, Furuta H, et al: Effects of mianserin on human sleep. Neuropsychobiology 24:198–204, 1990

Maggi A, Enna SJ: Regional alterations in rat brain neurotransmitter systems following chronic lithium treatment. J Neurochem 34:888–892, 1980

Maggi A, Perez J: Minireview: role of female gonadal hormones in the CNS: clinical and experimental aspects. Life Sci 37:893–906, 1985

Maitre L, Baltzer V, Mondadori C: Psychopharmacological and behavioural effects of anti-epileptic drugs in animals, in Anticonvulsants in Affective Disorders. Edited by Emrich HM, Okuma T, Muller AA. Amsterdam, Excerpta Medica, 1984, pp 3–13

Maj J, Rogoz Z, Skuza G, et al: Antidepressants given repeatedly increase the behavioural effect of dopamine D_2 agonist. J Neural Transm 78:1–8, 1989

Maj J, Rogoz Z, Skuza G: The effect of combined treatment with MK-801 and antidepressant drugs in the forced swimming test in rats. Polish Journal of Pharmacology and Pharmacy 44:217–226, 1992

Maj M, Pirozzi R, Kemali D: Long-term outcome of lithium prophylaxis in patients initially classified as complete responders. Psychopharmacol Bull 98:535–538, 1989

Majewska MD: Neurosteroids: endogenous bimodal modulators of the $GABA_A$ receptor: mechanisms of action and physiological significance. Prog Neurobiol 38:379–395, 1992

Majewska MD, Schwartz RD: Pregnenolone-sulfate: an endogenous antagonist of the γ-aminobutyric acid receptor complex in brain? Brain Res 404:355–360, 1987

Majewska MD, Harrison NL, Schwartz RD, et al: Steroid hormone metabolites are barbiturate-like modulators of the GABAa receptor. Science 232:1004–1007, 1986

Majewska MD, Ford-Rice F, Falkay G: Pregnancy-induced alterations of GABAa receptor sensitivity in maternal brain: an antecedent of post-partum "blues"? Brain Res 482:397–401, 1989

Majewska MD, Demirgoren S, Spivak CE, et al: Binding of pregenenolone sulfate to rat brain membranes suggests multiple sites of steroid action at the GABAa receptor. Eur J Pharmacol Mol Pharmacol 189:307–315, 1990

Malenka RC, Kauer JA, Perkel DJ, et al: The impact of postsynaptic calcium on synaptic transmission—its role in long-term potentiation. Trends Neurosci 12:444–450, 1989

Maletzky B, McFarland B, Burt A: Refractory obsessive-compulsive disorder and ECT. Convulsive Therapy 10:1:34–42, 1994

Malgaroli A: LTP expression: hanging like a yo-yo? Semin Cell Biol 5:231–241, 1994

Malizia AL, Bridges PK: The management of treatment-resistant affective disorder: clinical perspectives. J Psychopharmacol 6:145–155, 1992

Maller RA, Reiss S: Anxiety sensitivity in 1984 and panic attacks in 1987. J Anxiety Disord 6:241–247, 1992

Mallinger AG, Hanin I, Himmeloch JM, et al: Stimulation of cell membrane sodium transport activity by lithium: possible relationship to therapeutic action. Psychiatry Res 22:49–59, 1987

Mallya GK, White K, Waternaux C, et al: Short and long-term treatment of OCD with fluvoxamine. Ann Clin Psychiatry 4:77–80, 1992

Maltby N, Broe AA, Creasey H, et al: Efficacy of tacrine and lecithin in mild to moderate Alzheimer's disease: double blind trial. BMJ 308:879–893, 1994

Mamounas LA, Wilson MA, Axt KJ, et al: Morphological aspects of serotonergic innervation, in Serotonin, CNS Receptors and Brain Function (Advances in the Biosciences, Vol 85). Edited by Bradley PB, Handley SL, Cooper SJ, et al. Oxford, England, Pergamon, 1992, pp 97–118

Mandel MR, Welch CA, Mieske M, et al: Prediction of response to ECT in tricyclic-intolerant or tricyclic-resistant depressed patients. McLean Hospital Journal 2:203–209, 1977

Mandell AJ, Knapp S, Ehlers C, et al: The stability of constrained randomness: lithium prophylaxis at several neurobiological levels, in Neurobiology of Mood Disorders. Edited by Post RM, Ballenger JC. Baltimore, MD, Williams & Wilkins, 1984, pp 744–776

Manias B, Taylor DA: Inhibition of in vitro amine uptake into rat brain synaptosomes after in vivo administration of antidepressants. Eur J Pharmacol 95:305–309, 1983

Manier DH, Gillespie DD, Sulser E: Dual aminergic regulation of central beta adrenoceptors: effect of "atypical" antidepressants and 5-hydroxytryptophan. Neuropsychopharmacology 2:89–95, 1989

Manji HK: G proteins: implications for psychiatry. Am J Psychiatry 149:746–760, 1992

Manji HK, Lenox RH: Long-term action of lithium: a role for transcriptional and posttranscriptional factors regulated by protein kinase C. Synapse 16:11–28, 1994

Manji HK, Lenox RH: Protein kinase C signaling in the brain: molecular transduction of mood stabilization in the treatment of manic-depressive illness. Biol Psychiatry (in press)

Manji HK, Hsiao JK, Risby ED, et al: The mechanisms of action of lithium, I: effects on serotoninergic and noradrenergic systems in normal subjects. Arch Gen Psychiatry 48:505–512, 1991a

Manji HK, Bitran JA, Masana MI, et al: Signal transduction modulation by lithium: cell culture, cerebral microdialysis and human studies. Psychopharmacol Bull 27:199–208, 1991b

Manji HK, Etcheberrigaray R, Chen G, et al: Lithium dramatically decreases membrane-associated PKC in the hippocampus: selectivity for the alpha isozyme. J Neurochem 61:2303–2310, 1993

Manji HK, Chen G, Shimon H, et al: Guanine nucleotide-binding proteins in bipolar affective disorder: effects of long-term lithium treatment. Arch Gen Psychiatry 52:135–144, 1995

Manji HK, Bersudsky Y, Chen G, et al: Modulation of protein kinase C isozymes and substrates by lithium: the role of myo-inositol. Neuropsychopharmacology 15:370–381, 1996

Manji HK, Chen G, Hsiao JK, et al: Regulation of signal transduction pathways by mood stabilizing agents: implications for the pathophysiology and treatment of bipolar affective disorder, in Bipolar Medications: Mechanisms of Action. Edited by Manji HK, Bowden CL, Belmaker RH. Washington, DC, American Psychiatric Press (in press)

Manna V: [Bipolar affective disorders and role of intraneuronal calcium. Therapeutic effects of the treatment with lithium salts and/or calcium antagonist in patients with rapid polar inversion]. Minerva Med 82:757–763, 1991

Manzano JM, Llorca G, Ledesma A, et al: [Spanish adaptation of the Alzheimer's disease assessment scale (ADAS)]. Actas Luso Esp Neurol Psiquiatr Cienc Afines 22:64–70, 1994

Maragos WF, Greenamyre T, Penney JB, et al: Glutamate dysfunction in Alzheimer's disease: an hypothesis. Trends Neurosci 10:65–68, 1987

Marangell L, George MS, Bissette G, et al: Carbamazepine increases CSF thyrotropin-releasing hormone in affectively ill patients. Arch Gen Psychiatry 51:625–628, 1994

Marangos PJ, Daval JL, Weiss SRB, et al: Carbamazepine and brain adenosine receptors, in Neonatal Seizures. Edited by Wasterlain CG, Vert P. New York, Raven, 1990, pp 203–209

Marazziti D, Hollander E, Lensi P, et al: Peripheral markers of serotonin and dopamine function in OCD. Psychiatry Res 42:41–51, 1992

March JS, Kobak KS, Jefferson JW, et al: A double-blind placebo-controlled trial of fluvoxamine versus imipramine in outpatients with major depression. J Clin Psychiatry 51:1027–1033, 1990

Marcus EA, Carew JW: Developmental emergence of different forms of neuromodulation in Aplysia sensory neurons. Proc Natl Acad Sci U S A 95:4726–4731, 1998

Marder SR, Meibach RC: Risperidone in the treatment of schizophrenia. Am J Psychiatry 151:825–835, 1994

Marek GJ, McDougle CJ, Price LH, et al: A comparison of trazodone and fluoxetine: implications for a serotonergic mechanism of antidepressant action. Psychopharmacology 109:2–11, 1992

Margraf J, Ehlers A, Roth WT, et al: Sodium lactate infusions and panic attacks: a review and critique. Psychosom Med 48:23–51, 1986

Marin DB, Greenwald BS: Carbamazepine for aggressive agitation in demented patients. Am J Psychiatry 46:85, 1989

Markovitz PJ, Stagno SJ, Calabrese JR: Buspirone augmentation of fluoxetine in obsessive-compulsive disorder. Am J Psychiatry 147:798–800, 1990

Markowitz JS, Weissman PH, Ouelette R, et al: Quality of life in panic disorder. Arch Gen Psychiatry 46:984–992, 1989

Marks IM: The clarification of phobic disorders. Br J Psychiatry 116:377–386, 1970

Marks IM: Fears, Phobias, and Rituals. New York, Oxford University Press, 1987

Marks IM, Matthews AM: Brief standard self-rating for phobic patients. Behav Res Ther 17:263–267, 1982

Marks IM, Stern RS, Mawson D, et al: Clomipramine and exposure for obsessive compulsive rituals. Br J Psychiatry 136:1–25, 1980

Marley PD, Nagy JI, Emson PC, et al: Cholecystokinin in the rat spinal cord: distribution and lack of effect of neonatal capsaicin treatment and rhizotomy. Brain Res 238:494–498, 1982

Marley PD, Rehfeld JF, Emson PC: Distribution and chromatographic characterisation of gastrin and cholecystokinin in the rat central nervous system. J Neurochem 42:1523–1535, 1984

Marovitch S, Kumada M, Reis DJ: Role of parabrachialis in cardiovascular regulation in the cat. Brain Res 232:57–75, 1982

Martensson B, Aberg-Wistedt A: The use of selective serotonin reuptake inhibitors among Swedish psychiatrists. Nordic Journal of Psychiatry 50:443–450, 1996

Martin BR, Martin TJ, Fan F, et al: Central actions of nicotine antagonists. Med Chem Res 2:564–577, 1993

Martin KC, Casadio A, Zhu HEY, et al: Synapse specific long term facilitation of Aplysia sensory to motor synazases: a function for local protein synthesis in memory storage. Cell 91:927–938, 1997

Martin P, Laurent S, Massol J, et al: Effects of dihydropyridine drugs on reversal by imipramine of helpless behavior in rats. Eur J Pharmacol 162:185–188, 1989

Masana MI, Bitran JA, Hsiao JK, et al: Lithium effects on noradrenergic linked adenylate cyclase activity in intact rat brain: an in vivo microdialysis study. Brain Res 538:333–336, 1991

Masana MI, Bitran JA, Hsiao JK, et al: In vivo evidence that lithium inactivates Gi modulation of adenylate cyclase in brain. J Neurochem 59:200–205, 1992

Masana MI, Chen G, Shorts L, et al: Attenuation of PKC induced cyclic AMP increases by chronic lithium: an in vivo microdialysis study. (in press)

Mashford MH: Mianserin: an example of benefits and risks in therapy. Med J Aust 141:308–310, 1984

Maslanski JA, Leshko L, Busa WB: Lithium-sensitive production of inositol phosphates during amphibian embryonic mesoderm induction. Science 256:243–245, 1992

Mason BJ, Kocsis MD: Desipramine treatment of alcoholism. Psychopharmacol Bull 27:155–161, 1991

Masserman JH, Pechtel CT: Neuroses in monkeys: a preliminary report of experimental observations. Ann N Y Acad Sci 56:253, 1953

Mathe AA, Jousisto-Hanson J, Stenfors C, et al: Effect of lithium on tachykinins, calcitonin gene-related peptide, and neuropeptide Y in rat brain. J Neurosci Res 26:233–237, 1990

Mathews A, MacLeod C: Discrimination of threat cues without awareness in anxiety states. J Abnorm Psychol 95:131–138, 1986

Mathis M, Paul SM, Crawley JN: The neurosteroid pregnenolone sulfate blocks NMDA antagonist-induced deficits in a passive avoidance memory task. Psychopharmacology 116:201–206, 1994

Mathur C, Prasad VVK, Raju VS, et al: Steroids and their conjugates in the mammalian brain. Proc Natl Acad Sci U S A 90:85–88, 1993

Mattes JA: A pilot study of combined trazodone and tryptophan in obsessive-compulsive disorder. Int Clin Psychopharmacol 1:170–173, 1986

Mattson MP, Cheng B, Davis D, et al: Beta-amyloid peptides destabilize calcium homeostasis and render human cortical neurons vulnerable to excitotoxicity. J Neurosci 12:376–389, 1992

Matussek N: Neurobiologie und Depression. Medizinische Monatsschrift 3:109–112, 1968

Maura G, Andrioli SC, Cavazzani P: 5-hydroxytryptamine$_3$ receptor sites on cholinergic axon terminals of human cerebral cortex mediate inhibition of acetylcholine release. J Neurochem 58:2334–2337, 1992

Mavissakalian M, Turner SM, Michelson L, et al: Tricyclic antidepressants in obsessive-compulsive disorder: antiobsessional or antidepressant agents? II. Am J Psychiatry 142:572–576, 1985

Mawson D, Marks IM, Ramm L: Clomipramine for chronic obsessive compulsive rituals: two year follow-up and further findings. Br J Psychiatry 140:11–18, 1982

McAllister KH, Pratt JA: GR205171 blocks apomorphine and amphetamine-induced conditioned taste aversions. Eur J Pharmacol 353:141–148, 1998

McAuley JW, Reynolds IJ, Kroboth FJ, et al: Orally administered progesterone enhances sensitivity to triazolam in posmenopausal women. J Clin Psychopharmacol 1:3–11, 1995

McCall WV, Shelp FE, Weiner RD, et al: Convulsive threshold differences in right unilateral and bilateral ECT. Biol Psychiatry 34:606–611, 1993a

McCall WV, Reid S, Rosenquist P, et al: A reappraisal of the role of caffeine in ECT. Am J Psychiatry 150:1543–1545, 1993b

McCance SL, Cohen PR, Cowen PJ: Lithium increases 5-HT-mediated prolactin release. Psychopharmacology 99:276–281, 1989

McCann U, Hatzidimitriou G, Ridenour A, et al: Dexfenfluramine and serotonin neurotoxicity: further preclinical evidence that clinical caution is indicated. J Pharmacol Exp Ther 269:792–798, 1994

McCarley RW: REM sleep and depression: common neurobiological control mechanisms. Am J Psychiatry 139:565–570, 1982

McCarley RW, Hobson JA: Neuronal excitability modulation over the sleep cycle: a structural and mathematical model. Science 189:58–60, 1975

McCormick DA: Cellular mechanism of cholinergic control of neocortical and thalamic neuronal excitability, in Brain Cholinergic Systems. Edited by Steriade M, Biesold D. New York, Oxford University Press, 1990, pp 236–264

McCracken JT: A two-part model of stimulant action on attention-deficit hyperactivity disorder in children. J Neuropsychiatry Clin Neurosci 3:201–208, 1991

McDermott AB, Mayer ML, Westbrook GL: NMDA receptors activation increased cytoplasmatic calcium concentration in cultured spinal cord neurones. Nature 321:519–522, 1986

McDermut W, Pazzaglia PJ, Huggins T, et al: Use of single case analyses in off-on-off-on trials in affective illness: a demonstration of the efficacy of nimodipine. Depression 2:259–271, 1995

McDougle CJ, Price LH, Goodman WK: Fluvoxamine treatment of coincident autistic disorder and obsessive compulsive disorder: a case report. J Autism Dev Disord 20:537–543, 1990a

McDougle CJ, Goodman WK, Price LH, et al: Neuroleptic addition in fluvoxamine-refractory obsessive compulsive disorder: an open case series. Am J Psychiatry 147:652–654, 1990b

McDougle CJ, Price LH, Goodman WK, et al: A controlled trial of lithium augmentation in fluvoxamine-refractory obsessive-compulsive disorder: lack of efficacy. J Clin Psychopharmacol 11:175–184, 1991

McDougle CJ, Price LH, Volkmar FR, et al: Clomipramine in autism: preliminary evidence of efficacy. J Am Acad Child Adolesc Psychiatry 31:746–750, 1992

McDougle CJ, Goodman WK, Leckman JF, et al: The efficacy of fluvoxamine in obsessive compulsive disorder: effects of comorbid chronic tic disorder. J Clin Psychopharmacol 13:354–358, 1993a

McDougle CJ, Goodman WK, Leckman JF, et al: Limited therapeutic effect of addition of buspirone in fluvoxamine-refractory obsessive-compulsive disorder. Am J Psychiatry 150:647–649, 1993b

McDougle CJ, Goodman WK, Leckman JF, et al: Haloperidol addition in fluvoxamine-refractory obsessive compulsive disorder: a double-blind, placebo-controlled study in patients with and without tics. Arch Gen Psychiatry 51:302–308, 1994

McDougle CJ, Fleischmann RL, Epperson CN, et al: Risperidone addition in fluvoxamine-refractory obsessive-compulsive disorder: three cases [see comments]. J Clin Psychiatry 56:526–528, 1995

McElroy SL, Pope HG: Use of Anticonvulsants in Psychiatry: Recent Advances. Clifton, NJ, Oxford Health Care, 1988

McElroy SL, Keck PE Jr, Pope HG Jr: Sodium valproate: its use in primary psychiatric disorders. J Clin Psychopharmacol 7:16–24, 1987

McElroy SL, Pope HG Jr, Keck PE Jr, et al: Treatment of psychiatric disorders with valproate: a series of 73 cases. Psychiatr Psychobiol 3:81–85, 1988a

McElroy SL, Keck PE Jr, Pope HG Jr, et al: Valproate in primary psychiatric disorders: literature review and clinical experience in a private psychiatric hospital, in Use of Anticonvulsants in Psychiatry: Recent Advances. Edited by McElroy SL, Pope HG Jr. Clifton, NJ, Oxford Health Care, 1988b

McElroy SL, Keck PE Jr, Pope HG Jr, et al: Valproate in the treatment of rapid-cycling bipolar disorder. J Clin Psychopharmacol 8:275–279, 1988c

McElroy SL, Sessain EC, Pope HG Jr, et al: Clozapine in the treatment of psychotic mood disorders, schizoaffective disorder and schizophrenia. J Clin Psychiatry 52:411–414, 1991a

McElroy SL, Keck PE Jr, Pope HG Jr, et al: Correlates of antimanic response to valproate. Psychopharmacol Bull 27:127–133, 1991b

McElroy SL, Keck PE Jr, Pope HG Jr, et al: Clinical and research implications of the diagnosis of dysphoric or mixed mania or hypomania. Am J Psychiatry 149:1633–1644, 1992

McElroy SL, Keck PE Jr, Tugrul KC, et al: Valproate as a loading treatment in acute mania. Neuropsychobiology 27:146–149, 1993

McEntee WJ, Crook TH: Serotonin, memory and the aging brain. Psychopharmacology 103:143–149, 1991

McEntee WJ, Mair RG: Memory enhancement in Korsoff's psychosis with clonidine: further evidence for a noradrenergic deficit. Ann Neurol 7:466–470, 1980

McEwen BS: Non-genomic and genomic effects of steroids on neural activity. Trends Pharmacol Sci 12:141–147, 1991

McEwen BS, Angulo J, Cameron H, et al: Paradoxical effects of adrenal steroids on the brain: protection vs. degeneration. Biol Psychiatry 31:177–199, 1992

McGarvey K, Zis AP, Brown EE, et al: ECS-induced dopamine release: effects of electrode placement, anticonvulsant treatment and stimulus intensity. Biol Psychiatry 34:152–157, 1993

McGeer PL, Rogers J: Antiinflammatory agents as a therapeutic approach to Alzheimer's disease. Neurology 42:447–448, 1992

McGeer PL, McGeer EG, Rogers J, et al: Antiinflammatory drugs and Alzheimer's disease. Lancet 335:1037, 1990

McGeer PL, Harada M, Kimura H, et al: Prevalence of dementia amongst elderly Japanese with leprosy: apparent effect of chronic drug therapy. Dementia 3:146–149, 1992

McGehee DS, Heath MJ, Gelber S, et al: Nicotine enhancement of fast excitatory synaptic transmission in CNS by presynaptic receptors. Science 269:1692–1696, 1995

McGrath PJ, Stewart JW, Harrison W, et al: Treatment of tricyclic refractory depression with a monoamine oxidase inhibitor. Psychopharmacol Bull 23:169–172, 1987

McGurk SR, Levin ED, Butcher LL: Nicotinic-dopaminergic relationships and radial-arm maze performance in rats. Behav Neural Biol 52:78–86, 1989

McLean JH, Darby-King A, Sullivan RM, et al: Serotonergic influence on olfactory learning in the neonate rat. Behav Neural Biol 60:152–162, 1993

McNally RJ, Calamari JE: Obsessive-compulsive disorder in a mentally retarded woman. Br J Psychiatry 155:116–117, 1989

McNamara RK, Lenox RH: Comparative distribution of myristoylated alanine-rich C kinase substrate (MARCKS) and F1/GAP-43 gene expression in the adult rat brain. J Comp Neurol 379:48–71, 1997

McNamara RK, Lenox RH: Distribution of protein kinase C substrates MARCKS and MRP in the postnatal developing rat brain. J Comp Neurol 397:337–356, 1998

McNamara RK, Stumpo DJ, Morel LM, et al: Effects of reduced myristoylated alanine rich C-kinase substrate expression on spatial learning in mutant mice: transgenic rescue and interaction with gene background. Proc Natl Acad Sci U S A 95:14517–14522, 1998

McNamara RK, Hyde TM, Kleinman JE, et al: Expression of the myristoylated alanine-rich C kinase substrate (MARCKS) and MARCKS-related protein (MRP) in the hippocampus and prefrontal cortex of suicide victims. J Clin Psychiatry 60:21–26, 1999

McTavish D, Benfield P: Clomipramine: an overview of its pharmacological properties and a review of its therapeutic use in obsessive compulsive disorder and panic disorder. Drugs 39:136–153, 1990

Meco G, Alessandria A, Bonifati V, et al: Risperidone for hallucinations in levodopa-treated Parkinson's disease patients. Lancet 343:1370–1371, 1994

Medical Research Council: Clinical trial of the treatment of depressive illness. BMJ 5439:881–886, 1965

Meglio M, Ianelli A, Anile C, et al: Interaction of epileptic activities of bilateral deep temporal origin: an experimental study. Epilepsia 17:437–448, 1976

Meguro H, Mori H, Araki K, et al: Functional characterization of a heteromeric NMDA receptor channel from cloned cDNAs. Nature 357:70–74, 1992

Meichenbaum D, Turk DC: Facilitating treatment adherence. New York, Plenum, 1987

Meisel SR, Kutz I, Dayan KI, et al: Effect of Iraqi missile war on incidence of acute myocardial infarction and sudden death in Israeli civilians. Lancet 338:660–661, 1991

Melcangi RM, Celotti, F, Martini L: Progesterone 5a-reduction in neuronal and in different types of glial cell cultures: type 1 and 2 and oligodendrocytes. Brain Res 639:202–206, 1994

Melchior CL, Ritzmann RF: Dehydroepiandrosterone is an anxiolytic in mice on the plus maze. Pharmacol Biochem Behav 47:437–441, 1994a

Melchior CL, Ritzmann RF: Pregnenolone and pregnenolone sulfate, alone and with ethanol, in mice on the plus-maze. Pharmacol Biochem Behav 48:893–897, 1994b

Melia PI: Prophylactic lithium: a double-blind trial in recurrent affective disorders. Br J Psychiatry 116:621–624, 1970

Meller E, Goldstein M, Geyer MA: Receptor reserve for 5-hydroxytryptamine 1A-mediated inhibition of serotonin synthesis: possible relationship to anxiolytic properties of 5-hydroxitryptamine 1A agonists. Mol Pharmacol 37:231–237, 1990

Mellinger GD, Balter MB, Uhlenhuth EH: Insomnia and its treatment: prevalence and correlates. Arch Gen Psychiatry 42:225–232, 1985

Mellman LA, Gorman JM: Successful treatment of obsessive-compulsive disorder with ECT. Am J Psychiatry 141:596–597, 1984

Mellman LA, Gorman JM: Successful treatment of OCD. Psychiatry 141:596–597, 1992

Mellman TA, Uhde WT: Electroencephalographic sleep in panic disorder. Arch Gen Psychiatry 46:178–184, 1989

Mellon SH: Neurosteroids: biochemistry, modes of action, and clinical relevance. J Clin Endocrinol Metab 78:1003–1008, 1994

Mellon SH, Deschepper CF: Neurosteroid biosynthesis: genes for adrenal steroidogenic enzymes are expressed in the brain. Brain Res 629:283–292, 1993

Melloni P, Carniel G, Della Toree A, et al: Potential antidepressant agents. α-aryloxy-benzyl derivatives of ethanolamine and morpholine. Eur J Med Chem Chim Ther 19:235–242, 1984

Mellow AM, Solano-López C, Davis S: Sodium valproate in the treatment of behavioral disturbance in dementia. J Geriatr Psychiatry Neurol 6:28–32, 1993

Meltzer HL: Mode of action of lithium in affective disorders: an influence on intracellular calcium functions. Pharmacol Toxicol 66:84–99, 1990

Meltzer HL, Kassir S, Dunner DL, et al: Repression of a lithium pump as a consequence of lithium ingestion by manic-depressive subjects. Psychopharmacology 54:113–118, 1982

Meltzer HY: Role of the serotonergic system in pituitary hormone secretion: the pharmacological challenge paradigm in man, in Serotonin From Cell Biology to Pharmacology and Therapeutics. Edited by Vanhoutte PM, Saxena PR, Paoletti R, et al. Dordrecht, The Netherlands, Kluwer, 1990, pp 239–247

Meltzer HY, Lowy MT: The serotonin hypothesis of depression, in Psychopharmacology: The Third Generation of Progress. Edited by Meltzer HY. New York, Raven, 1987, pp 513–526

Meltzer HY, Simonovic M, Sturgeon RD, et al: Effect of antidepressants, lithium and electroconvulsive treatment on rat serum prolactin levels. Acta Psychiatr Scand Suppl 290:100–121, 1981

Meltzer HY, Arora RC, Goodnick P: Effect of lithium carbonate on serotonin uptake in blood platelets of patients with affective disorders. J Affect Disord 5:215–221, 1983

Meltzer HY, Lowy M, Robertson A, et al: Effect of 5-hydroxytryptophan on serum cortisol levels in major affective disorders: III. Effect of antidepressants and lithium carbonate. Arch Gen Psychiatry 41:391–397, 1984

Mendels J: The prediction of response to electroconvulsive therapy. Am J Psychiatry 124:153–159, 1967

Mendels J: Lithium in the treatment of depression. Am J Psychiatry 133:373–378, 1976

Mendels J, Reimherr F, Roberts D, et al: A double-blind comparison of nefazadone and imipramine in the treatment of depressed patients. Proceedings of the Annual Congress of the American College of Neuropsychopharmacology 1:451–452, 1991

Mendels J, Reimherr F, Marcus RN, et al: A double-blind placebo-controlled trial of two ranges of nefazodone in the treatment of depressed outpatients. J Clin Psychiatry 56 (suppl 6):30–36, 1995

Mendelson SD, Quartermain D, Francisco T, et al: 5-HT$_{1A}$ agonists induce anterograde amnesia in mice through a post synaptic mechanism. Eur J Pharmacol 236:177–182, 1993

Mendelson WB, Gillin JC, Wyatt RJ (eds): Human Sleep and Its Disorders. New York, Plenum, 1977

Mendelson WB, Sack DA, James SP, et al: Frequency analysis of the sleep EEG in depression. Psychiatry Res 21:89–94, 1987a

Mendelson WB, Martin JW, Perlis M, et al: Sleep induction by an adrenal steroid in the rat. Psychopharmacology 93:226–229, 1987b

Mendlewicz J, Kerkhofs M: Sleep electroencephalography in depressive illness: a collaborative study by the World Health Organization. Br J Psychiatry 159:505–509, 1991

Mendlewicz J, Dunbar GC, Hoffiman G: Changes in sleep EEG architecture during the treatment of depressed patients with mianserin. Acta Psychiatr Scand 72:26–29, 1985

Mendlewicz J, Kempenaers C, de Maertelaer V: Sleep EEG and amitriptyline treatment in depressed inpatients. Biol Psychiatry 30:691–702, 1991

Meneses A, Hong E: Effect of fluoxetine on learning and memory involves multiple 5-HT systems. Pharmacol Biochem Behav 52:341–346, 1995

Meneses A, Hong E: 5-HT1A receptors modulate the consolidation of learning in normal and cognitively impaired rats. Neurobiol Learn Mem 71(2):207–218, 1999

Mennini T, Mocaer E, Garattini S: Tianeptine, a selective enhancer of serotonin uptake in rat brain. Naunyn Schmiedebergs Arch Pharmacol 336:478–482, 1987

Mensah-Niagan AG, Feuilloley M, Dupont E, et al: Immunocytochemical localization and biological activity of 3β-hydroxysteroid dehydrogenase in the central nervous system of the frog. J Neurosci 14:7306–7318, 1994

Menzaghi F, Howard RL, Heinrichs SC, et al: Characterization of a novel and potent corticotropin-releasing factor antagonist in rats. J Pharmacol Exp Ther 269:564–572, 1994

Mesulam MM, Mufson EJ, Levey AI, et al: Atlas of cholinergic neurons in the forebrain and upper brainstem of the macaque based on monoclonal choline acetyltransferase immuno histochemistry and acetylcholinesterase histochemistry. Neuroscience 12:669–686, 1984

Metz A, Shader RI: Combination of fluoxetine with pemoline in the treatment of major depressive disorders. Int Clin Psychopharmacol 6:93–96, 1991

Metz A, Evoniuk G, De Veaugh-Geiss J: Multicentre trial of a 5-HT$_3$ antagonist, ondansetron, in panic disorder (abstract). Paper presented at the 33rd annual meeting of the American College of Neuropsychopharmacology, San Juan, Puerto Rico, 1994, p 165

Metzger ED, Friedman RS: Treatment-related depression. Psychiatric Annals 24:540–544, 1994

Meyer A: Psychobiology: A Science of Man. Springfield, IL, Charles C Thomas, 1957

Meyer EM, de Fiebre CM, Hunter BE, et al: Effects of anabaseine-related analogs on rat brain nicotinic receptor binding and on avoidance behaviors. Drug Dev Res 31:127–134, 1994

Meyer FB, Tally PW, Anderson RE, et al: Inhibition of electrically induced seizures by a dihydropyridine calcium channel blocker. Brain Res 384:180–183, 1986

Meyer HH, Gottlieb R: Theory of narcosis, in Experimental Pharmacology as a Basis for Therapeutics, 2nd Edition. Translated by Henderson VE. Philadelphia, PA, JB Lippincott, 1926, pp 116–29

Meyer JS, Welch KM, Deshmukh VD: Neurotransmitter precursor amino acids in the treatment of multi infarct dementia and Alzheimer's disease. J Am Geriatr Soc 25:289–298, 1977

Mhatre M, Mehta AK, Ticku MK: Chronic ethanol administration increases the binding of the benzodiazepine inverse agonist and alcohol antagonist (H) RO 15–4513 in rat brain. Eur J Pharmacol 153:141–145, 1988

Michael C, Kantor H, Shore H: Further psychometric evaluation of older women—the effect of estrogen administration. J Gerontol 25:337–341, 1970

Michaelis R, Hofmann E: Zur phanomenologie und atiopathogenese der hypersomnie bei endogen-phasischen depressionen, in The Nature of Sleep. Edited by Jovanovic UJ. Stuttgart, Gustav Fischer Verlag, 1973, pp 190–193

Michelson D, Lydiard B, Pollack MH, et al: Outcome assessment and clinical improvement in panic disorder: evidence from a randomized controlled trial of fluoxetine and placebo. Am J Psychiatry 155:1570–1577, 1998

Middlemiss DN, Palmer AM, Edel N, et al: Binding of the novel serotonin agonist 8-hydroxy-2-(di-n-propylamino) tetralin in normal and Alzheimer brain. J Neurochem 46:993–996, 1986

Migliorelli R, Starkstein SE, Teson A, et al: SPECT findings in patients with primary mania. J Neuropsychiatry Clin Neurosci 5:379–383, 1993

Miller HL, Delgado PL, Salomon RM, et al: Clinical and biochemical effects of catecholamine depletion on antidepressant-induced remission of depression. Arch Gen Psychiatry 53:117–128, 1996a

Miller HL, Delgado PL, Salomon RM, et al: Effects of alpha-methyl-para-tyrosine (AMPT) in drug-free depressed patients. Neuropsychopharmacology 14: 151–157, 1996b

Miller TP, Grogan TM, Dalton WS, et al: P-glycoprotein expression in malignant lymphoma and reversal of clinical drug resistance with chemotherapy plus high-dose verapamil. J Clin Oncol 9:17–24, 1991

Milne RJ, Goa KL: Citaolpram: a review of its pharmacodynamic and pharmacokinetic properties, and therapeutic potential in depressive illness. Drugs 41:450–477, 1991

Mindus P, Jenike MA: Neurosurgical treatment of malignant OCD. Psychiatr Clin North Am 15:921–938, 1992

Mindus P, Rasmussen SA, Lindquist C: Neurosurgical treatment for refractory obsessive-compulsive disorder: implications for understanding frontal lobe function. J Neuropsychiatry 6:467–477, 1994

Minot R, Luthringer R, Macher JP: Effect of moclobemide on the psychophysiology of sleep/wake cycles: a neuroelectrophysiological study of depressed patients administered with moclobemide. Int Clin Psychopharmacol 7:181–189, 1993

Minter RE, Mandel MR: The treatment of psychotic major depressive disorder with drugs and electroconvulsive therapy. J Nerv Ment Dis 167:726–733, 1979

Miquel MC, Hamon M: 5-HT1 receptor subtypes: pharmacological heterogeneity, in Serotonin Receptor Subtypes: Pharmacological Significance and Clinical Implications. Edited by Langer SZ, Brunello N, Racagni G, et al. International Academy for Biomedical and Drug Research. Basel, Switzerland, Karger, 1992, pp 44–55

Misane I, Johansson C, Ögren SO: Analysis of the 5-HT$_{1A}$ receptor involvement in passive avoidance in the rat. Br J Pharmacol 125:499–509, 1998

Mita T, Hanada S, Nighino N, et al: Decreased serotonin S2 and increased dopamine D2 receptors in chronic schizophrenia. Biol Psychiatry 21:1407–1414, 1986

Mitchell P, Selbie L, Waters B, et al: Exclusion of close linkage of bipolar disorders to dopamine D$_1$ and D$_2$ receptor gene markers. J Affect Disord 25:1–12, 1992

Mitchell P, Waters B, Vivero C, et al: Exclusion of close linkage of bipolar disorders to the dopamine D3 receptor gene in nine Australian pedigrees. J Affect Disord 27:213–224, 1993

Mitsushima D, Hei DL, Terasawa E: GABA is an inhibitory neurotransmitter restricting the release of luteinizing hormone-releasing hormone before the onset of puberty. Proc Natl Acad Sci U S A 91:395–399, 1994

Miura N, Nakata N, Tanaka Y, et al: Improving effects of FG-7080 a serotonin reuptake inhibitor on scopolamine-induced performance deficits of memory tasks in rats. Jpn J Pharmacol 62:203–206, 1993

Mizuta T, Segawa T: Chronic effects of imipramine and lithium on 5-HT receptor subtypes in rat frontal cortex, hippocampus and choroid plexus: quantitative receptor autoradiographic analysis. Jpn J Pharmacol 50:315–326, 1989

Mocaer E, Retori MC, Kamoun A: Pharmacological antidepressive effects and tianeptine-induced 5-HT uptake increase. Clin Neuropharmacol 11 (suppl 2):S32–S42, 1988

Modigh K: Antidepressant drugs in anxiety disorders. Acta Psychiatr Scand 76 (suppl 335):57–71, 1989

Modigh K, Westberg P, Eriksson E: Superiority of clomipramine over imipramine in the treatment of panic disorder: a placebo controlled trial. J Clin Psychopharmacol 12:251–261, 1992

Mogilnicka E, Czyrak A, Maj J: Dihydropyridine calcium channel antagonists reduce immobility in the mouse behavioral despair test; antidepressants facilitate nifedipine action. Eur J Pharmacol 138:413–416, 1987

Mogilnicka E, Czyrak A, Maj J: BAY K 8644 enhances immobility in the mouse behavioral despair test, an effect blocked by nifedipine. Eur J Pharmacol 151:307–311, 1988

Mohr E, Schleger J, Fabbrini G, et al: Clonidine treatment of Alzheimer's disease. Arch Neurol 46:376–378, 1989

Moll H: The treatment of postencephalitic parkinsonism by nicotine. BMJ 1:1079–1081, 1926

Moller HJ, Schmid-Bode W, Cording-Tommel C, et al: Psychopathological and social outcome in schizophrenia versus affective/schizoaffective psychoses and prediction of poor outcome in schizophrenia. Acta Psychiatr Scand 77:379–389, 1988

Moller HJ, Kissling W, Riehl T, et al: Double blind evaluation of the antimanic properties of carbamazepine as a comedication to haloperidol. Prog Neuropsychopharmacol Biol Psychiatry 13:127–136, 1989

Molloy DW, Guyatt GH, Wilson DB, et al: Effect of tetrahydroaminoacridine on cognitive function and behaviors in Alzheimer's disease. Canadian Medical Association Journal 144(1):29–34, 1991

Monroe RR: Maintenance electroconvulsive therapy. Psychiatr Clin North Am 14:947–960, 1991

Montenegro R, Comide E, Castro JM, et al: Nimodipine in the treatment of involutional depressive syndrome, in Nimodipine: Pharmacological and Clinical Studies. Edited by Betz E, Deck K, Hoffmeister F. Stuttgart, Germany, Schattauer, 1985, pp 345–358

Montero RF, Berger M: Antidepressant and antimanic drugs, in Handbook of Experimental Pharmacology: Pharmacology of Sleep. Edited by Kales A. Berlin, Springer-Verlag, 1995

Montgomery I, Oswald I, Morgan K, et al: Trazodone enhances sleep in subjective quality but not in objective duration. Br J Clin Pharmacol 16:139–144, 1983

Montgomery SA: CMI in obsessional neurosis: a placebo controlled trial. Pharm Med 1:89, 1980

Montgomery SA: The advantages of paroxetine in different subgroups of depression. Int Clin Psychopharmacol 6 (suppl 4):91–100, 1992a

Montgomery SA: The diagnostic place of OCD and panic disorders as serotonergic illnesses, in Serotonin, CNS Receptors and Brain Function (Advances in the Biosciences, Vol 85). Edited by Bradley PB, Handley SL, Cooper SJ, et al. Oxford, England, Pergamon, 1992b, pp 325–334

Montgomery SA: Pharmacological treatment of obsessive compulsive disorder, in Current Insights in Obsessive Compulsive Disorder. Edited by Hollander E, Zohar A, Marazziti D, et al. Chichester, England, Wiley, 1994, pp 215–225

Montgomery SA: Are 2 week trials sufficient to indicate efficacy? Psychopharmacol Bull 31:41–44, 1995a

Montgomery SA: Rapid onset of action of venlafaxine. Int Clin Psychopharmacol 10 (suppl 2):21–27, 1995b

Montgomery SA: Safety of mirtazapine: a review. Int Clin Psychopharmacol 10 (suppl 4):37–45, 1995c

Montgomery SA: Selective serotonin reuptake inhibitors in the acute treatment of depression, in Psychopharmacology: The Fourth Generation of Progress. Edited by Bloom FE, Kupfer DJ. New York, Raven, 1995d, pp 1043–1051

Montgomery SA: The efficacy of mirtazapine. Paper presented at the European College of Neuropsychopharmacology Congress, Amsterdam, September 1996

Montgomery SA, Åsberg M: A new depression scale designed to be sensitive to change. Br J Psychiatry 134:382–389, 1979

Montgomery SA, Dunbar G: Paroxetine is better than placebo in relapse prevention and prophylaxis of recurrent depression. Int Clin Psychopharmacol 8(3):189–195, 1993

Montgomery SA, Kasper S: Comparison of compliance between serotonin reuptake inhibitors and tricyclic antidepressants: a meta-analysis. Int Clin Psychopharmacol 9 (suppl 4):33–40, 1995

Montgomery SA, Mancaux A: Fluvoxamine in the treatment of obsessive compulsive disorder. Int Clin Psychopharmacol 7 (suppl 1):5–9, 1992

Montgomery SA, McAulay R, Rani SJ, et al: A double-blind comparison of zimelidine and amitriptyline in endogenous depression. Acta Psychiatr Scand 63 (suppl 290):314–327, 1981

Montgomery SA, Dufour H, Brion S, et al: Prophylactic efficacy of fluoxetine in unipolar depression. Br J Psychiatry 153 (suppl):69–76, 1988

Montgomery SA, Baldwin D, Priest RG, et al: Minaprine and dose response in depression: an investigation of two fixed doses of minaprine compared with imipramine Pharmacopsychiatry 24:168–174, 1991

Montgomery SA, Fineberg NA, Montgomery DB, et al: L-Tryptophan in obsessive compulsive disorder—a placebo controlled study. Eur Neuropsychopharmacol 2 (suppl 2):384, 1992

Montgomery SA, Rasmussen JGC, Tanghoj P: A 24 week study of 20mg citalopram, 40mg citalopram and placebo in the prevention of relapse of major depression. Int Clin Psychopharmacol 8:181–188, 1993a

Montgomery SA, McIntyre A, Osterheider M, et al: A double blind, placebo-controlled study of fluoxetine in patients with DSM-III-R obsessive compulsive disorder. Eur Neuropsychopharmacol 3:143–152, 1993b

Montgomery SA, Pedersen V, Tanghoj P, et al: The optimal dosing regimen for citalopram—a meta-analysis of nine placebo-controlled studies. Int Clin Psychopharmacol 9 (suppl 1):35–40, 1994a

Montgomery SA, Henry J, McDonald G, et al: Selective serotonin reuptake inhibitors: meta-analysis of discontinuation rates. Int Clin Psychopharmacol 9:47–53, 1994b

Montgomery SA, Dunner DL, Dunbar GC: Reduction of suicidal thoughts with paroxetine in comparison with reference antidepressants and placebo. Eur Neuropsychopharmacol 5:5–13, 1995

Montgomery SA, Brown RE, Clark M: Economic analysis of treating depression with nefazodone v. imipramine. Br J Psychiatry 168:768–771, 1996

Monti JM: Effect of a reversible monoamine oxidase-A inhibitor (moclobemide) on sleep of depressed patients. Br J Psychiatry Suppl 155:61–65, 1989

Monti JM, Alterwain P, Monti D: The effects of moclobemide on nocturnal sleep of depressed patients. J Affect Disord 20:201–208, 1990

Montkowski A, Holsboer F: Absence of cognitive and memory deficits in transgenic mice with heterozygous disrupt of the brain-derived neurotrophic factor gene. J Psychiatr Res (in press)

Montkowski A, Barden N, Wotjak C, et al: Long-term antidepressant treatment reduces behavioural deficits in transgenic mice with impaired glucocorticoid receptor function. J Neuroendocrinol 7:841–845, 1995

Moran TH, Robinson PH, Goldrich MS, et al: Two brain cholecystokinin receptors: implications for behavioral actions. Brain Res 362:175–179, 1986

Moret C, Charveron M, Finberg JPM, et al: Biochemical profile of midalcipran (F2207), 1-phenyl-1-diethyl-aminocarbonyl-2-aminomethyl-cyclopropane(Z) hydrochloride, a potential fourth generation antidepressant drug. Neuropharmacology 24:1211–1219, 1985

Morgan K, Oswald I, Borrow S: Effects of a single dose of mianserin on sleep. Br J Clin Pharmacol 10:525–527, 1980

Morgan MJ: Memory deficits associated with recreational use of "Ecstasy" (MDMA). Psychopharmacology 141:30–36, 1999

Mork A, Geisler A: Mode of action of lithium on the catalytic unit of adenylate cyclase from rat brain. Pharmacol Toxicol 60:241–248, 1987

Mork A, Geisler A: Effects of GTP on hormone-stimulated adenylate cyclase activity in cerebral cortex, striatum, and hippocampus from rats treated chronically with lithium. Biol Psychiatry 26:279–288, 1989a

Mork A, Geisler A: Effects of lithium ex vivo on the GTP-mediated inhibition of calcium-stimulated adenylate cyclase activity in rat brain. Eur J Pharmacol 168:347–354, 1989b

Mork A, Geisler A: The effects of lithium in vitro and ex vivo on adenylate cyclase in brain are exerted by distinct mechanisms. Neuropharmacology 28:307–311, 1989c

Mork A, Klysner R, Geisler A: Effects of treatment with a lithium-imipramine combination on components of adenylate cyclase in the cerebral cortex of the rat. Neuropharmacology 29:261–267, 1990

Mork A, Geisler A, Hollund P: Effects of lithium on second messenger systems in the brain. Pharmacol Toxicol 71 (suppl 1):4–71, 1992

Morris LS, Schultz RM: Patient compliance: an overview. J Clin Pharm Ther 17:283–295, 1992

Morris PLP, Mayberg HS, Bolla K, et al: A preliminary study of cortical S2 serotonin receptors and cognitive performance following stroke. J Neuropsychiatry Clin Neurosci 5:395–400, 1993

Morrow LA, Pace JR, Purdy RH, et al: Characterization of steroid interactions with g-aminobutyric acid receptor-gated chloride ion channels: evidence for multiple steroid recognition sites. Mol Pharmacol 37:226–229, 1990

Morselli PL: On the therapeutic action of alpidem in anxiety disorders: an overview of the European data. Pharmacopsychiatry 23:129, 1990

Mortola JF: The use of psychotropic agents in pregnancy and lactation. Psychiatr Clin North Am 12:69–87, 1989

Moshe S, Albala BJ: Maturational changes in postictal refractoriness and seizure susceptibility in developing rats. Ann Neurol 13:552–557, 1983

Mosolov SN: [Comparative effectiveness of preventive use of lithium carbonate, carbamazepine and sodium valproate in affective and schizoaffective psychoses]. Zh Nevrol Psikhiatr Im S S Korsakova 91:78–83, 1991

Mota de Freitas DE, Espanol MT, Dorus E: Lithium transport in red blood cells of bipolar patients, in Lithium and the Blood. Edited by Gallicchio VS. Farmington, CT, Karger, 1991, pp 96–120

Mountjoy CQ, Roth M, Garside RF, et al: A clinical trial of phenelzine anxiety, depressive and phobic neurosis. Br J Psychiatry 131:468–492, 1977

Mouradian MM, Blin J, Giuffra M: Somatostatin replacement therapy of Alzheimer's dementia. Ann Neurol 30:610–613, 1991

Mouret J, Lemoine P, Minuit MP, et al: Effects of trazodone on the sleep of depressed subjects, a polygraphic study. Psychopharmacology 95 (suppl):S37–S43, 1988

Mrazek DA: Psychiatric complications of pediatric asthma. Annals of Allergy 69:285–290, 1992

Mucha RF, Herz A: Motivational properties of kappa and mu opioid receptor agonists studied with place and taste preference conditioning. Psychopharmacology 86:274–280, 1995

Mucha RF, Pineal JPJ: Post seizure inhibition of kindled seizures. Exp Neurol 18:1–13, 1968

Mufson EJ, Cochran E, Benzing W, et al: Galaninergic innervation of the cholinergic vertical limb of the diagonal band (Ch2) and bed nucleus of the stria terminalis in aging, Alzheimer's disease and Down's syndrome. Dementia 4:237–250, 1993

Muhlbauer HD: The influence of fenfluramine stimulation on prolactin plasma levels in lithium long-term-treated manic-depressive patients and healthy subjects. Pharmacopsychiatry 17:191–193, 1984

Muhlbauer HD, Muller-Oerlinghausen B: Fenfluramine stimulation of serum cortisol in patients with major affective disorders and healthy controls: further evidence for a central serotonergic action of lithium in man. J Neural Transm 61:81–94, 1985

Muir JL, Dunnett SB, Robbins TW, et al: Attentional functions of the forebrain cholinergic systems: effects of intraventricular hemicholinium, physostigmine, basal forebrain lesions and intracortical grafts on a multiple-choice serial reaction time task. Exp Brain Res 89:611–622, 1992

Mukherjee S: Mechanisms of the antimanic effect of electroconvulsive therapy. Convulsive Therapy 5:227–243, 1989

Mukherjee S, Sackeim HA, Lee C: Unilateral ECT in the treatment of manic episodes. Convulsive Therapy 4:74–80, 1988

Mukherjee S, Sackeim HA, Schnur DB: Electroconvulsive therapy of acute manic episodes: a review of 50 years' experience. Am J Psychiatry 151:169–176, 1994

Muller AA, Stoll K-D: Carbamazepine and oxcarbamazepine in the treatment of manic syndromes: studies in Germany, in Anticonvulsants in Affective Disorders. Edited by Emrich HM, Okuma T, Muller AA. Amsterdam, Excerpta Medica, 1984, pp 139–147

Muller D, Buchs PA, Stoppini L, et al: Long-term potentiation, protein kinase C, and glutamate receptors. Mol Neurobiol 5:277–288, 1991

Mullin JM, Pandita-Gunawardena VR, Whitehead AM: A double-blind comparison of fluvoxamine and dothiepin in the treatment of major affective disorder. British Journal of Clinical Practice 42:51–55, 1988

Mullins LJ, Brinley FJ: Calcium binding and regulation in nerve fibers, in Calcium Binding Protein and Calcium Function. Edited by Wasserman RH, Corradino RA, Carafoli E. New York, North-Holland, 1977, pp 87–95

Munjack DJ, Baltazar PL, Bohn PB, et al: Clonazepam in the treatment of social phobia: a pilot study. J Clin Psychiatry 51:35–40, 1990

Munjack D, Bruns J, Baltazar PL, et al: A pilot study of buspirone in the treatment of social phobia. J Anxiety Disord 5:87–98, 1991

Muramoto O, Sugishita M, Ando K: Cholinergic system and constructional praxis: a further study of physostigmine in Alzheimer's disease. J Neurol Neurosurg Psychiatry 47:485–491, 1984

Murasaki M: Overview of serotonin 1A receptor selective agents in anxiety disorders—the developmental situation in Japan. International Review of Psychiatry 7:105–113, 1995

Murasaki M, Mori A, Endo S, et al: Late phase 2 study of a new anxiolytic SM-3997 (tandospirone) on neurosis. Clinical Evaluation 20:259–293, 1992

Murase K, Randic M, Shirasaki T, et al: Serotonin suppresses N-methyl-D-aspartate responses in acutely isolated spinal dorsal horn neurones of the rat. Brain Res 525:84–91, 1990

Murphy BEP, Wolkowitz OM: The pathophysiologic significance of hypercorticism; antiglucocorticoid strategies. Psychiatr Ann 23:682–690, 1993

Murphy BEP, Dhar V, Ghadirian AM, et al: Response to steroid suppression in major depression resistant to antidepressant therapy. J Clin Psychopharmacol 11:121–126, 1991

Murphy DL: Neuropsychiatric disorders and the multiple human brain serotonin receptor subtypes and subsystems. Neuropsychopharmacology 3:457, 1990

Murphy DL, Beigel A, Weingartner H, et al: The quantification of manic behavior, in Psychological Measurements in Psychopharmacology. Edited by Pichot P. Basel, Switzerland, Karger, 1974a, pp 203–220

Murphy DL, Donnelly C, Moskowitz J: Inhibition by lithium of prostaglandin E1 and norepinephrine effects on cyclic adenosine monophosphate production in human platelets. Clin Pharmacol Ther 14:810–814, 1974b

Murphy DL, Lake CR, et al: Psychoactive drug effects on plasma norepinephrine and plasma dopamine B-hydroxylase in man, in Catecholamines: Basic and Clinical Frontiers. Edited by Usdin E, Kopin IJ, Barchas J. Elmsford, NY, Pergamon, 1979, pp 918–920

Murphy DL, Siever LJ, Insel TR: Therapeutic responses to TCA and related drugs in non-affective disorder patient population. Prog Neuropsychopharmacol Biol Psychiatry 9:3–13, 1985

Murphy DL, Piggott TA, Grady TA, et al: Neuropharmacological investigations of brain serotonin subsystem functions in obsessive-compulsive disorder, in Serotonin, CNS Receptors and Brain Function (Advances in the Biosciences, Vol 85). Edited by Bradley PB, Handley SL, Cooper SJ, et al. Oxford, England, Pergamon, 1992, pp 271–285

Murphy DL, Mitchell PB, Potter WZ: Novel pharmacological approaches to the treatment of depression, in Psychopharmacology: The Fourth Generation of Progress, Vol 96. Edited by Bloom FE, Kupfer DJ. New York, Raven, 1995, pp 1143–1153

Murphy TH, Worley PF, Baraban JM: L-type voltage-sensitive calcium channels mediate synaptic activation of immediate early genes. Neuron 7:625–635, 1991

Murtha SJ, Pappas BA: Neurochemical, histopathological and mnemonic effects of combined lesions of the medial septal and serotonin afferents to the hippocampus. Brain Res 651:16–26, 1994

Muscat R, Towell A, Willner P: Changes in dopamine autoreceptor sensitivity in an animal model of depression. Psychopharmacology 94:545–550, 1988

Muscat R, Papp M, Willner P: Antidepressant-like effects of dopamine agonists in an animal model of depression. Biol Psychiatry 31:937–946, 1992

Myers ED, Calvert EJ: Information, compliance and side effects: a study of patients on antidepressant medication. Br J Clin Pharmacol 17:21, 1984

Myers RD, Swartzwelder HS, Peinado JM, et al: CCK and other peptides modulate hypothalamic norepinephrine release in the rat: dependence on hunger or satiety [published erratum appears in Brain Res Bull 18:65, 1987]. Brain Res Bull 17:583–597, 1986

Myrsten A, Post B, Frankenhaeuser M, et al: Changes in behavioral and physiological activation induced by cigarette smoking in habitual smokers. Psychopharmacology 76:232–235, 1972

Myslobodsky MS: Pro- and anticonvulsant effects of stress: the role of neuroactive steroids. Neurosci Biobehav Rev 17:129–139, 1993

Nagaki S, Kato N, Minatogawa Y, et al: Effects of anticonvulsants and gamma-aminobutyric acid (GABA)-mimetic drugs on immunoreactive somatostatin and GABA contents in the rat brain. Life Sci 46:1587–1595, 1990

Nagy A, Johansson R: The demethylation of imipramine and clomipramine and desipramine in plasma and spinal fluid. Arch Gen Psychiatry 54:125–131, 1977

Nahorski SR, Ragan CI, Challiss RAJ: Lithium and the phosphoinositide cycle: an example of uncompetitive inhibition and its pharmacological consequences. Trends Pharmacol Sci 12:297–303, 1991

Nahorski SR, Jenkinson S, Challiss RA: Disruption of phosphoinositide signalling by lithium. Biochem Soc Trans 20:430–434, 1992

Naiman IF, Muniz DE, Stewart RB, et al: Practicality of a lithium dosing guide. Am J Psychiatry 138:1369–1371, 1981

Nalepa I, Vetulani J: Enhancement of the responsiveness of cortical adrenergic receptors by chronic administration of the 5-hydroxytryptamine uptake inhibitor citalopram. J Neurochem 60:2029–2035, 1993

Nalepa I, Vetulani J: The responsiveness of cerebral cortical adrenergic receptors after chronic administration of atypical antidepressant mianserin. J Psychiatry Neurosci 19(2):120, 1994

Nasrallah HA, Varney N, Coffman JA, et al: Opiate antagonism fails to reverse post-ECT cognitive deficits. J Clin Psychiatry 47:555–556, 1986

Nasrallah HA, Coffman JA, Olson SC: Structural brain-imaging findings in affective disorders: an overview. J Neuropsychiatry Clin Neurosci 1:21–26, 1989

Naylor GJ, Smith AHW: Defective genetic control of sodium-pump density in manic depressive psychosis. Psychol Med 11:257–263, 1981

Naylor GJ, McNamee HB, Moody JP: Erythrocyte sodium and potassium in depressive illness. J Psychosom Res 14:173–177, 1970

Naylor GJ, McNamee HB, Moody JP: Changes in erythrocyte sodium and potassium on recovery from depressive illness. Br J Psychiatry 118:219–223, 1971

Naylor GJ, Dick DAT, Dick EG, et al: Lithium therapy and erythrocyte membrane cation carrier. Psychopharmacologia 37:81–86, 1974

Naylor GJ, Smith AHW, Dick EG, et al: Erythrocyte membrane cation carrier in manic-depressive psychosis. Psychol Med 10:521–525, 1980

Nedergaard S, Engberg I, Flatman JA: Serotonin facilitates NMDA responses of cat neocortical neurones. Acta Physiol Scand 128:323–325, 1986

Nedergaard S, Engberg I, Flatman JA: The modulation of excitatory amino acid responses by serotonin in the cat neocortex in vitro. Cell Mol Neurobiol 7:367–379, 1987

Neil JF, Merikangas JR, Foster FG, et al: Waking and all-night sleep EEG's in anorexia nervosa. Clin Electroencephalogr 11:9–15, 1980

Nelsen MR, Dunner DL: Treatment resistance in unipolar depression and other disorders: diagnostic concerns and treatment possibilities. Psychiatr Clin North Am 16:541–566, 1993

Nelson JC, Bowers MB: Delusional unipolar depression. Arch Gen Psychiatry 35:1321–1328, 1978

Nelson JC, Mazure CM: Lithium augmentation in psychotic depression refractory to combined drug treatment. Am J Psychiatry 143:363–366, 1986

Nelson JC, Mazure CM, Bowers MB, et al: A preliminary, open study of the combination of fluoxetine and desipramine for rapid treatment of major depression. Arch Gen Psychiatry 48:303–307, 1991

Nelson SC, Herman MM, Bensch KG, et al: Localization and quantitation of lithium in rat tissue following intraperitoneal injections of lithium chloride, II: brain. J Pharmacol Exp Ther 212:11–15, 1980

Nelson WH, Khan A, Orr WW: Delusional depression, phenomenology, neuro-endocrine function and tricyclic antidepressant response. J Affect Disord 6: 297–306, 1984

Nemeroff CB: Corticotropin-releasing factor, in Neuropeptides and Psychiatric Disorders. Edited by Nemeroff CB. Washington, DC, American Psychiatric Press, 1991a, pp 75–92

Nemeroff CB: Neuropeptides and Psychiatric Disorders. Washington, DC, American Psychiatric Press, 1991b

Nemeroff CB: New vistas in neuropeptide research in neuropsychiatry: focus on corticotropin-releasing factor. Neuropsychopharmacology 6:69–75, 1992

Nemeroff CB, Evans DL: Correlation between the dexamethasone suppression test in depressed patients and clinical response. Am J Psychiatry 141:247–249, 1984

Nemeroff CB, Bissette G, Martin JB, et al: Effect of chronic treatment with thyrotropin-releasing hormone (TRH) or an analog of TRH (linear-beta-alanine TRH) on the hypothalamic-pituitary-thyroid axis. Neuroendocrinology 30:193–199, 1980

Nemeroff CB, Widerlov E, Bissette G, et al: Elevated concentrations of CSF corticotropin-releasing factor-like immunoreactivity in depressed patients. Science 226:1342–1344, 1984

Nemeroff CB, Owens MJ, Bissette G, et al: Reduced corticotropin-releasing factor (CRF) binding sites in the frontal cortex of suicides. Arch Gen Psychiatry 45:577–579, 1988

Nemeroff CB, Krishnan KRR, Reed D, et al: Adrenal gland enlargement in major depression: a computed tomographic study. Arch Gen Psychiatry 49:384–387, 1992

Nestler EJ, Terwilliger RZ, Duman RS: Chronic antidepressant administration alters the subcellular distribution of cyclic AMP-dependent protein kinase in rat frontal cortex. J Neurochem 53:1644–1647, 1989

Nestor PG, Parasuraman R, Haxby JV, et al: Divided attention and metabolic brain dysfunction in mild dementia of the Alzheimer's type. Neuropsychologia 29(5):379–387, 1991

Neubig RR, Gantzos RD, Thomsen WJ: Mechanism of agonist and antagonist binding to alpha-2-adrenergic receptors; evidence for a precoupled receptor-guanine nucleotide protein complex. Biochemistry 27:2374–2384, 1988

Neuvonen PJ, Pohjola-Sintonen F, Tacke U, et al: Five fatal cases of serotonin syndrome after moclobemide-citalopram or moclobemide-clomipramine overdoses. Lancet 342:1419, 1993

Nevins ME, Anthony EW: Antagonists at the serotonin-3 receptor can reduce the fear-potentiated startle response in the rat: evidence for different types of anxiolytic activity? J Pharmacol Exp Ther 268:248, 1994

Newhouse PA, Sunderland T, Tariot PN: The effects of acute scopolamine in geriatric depression. Arch Gen Psychiatry 45:906–912, 1988a

Newhouse PA, Sunderland T, Tariot PN, et al: Intravenous nicotine in Alzheimer's disease: a pilot study. Psychopharmacology 95:171–175, 1988b

Newhouse PA, Sunderland T, Narang PK, et al: Neuroendocrine, physiologic, and behavioral responses following intravenous nicotine in nonsmoking healthy volunteers and in patients with Alzheimer's disease. Psychoneuroendocrinology 15:471–484, 1990

Newhouse PA, Potter A, Corwin J, et al: Acute nicotinic blockade produces cognitive impairment in normal humans. Psychopharmacology 108:480–484, 1992a

Newhouse PA, Penetar D, Fertig J: Stimulant drug effects after prolonged total sleep deprivation: a comparison of amphetamine, nicotine, and deprenyl. Mil Psychol 4:207–234, 1992b

Newhouse PA, Potter A, Lenox RH: Effects of nicotinic agents on human cognition: possible therapeutic applications in Alzheimer's and Parkinson's diseases. Med Chem Res 2:628–642, 1993

Newhouse PA, Potter A, Corwin J, et al: Age-related effects of the nicotinic antagonist mecamylamine on cognition and behavior. Neuropsychopharmacology 10:93–107, 1994

Newhouse PA, Potter A, Corwin J, et al: Acute cognitive effects of nicotine in Alzheimer's and Parkinson's disease. Paper presented at the 34th annual meeting of the American College of Neuropsychopharmacology, San Juan, Puerto Rico, December 11–15, 1995

Newman ME, Belmaker RH: Effects of lithium in vitro and ex vivo on components of the adenylate cyclase system in membranes from the cerebral cortex of the rat. Neuropharmacology 26:211–217, 1987

Newman M, Klein E, Birmaher B, et al: Lithium at therapeutic concentrations inhibits human brain noradrenaline sensitive cyclic AMP accumulation. Brain Res 278:380–381, 1983

Newman ME, Drummer D, Lerer B: Single and combined effects of desimipramine and lithium on serotonergic receptor number and second messenger function in rat brain. J Pharmacol Exp Ther 252:826–831, 1990

Newman ME, Lerer B, Lichtenberg P, et al: Platelet adenylate cyclase activity in depression and after clomipramine and lithium treatment. Psychopharmacology 109:231–234, 1992

Newman SC: The prevalence of depression in Alzheimer's disease and vascular dementia in a population sample. J Affect Disord 52:169–176, 1999

Nibuya M, Rydelek-Fitzgerald L, Russell DS, et al: Induction of BDNF and trkB by electroconvulsive seizure: regional regulation and role of CREB. Soc Neurosci 24:1312, 1994

Nicholson AN, Pascoe PA: 5-Hydroxytryptamine and noradrenaline uptake inhibition: studies on sleep in man. Neuropharmacology 25:1079–1083, 1986

Nicholson AN, Pascoe PA: Studies on the modulation of the sleep-wakefulness continuum in man by fluoxetine, a 5-HT uptake inhibitor. Neuropharmacology 27:597–602, 1988

Nicholson AN, Pascoe PA: Monoaminergic transmission and sleep in man, in Serotonin, Sleep and Mental Disorder. Edited by Idzikowski C, Cowen PJ. Petersfield, England, Wrightson Biomedical Publishing, 1991, pp 215–226

Nicholson AN, Pascoe PA, Stone BM: Modulation of catecholamine transmission and sleep in man. Neuropharmacology 25:271–274, 1986

Nicholson AN, Pascoe PA, Turner C: Modulation of sleep by trimipramine in man. Eur J Pharmacol 37:145–150, 1989a

Nicholson AN, Belyavin AJ, Pascoe PA: Modulation of rapid eye movement sleep in humans by drugs that modify monoaminergic and purinergic transmission. Neuropsychopharmacology 2:131–143, 1989b

Nicoll RA, Madison DV, Lancaster B: Noradrenergic modulation of neuronal excitability in mammalian hippocampus, in Psychopharmacology: The Third Generation of Progress. Edited by Meltzer HY. New York, Raven, 1987, pp 105–112

Nierenberg AA: The treatment of severe depression: is there an efficacy gap between SSRI and TCA antidepressant generations? J Clin Psychiatry 55:55–59 [discussion 60–61, 98–100], 1994

Nierenberg AA, Amsterdam JD: Resistant depression: definition and treatment approaches. J Clin Psychiatry 51 (suppl):39–47, 1990

Nierenberg AA, Adler LA, Peselow E, et al: Trazodone for antidepressant-associated insomnia. Am J Psychiatry 151:1069–1072, 1994a

Nierenberg AA, Feighner JP, Rudolph R, et al: Venlafaxine for treatment-resistant unipolar depression. J Clin Psychopharmacol 14:419–423, 1994b

NIMH/NIH Consensus Development Panel: Mood disorders: pharmacologic prevention of recurrences (NIMH/NIH Consensus Development Conference Statement). Am J Psychiatry 42:469–476, 1985

Nishi M, Whitaker-Azmitia PM, Azmitia EC: Enhanced synaptophysin immunoreactivity in rat hippocampal culture by 5-HT$_{1A}$ agonist S100B, and corticosteroid receptor agonists. Synapse 23:1–9, 1996

Nishizuka Y: Intracellular signaling by hydrolysis of phospholipids and activation of protein kinase C. Science 258:607–614, 1992

Nitsch RM, Growden JH: Commentary: Role of cholinergic transmission in the regulation of amyloid b-protein precursor processing. Biochem Pharmacol 47(8):1275–1284, 1994

Nobler MS, Sackeim HA: Augmentation strategies in electroconvulsive therapy: a synthesis. Convulsive Therapy 9:331–351, 1993

Nobler MS, Sackeim HA: Electroconvulsive therapy: clinical and biological aspects, in Prediction of Treatment Response in Mood Disorders. Edited by Goodnick P. Washington, DC, American Psychiatric Press, 1996, pp 177–198

Nobler MS, Sackeim HA, Solomou M, et al: EEG manifestations during ECT: effects of electrode placement and stimulus intensity. Biol Psychiatry 34:321–330, 1993

Nobler MS, Sackeim HA, Prohovnik I, et al: Regional cerebral blood flow in mood disorders, III: treatment and clinical response. Arch Gen Psychiatry 51:884–897, 1994

Nolen WA, Haffmans PMJ, Bouvy PF, et al: Monoamine oxidase inhibitors in resistant major depression. J Affect Disord 28:189–197, 1993

Nomikos GC, Damsma G, Wenkstern D, et al: Chronic desipramine enhances amphetamine-induced increases in interstitial concentrations of dopamine in the nucleus accumbens. Eur J Pharmacol 195:63–73, 1991

Nomikos GC, Damsma D, Wenkstern D, et al: Effects of chronic bupropion on interstitial concentrations of dopamine in rat nucleus accumbens and striatum. Neuropsychopharmacology 7:7–14, 1992

Nora JJ, Nora HA, Toews WH: Lithium, Ebstein's anomaly, and other congenital heart defects. Lancet 2:594–595, 1974

Norberg L, Wahlström G, Bäckström T: The anaesthetic potency of 3a-hydroxy-5a-pregnan-20-one and 3a-hydroxy-5b-pregnan-20-one determined with an intravenous EEG-threshold method in male rats. Pharmacol Toxicol 61:42–47, 1987

Nordberg A: Human nicotinic receptors-their role in aging and dementia. Neurochem Int 25:93–97, 1994

Nordin C: The CSF/plasma ratio of 10-hydroxynortriptyline is influenced by sex and body height. Psychopharmacology 113:222–224, 1993

Normile HJ, Altman HJ, Galloway M: Facilitation of discrimination learning in aged rats following depletion of brain serotonin. American Geriatrics Society Abstracts 43:549, 1986

Nowak G, Zak J: Effects of repeated treatment with antidepressant drugs and electroconvulsive shocks on the D_2 dopaminergic receptor turnover in the rat brain. Pharmacol Toxicol 69:87–89, 1991

Nowak G, Paul IA, Popik P, et al: Ca^{2+} antagonists effect an antidepressant-like adaptation of the NMDA receptor complex. Eur J Pharmacol 247:101–102, 1993

Noyes R, Dempsey GM, Blum A, et al: Lithium treatment of depression. Compr Psychiatry 15:187–193, 1974

Noyes R, Clancey J, Woodman CO, et al: Environmental factors related to the outcome of panic disorder: a seven-year follow-up study. J Nerv Dis 181:529–538, 1993

Nurnberger J Jr, Jimerson DC, Allen JR, et al: Red cell ouabain-sensitive Na^+-K^+-adenosine triphosphatase: a state marker in affective disorder inversely related to plasma cortisol. Biol Psychiatry 17:981–992, 1982

Nutt D, Montgomery SA: Moclobemide in the treatment of social phobia. Int Clin Psychopharmacol 11 (suppl 3):77–82, 1996

Nutt DJ, Glue P, Lawson CW, et al: Flumazenil provocation of panic attacks: evidence for altered benzodiazepine receptor sensitivity ion panic disorder. Arch Gen Psychiatry 47:917–925, 1990

Nystrom S: On relation between clinical factors and efficacy of ECT in depression. Acta Psychiatrica et Neurologica Scandinavica Supplementum 181:11–135, 1964

Oberholzer AF, Hendriksen C, Monsch AU, et al: Safety and effectiveness of low-dose clozapine in psychogeriatric patients: a preliminary study. Int Psychogeriatr 4:187–195, 1992

Odagaki Y, Koyama T, Matsubara S, et al: Effects of chronic lithium treatment on serotonin binding sites in rat brain. J Psychiatr Res 24:271–277, 1990

O'Dwyer AM, Lightman SL, Marks MN, et al: Treatment of major depression with metyrapone and hydrocortisone. J Affect Disord 33:123–128, 1995

Oehrberg S, Christiansen PE, Behnke K, et al: Paroxetine in the treatment of panic disorder: a randomised, double-blind, placebo-controlled study. Br J Psychiatry 167(3)374–379, 1995

Offord D, Boyle MH, Racine Y: Ontario Child Health Study: correlates of disorder. J Am Acad Child Adolesc Psychiatry 28:856–860, 1989

Ogren S-O: Forebrain serotonin and avoidance learning: behavioural and biochemical studies on the acute effect of p-chloroamphetamine on one-way active avoidance learning in the rat. Pharmacol Biochem Behav 16:881–895, 1982

Ogren S-O: Central serotonin neurons in avoidance learning interactions with noradrenaline and dopamine neurons. Pharmacol Biochem Behav 23:107–124, 1985

Ogren S-O: Analysis of the avoidance learning deficit induced by the serotonin releasing compound p-chloroamphetamine. Brain Res Bull 16:645–660, 1986

Ogren S-O, Johansson C: Separation of the associative and non-associative effects of brain serotonin released by p-chloramphetamine dissociable serotonergic involvement in avoidance learning, pain and motor function. Psychopharmacology 86:12–26, 1985

Ogren S-O, Ross SB, Holm AC, et al: 5-Hydroxytryptamine and avoidance performance in the rat: antagonism of the acute effect of p-chloroamphetamine by zimetidine, an inhibitor of 5-hydroxytryptamine uptake. Neurosci Lett 7:331–336, 1977

Ogren S-O, Hokfelt T, Kask K, et al: Evidence for a role of the neuropeptide galanin in spatial learning (letter). Neuroscience 51:1–5, 1992

Ohkura T, Isse K, Akazawa K, et al: Low-dose estrogen replacement therapy for Alzheimer disease in women. Menopause: The Journal of the North American Menopause Society 1(3):125–130, 1994

Ohno M, Watanabe S: Differential effects of 5-HT$_3$ receptor antagonism on working memory failure due to deficiency of hippocampal cholinergic and glutamatergic transmission in rats. Brain Res 62:211–215, 1997

Ohno M, Yamamoto T, Watanabe S: Blockade of 5-HT$_2$ receptors against impairment of working memory following transient forebrain ischemia in the rat. Neurosci Lett 129:185–188, 1991

Ohno M, Yamamoto T, Watanabe S: Working memory deficits induced by intrahippocampal administration of 8-OH-DPAT a 5-HT$_{1A}$ receptor agonist in the rat. Eur J Pharmacol 234:29–34, 1993

Ohno M, Kishi A, Watanabe S: Effect of cholinergic activation by physostigmine on working memory failure caused in rats by pharmacological manipulation of hippocampal glutamatergic and 5-HTergic neurotransmission. Neurosci Lett 217:21–24, 1996

Ohouha DC, Hyde TM, Kleinman JE: The role of serotonin in schizophrenia: an overview of the nomenclature, distribution and alterations of serotonin receptors in the central nervous system. Psychopharmacology 112:S5–S15, 1993

Okamoto Y, Kagaya A, Shinno H, et al: Serotonin-induced platelet calcium mobilization is enhanced in mania. Life Sci 56:327–332, 1995

Oken BS, Kishiyama SS, Kaye JA, et al: Attention deficit in Alzheimer's disease is not stimulated by an anticholinergic/antihistaminergic drug and is distinct from deficits in healthy aging. Neurology 44:657–662, 1994

Okuma T, Inanaga K, Otsuki S, et al: Comparison of the antimanic efficacy of carbamazepine and chlorpromazine: a double-blind controlled study. Psychopharmacology 66:211–217, 1979

Okuma T, Inanaga K, Otsuki S, et al: A preliminary double-blind study of the efficacy of carbamazepine in prophylaxis of manic-depressive illness. Psychopharmacology 73:95–96, 1981

Okuma T, Yamashita I, Takahashi R, et al: Double-blind controlled studies on the therapeutic efficacy of carbamazepine in affective and schizophrenic patients (abstract). Psychopharmacology 96:102, 1988

Okuma T, Yamashita I, Takahashi R, et al: Comparison of the antimanic efficacy of carbamazepine and lithium carbonate by double-blind controlled study. Pharmacopsychiatry 23:143–150, 1990

Olajide D, Lader M: A comparison of buspirone, diazepam and placebo in patients with chronic anxiety states. J Clin Psychopharmacol 7:148–152, 1987

Old Age Depression Interest Group: How long should the elderly take antidepressants? A double-blind placebo-controlled study of continuation/prophylaxis therapy with diothepin. Br J Psychiatry 162:175–182, 1993

Olenik C, Gotz E, Uhl A, et al: Evidence for a role of noradrenergic neurons in the increase in concentration of preprocholecystokinin-mRNA after cerebral cortex injury in rats. Neuropeptides 24:145–150, 1993

Olfson M, Marcus S, Sackeim HA, et al: Use of ECT for the inpatient treatment of recurrent major depression. Am J Psychiatry 155:22–29, 1998

Olianas MC, Onali P: Phorbol esters increase GTP-dependent adenylate cyclase activity in rat brain striatal membranes. J Neurochem 47:890–897, 1986

Olney JW, Collins RC, Sloviter RS: Excitotoxic mechanism of epileptic brain damage. Adv Neurol 44:857–877, 1986

Olpe H, Kolb CN, Hausdorf A, et al: 4-Aminopyridine and barium chloride attenuate the anti-epileptic effect of carbamazepine in hippocampal slices. Experientia 47:254–257, 1991

Olson L, Nordberg A, von Holst H, et al: Nerve growth factor affects 11-C-nicotine binding, blood flow, EEG, and verbal episodic memory in Alzheimer patient (case report). J Neural Transm 4:79–95, 1992

Oppenheim G: Estrogen in the treatment of depression: neuropharmacological mechanisms. Arch Gen Psychiatry 43:569–573, 1986

Oren DA, Moul DE, Schwartz PJ, et al: A controlled trial of levodopa plus carbidopa in the treatment of winter seasonal affective disorders: a test of the dopamine hypothesis. J Clin Psychopharmacol 14:196–200, 1994

Ormandy G, Jope RS: Analysis of the convulsant-potentiating effects of lithium in rats. Exp Neurol 111:356–361, 1991

Osman OT, Rudorfer MV, Potter WZ: Idazoxan: a selective α_2 antagonist and effective sustained antidepressant in two bipolar depressed patients (letter). Arch Gen Psychiatry 46:958–959, 1989

Oswald I, Adam K: Effects of paroxetine on human sleep. Br J Clin Pharmacol 22:97–99, 1986

Ottevanger EA: The efficacy of fluvoxamine in patients with severe depression. British Journal of Clinical Research 2:125–132, 1991

Ottosson J: Experimental studies of the mode of action of electroconvulsive therapy. Acta Psychiatr Scand Suppl 145:1–141, 1960

Overall JE, Gorham DR: The Brief Psychiatric Rating Scale. Psychol Rep 10:799–812, 1962

Owens MJ, Nemeroff CB: Physiology and pharmacology of corticotropin-releasing factor. Pharmacol Rev 43:425–473, 1991

Owens MJ, Vargas AM, Nemeroff CB: The effects of alprazolam on corticotropin-releasing factor neurons in the rat brain: implications for a role for CRF in the pathogenesis of anxiety disorder. J Psychiatr Res 27 (suppl 1):209, 1993

Ozaki N, Chuang DM: Lithium increases transcription factor binding to AP-1 and cyclic AMP-responsive element in cultured neurons and rat brain. J Neurochem 69:2336–2344, 1997

Paczynski RP, Meyer FB, Anderson RE: Effects of the dihydropyridine Ca^{2+} channel antagonist nimodipine on kainic acid-induced limbic seizures. Epilepsy Res 6:33–38, 1990

Paetsch RR, Greenshaw AJ: Effect of chronic antidepressant treatment on dopamine-related [^{3}H] SCH23390 and [^{3}H] spiperone binding in the rat striatum. Cell Mol Neurobiol 12:597–606, 1992

Palacios JM, Waeber C, Mengod G, et al: Molecular neuroanatomy of 5-HT receptors, in Serotonin: Molecular Biology, Receptors and Functional Effects. Edited by Fozard JR, Saxena PR. Basel, Switzerland, Birkhäuser, 1991, pp 5–20

Palmour RM, Bradwejn J, Ervin FR: The anxiogenic effects of CCK-4 in monkeys are reduced by CCK-B antagonists, benzodiazepines or adenosine A2 agonists. Eur Neuropsychopharmacol 2(3):193–195, 1992a

Palmour R, Bradwejn J, Ervin F: The anxiogenic effects of CCK_4 in monkeys are reduced by CCK-B antagonists, benzodiazepines or adenosine A2 agonists. Clin Neuropharmacol 15 (suppl 1):489B, 1992b

Pancheri P, Bressa GM, Borghi C: Double blind randomised studies on the therapeutic action of alpidem in generalised anxiety disorders, in Imidazopyridines in Anxiety Disorders: A Novel Experimental and Therapeutic Approach. Edited by Bartholini G, Garreau M, Morselli PL. New York, Raven, 1993, pp 155–164

Pande AC, Sayler ME: Adverse events and treatment discontinuations in fluoxetine clinical trials. Int Clin Psychopharmacol 8:267–270, 1993

Pande AC, Krugler T, Haskett RF, et al: Predictors of response to electroconvulsive therapy in major depressive disorder. Biol Psychiatry 24:91–93, 1988

Pande AC, Grunhaus LJ, Haskett RF, et al: Electroconvulsive therapy in delusional and non-delusional depressive disorder. J Affect Disord 19:215–219, 1990

Pande AC, Calarco MM, Grunhaus LJ: Combined MAOI-TCA treatment in refractory depression, in Refractory Depression. Edited by Amsterdam J. New York, Raven, 1991, pp 115–121

Pandey GN, Janicak PG, Javaid JI, et al: Increased 3H-clonidine binding in the platelets of patients with depressive and schizophrenic disorders. Psychiatry Res 28:73–88, 1989

Pandya PK, Huang SC, Talkad VD, et al: Biochemical regulation of the three different states of the cholecystokinin (CCK) receptor in pancreatic acini. Biochim Biophys Acta 1224:117–126, 1994

Pani L, Kuzmin A, Diana M, et al: Calcium receptor antagonists modify cocaine effects in the central nervous system differently. Eur J Pharmacol 190:217–221, 1990

Papadimitriou GN, Kerkhofs M, Kempenaers C, et al: EEG sleep in patients with generalized anxiety disorder. Psychiatry Res 26:183–190, 1988

Papadimitriou GN, Christodoulou GN, Katsouyanni K, et al: Therapy and prevention of affective illness by total sleep deprivation. J Affect Disord 27:107–116, 1993

Papp M, Muscat R, Willner P: Additive effects of chronic treatment with antidepressant drugs and intermittent treatment with a dopamine agonist. Eur Neuropsychopharmacol 2:121–125, 1992

Papp LA, Klein DF, Gorman JM: Carbon dioxide hypersensitivity, hyperventilation, and panic disorder. Am J Psychiatry 150:1149–1157, 1993

Papp M, Klimek V, Willner P: Parallel changes in dopamine D_2 receptor binding in limbic forebrain associated with chronic mild stress-induced anhedonia and its reversal by imipramine. Psychopharmacology 115:441–446, 1994

Parasuraman R, Haxby JV: Attention and brain function in Alzheimer's disease. Neuropsychology 7:242–272, 1993

Parasuraman R, Greenwood PM, Haxby JV, et al: Visuospatial attention in dementia of the Alzheimer type. Brain 115:711–733, 1992

Parks RW, Young CS, Rippey RF, et al: Nicotinic stimulation of anterior regional glucose metabolism in Alzheimer's disease: preliminary study with transdermal patches, in Alzheimer's Disease: Therapeutic Strategies. Edited by Giacobini E, Becker R. Boston, MA, Birkhäuser, 1994, pp 424–427

Parrott AC, Craig D: Cigarette smoking and nicotine gum (0, 2 and 4 mg): effects upon four visual attention tasks. Neuropsychobiology 25:34–43, 1992

Parsa MA, Ramirez LF, Loula EC, et al: Effect of clozapine on psychotic depression and parkinsonism (letter). J Clin Psychopharmacol 11:330–331, 1991

Pascual J, del Arco C, Gonzalez A, et al: Quantitative light microscopic autoradiographic localization of α_2 adrenoceptors in the human brain. Brain Res 585:116–127, 1992

Pascual-Leone A, Houser CM, Reese K, et al: Safety of rapid-rate transcranial magnetic stimulation in normal volunteers. Electroencephalogr Clin Neurophysiol 89:120–130, 1993

Pascual-Leone A, Valls-Sole J, Wassermann EM, et al: Responsiveness to rapid-rate transcranial magnetic stimulation of the human motor cortex. Brain 117:847–858, 1994

Passouant P, Cadhilac J, Billiard M: Withdrawal of the paradoxal sleep by clomipramine: electrophysiological, histochemical and biochemical study. Int J Neurol 10:186–197, 1975

Patchev VK, Shoaib M, Holsboer F, et al: The neurosteroid tetrahydroprogesterone counteracts corticotropin-releasing hormone-induced anxiety and alters the release and gene expression of corticotropin-releasing hormone in the rat hypothalamus. Neuroscience 62:265–271, 1994

Patel B, Tandon R: Development of obsessive-compulsive symptoms during clozapine treatment. Am J Psychiatry 150:836, 1993

Patel J, Keith RA, Salama AI, et al: Role of calcium in regulation of phosphoinositide signaling pathway. J Mol Neurosci 3:1–9, 1991

Patil VJ: Development of transient obsessive-compulsive symptoms during treatment with clozapine. Am J Psychiatry 149:272, 1992

Pato MT, Zohar-Kadouch R, Zohar J, et al: Return of symptoms after discontinuation of CMI in patients with OCD. Am J Psychiatry 145:1521–1522, 1988

Pato PT, Pigott TA, Hill JL, et al: Controlled comparison of buspirone and CMI in OCD. Am J Psychiatry 148:127–129, 1991

Patterson JF: Treatment of acute mania with verapamil (letter). J Clin Psychopharmacol 7:206–207, 1987

Patwardhan RV, Mitchell MC, Johnson RF, et al: Differential effects of oral contraceptive steroids on the metabolism of benzodiazepines. Hepatology 3(2): 248–253, 1983

Paudice P, Raiteri M: Cholecystokinin release mediated by 5-HT3 receptors in rat cerebral cortex and nucleus accumbens. Br J Pharmacol 103:1790–1794, 1991

Paul IA, Trullas R, Skolnick P, et al: Down-regulation of cortical β-adrenoceptors by chronic treatment with functional NMDA antagonists. Psychopharmacology 106:285–287, 1992

Paul IA, Layer RT, Skolnick P, et al: Adaptation of the N-methyl-D-aspartate receptor complex in rat front cortex following chronic treatment with electroconvulsive shock or imipramine. Eur J Pharmacol 247:305–312, 1993

Paul SM, Purdy RH: Neuroactive steroids. FASEB J 6:2311–2322, 1992

Paul V, Balasubramaniam E, Kazi M: The neurobehavioural toxicity of endosulfan in rats: a serotonergic involvement in learning impairment. Eur J Pharmacol 270:1–7, 1994

Pauls DL, Towbin KE, Leckman JF, et al: Gilles de la Tourette's syndrome and obsessive-compulsive disorder: evidence supporting a genetic relationship. Arch Gen Psychiatry 43:1180–1182, 1986

Pavlasevic S, Bednar I, Qureshi GA, et al: Brain cholecystokinin tetrapeptide levels are increased in a rat model of anxiety. Neuroreport 5:225–228, 1993

Paykel ES: Clinical efficacy of reversible and selective inhibitors of monoamine oxidase A in major depression. Acta Psychiatr Scand Suppl 386:22–27, 1995

Paykel ES, Myers JK, Deinelt MN, et al: Life events and depression: a controlled study. Arch Gen Psychiatry 21:753–760, 1969

Pazos A, Palacios JM: Quantitative autoradiographic mapping of serotonin receptors in the rat brain, I: serotonin-1 receptors. Brain Res 346:205–230, 1985

Pazzaglia PJ, Post RM: Contingent tolerance and reresponse to carbamazepine: a case study in a patient with trigeminal neuralgia and bipolar disorder. J Neuropsychiatry Clin Neurosci 4:76–81, 1992

Pazzaglia PJ, Post RM, Ketter TA, et al: Preliminary controlled trial of nimodipine in ultra-rapid cycling affective dysregulation. Psychiatry Res 49:257–272, 1993

Pazzaglia PJ, Post RM, Ketter TA, et al: Nimodipine monotherapy and carbamazepine augmentation in patients with refractory recurrent affective illness. J Clin Psychopharmacol 18:404–413, 1998

Peabody C, Thiemann S, Pigache R, et al: Desglycinamide-9-arginine-8-Vasopressin (Org 5667) in patients with dementia. Neurobiol Aging 6:95–100, 1985

Pearlson GD, Garbacz DJ, Tompkins RH, et al: Clinical correlates of lateral ventricular enlargement in bipolar affective disorder. Am J Psychiatry 141:253–256, 1984

Pecknold JC, Matas M, Howarth BG, et al: Evaluation of buspirone as an antianxiety agent: buspirone and diazepam versus placebo. Can J Psychiatry 34:766–771, 1989

Pecknold JC, Lathe L, Iny L, et al: Platelet [3H] paroxetine and [3H] imipramine binding in zacopride treated patients with generalized anxiety disorder: preliminary results, in New Concepts of Anxiety (Pierre Fabre Monograph Series). Edited by Briley M, File SE. London, Macmillan, 1991, p 168

Pecknold JC, Luthe L, Scott-Fleury MH, et al: Gepirone and the treatment of panic disorder: an open study. J Clin Psychopharmacol 13:145–149, 1993

Pedersen CA: The psychiatric significance in oxytocin, in Neuropeptides and Psychiatric Disorders. Edited by Nemeroff CB. Washington, DC, American Psychiatric Press, 1991, pp 131–148

Pereira EFR, Reinhardt-Maelicke S, Schrattenholz A, et al: Identification and functional characterization of a new agonist site on nicotinic acetylcholine receptors of cultured hippocampal neurons. J Pharmacol Exp Ther 265:1474–1491, 1993

Perez de la Mora N, Hernandez-Gomez AM, et al: Cholecystokinin-8 increases K^+-evoked [^{3}H]gamma-aminobutyric acid release in slices from various brain areas. Eur J Pharmacol 250:423–430, 1993

Perez V, Gilaberte I, Faries D, et al: Randomised, double blind, placebo-controlled trial of pindolol in combination with fluoxetine antidepressant treatment. Lancet 349(9065):1594–1597, 1997

Perna G, Marconi C, Battaglia M, et al: Subclinical impairment of lung airways in patients with panic disorder. Biol Psychiatry 36:601–605, 1994

Perna G, Cocchi S, Bertani A, et al: Sensitivity to 35% CO_2 in healthy first-degree relatives of patients with panic disorder. Am J Psychiatry 152:623–625, 1995

Peroutka SJ, Howell TA: The molecular evolution of G protein-coupled receptors: focus on 5-hydroxytryptamine receptors. Neuropharmacology 33:319–324, 1994

Perrin MH, Donaldson CJ, Chen R, et al: Cloning and functional expression of a rat brain corticotropin releasing factor (CRF) receptor. Endocrinology 133:3058–3061, 1993

Perry EK: The cholinergic hypothesis—ten years on. Br Med Bull 42(1):63–69, 1986

Perry EK, Perry RH, Blessed G, et al: Necropsy evidence of central cholinergic deficits in senile dementia. Lancet 1:189, 1977

Perry EK, Tomlinson BE, Blessed G, et al: Correlation of cholinergic abnormalities with senile plaques and mental test scores in senile dementia. BMJ 2:1457–1459, 1978

Perry EK, Perry RH, Candy JM, et al: Cortical serotonin–S2 receptor binding abnormalities in patients with Alzheimer's disease: comparison with Parkinson's disease. Neurosci Lett 51:353–357, 1984

Perry EK, Curtis M, Dick DJ, et al: Cholinergic correlates of cognitive impairment in Parkinson's disease: comparisons with Alzheimer's disease. J Neurol Neurosurg Psychiatry 48:413–421, 1985

Perry PJ, Garvey MJ, Noyes R: Benzodiazepine treatment of generalized anxiety disorder, in Handbook of Anxiety, Vol 4: The Treatment of Anxiety. Edited by Noyes R, Burroughs GD. Amsterdam, Elsevier, 1990, pp 111–145

Perse TL, Greist JH, Jeffersen JW, et al: Fluvoxamine treatment of obsessive-compulsive disorder. Am J Psychiatry 144:1543–1548, 1987

Persinger MA, Makarec K, Bradley JC: Characteristics of limbic seizures evoked by peripheral injections of lithium and pilocarpine. Physiol Behav 44:27–37, 1988

Pert A, Rosenblatt JE, Sivit C, et al: Long-term treatment with lithium prevents the development of dopamine receptor supersensitivity. Science 201:171–173, 1978

Pert CB, Pert A, Rosenblatt JE, et al: Catecholamine receptor stabilization. A possible mode of lithium's antimanic action, in Catecholamines: Basic and Clinical Frontiers. Edited by Usdin E, Kopin IJ, Barchas JD. New York, Pergamon, 1979, pp 583–585

Peters BH, Levin HS: Memory enhancement after physostigmine treatment in the amnesic syndrome. Arch Neurol 34:215–219, 1977

Peterson R: Scopolamine-induced learning failures in man. Psychopharmacology 52:283–289, 1977

Petkov VD, Kehayov R: Effects of agonists and antagonists of some serotonin receptor subtypes on memory and their modulation by the 5-HT uptake inhibitor fluoxetine. Acta Physiol Pharmacol Bulg 20:83–90, 1994

Petkov VD, Belcheva S, Konstantinova E, et al: Participation of different 5-HT receptors in the memory process in rats and its modulation by the serotonin depletor p-chlorohenylalinine. Acta Neurobiol Exp (Warsz) 55:243–252, 1995

Petrie WM, Ban TA, Berney S, et al: Loxapine in psychogeriatrics: a placebo and standard-controlled clinical investigation. J Clin Psychopharmacol 2:122–126, 1982

Petterson U, Fyro B, Sedvall G: A new scale for the longitudinal rating of manic states. Acta Psychiatr Scand 49:248–256, 1973

Pettinati HM, Stephens SM, Willis KM, et al: Evidence for less improvement in depression in patients taking benzodiazepines during unilateral ECT. Am J Psychiatry 147:1029–1035, 1990

Petty F: GABA and mood disorders: a brief review and hypothesis. J Affect Disord 34:275–281, 1995

Pfaff DW: Molecular strategies for identifying the roles of steroids in behavior. Paper presented at the annual meeting of the Society of Biological Psychiatry, New York, May 1–5, 1996

Pfeiffer A, Veilleux S, Barden N: Antidepressant and other centrally acting drugs regulate glucocorticoid receptor messenger RNA levels in rat brain. Psychoneuroendocrinology 16:505–515, 1991

Pflug B, Tolle R: Disturbance of 24 hour rhythm, endogenous depression, and the treatment of endogenous depression. International Pharmacopsychiatry 6:187–196, 1971

Pfohl B, Stangl D, Zimmerman M: The implications of DSM III personality disorders for patients with major depression. J Affect Disord 7:309–318, 1984

Phelps ME, Mazziotta JC, Baxter, L, et al: Positron emission tomographic study of affective disorders: problems and strategies. Ann Neurol 15 (suppl):149–156, 1984

Phillip E, Wilckens T, Friess E, et al: Cholecystokinin, gastrin and stress hormone response in marathon runners. Peptides 13:125–128, 1992

Phillips SM, Sherwin BB: Effects of estrogen on memory function in surgically menopausal women. Psychoneuroendocrinology 17:485–495, 1992

Piazza PV, Deminiere JM, Le Moal M, et al: Factors that predict individual vulnerability to AMPH self-administration. Science 245:1511–1513, 1989

Pickar D, Owen RR, Litman RE, et al: Clinical and biologic response to clozapine in patients with schizophrenia. Arch Gen Psychiatry 49:345–353, 1992

Pigott TA, Murphy DL: In reply to "Are effective antiobsessional drugs interchangeable?" (letter). Arch Gen Psychiatry 48:858–859, 1991

Pigott TA, Pato MT, Bernstein SE, et al: Controlled comparisons of clomipramine and fluoxetine in the treatment of obsessive-compulsive disorder: behavioral and biological results [see comments]. Arch Gen Psychiatry 47:926–932, 1990

Pigott TA, Pato MT, L'Heureux F, et al: A controlled comparison of adjuvant lithium carbonate or thyroid hormone in clomipramine-treated patients with obsessive-compulsive disorder. J Clin Psychopharmacol 11:242–248, 1991a

Pigott TA, Zohar J, Hill JL, et al: Meterogoline blocks the behavioral and neuroendocrine effects of orally administered m-chlorophenylpiperazine in patients with obsessive-compulsive disorder. Biol Psychiatry 29:418–26, 1991b

Pigott TA, L'Heureux F, Hill JL, et al: A double-blind study of adjuvant buspirone hydrochloride in clomipramine-treated patients with obsessive-compulsive disorder. J Clin Psychopharmacol 12:11–18, 1992a

Pigott TA, L'Heureux F, Rubenstein CS, et al. A double-blind, placebo-controlled study of trazodone in patients with obsessive-compulsive disorder. J Clin Psychopharmacol 12:156–162, 1992b

Pigott TA, Hill JL, Gardy TA, et al: A comparison of the behavioral effects of oral versus intravenous mCPP administration in OCD patients and the effect of metergoline prior to i.v. mCPP [see comments]. Biol Psychiatry 33:3–14, 1993

Pilowsky R, West M, Chalmers J: Renal sympathetic nerve responses to stimulation, inhibition and destruction of the ventrolateral medulla in the rabbit. Neurosci Lett 60:51–55, 1985

Pinder RM, Fink M: Mianserin. Mod Probl Pharmacopsychiatry 18:70–101, 1982

Pinder RM, Wieringa JH: Third generation antidepressants. Med Res Rev 13:259–325, 1993

Pine DS, Weese-Mayer DW, Silvestri JM, et al: Anxiety and congenital central hypoventilation syndrome. Am J Psychiatry 151:864–870, 1994

Pine DS, Cohen P, Brook J: Emotional problems during youth as predictors of stature during early adulthood: results from a prospective epidemiologic study. Pediatrics 97:856–863, 1996a

Pine DS, Wasserman G, Coplan J, et al: Serotonergic and cardiac correlates of aggression in children. Ann N Y Acad Sci 794:391–393, 1996b

Pinget M, Straus E, Yalow RS: Localization of cholecystokinin-like immunoreactivity in isolated nerve terminals. Proc Natl Acad Sci U S A 75:6324–6326, 1978

Pinner E, Rich CL: Effects of trazodone on aggressive behavior in seven patients with organic mental disorders. Am J Psychiatry 145:1295–1296, 1988

Pisegna JR, de Weerth A, Huppi K, et al: Molecular cloning of the human brain and gastric cholecystokinin receptor: structure, functional expression and chromosomal localization. Biochem Biophys Res Commun 189:296–303, 1992

Pitman RK: Animal models of compulsive behavior. Biol Psychiatry 26:189–198, 1989

Pitsikas N, Borsini F: Itasetron (DAU 6215) prevents age-related memory deficits in the rat in a multiple choice avoidance task. Eur J Pharmacol 12:115–119, 1996

Pitsikas N, Borsini F: Differential effects of tropisetron and ondansetron in learning and memory paradigms. Pharmacol Biochem Behav 56:571–576, 1997

Pitsikas N, Brambilla A, Borsini F: Effect of DAU6215, a novel 5-HT$_3$ receptor antagonist, on scopolamine induced amnesia in the rat in a spatial learning task. Pharmacol Biochem Behav 47:95–99, 1994

Pitts CD, Oakes R, Gergel IP: Effectiveness of paroxetine in the treatment of generalized social phobia. Paper presented at the 35th annual meeting of the American College of Neuropsychopharmacology, San Juan, Puerto Rico, 1996

Placidi GF, Lenzi A, Lazzerini F, et al: The comparative efficacy and safety of carbamazepine versus lithium: a randomized, double-blind 3-year trial in 83 patients. J Clin Psychiatry 47:490–494, 1986

Plotsky PM, Meaney MJ: Early, postnatal experience alters hypothalamic corticotropin-releasing factor (CRF) mRNA, median eminence CRF content and stress-induced release in adult rats. Mol Brain Res 18:195–200, 1993

Plotsky PM, Otto S, Sutta S: Neurotransmitter modulation of corticotropin-releasing factor secretion into hypophysial-portal secretion. Life Sci 41:1311–1317, 1987

Plum F, Posner JB, Troy B: Cerebral metabolic and circulatory responses to induced convulsions in animals. Arch Neurol 16:1–13, 1968

Pohl R, Yeragani V, Balon R, et al: The jitterines syndrome in panic disorder patients treated with antidepressants. J Clin Psychiatry 49:100–104, 1988

Pohl R, Balon R, Yeragani VK, et al: Serotonergic anxiolytics in the treatment of panic disorder: a controlled study with buspirone. Psychopathology 22 (suppl 1):60–67, 1989

Pohl RB, Wolkow RM, Clary CM: Sertraline in the treatment of panic disorder: a double-blind multicenter trial. Am J Psychiatry 155:1189–1195, 1998

Poirer MF, Galzin AM, et al: Short-term lithium administration to healthy volunteers produces long-lasting pronounced changes in platelet serotonin uptake but not imipramine binding. Psychopharmacology 94:521–526, 1988

Poirier-Littre MF, Loo H, Dennis T, et al: Lithium treatment increases norepinephrine turnover in the plasma of healthy subjects (letter). Arch Gen Psychiatry 50:72–73, 1993

Poitou P, Bohuon C: Catecholamine metabolism in the rat brain after short and long term lithium administration. J Neurochem 25:535–537, 1975

Pollack MH, Hammerness P: Adjunctive yohimbine for treatment of refractory depression. Biol Psychiatry 33:220–221, 1993

Pollack MH, Rosenbaum JF: Verapamil in the treatment of recurrent unipolar depression. Biol Psychiatry 22:779–782, 1987

Pollack MH, Otto MW, Worthington JJ, et al: Sertraline in the treatment of panic disorder—a flexible-dose multicenter trial. Arch Gen Psychiatry 55:1010–1016, 1998

Pollock BG: Recent developments in drug metabolism of relevance to psychiatrists. Harv Rev Psychiatry 2:204–213, 1994

Pontzer NJ, Crews FT: Desensitization of muscarinic stimulated hippocampal cell firing is related to phosphoinositide hydrolysis and inhibited by lithium. J Pharmacol Exp Ther 253:921–929, 1990

Pope HG Jr, McElroy SL, Satlin A, et al: Head injury, bipolar disorder, and response to valproate. Compr Psychiatry 29:34–38, 1988

Pope HG Jr, McElroy SL, Keck PE Jr, et al: Valproate in the treatment of acute mania: a placebo-controlled study. Arch Gen Psychiatry 48:62–68, 1991

Porges SW: Vagal tone: a mediator of affects, in The Development of Affect Regulation and Dysregulation. Edited by Garber JA, Dodge KA. New York, Cambridge University Press, 1991

Porsolt RD, Bertin A, Jalfre M: Behavioral despair in mice: a primary screening test for antidepressants. Archives Internationales de Pharmacodynamie et de Therapie 229:327–336, 1977

Porsolt RD, Bertin A, Blavet N: Immobility induced by swimming in rats: effects of agents which modify central catecholamine and serotonin activity. Eur J Pharmacol 57:201–220, 1979

Porsteinsson AP, Tariot PN, Erb R, et al: An open trial of valproate for agitation in geriatric neuropsychiatric disorders. Am J Geriatr Psychiatry 5:344–351, 1997

Posener JA, Schildkraut JJ, Williams GH, et al: Acute and delayed effects of corticotropin-releasing hormone on dopamine activity in man. Biol Psychiatry 36:616–621, 1994

Posner MI: Orienting of attention. Q J Exp Psychol 32:3–25, 1980

Post RM: Alternatives to lithium for bipolar affective illness, in American Psychiatric Press Review of Psychiatry, Vol 9. Edited by Tasman A, Goldfinger SM, Kaufmann C. Washington, DC, American Psychiatric Press, 1990a, pp 170–202

Post RM: Prophylaxis of bipolar affective disorder. International Review of Psychiatry 2:277–320, 1990b

Post RM: Transduction of psychosocial stress into the neurobiology of recurrent affective disorder. Am J Psychiatry 149:999–1010, 1992

Post RM: Mechanisms underlying the evolution of affective disorders: implications for long-term treatment, in Progress in Psychiatry: Severe Depressive Disorders. Edited by Grunhaus L, Greden JF. Washington, DC, American Psychiatric Press, 1994, pp 23–65

Post RM, Chuang D-M: Mechanism of action of lithium: comparison and contrast with carbamazepine, in Lithium and the Cell: Pharmacology and Biochemistry. Edited by Birch NJ. London, Academic Press, 1991, pp 199–241

Post RM, Weiss SRB: The neurobiology of treatment-resistant mood disorders, in Psychopharmacology: The Fourth Generation of Progress. Edited by Bloom FE, Kupfer DJ. New York, Raven, 1995

Post RM, Weiss SRB: A speculative model of affective illness cyclicity based on patterns of drug tolerance observed in amygdala-kindled seizures. Mol Neurobiol 13:33–60, 1996

Post RM, Kotin J, Goodwin FK, et al: Psychomotor activity and cerebrospinal fluid amine metabolites in affective illness. Am J Psychiatry 130:67–72, 1973

Post RM, Stoddard FJ, Gillin JC, et al: Alterations in motor activity, sleep, and biochemistry in a cycling manic-depressive patient. Arch Gen Psychiatry 34:470–477, 1977

Post RM, Ballenger JC, Hare TA, et al: Cerebrospinal fluid GABA in normals and patients with affective disorders. Brain Res Bull 5 (suppl 2):755–759, 1980

Post RM, Uhde TW, Ballenger JC, et al: Prophylactic efficacy of carbamazepine in manic-depressive illness. Am J Psychiatry 140:1602–1604, 1983

Post RM, Ballenger JC, Uhde TW, et al: Efficacy of carbamazepine in manic-depressive illness: implications for underlying mechanisms, in Neurobiology of Mood Disorders. Edited by Post RM, Ballenger JC. Baltimore, MD, Williams & Wilkins, 1984, pp 777–816

Post RM, Rubinow DR, Ballenger JC: Conditioning and sensitisation in the longitudinal course of affective illness. Br J Psychiatry 149:191–201, 1986a

Post RM, Rubinow DR, Uhde TW, et al: Dopaminergic effects of carbamazepine: relationship to clinical response in affective illness. Arch Gen Psychiatry 43:392–397, 1986b

Post RM, Putnam F, Uhde TW: Electroconvulsive therapy as an anticonvulsant: implications for its mechanism of action in affective illness. Ann N Y Acad Sci 462:376–388, 1986c

Post RM, Uhde TW, Roy-Byrne PP, et al: Correlates of antimanic response to carbamazepine. Psychiatry Res 21:71–83, 1987

Post RM, Roy-Byrne PP, Uhde TW: Graphic representation of the life course of illness in patients with affective disorder. Am J Psychiatry 145:844–848, 1988

Post RM, Leverich GS, Rosoff AS, et al: Carbamazepine prophylaxis in refractory affective disorders: a focus on long-term follow-up. J Clin Psychopharmacol 10:318–327, 1990

Post RM, Weiss, SRB, Chuang D-M: Mechanisms of action of anticonvulsants in affective disorders: comparisons with lithium. J Clin Psychopharmacol 12:23S–35S, 1992

Post RM, Ketter TA, Denicoff K, et al: Assessment of anticonvulsant drugs in patients with bipolar illness, in Human Psychopharmacology, Vol 4. Edited by Hindmarch I, Stonier PD. Chichester, England, Wiley, 1993a, pp 211–245

Post RM, Leverich GS, Pazzaglia PJ, et al: Lithium tolerance and discontinuation as pathways to refractoriness, in Lithium in Medicine and Biology. Edited by Birch NJ, Padgham C, Hughes MS. Lancashire, England, Marius Press, 1993b, pp 71–84

Post RM, Ketter TA, Pazzaglia PJ, et al: New developments in the use of anticonvulsants as mood stabilizers. Neuropsychobiology 27:132–137, 1993c

Post RM, Ketter TA, Pazzaglia PJ, et al: Anticonvulsants in refractory mood disorders, in Refractory Depression: Current Strategies and Future Directions. Edited by Nolen WA, Zohar J, Roose SP, et al. Chichester, England, Wiley, 1994a, pp 97–114

Post RM, Weiss SRB, Chuang D, et al: Mechanisms of action of carbamazepine in seizure and affective disorders, in Anticonvulsants in Mood Disorders. Edited by Joffe RT, Calabrese JR. New York, Marcel Dekker, 1994b, pp 43–92

Potokar J, Nutt DJ: Anxiolytic potential of benzodiazepine receptor partial agonists. CNS Drugs 1:305–315, 1994

Potter E, Behan DP, Linton EA, et al: The central distribution of a corticotropin-releasing factor (CRF)-binding protein predicts multiple sites and modes of interaction with CRF. Proc Natl Acad Sci U S A 89:4192–4196, 1992

Potter WZ, Rudorfer MV: Electroconvulsive therapy—a modern medical procedure. N Engl J Med 328:882–883, 1993

Potter WZ, Scheinin M, Golden RN, et al: Selective antidepressants lack specificity on norepinephrine and serotonin metabolites in cerebrospinal fluid. Arch Gen Psychiatry 42:1171–1177, 1985

Potter WZ, Rudorfer MV, Manji HK: Potential new pharmacotherapies for refractory depression, in American Psychiatric Press Review of Psychiatry, Vol 9. Edited by Tasman A, Goldfinger SM, Kaufmann C. Washington, DC, American Psychiatric Press, 1990, pp 145–169

Potter WZ, Rudorfer MV, Manji HK: The pharmacological treatment of depression. N Engl J Med 325:633–642, 1991

Potter WZ, Manji HK, Rudorfer M: Tricyclics and tetracyclics, in the American Psychiatric Press Textbook of Psychopharmacology. Edited by Schatzberg AF, Nemeroff CB. Washington, DC, American Psychiatric Press, 1995

Pough TF, Jerath BK, Smith WM, et al: Rates of mental disease related to child bearing. N Engl J Med 268:1224–1228, 1963

Powell GF, Raiti S, Blizzard RM: Emotional deprivation and growth retardation simulating idiopathic hypopituitarism, II: endocrinologic evaluation of the syndrome. N Engl J Med 276:1279–1283, 1967

Powell KR, Barrett JE: Evaluation of the effects of PD 134308 (CI-988), a CCK-B antagonist, on the punished responding of squirrel monkeys. Neuropeptides 19 (suppl):75–78, 1991

Powers JS, Decoskey D, Kahrillas PJ: Physostigmine for the treatment of delirium tremens. J Clin Pharmacol 21:57–60, 1981

Prange AJ Jr: Paroxysmal auricular tachycardia apparently resulting from combined thyroid-imipramine treatment. Am J Psychiatry 119:994–995, 1963

Prange AJ: Estrogen may well affect response to antidepressant. JAMA 219:143–144, 1972

Prange AJ: Hormones as antidepressants: the thyroid model, in Endocrine Psychopharmacology. Edited by Halbreich U. Washington, DC, American Psychiatric Press (in press)

Prange AJ, Wilson IC, Rabon AM, et al: Enhancement of imipramine antidepressant activity by thyroid hormone. Am J Psychiatry 126:457–468, 1969

Prange AJ Jr, Wilson IC, Lara PP, et al: Effects of thyrotropin-releasing hormone in depression. Lancet 2:999–1002, 1972

Prange AJ Jr, Wilson IC, Breese GR, et al: Hormonal alteration of imipramine response: a review, in Hormones Behavior and Psychopathology. Edited by Sachar EJ. New York, Raven, 1976, p 41

Prange AJ Jr, Loosen PT, Wilson IC, et al: The therapeutic use of hormones of the thyroid axis in depression, in Neurobiology of Mood Disorders (Frontiers of Clinical Neuroscience, Vol 1). Edited by Post RM, Ballenger JC. Baltimore, MD, Williams & Wilkins, 1984, p 311

Prange AJ, Mason GA, Garbutt JC: Thyroid axis syndromes in depression: definitions and interpretations, in Pharmacotherapy of Depression: Applications for the Outpatient Practitioner. Edited by Amsterdam JD. New York, Marcel Dekker, 1990, pp 35–55

Pranzatelli MR: Benzodiazepine-induced shaking behavior in the rat: structure-activity and relation to serotonin and benzodiazepine receptors. Exp Neurol 104:241–250, 1989

Preskorn SH: Pharmacokinetics of antidepressants: why and how they are relevant to treatment (review). J Clin Psychiatry 54 (suppl):14–34, 1993

Preskorn SH: Should rational drug development in psychiatry target more than one mechanism of action in a single molecule? Int Rev Psychiatry 7:17–28, 1995

Preskorn SH, Mac DS: Plasma levels of amitriptyline: effects of age and sex. J Clin Psychiatry 46:276–277, 1985

Preston GC: 5-HT$_3$ antagonists and disorders of cognition, in Recent Advances in the Treatment of Neurodegenerative Disorders and Cognitive Dysfunction. Edited by Racagni G, Brunelo N, Langer SZ. Basel, Switzerland, Karger, 1994, pp 89–93

Preston GC, Millson DS, Ceuppens PR, et al: Effects of the 5-HT$_3$ receptor antagonist GR68755 on a scopolamine-induced cognitive deficit in healthy subjects. Br J Clin Pharmacol 32:546P, 1991

Price H, Goddard AW, Barr LC, et al: Pharmacological challenges in anxiety disorders, in Psychopharmacology: The Fourth Generation of Progress. Edited by Bloom FE, Kupfer DJ. New York, Raven, 1995, pp 1331–1325

Price LH, Charney DS, Heninger GR: Variability of response to lithium augmentation in refractory depression. Am J Psychiatry 143:1387–1392, 1986

Price LH, Charney DS, Delgado PL, et al: Lithium treatment and serotoninergic function. Arch Gen Psychiatry 46:13–19, 1989

Price LH, Charney DS, Delgado PL, et al: Lithium and serotonin function: implications for the serotonin hypothesis of depression. Psychopharmacology 100:3–12, 1990

Prien RF, Gelenberg AJ: Alternatives to lithium for preventive treatment of bipolar disorder. Am J Psychiatry 146:840–848, 1989

Prien RF, Kocsis JH: Long-term treatment of mood disorders, in Psychopharmacology: The Fourth Generation of Progress. Edited by Bloom FA, Kupfer DJ. New York, Raven, 1995

Prien RF, Kupfer DJ: Continuation drug therapy for major depressive episodes: how long should it be maintained? Am J Psychiatry 143:18–23, 1986

Prien RF, Klett J, Caffey EM Jr: Lithium carbonate and imipramine in prevention of affective episodes: a comparison in recurrent affective illness. Report of the Veterans Administration and National Institute of Mental Health Collaborative Study. Arch Gen Psychiatry 29:420–425, 1973a

Prien RF, Caffey EM Jr, Klett CJ: Prophylactic efficacy of lithium carbonate in manic-depressive illness. Arch Gen Psychiatry 28:337–341, 1973b

Prien RF, Klett J, Caffey EM Jr: Lithium carbonate and imipramine in prevention of affective episodes: report from the VA-NIMH collaborative study of lithium therapy. Arch Gen Psychiatry 29:420–425, 1978

Prien RF, Kupfer DJ, Mansky PA, et al: Drug therapy in the prevention of recurrences in unipolar and bipolar affective disorders. Report of the NIMH Collaborative Study Group Comparing Lithium Carbonate, Imipramine, and a Lithium Carbonate-Imipramine Combination. Arch Gen Psychiatry 41:1096–1104, 1984

Prien RF, Himmelhoch JM, Kupfer DF: Treatment of mixed mania. J Affect Disord 15:9–15, 1988

Prince DA, Wilder BJ: Cortical mechanisms in cortical epileptogenic foci "surrounded" inhibition. Arch Neurol 16:194–202, 1967

Prinz PN, Vitaliano PP, Vitiello MV, et al: Sleep, EEG and mental function changes in senile dementia of the Alzheimer's type. Neurobiol Aging 3:361–370, 1982

Pritchett DB, Seeburg PH: GABAa receptor alpha-5 subunit creates novel type II benzodiazepine receptor pharmacology. J Neurochem 54:1802–1804, 1990

Prohovnik I, Mayeux R, Sackheim HA, et al: Cerebral profusion as a diagnostic marker of early Alzheimer's disease. Neurology 38:931–937, 1988

Provost SC, Woodward R: Effects of nicotine gum on repeated administration of the Stroop test. Psychopharmacology 104:536–540, 1991

Prudic J, Sackeim HA, Devanand DP: Medication resistance and clinical response to electroconvulsive therapy. Psychiatry Res 31:287–296, 1990

Prudic J, Haskett RF, Mulsant B, et al: Resistance to antidepressant medications and short-term clinical response to ECT. Am J Psychiatry 153:985–992, 1996

Prudic J, Fitzsimons L, Nobler MS, et al: Naloxone in the prevention of the adverse cognitive effects of ECT: a within-subject, placebo controlled study. Neuropsychopharmacology (in press)

Przegalinski E, Jurkowska T: Repeated treatment with antidepressants does not modify the locomotor effect of dopaminergic stimulants injected into the rat hippocampus. Archives Internationales de Pharmacodynamie et de Therapie 305:152–162, 1990

Puia G, Santi MR, Vincini S, et al: Neurosteroids act on recombinant human GABAa receptors. Neuron 39:759–765, 1990

Puia G, Ducic I, Vincini S, et al: Does neurosteroid modulatory efficacy depend on GABAa receptor subunit composition? Receptors Channels 1:135–142, 1993

Pulsinelli WA, Brierly JB, Plum F: Temporal profile of neuronal damage in a model of transient forebrain ischemia. Ann Neurol 11:491–498, 1982

Purba JS, Hoogendijk WJG, Hofman MA, et al: Increased number of vasopressin and oxytocin-expressing neurons in the paraventricular nucleus of the human hypothalamus in depression. Arch Gen Psychiatry 53:137–143, 1996

Purdy RH, Morrow AL, Blin JR, et al: Synthesis, metabolism, and pharmacological activity of 3a-hydroxysteroids which potentiate GABA receptor-mediated chloride ion uptake in rat cerebral cortical synaptoneurosomes. J Med Chem 33:1572–1581, 1990

Purdy RH, Morrow AL, Moore PH, et al: Stress-induced elevations of g-aminobutyric acid type A receptor active steroids in the rat brain. Proc Natl Acad Sci U S A 88:4553–4557, 1991

Quartermain D, Clement J, Schemer A: 5-HT$_{1A}$ agonists disrupt memory of fear conditioning in mice. Biol Psychiatry 33:247–254, 1993

Quartermain D, Clement J, Schemer A: The 5-HT$_{1A}$ agonist tandospirone disrupts retention but not acquisition of active avoidance learning. Pharmacol Biochem Behav 48:805–807, 1994

Quera-Salva MA, Orluc A, Goldenberg F, et al: Insomnia and use of hypnotics: study of a French population. Sleep 14(5):386–391, 1991

Quirion R, Richard J, Wilson A: Muscarinic and nicotinic modulation of cortical acetylcholine release monitored by in vivo microdialysis in freely moving rats. Synapse 17:92–100, 1994

Quitkin FM: The importance of dosage in prescribing antidepressants. Br J Psychiatry 147:593–597, 1985

Quitkin FM, Rabkin JG, Ross D, et al: Duration of antidepressant drug treatment: what is an adequate trial? Arch Gen Psychiatry 41:238–245, 1984

Quitkin FM, Stewart JW, McGrath PJ, et al: Phenelzine versus imipramine in the treatment of probably atypical depression: defining syndrome boundaries of selective MAOI responders. Am J Psychiatry 145:306–311, 1988

Quitkin FM, Harrison W, Stewart JW, et al: Response to phenelzine and imipramine in placebo nonresponders with atypical depression: a new application of the crossover design. Arch Gen Psychiatry 48:319–323, 1991

Qureshi GA, Hansen S, Sodersten P: Offspring control of cerebrospinal fluid GABA concentrations in lactating rats. Neurosci Lett 75:85–88, 1987

Raadsheer FC, Hoogendijk WJG, Stam FC, et al: Increased numbers of corticotropin-releasing hormone expressing neurons in the hypothalamic paraventricular nucleus of depressed patients. Clin Neuroendocrinol 60:436–444, 1994

Radja F, Laporte AM, Daval G, et al: Autoradiography of serotonin receptor subtypes in the central nervous system. Neurochem Int 18:1–15, 1992

Raffaele KC, Berardi A, Asthana S, et al: Effects of long-term continuous infusion of the muscarinic agonist arecoline on verbal memory in dementia of the Alzheimer type. Psychopharmacol Bull 27:315–319, 1991

Rahman MK, Akhtar MJ, Salva NC, et al: A double-blind randomized comparison of fluvoxamine with dothiepin in the treatment of depression in elderly patients. British Journal of Clinical Practice 45:255–258, 1991

Raiteri M, Maura G, Folghera S, et al:Modulation of 5-hydroxytryptamine release by presynaptic inhibitory alpha 2-adrenoceptors in the human cerebral cortex. Naunyn Schmiedebergs Arch Pharmacol 342:508–512, 1990

Raiteri M, Paudice P, Vallebuona F: Inhibition by 5-HT$_3$ receptor antagonists of release of cholecystokinin-like immunoreactivity from the frontal cortex of freely moving rats. Naunyn Schmiedebergs Arch Pharmacol 347:111–114, 1993a

Raiteri M, Paudice P, Vallebuona F: Release of cholecystokinin in the central nervous system. Neurochem Int 22(6):519–527, 1993b

Ramakers GMJ, McNamara RK, Lenox RH, et al: Differential changes in the phosphorylation of the protein kinase C substrates MARCKS and GAP-43/B-50 during long-term potentiation and long-term depression in the CA1 field of the hippocampus. J Neurochem (in press)

Ramaprasad S, Newton JEO, Cardwell D, et al: In vivo ^{7}Li NMR imaging and localized spectroscopy of rat brain. Magn Reson Med 25:308–318, 1992

Rampello L, Nicoletti G, Raffaele R: Dopaminergic hypothesis for retarded depression: a symptom profile for predicting therapeutic responses. Acta Psychiatr Scand 84:552–554, 1991

Rana RS, Hopkin LE: Role of phosphoinositides in transmembrane signaling. Physiol Rev 70:115–164, 1990

Randrup A, Braestrup C: Uptake inhibition of biogenic amines by newer antidepressant drugs: relevance to the dopamine hypothesis of depression. Psychopharmacology 53:309–314, 1977

Randrup A, Munkvad I, Fog R, et al: Mania, depression and brain dopamine, in Current Developments in Psychopharmacology, Vol 2. Edited by Essmann WB, Valzelli L. New York, Spectrum Publications, 1975, pp 206–248

Rapee RM: Psychological factors influencing the affective response to biological challenge procedures in panic disorder. J Anxiety Disord 9:59–74, 1995

Rapee RM, Medoro L: Fear of physical sensations and trait anxiety as mediators of the response to hyperventilation in nonclinical subjects. J Abnorm Psychol 103:693–699, 1994

Rapee RM, Brown TA, Antony MM, et al: Response to hyperventilation and inhalation of 5.5% carbon-dioxide enriched air across the DSM-III-R anxiety disorders. J Abnorm Psychol 101:538–552, 1992

Rapier C, Lunt GG, Wonnacott S: Nicotinic modulation of [^{3}H]dopamine release from striatal synaptosomes: pharmacological characterisation. J Neurochem 54:937–945, 1990

Raskin A: Age-sex differences in response to antidepressant drugs. J Nerv Ment Dis 159:120–130, 1974

Raskin A, Schulterbrandt J, Reatig N, et al: Replication of factors of psychopathology in interview, ward behavior and self-report ratings of hospitalized depressives. J Nerv Ment Dis 148:87–98, 1969

Raskind MA: Alzheimer's disease: treatment of noncognitive behavioral abnormalities, in Psychopharmacology: The Fourth Generation of Progress. Edited by Bloom FE, Kupfer DJ. New York, Raven, 1995, pp 1427–1435

Rasmussen SA: Lithium and tryptophan augmentation in clomipramine resistant obsessive-compulsive disorder. Am J Psychiatry 141:1283–1285, 1984

Rasmussen SA, Eisen JL, Pato MT: Current issues in the pharmacologic management of obsessive compulsive disorder [published erratum appears in J Clin Psychiatry 54:491, 1993]. J Clin Psychiatry 54 (suppl):4–9, 1993

Rattray M, Singhvi S, Wu PY, et al: Benzodiazepines increase preprocholecystokinin messenger RNA levels in rat brain. Eur J Pharmacol 245:193–196, 1993

Ravaris CL, Nies A, Robinson D, et al: A multiple-dose, controlled study of phenelzine in depression-anxiety states. Arch Gen Psychiatry 33:347–350, 1976

Ravindran AV, Chudzik J, Bialik RJ, et al: Platelet serotonin measures in primary dysthymia. Am J Psychiatry 151:1369–1371, 1994a

Ravindran AV, Bialik RJ, Lapierre YD: Primary early onset dysthymia, biochemical correlates of the therapeutic response to fluoxetine, I: platelet monoamine oxidase and the dexamethasone suppression test. J Affect Disord 31:111–117, 1994b

Ravindran AV, Bialik RJ, Lapierre YD: Therapeutic efficacy of specific serotonin reuptake inhibitors (SSRIs) in dysthymia. Can J Psychiatry 39(1): 21–26, 1994c

Ravindran AV, Bialik RJ, Lapierre YD: Primary early onset dysthymia, biochemical correlates of the therapeutic response to fluoxetine, II: urinary metabolites of serotonin, norepinephrine and melatonin. J Affect Disord 31:119–123, 1994d

Razani J, White KL, White J, et al: The safety and efficacy of combined amitryptiline and tranylcypromine antidepressant treatment—a controlled trial. Arch Gen Psychiatry 40:657–661, 1983

Read HL, Kiraly M, Dun NJ: Serotonin differentially affects synaptic potentials evoked in the rat cerebral cortical slice. Eur J Pharmacol 183:1383P, 1990

Reading PJ: Frontal lobe dysfunction in schizophrenia and Parkinson's disease—a meeting point for neurology, psychology and psychiatry: discussion paper. J R Soc Med 84:349–353, 1991

Rechtschaffen A, Kales A: A manual for standardized terminology, techniques and scoring system for sleep stages of human subjects. Los Angeles, CA, Brain Information Service, Brain Research Institute, 1968

Reddy PL, Khanna S, Subhash MN, et al: Erythrocyte membrane Na-K ATPase activity in affective disorder. Biol Psychiatry 26:533–537, 1989

Redei E, Hilderbrand H, Aird F: Corticotropin release-inhibiting factor is preprothyrotropin-releasing hormone-(178–199). Endocrinology 136:3557–3563, 1995

Redmond DE: Studies of the nucleus locus coeruleus in monkeys and hypotheses for neuropsychopharmacology, in Psychopharmacology: The Third Generation of Progress. Edited by Meltzer HY. New York, Raven, 1988

Redmond DE, Huang YH: New evidence for a locus ceruleus-norepinephrine connection with anxiety. Life Sci 25:2149, 1979

Regier DA, Narrow WE, Rae DS: The epidemiology of anxiety disorders: the Epidemiologic Catchment Area (ECA) experience. J Psychiatr Res 24:3–14, 1990

Rehfeld JF: Immunochemical studies on cholecystokinin, II: distribution and molecular heterogeneity in the central nervous system and small intestine of man and hog. J Biol Chem 253:4022–4030, 1978

Rehfeld JF: Tetrin, in Gut Hormones. Edited by Bloom SR, Polak JM. New York, Churchill Livingstone, 1981, pp 240–247

Rehfeld JF: CCK and anxiety: introduction, in Multiple Cholecystokinin Receptors in Man. Edited by Iversen S, Dourish C, Cooper F. Oxford, England, Oxford University Press, 1992a, pp 117–120

Rehfeld JF: Cholecystokinin expression in the central nervous system. Eur Neuropsychopharmacol 2(3):189–191, 1992b

Rehfeld JF: The molecular nature of cholecystokinin in plasma—an in vivo immunosorption study in rabbits. Scand J Gastroenterol 29:110–121, 1994

Rehfeld JF, Hansen HF: Characterization of preprocholecystokinin products in the porcine cerebral cortex: evidence of different processing pathways. J Biol Chem 261:5832–5840, 1986

Rehfeld JF, Nielsen FC: Molecular forms and regional distribution of cholecystokinin in the central nervous system, in Cholecystokinin and Anxiety: From Neuron to Behavior. Edited by Bradwejn J, Vasar E. Austin, TX, RG Landes, 1995, pp 33–56

Rehm LP: Behavior Therapy for Depression. New York, Academic Press, 1979

Reich JR, Yates W: A pilot study of treatment of social phobia with alprazolam. Am J Psychiatry 145:590–594, 1988

Reid WGJ, Broe GA, Morris JGL, et al: The role of cholinergic deficiency in neuropsychological deficits in idiopathic Parkinson's disease. Dementia 3:114–120, 1990

Reifler BV, Larson E, Teri L, et al: Alzheimer's disease and depression. J Am Geriatr Soc 14:855–859, 1986

Reifler BV, Teri L, Raskind M, et al: Double-blind trial of imipramine in Alzheimer's disease patients with and without depression. Am J Psychiatry 146:45–49, 1989

Reisberg B, Ferris SH, DeLean MJ, et al: The Global Deterioration Scale for Assessment of Primary Degenerative Dementia. Am J Psychiatry 139:1136–1139, 1982

Reisine T, Zatz M: Interactions between lithium, calcium, diacylglycerides and phorbol esters in the regulation of ACTH release from AtT-20 cells. J Neurochem 49:884–889, 1987

Reiss S, Peterson R, Gorsky D, et al: Anxiety sensitivity, anxiety frequency and the prediction of fearfulness. Behav Res Ther 24:1–8, 1986

Reiter RJ: The neurohormone melatonin: neuropharmacological actions and implications, in Endocrine Psychopharmacology. Edited by Halbreich U. Washington, DC, American Psychiatric Press (in press a)

Reiter RJ: The pineal gland and its neurohormone melatonin: basic aspects, in Hormonal Modulation of Brain and Behavior. Edited by Halbreich U. Washington, DC, American Psychiatric Press (in press b)

Reiter RJ, Melchiorri D, Sewerynek E: A review of the evidence supporting melatonin's role as an antioxidant. J Pineal Res 18:1–11, 1995

Reiter SR, Pollack S, Rosenbaum JF, et al: Clonazepam for the treatment of social phobia. J Clin Psychiatry 51:470–472, 1990

Remington G, Adams M: Risperidone and obsessive-compulsive symptoms (letter). J Clin Psychopharmacol 14:358–359, 1994

Rennel ML, Gregory TF, Blaumanis OR, et al: Evidence for a paravascular fluid circulation in the mammalian central nervous system, provided by the rapid distribution of tracer protein throughout the brain from subarachnoid space. Brain Res 326:47–63, 1985

Renynghe de Voxrie GV: G34586 (CMI) in obsessive compulsive neurosis. Acta Neurologica Belgica 68:787–792, 1968

Reppert SM, Godson C, Mahle CD: Molecular characterization of a second melatonin receptor expressed in the human retina and brain: the Mel_{1b} melatonin receptor. Proc Natl Acad Sci U S A 92:8734–8736, 1995

Reul JMHM, Stec I, Söder M, et al: Chronic treatment of rats with the antidepressant amitriptyline attenuates the activity of the hypothalamic-pituitary-adrenocortical system. Endocrinology 133:312–320, 1993

Reul JMHM, Labeur MS, Grigoriadis DE, et al: Hypothalamic-pituitary-adrenocortical axis changes in the rat after long-term treatment with the reversible monoamine oxidase A inhibitor moclobemide. Neuroendocrinology 60: 509–519, 1994a

Reul JMHM, Stec I, Wiegers GJ, et al: Prenatal immune challenge alters the hypothalamic-pituitary-adrenocortical axis in adult rats. J Clin Invest 93:2600–2607, 1994b

Reus VI: Psychiatric aspects of thyroid disease, in The Thyroid Axis and Psychiatric Illness. Edited by Joffe RT, Levitt AJ. Washington, DC, American Psychiatric Press, 1993, pp 171–194

Reus VI, Berlant JR: Behavioral disturbances associated with disorders of the hypothalamic-pituitary-adrenal system, in Medical Mimics of Psychiatric Disorders. Edited by Extein I, Gold MS. Washington, DC, American Psychiatric Press, 1986, pp 111–130

Rex A, Fink H, Marsden CA: Effects of BOC-CCK-4 and L 365,260 and cortical 5-HT release in guinea-pigs on exposure to the elevated plus maze. Neuropharmacology 33:559–565, 1994a

Rex A, Barth T, Voigt JP, et al: Effects of cholecystokinin tetrapeptide and sulfated cholecystokinin octapeptide in rat models of anxiety. Neurosci Lett 172:139, 1994b

Reyneke L, Allin R, Russell V, et al: Lack of effect of chronic desipramine treatment on dopaminergic activity in the nucleus accumbens of the rat. Neurochem Res 14:661–665, 1989

Reynolds CF, Kupfer DJ: Sleep research in affective illness: state of the art circa 1987. Sleep 10:199–215, 1987

Reynolds CF III, Shaw DH, Newton TF, et al: EEG sleep in outpatients with generalized anxiety: a preliminary comparison with depressed outpatients. Psychiatry Res 8:81–89, 1983

Reynolds JN, Baskys A, Carlen PL: The effects of serotonin on N-methyl-D-aspartate and synaptically evoked depolarisations in rat neocortical neurones. Brain Res 456:286–292, 1988

Reznikoff GA, Manaker S, Rhodes H, et al: Localization and quantification of β-adrenergic receptors in human brain. Neurology 36:1067–1073, 1986

Ribeiro SCM, Tandon R, Grunhaus L, et al: The DST as a predictor of outcome in depression: a meta-analysis. Am J Psychiatry 150:1618–1629, 1993

Ricaurte GA, Markowska AL, Wenk GL, et al: 3,4-Methylene dioxyamphetamine, serotonin and memory. J Pharmacol Exp Ther 266:1097–1105, 1993

Rice EH, Sombrotto LB, Markowitz, et al: Cardiovascular morbidity in high-risk patients during ECT. Am J Psychiatry 151:1637–1641, 1994

Rich CL, Spiker DG, Jewell SW, et al: The efficiency of ECT, I: response rate in depressive episodes. Psychiatry Res 11:167–176, 1984

Rich CL, Spiker DG, Jewell SW, et al: ECT response in psychotic versus nonpsychotic unipolar depressives. J Clin Psychiatry 47:123–125, 1986

Rich JB, Rasmussen AX, Folstein MF, et al: Nonsteroidal antiinflamatory drugs in Alzheimer's disease. Neurology 45:51–55, 1995

Richards G, Schoch P, Jenck F: Benzodiazepine receptors and their ligands, in 5-HT$_{1A}$ Agonists, 5-HT$_3$ Antagonists and Benzodiazepines: Their Comparative Behavioural Pharmacology. Edited by Rodgers RJ, Cooper SJ. Chichester, England, Wiley, 1991, pp 1–30

Richelson E, Nelson A: Antagonism by neuroleptics of neurotransmitter receptors of normal brain in vitro. Eur J Pharmacol 103:197–204, 1984

Rickels K, Schweizer E: The treatment of generalized anxiety disorder in patients with depressive symptomatology. J Clin Psychiatry 54 (suppl):20–23, 1993

Rickels K, Weisman K, Norstad N, et al: Buspirone and diazepam in anxiety: a controlled study. J Clin Psychiatry 43(12 pt 2):81–86, 1982

Rickels K, Feighner JP, Smith WT: Alprazolam, amitriptyline, doxepin, and placebo in the treatment of depression. Arch Gen Psychiatry 42:134–141, 1985

Rickels K, Schweizer E, Weiss S, et al: Maintenance drug treatment for panic disorder, II: short- and long-term outcome after drug taper. Arch Gen Psychiatry 50:61–68, 1993

Rickels K, Schweizer E, Clary C, et al: Nefazodone and imipramine in major depression: a placebo-controlled trial. Br J Psychiatry 164:802–805, 1994

Riddell FG: Studies on Li$^+$ transport using 7Li and 6Li nuclear magnetic resonance, in Lithium and the Cell. Edited by Birch NJ. San Diego, CA, Academic Press, 1991, pp 85–98

Riddle MA, Leckman JF, Hardin MT, et al: Fluoxetine treatment of obsessions and compulsions in patients with Tourette's syndrome. Am J Psychiatry 145:1173–1174, 1988

Riddle WJR, Scott AIF, Bennie J, et al: Current intensity and oxytocin release after electroconvulsive therapy. Biol Psychiatry 33:839–841, 1993

Riedel WJ, Klaassem T, Deutz NE, et al: Tryptophan depletion in normal volunteers produces selective impairment in memory consolidation. Psychopharmacology 141:362–369, 1999

Rieder RO, Mann LS, Weinberger DR, et al: Computed tomographic scans in patients with schizophrenia, schizoaffective and bipolar affective disorder. Arch Gen Psychiatry 40:735–739, 1983

Riekkinen M, Sirvio J, Toivanen T, et al: Combined treatment with a 5-HT$_{1A}$ receptor agonist and a muscarinic acetylcholine receptor antagonist disrupts water maze navigation behaviour. Psychopharmacology 122:137–146, 1995

Riemann D, Berger M: The effects of total sleep deprivation and subsequent treatment with clomipramine on depressive symptoms and sleep electroencephalography in patients with a major depressive disorder. Acta Psychiatr Scand 81:24–31, 1990

Riemann DS, Velthaus S, Laubenthal S, et al: REM-suppressing effects of amitriptyline and amitriptyline-N-oxide after acute medication in healthy volunteers: results of two uncontrolled pilot trials. Pharmacopsychiatry 23:253–258, 1990

Riemann D, Gann H, Fleckenstein P, et al: Effect of RS 86 on REM latency in schizophrenia. Psychiatry Res 38:89–92, 1991

Riemann D, Hohagen F, Bahro M, et al: Cholinergic neurotransmission, REM sleep and depression. J Psychosom Res 38 (suppl 1):15–25, 1994

Rihmer Z, Arato M, Szadoczky E, et al: The dexamethasone suppression test in psychotic versus nonpsychotic endogenous depression. Br J Psychiatry 145:508–511, 1984

Ringold AL: Paroxetine efficacy in social phobia. J Clin Psychiatry 55:363–364, 1994

Risby ED, Hsiao JK, Manji HK, et al: The mechanisms of action of lithium, II: effects on adenylate cyclase activity and β-adrenergic receptor binding in normal subjects. Arch Gen Psychiatry 48:513–524, 1991

Risch SC: Beta-endorphin hypersecretion in depression: possible cholinergic mechanism. Biol Psychiatry 17:1071–1079, 1982

Riva M, Brunello N, Rovescalli AC, et al: Effect of reboxetine, a new antidepressant drug, on the central noradrenergic system: behavioral and biochemical studies. Journal of Drug Development 1:243–253, 1989

Robbins TW, Brown VJ: The role of the striatum in the mental chronometry of action: a theoretical review. Rev Neurosci 2:181–213, 1990

Robbins TW, Everitt BJ, Marston HM, et al: Comparative effects of ibotenic acid- and quisqualic acid-induced lesions of the substantia innominata on attentional function in the rat: further implications for the role of the cholinergic neurons of the nucleus basalis in cognitive processes. Behav Brain Res 35:221–224, 1989

Robel P, Bourreau E, Corpéchot C, et al: Neurosteroids: 3β-hydroxy-δ-5-derivatives in rat and monkey brain. J Steroid Biochem 27:649–655, 1987

Roberts JM: Prognostic factors in the electroshock treatment of depressive states: (1) clinical features from history and examination. Journal of Mental Science 105:693–702, 1959

Roberts RK, Desmond PV, Wilkinson GR, et al: Disposition of chlordiazepoxide: sex differences and effects of oral contraceptives. Clin Pharmacol Ther 25:826–831, 1979

Robertson MM, Trimble MR: Major tranquillisers used as antidepressants: a review. J Affect Disord 4:173–193, 1982

Robin A, Binnie CD, Copas JB: Electrophysiological and hormonal responses to three types of electroconvulsive therapy. Br J Psychiatry 147:707–712, 1985

Robins LN, Helzer JE, Weissman MM, et al: Lifetime prevalence of specific psychiatric disorders in three sites. Arch Gen Psychiatry 41:949–958, 1984

Robinson DG, Spiker DG: Delusional depression: a one year follow-up. J Affect Disord 9:79–83, 1985

Robinson DR, Shrotriya RC, Alms DR, et al: Treatment of panic disorder: nonbenzodiazepine anxiolytics, including buspirone. Psychopharmacol Bull 25:21–26, 1989

Robinson DS, Nies A, Avaris CL, et al: Clinical pharmacology of phenelzine. Arch Gen Psychiatry 35:629–635, 1978

Robinson DS, Lerfald SC, Bennett B, et al: Continuation and maintenance treatment of major depression with the monoamine oxidase inhibitor phenelzine: a double-blind placebo-controlled discussion study. Psychopharmacol Bull 27:31–39, 1991

Robinson RG, Boston JD, Starkstein SE, et al: Comparison of mania and depression after brain injury: causal factors. Am J Psychiatry 145:172–178, 1988

Robinson SE: Effect of specific serotonergic lesions on cholinergic neurons in the hippocampus, cortex and striatum. Life Sci 32:345–353, 1983

Rodriguez-Sierra JF, Hagley MT, Hendricks SE: Anxiolytic effects of progesterone are sexually dimorphic. Life Sci 38:1841–1845, 1986

Roemer RA, Dubin WR, Jaffe R, et al: An efficacy study of single- versus double-seizure induction with ECT in major depression. J Clin Psychiatry 51:473–478, 1990

Rogeness GA, Javors MA, Pliszka SR: Neurochemistry and child and adolescent psychiatry. J Am Acad Child Adolesc Psychiatry 31:765–781, 1992

Roger SL, Farlow MR, Mohs RC: A 24-week double blind, placebo-controlled trial of donepezil in patients with Alzheimer's disease. Neurology 50:136–145, 1998

Rogers J, Luber-Narod J, Styren SD, et al: Expression of immune system-associated antigens by cells of the human nervous system: relationship to the pathology of Alzheimer's disease. Neurobiol Aging 9:339–349, 1988

Ronai AZ, Vizi SF: The effect of lithium treatment on the acetylcholine content of rat brain. Biochem Pharmacol 24:1819–1820, 1975

Rooney TA, Nahorski SR: Regional characterization of agonist and depolarization-induced phosphoinositide hydrolysis in rat brain. J Pharmacol Exp Ther 239:873–880, 1986

Roose SP, Glassman AH, Walsh BT, et al: Tricyclic nonresponders: phenomenology and treatment. Am J Psychiatry 143:345–348, 1986

Roose SP, Glassman AH, Attia E, et al: Comparative efficacy of selective serotonin reuptake inhibitors and tricyclics in the treatment of melancholia. Am J Psychiatry 151:1735–1739, 1994

Rosen JB, Weiss SRB, Post RM: Contingent tolerance to carbamazepine: alterations in TRH mRNA and TRH receptor binding in limbic structures. Brain Res 651:252–260, 1994

Rosen WG, Mohs RC, Davis KL: A new rating scale for Alzheimer's disease. Am J Psychiatry 141:1356–1364, 1984

Rosenberg C, Damsbo N, Fuglum E, et al: Citalopram and clomipramine in the treatment of depressive patients in general practice: a Nordic multicentre clinical study. Int Clin Psychopharmacol 9 (suppl 1):41–48, 1994

Rosenblatt JE, Pert CB, Tallman JF, et al: The effect of imipramine and lithium on alpha- and beta-receptor binding in rat brain. Brain Res 160:186–191, 1979

Rosenblatt JE, Pert A, Layton B, et al: Chronic lithium reduced ^{3}H-spiroperidol binding in rat striatum. Eur J Pharmacol 67:321–322, 1980

Rosenblum LA, Coplan JD, Friedman S, et al: Dose-response effects of oral yohimbine in unrestrained primates. Biol Psychiatry 28:647–657, 1991

Rosenstein DL, Takeshita J, Nelson JC: Fluoxetine-induced elevation and prolongation of tricyclic levels in overdose (letter). Am J Psychiatry 148:807, 1991

Rosenthal NE, Sack DA, Gillin JC, et al: Seasonal affective disorder: a description of the syndrome and preliminary findings with light therapy. Arch Gen Psychiatry 41:72–80, 1984

Roskos LK, Boudinot FD: Effects of dose and sex on the pharmacokinetics of piroxicam in the rat. Biopharm Drug Dispos 11:215–225, 1990

Rösler M, Anand R, Cici-Sain A, et al: Efficacy and safety of rivastigmine in patients with Alzheimer's disease: international randomized controlled trial. BMJ 318:633–640, 1999

Rossetti ZL, Pani L, Kuzmin A, et al: Dihydropyridine calcium antagonists prevent cocaine-, but not amphetamine-, induced dopamine release and motor activity in rats. Acta Physiol Hung 75 (suppl):249–250, 1990

Rossetti ZL, Lai M, Hmaidan Y, et al: Depletion of mesolimbic dopamine during behavioural despair: partial reversal by chronic imipramine. Eur J Pharmacol 242:313–315, 1993

Rossor M: The neurochemistry of cortical dementias, in Cognitive Neurochemistry. Edited by Stahl SM, Iversen SD, Goodman EC. Oxford, England, Oxford Science Publications, 1987, pp 233–247

Roth T, Zorick F, Wittig R, et al: The effects of doxepine HCL on sleep and depression. J Clin Psychiatry 43:366–368, 1982

Rothschild AJ: Delusional depression: a review of the literature and current perspectives. McLean Hospital Journal 2:68–83, 1985

Rothschild AJ, Samson JA, Bessette MP, et al: Efficacy of the combination of fluoxetine and perphenazine in the treatment of psychotic depression. J Clin Psychiatry 54:338–342, 1993

Rouillon F, Serrurier D, Miller H, et al: Prophylactic efficacy of maprotiline on unipolar depression relapse. J Clin Psychiatry 52:423–431, 1991

Rowan MJ, Cullen WK, Moulton B: Buspirone impairment of performance of passive avoidance and spatial learning tasks in the rat. Psychopharmacology 100:393–398, 1990

Rowell PP, Winkler DL: Nicotinic stimulation of [³H]acetylcholine release from mouse cerebral cortical synaptosomes. J Neurochem 43:1593–1598, 1984

Roy A, Karoum F, Pollack S: Marked reduction in indexes of dopamine metabolism among patients with depression who attempt suicide. Arch Gen Psychiatry 49:447–450, 1992

Roy MA, Crowe RR: Validity of the familial sporadic subtypes of schizophrenia. Am J Psychiatry 151:805–814, 1994

Roy-Byrne P, Post RM, Uhde TW, et al: The longitudinal course of recurrent affective illness: life chart data from research patients at the NIMH. Acta Psychiatr Scand Suppl 317:1–34, 1985

Roy-Byrne PP, Uhde TW, Post RM, et al: The corticotropin-releasing hormone stimulation test in patients with panic disorder. Am J Psychiatry 143:896–899, 1986

Ruberg M, Ploska F, Javoy-Agid F, et al: Muscarinic binding and choline acetyltransferase activity in Parkinsonian subjects with reference to dementia. Brain Res 232:129–139, 1982

Rubin RT, Gouin PR, Arenander AT, et al: Human growth hormone release during sleep following prolonged flurazepam administration. Research Communications in Chemical Pathology and Pharmacology 6:331–334, 1973

Rubin RT, Poland RE, Lesser IM, et al: Neuroendocrine aspects of primary endogenous depression, I: cortisol secretory dynamics in patients and matched controls. Arch Gen Psychiatry 44:328–336, 1987

Rubin RT, Phillips JJ, Sadow TF, et al: Adrenal gland volume in major depression: increase during the depressive episode and decrease with successful treatment. Arch Gen Psychiatry 52:213–218, 1995

Rubinow DR: Cerebrospinal fluid somatostatin and psychiatric illness. Biol Psychiatry 21:341–365, 1986

Rudolph R, Entsuah R, Derivan A: Early clinical response in depression to venlafaxine hydrochloride (abstract). Biol Psychiatry 29:630S, 1991

Rudorfer MV, Hau HG, Clayton PJ: Dexamethasone suppression test in primary depression: significance of family history and psychosis. Biol Psychiatry 17:41–48, 1982

Rudorfer MV, Skwerer RG, Rosenthal NE: Biogenic amines in seasonal affective disorders: effects of light therapy. Psychiatry Res 46:19–28, 1993

Rudorfer MV, Manji HK, Potter WZ: Comparative tolerability profiles of the newer versus older antidepressants. Drug Saf 10(1):18–46, 1994

Ruegg RG, Evans DL, Comer WS, et al: Lithium plus fluoxetine treatment of obsessive compulsive disorder (NR92), in 1990 New Research Program and Abstracts, American Psychiatric Association 143rd Annual Meeting, New York, NY, May 12–17, 1990. Washington, DC, American Psychiatric Association, 1990, p 81

Ruotsalainen S, MacDonald E, Miettinen R, et al: Additive deficits in the choice accuracy of rats in the delayed non-matching to position task after cholinolytics and serotonergic lesions are non-mnenonic in nature. Psychopharmacology 130:303–312, 1997

Ruotsalainen S, Miettinen R, MacDonald E, et al: The role of the dorsal raphe-serotonergic system and cholinergic receptors in the modulation of working memory. Neurosci Biobehav Rev 22:21–31, 1998

Rupprecht R, Reul JMHM, Trapp T, et al: Progesterone receptor-mediated effects of neuroactive steroids. Neuron 11:523–530, 1993

Rush AJ, Beck AT, Kovacs M, et al: Comparative efficacy of cognitive therapy and pharmacotherapy in the treatments of depressed outpatients. Cognitive Therapy Research 1:17–37, 1977

Rush AJ, Schlesser MA, Stokely EM, et al: Cerebral blood flow in depression and mania. Psychopharmacol Bull 18:6–8, 1982

Rush AJ, Ermann MK, Giles DE, et al: Polysomnographic findings in recently drug-free and clinically remitted depressed patients. Arch Gen Psychiatry 43:878–884, 1986

Russell RW, Pechnick R, Jope RS: Effects of lithium on behavioral reactivity: relation to increases in brain cholinergic activity. Psychopharmacology 73:120–125, 1981

Russell VA, Lamm MC, Taljaard JJ: Lack of interaction between alpha 2-adrenoceptors and dopamine D2-receptors in mediating their inhibitory effects on [^{3}H] dopamine release from rat nucleus accumbens. Neurochem Res 18:285–289, 1993

Rusted JM: Dissociative effects of scopolamine on working memory in healthy young volunteers. Psychopharmacology 96:487–492, 1988

Rusted JM, Warburton DM: The effects of scopolamine on working memory in healthy young volunteers. Psychopharmacology 96:145–152, 1988

Rusted JM, Warburton DM: Cognitive models and cholinergic drugs. Neuropsychobiology 21:31–36, 1989

Rusted J, Graupner L, O'Connell N, et al: Does nicotine improve cognitive function? Psychopharmacology 115:547–549, 1994

Ryan ND, Dahl RE: The biology of depression in children and adolescents, in Biology of Depressive Disorders, Part B: Subtypes of Depression and Comorbid Disorders. Edited by Mann JJ, Kupfer D. New York, Plenum, 1994

Rybakowski J, Frazer A, Mendels J: Lithium efflux from erythrocytes incubated in vitro during lithium carbonate administration. Communications in Psychopharmacology 2:105–112, 1978

Sachar EJ, Hellman L, Roffwarg HP, et al: Disrupted 24 hour patterns of cortisol secretion in psychotic depressives. Arch Gen Psychiatry 28:19–24, 1973

Sack RL, Blood ML, Lewy AJ: Melatonin administration to night shift workers: an update. Sleep Research 24:539, 1995

Sackeim HA: The cognitive effects of electroconvulsive therapy, in Cognitive Disorders: Pathophysiology and Treatment. Edited by Moos WH, Gamzu ER, Thal LJ. New York, Marcel Dekker, 1992, pp 183–228

Sackeim HA: Central issues regarding the mechanisms of action of electroconvulsive therapy: directions for future research. Psychopharmacol Bull 30:281–308, 1994a

Sackeim HA: Continuation therapy following ECT: directions for future research. Psychopharmacol Bull 30:501–521, 1994b

Sackeim HA, Decina P, Prohovnik I, et al: Anticonvulsant and antidepressant properties of electroconvulsive therapy: a proposed mechanism of action. Biol Psychiatry 18:1301–10, 1983

Sackeim HA, Decina P, Prohovnik I, et al: Dosage, seizure threshold and the antidepressant efficacy of electroconvulsive therapy. Ann N Y Acad Sci 462:398–410, 1986

Sackeim HA, Decina P, Kanzler M, et al: Effects of electrode placement on the efficacy of titrated, low-dose ECT. Am J Psychiatry 144:1449–1455, 1987a

Sackeim HA, Decina P, Prohovnik I, et al: Seizure threshold in electroconvulsive therapy. Effects of sex, age, electrode placement, and number of treatments. Arch Gen Psychiatry 44:355–360, 1987b

Sackeim HA, Decina P, Portnoy S, et al: Studies of dosage, seizure threshold, and seizure duration in ECT. Biol Psychiatry 22:249–268, 1987c

Sackeim HA, Prudic J, Devanand DP, et al: The impact of medication resistance and continuation pharmacotherapy on relapse following response to electroconvulsive therapy in major depression. J Clin Psychopharmacol 10:96–104, 1990

Sackeim HA, Devanand DP, Prudic J: Stimulus intensity, seizure threshold, and seizure duration: impact on the efficacy and safety of electroconvulsive therapy. Psychiatr Clin North Am 14:803–843, 1991

Sackeim HA, Prudig J, Devanand DP, et al: Effects of stimulus intensity and electrode placement on the efficacy and cognitive effects of electroconvulsive therapy. N Engl J Med 328:839–846, 1993

Sackeim HA, Long J, Luber B, et al: Physical properties of the ECT stimulus, I: basic principles. Convulsive Therapy 10:93–123, 1994

Sackeim HA, Devanand DP, Nobler MS: Electroconvulsive therapy, in Psychopharmacology: The Fourth Generation of Progress. Edited by Bloom F, Kupfer D. New York, Raven, 1995, pp 1123–1141

Sackeim HA, Luber B, Kutzman GP, et al: The effects of electroconvulsive therapy on quantitative electroencephalograms: relationship to clinical outcome. Arch Gen Psychiatry 53:814–824, 1996

Sagi-Eisenberg R: GTP binding proteins as possible targets for protein kinase C action. Trends Biochem Sci 14:355–357, 1989

Sahakian BJ, Coull JT: Nicotine and THA: Evidence for improved attention in patients with dementia of the Alzheimer type. Drug Development Research 31:80–88, 1994

Sahakian B, Jones G, Levy R, et al: The effects of nicotine on attention, information processing and short-term memory in patients with dementia of the Alzheimer type. Br J Psychiatry 154:797–800, 1989

Sahgal A, Keith AB: Combined serotonergic-cholinergic lesions do not disrupt memory in rats. Pharmacol Biochem Behav 45(4)995–1001, 1993

Saito N, Guitart X, Hayward M, et al: Corticosterone differentially regulates the expression of $G_s a$ and $G_i a$ messenger RNA and protein in rat cerebral cortex. Proc Natl Acad Sci U S A 86:3906–3910, 1989

Sakauye KM, Camp CJ, Ford PA: Effects of buspirone on agitation associated with dementia. Am J Geriatr Psychiatry 1:82–84, 1993

Sakkas PN, Soldatos CR, Bergiannaki JD, et al: In search of the adaptation effect: sleep patterns of normal individuals and depressed patients, in Psychiatry: A World Perspective, Vol 2: Neuroscience in Psychiatry: Biological Correlates of Mental Disorders. Edited by Stefanis CN, Soldatos CR, Rabavilas AD. New York, Excerpta Medica, 1990, pp 380–385

Saletu B, Frey R, Krupka M, et al: Sleep laboratory studies on the single-dose effects of serotonin uptake inhibitors paroxetine and fluoxetine on human sleep and waking qualities. Sleep 14:439–447, 1991

Salzman L, Thaler FH: OCD: a review of the literature. Am J Psychiatry 138: 286–296, 1981

Samorajski T: Central neurotransmitter substances and aging: a review. Journal of the American Psychiatric Society 25:337–348, 1977

Sampson D, Willner P, Muscat R: Reversal of antidepressant action by dopamine antagonists in an animal model of depression. Psychopharmacology 104:491–495, 1991

Sanderson WC, Rapee RM, Barlow DH: The influence of perceived control on panic attacks induced via inhalation of 5.5% carbon-dioxide enriched air. Arch Gen Psychiatry 46:157–162, 1989

Sandford JJ, D'Orlando KJ, Gammans RE, et al: Pilot crossover trial of pagoclone and placebo in patients with DSM-IV panic disorder. Poster presented at the CINP Congress, Glasgow, Scotland, 1998

Sandor P, Shapiro CM: Sleep patterns in depression and anxiety: theory and pharmacological effects. J Psychosom Res 38 (suppl 1):125–139, 1994

Sapolsky RM: Stress in the wild. Sci Am 262:116–123, 1990

Sarantidis D, Waters B: Predictors of lithium prophylaxis effectiveness. Prog Neuropsychopharmacol 5:507–510, 1981

Sargent PB: The diversity of neuronal nicotine acetylcholine receptors. Annu Rev Neurosci 16:403–443, 1993

Saridaki E, Carter DA, Lightman SL: g-Aminobutyric acid regulation of neurohypophysial hormone secretion in male and female rats. J Endocrinol 121:343–349, 1989

Sarkadi B, Alifimoff JK, Gunn RB, et al: Kinetics and stoichiometry of Na-dependent Li transport in human red blood cells. J Gen Physiol 72:249–265, 1978

Savino M, Perugi G, Simmonini E, et al: Affective comorbidity in panic disorder: is there a bipolar connection? J Affect Disord 28:155–163, 1993

Savolainen KM, Hirvonen MR, Tarhanen J, et al: Changes in cerebral inositol-1-phosphate concentrations in LiCl-treated rats: regional and strain differences. Neurochem Res 15:541–545, 1990

Scavone JM, Greenblatt DJ, Locniskar A, et al: Alprazolam pharmacokinetics in women on low-dose oral contraceptives. J Clin Pharmacol 28:454–457, 1988

Schatzberg AF, Ballenger JC: Decisions for the clinician in the treatment of panic disorder: when to treat, which treatment to use, and how long to treat. J Clin Psychiatry 52 (suppl):26–31, 1991

Schatzberg AF, Cole JO: Manual of Clinical Psychopharmacology, 2nd Edition. Washington, DC, American Psychiatric Press, 1991

Schatzberg AF, Rothschild AJ: Psychotic (delusional) major depression: should it be included as a distinct syndrome in DSM-IV? Am J Psychiatry 149:733–745, 1992

Schatzberg AF, Cole JO, Cohen BM, et al: Survey of depressed patients who have failed to respond to treatment, in The Affective Disorders. Edited by Davis JM, Maas JW. Washington, DC, American Psychiatric Press, 1983, pp 73–85

Schatzberg AF, Rothschild AJ, Langlais PJ, et al: A corticosteroid/dopamine hypothesis for psychotic depression and related states. J Psychiatry Res 19:57–64, 1985

Schatzberg AF, Cole JO, Elliott GR: Recent views of treatment-resistant depression, in Psychosocial Aspects of Nonresponse to Antidepressant Drugs. Edited by Halbreich U, Feinberg SS. Washington, DC, American Psychiatric Press, 1986, pp 95–109

Schatzberg AF, Kornstein S, Keitner G, et al: Gender and treatment response in chronic depression. Paper presented at the 34th annual meeting of the American College of Neuropsychopharmacology, San Juan, Puerto Rico, December 11–15, 1995, Scientific Abstracts, p 247

Schedlowski M, Fluge T, Richter S, et al: Beta-endorphin, but not substance-P, is increased by acute stress in humans. Psychoneuroendocrinology 20:103–110, 1995

Schildkraut JJ: The catecholamine hypothesis of affective disorder: a review of supporting evidence. Am J Psychiatry 122:509–522, 1965

Schildkraut JJ: The effects of lithium on norepinephrine turnover and metabolism: basic and clinical studies, in Lithium: Its Role in Psychiatric Research and Treatment. Edited by Gershon S, Shopsin B. New York, Plenum, 1973, pp 51–73

Schildkraut JJ: The effects of lithium on norepinephrine turnover and metabolism: basic and clinical studies. J Nerv Ment Dis 158:348–360, 1974

Schildkraut JJ, Schanberg SM, Kopin IJ: The effects of lithium ion on 3H-norepinephrine metabolism in brain. Life Sci 16:1479–1483, 1966

Schildkraut JJ, Logue MA, Dodge GA: The effect of lithium salts on the turnover and metabolism of norepinephrine in rat brain. Psychopharmacologia 14:135–141, 1969

Schlegel S, Kretzschmar K: Computed tomography in affective disorders, part I: ventricular and sulcal measurements. Biol Psychiatry 22:4–14, 1987

Schmauss M, Laakmann G, Dieterle D: Effects of α_2-receptor blockade in addition to tricyclic antidepressants in therapy-resistant depression. J Clin Psychopharmacol 8:108–111, 1988

Schmidt CJ, Fadayel GM: The selective 5-HT$_{2A}$ antagonist, MDL 100,907, increases dopamine efflux in the prefrontal cortex of the rat. Eur J Pharmacol 273:273–279, 1995

Schmidt PJ, Purdy RH, Moore PH, et al: Circulating levels of anxiolytic steroids in the luteal phase in women with premenstrual syndrome and in control subjects. J Clin Endocrinol Metab 79:1256–1260, 1994

Schmutz M, David J, Grewal RS, et al: Pharmacological and neurochemical aspects of tolerance, in Tolerance to Beneficial and Adverse Effects of Antiepileptic Drugs. Edited by Koella WP. New York, Raven, 1986, pp 25–36

Schneider MA, Brotherton PL, Hailes J: The effect of exogenous oestrogens on depression in menopausal women. Med J Aust 2:162–165, 1977

Schneier FR, Liebowitz MR, Davies SO, et al: Fluoxetine in panic disorder. J Clin Psychopharmacol 10:119–121, 1990

Schneier, FR, Chin SJ, Hollander E, et al: Fluoxetine in social phobia. J Clin Psychopharmacol 12:62–64, 1992

Schneier FR, Saoud JB, Campeas R, et al: Buspirone in social phobia. J Clin Psychopharmacol 13:251–256, 1993

Schnizer RA, McNamara RK, Streit WJ, et al: Differential expression of MARCKS, MRP & GAP-43 mRNA in the facial nucleus during neuronal regeneration and degeneration. Society for Neuroscience Abstracts 23:612, 1997

Schou M: Lithium research at the Psychopharmacology Research Unit, Risskov, Denmark: a historical account, in Origin, Prevention and Treatment of Affective Disorders. Edited by Schou M, Stromgren E. London, Academic Press, 1979, pp 1–8

Schou M, Juel-Nielson N, Strömgren E, et al: The treatment of manic psychoses by administration of lithium salts. J Neurol Neurosurg Psychiatry 17:250–260, 1954

Schousboe A, Frandsen A, Wahl P, et al: Neurotoxicity and excitatory amino acid antagonists. Neurotoxicology 15:477–481, 1994

Schreiber W, Laver C, Krieg J, et al: REM sleep disinhibition after cholinergic challenge in subjects at high risk for psychiatric disorders. Biol Psychiatry 330:79–90, 1992

Schubert W, Prior R, Weidemann A: Localization of Alzheimer betaA4 amyloid precursor protein at central and peripheral synaptic sites. Brain Res 563:184–194, 1991

Schuckit MA: Clinical studies of buspirone. Psychopathology 17 (suppl 3):61–68, 1984

Schultz JE, Siggins GR, Schocker FW, et al: Effects of prolonged treatment with lithium and tricyclic antidepressants on discharge frequency, norepinephrine responses and beta receptor binding in rat cerebellum: electrophysiological and biochemical comparison. J Pharmacol Exp Ther 216:28–38, 1981

Schwartz BL, Hashtroudis S, Herting RL, et al: d-Cycloserine enhances implicit memory in Alzheimer patients. Neurology 46:420–424, 1996

Schwartz RD, Lehmann J, Kellar KJ: Presynaptic nicotinic cholinergic receptors labeled by [3H]acetylcholine on catecholamine and serotonin receptors in brain. J Neurochem 42:1495–1498, 1984

Schwarz RD, Callahan MJ, Davis RE, et al: Selective muscarinic agonists for Alzheimer disease treatment, in Alzheimer Disease: Therapeutic Strategies. Edited by Giacobini E, Becker R. Boston, MA, Birkhäuser, 1994, pp 224–228

Schwarz S, Pohl P: Steroids and opioid receptors. J Steroid Biochem Mol Biol 48:391–404, 1994

Schweizer E, Rickels K: Buspirone in the treatment of panic disorder: a controlled pilot comparison with clorazepate. J Clin Psychopharmacol 8:303, 1988

Schweizer E, Rickels K, Amsterdam JD, et al: What constitutes an adequate antidepressant trial of fluoxetine? J Clin Psychiatry 51:8–11, 1990

Schweizer E, Case WG, Garcia-Espana F, et al: Progesterone co-administration in patients discontinuing long-term benzodiazepine therapy: effects on withdrawal severity and taper outcome. Psychopharmacology 117:424–429, 1995

Scolnick P, Moncada V, Barker J, et al: Pentobarbital has dual actions to increase brain benzodiazepine receptor affinity. Science 211:1448–1450, 1981

Scott AI, Whalley LJ, Legros JJ: Treatment outcome, seizure duration, and the neurophysin response to ECT. Biol Psychiatry 25:585–597, 1989

Scott AI, Shering PA, Legros JJ, et al: Improvement in depressive illness is not associated with altered release of neurophysins over a course of ECT. Psychiatry Res 36:65–73, 1991

Secunda SK, Katz MM, Koslow SH, et al: Mania: diagnosis, state measurement and prediction of treatment response. J Affect Disord 8:113–121, 1985

Seeman MV: Neuroleptic prescription for men and women. Social Pharmacology 3(3):219–236, 1989

Seeman P, Van Tol HHM: Dopamine receptor pharmacology. Trends Pharmacol Sci 15:264–270, 1994

Segal DS, Callaghan M, Mandell AJ: Alterations in behaviour and catecholamine biosynthesis induced by lithium. Nature 254:58–59, 1975

Seguela P, Wadiche J, Dineley-Miller K, et al: Molecular cloning, functional properties, and distribution of rat brain $\alpha7$: a nicotinic cation channel highly permeable to calcium. J Neurosci 13:596–604, 1993

Sellers EM: Drug interactions, in Principles of Medical Pharmacology, 4th Edition. Edited by Kalant H, Roschlau WHE, Sellers EM. New York, Oxford University Press, 1985, pp 129–140

Sellers EM, Busto V, Kaplan HL, et al: Clinical abuse liability of partial and full agonist benzodiazepines: a comparison of bretazenil, diazepam and alprazolam, in Biological Psychiatry: Proceedings of the 5th World Congress of Biological Psychiatry, Florence, Italy, June 9–14, 1991. Edited by Racagni G, Brunello N, Fukuda T. New York, Excerpta Medica, 1991, pp 709–712

Selye H: The anesthetic effect of steroid hormones. Proc Soc Exp Biol Med 46:116–121, 1941

Sernyak MJ, Griffin RA, Johnson RM, et al: Neuroleptic exposure following inpatient treatment of acute mania with lithium and neuroleptic. Am J Psychiatry 151:133–135, 1994

Serra G, Forgioni A, D'Aquila PS, et al: Possible mechanism of antidepressant effect of L-sulpiride. Clin Neuropharmacol 13 (suppl 1):576–583, 1990a

Serra G, Colln M, D'Aquila PS, et al: Possible role of dopamine D1 receptor in the behavioral supersensitivity to dopamine agonists induced by chronic treatment with antidepressants. Brain Res 527:234–243, 1990b

Sershen H, Hashim, A, Lajtha A: Behavioral and biochemical effects of nicotine in an MPTP-induced mouse model of Parkinson's disease. Pharmacol Biochem Behav 28:299–303, 1987

Service RF: Will a new type of drug make memory-making easier? Science 266:218–219, 1994

Sevringhaus EL: Use of folliculin in involutional states. Am J Obstet Gynecol 25:361–368, 1933

Seyfried CA, Boettcher H: Central D_2-autoreceptor agonists, with special reference to indolylbutylamines. Drugs of the Future 15:819–832, 1990

Seyfried CA, Greiner, HE, Haase AF: Biochemical and functional studies on EMD 49980: a potent, selectively presynaptic D_2 dopamine agonist with actions on serotonin systems. Eur J Pharmacol 160:31–41, 1989

Shankel LW, Dimassimo DA, Whittier JR: Changes with age in electrical reactions in mental patients. Psychiatr Q 34:284–292, 1960

Shapira B, Oppenheim G, Zohar J, et al: Lack of efficacy of estrogen supplementation to imipramine in resistant female depressives. Biol Psychiatry 20:76–578, 1985

Shapira B, Gorfine M, Lerer B: A prospective study of lithium continuation therapy in depressed patients who have responded to electroconvulsive therapy. Convulsive Therapy 11:80–85, 1995

Shapiro E, Shapiro AK, Fulop GK, et al: Controlled study of haloperidol, pimozide and placebo for the treatment of Gilles de la Tourette's syndrome. Arch Gen Psychiatry 46:722–730, 1989

Sharp T, Bramwell SR, Lambert P, et al: Effect of short- and long-term administration of lithium on the release of endogenous 5-HT in the hippocampus of the rat in vivo and in vitro. Neuropharmacology 30:977–984, 1991

Sharpley AL, Cowen PJ: Effect of the pharmacological treatment on sleep of depressed patients. Biol Psychiatry 37:85–98, 1995

Sharpley AL, Walsh AES, Cowen PJ: Nefazodone—a novel antidepressant—may increase REM sleep. Biol Psychiatry 31:1070–1073, 1992

Shaw DM, Harris B, Lloyd AT, et al: A comparison of the antidepressant action of citalopram and amitriptyline. Br J Psychiatry 149:515–517, 1986

Shaw PJ, Ince PG: A quantitative autoradiographic study of H-3-Kainate binding sites in the normal human spinal-cord, brain stem, motor cortex. Brain Res 641:39–45, 1994

Shea MT, Pilkonis PA, Beckham E, et al: Personality disorders and treatment outcome in the NIMH treatment of depression collaborative research program. Am J Psychiatry 147:711–718, 1990

Sheehan DV: The Anxiety Disease. New York, Bantam Books, 1986, p 38

Sheehan DV, Ballenger JC, Jacobsen G: Treatment of endogenous anxiety with phobic, hysterical and hypochondriacal symptoms. Arch Gen Psychiatry 37:51–59, 1980

Sheehan DV, Raj AB, Sheehan KH, et al: The relative efficacy of buspirone, imipramine and placebo in panic disorder: a preliminary report. Pharmacol Biochem Behav 29:815–817, 1988

Sheehan M, de Belleroche J: Facilitation of GABA release by cholecystokinin and caerulein in rat cerebral cortex. Neuropeptides 3:429–434, 1983

Sherman AD, Petty F: Additivity of neurochemical changes in learned helplessness and imipramine. Behav Neural Biol 35:344–353, 1982

Sherman WR: Lithium and the phosphoinositide signaling system, in Lithium and the Cell. Edited by Birch NJ. London, Academic Press, 1991, pp 121–157

Sherman WR, Munsell LY, Gish BG, et al: Effects of systemically administered lithium on phosphoinositide metabolism in rat brain, kidney, and testis. J Neurochem 44:798–807, 1985

Sherman WR, Gish BG, Honchar MP, et al: Effects of lithium on phosphoinositide metabolism in vivo. Federation Proceedings 45:2639–2646, 1986

Shingai R, Sutherland ML, Barnard EA: Effects of subunit types of the cloned GABAa receptor on the response to a neurosteroid. Eur J Pharmacol 206:77–80, 1991

Shipley JE, Kupfer DJ, Griffin SJ, et al: Comparison of effects of desipramine and amitriptyline on EEG sleep of depressed patients. Psychopharmacology 85:14–22, 1985

Shipley JE, Kupfer DJ, Griffith R, et al: Computer analysis of EEG sleep delta waves and rapid eye movements: a comparison of two techniques. Sleep Res 17:353, 1988

Shipley MT: Transport of molecules from nose to brain: transneuronal anterograde and retrograde labeling in the rat olfactory system by wheat germ agglutinin–horseradish peroxidase applied to the nasal epithelium. Brain Res Bull 15:129–142, 1985

Shippenberg TS, Herz A: Influence of chronic lithium treatment upon the motivational effects of opioids: alteration in the effects of mu- but not kappa-opioid receptor ligands. J Pharmacol Exp Ther 256:1101–1106, 1991

Shippenberg TS, Millan MJ, Mucha RF, et al: Involvement of beta-endorphin and mu-opioid receptors in mediating the aversive effect of lithium in the rat. Eur J Pharmacol 154:135–144, 1988

Shively J, Reeve JR, Eysselein V, et al: CCK-5: sequence analysis of a small cholecystokinin from canine brain and intestine. Am J Physiol 252:G272–G275, 1987

Shukla GS: Combined lithium and valproate treatment and subsequent withdrawal: serotonergic mechanism of their interaction in discrete brain regions. Prog Neuropsychopharmacol Biol Psychiatry 9:153–156, 1985

Shute CCD, Lewis PR: The ascending cholinergic reticular system: neocortical, olfactory and subcortical projections. Brain 90:521–540, 1967

Sibley DR, Monsma FJ: Molecular biology of dopamine receptors. Trends Pharmacol Sci 13:61–69, 1992

Siegfried K: First impressions with an ACTH analog (HOE 427) in the treatment of Alzheimer's disease. Ann N Y Acad Sci 640:280–283, 1991

Siegfried K: Der heuristische Wert der Hypothese eines zentralen cholinergen Defizits beim Morbus Alzheimer als Ausgangspunkt einer pharmakologischen Behandlungsstrategie, in Pharmakopsychologie. Edited by Oldigs-Kerber J, Leonard J. Jena-Stuttgart, Gustav Fischer Verlag, 1992, pp 459–470

Siegfried K: The cholinergic hypothesis in Alzheimer's disease—clinical evidence gained with velnacrine, in Alzheimer's Disease. Clinical and Treatment Perspectives. Edited by Cutler NR, Gottfried CG, Siegfried K. Chichester, England, Wiley, 1995a, pp 53–73

Siegfried K: The efficacy of cholinergic drugs in patients with Alzheimer's disease—focus on the aminoacridines. Human Psychopharmacology 10:89–96, 1995b

Siegfried K: Neurotransmitter-based treatment of Alzheimer's disease: the example of velnacrine, in Developments in Dementia and Functional Disorders in the Elderly. Edited by Levy R, Howard R. Bristol, PA, Wrightson Biomedical Publishing, 1995c, pp 77–83

Siegfried K, Civil R: Clinical update of velnacrine research, in Alzheimer Disease: Therapeutic Strategies. Edited by Giacobini E, Becker R. Boston, MA, Birkhäuser, 1994, pp 150–154

Sierles FS, Chen J-J, McFarland RE, et al: Post traumatic stress disorder and concurrent psychiatric illness: a preliminary report. Am J Psychiatry 140:1177–1179, 1983

Siever LJ, Davis KL: Overview: toward a dysregulation hypothesis of depression. Am J Psychiatry 142:1017–1031, 1985

Siitonen L, Sonck T, Janne J: Effect of beta-blockade on performance: use of beta-blockade in bowling and in shooting competitions. J Int Med Res 5:395–366, 1977

Sikdar S, Kulhara P, Avasthi A, et al: Combined chlorpromazine and electroconvulsive therapy in mania. Br J Psychiatry 164:806–810, 1994

Simeon JG, Thatte S, Wiggins D: Treatment of adolescent obsessive-compulsive disorder with a clomipramine-fluoxetine combination. Psychopharmacol Bull 26:285–290, 1990

Simon JR, Kuhar MJ: High affinity choline uptake: ionic and energy requirement. J Neurochem 27:93–99, 1976

Simpson DM, Foster D: Improvement in organically disturbed behavior with trazodone treatment. J Clin Psychiatry 47:191–193, 1986

Simpson GM, Lee JH, Cuculica A, et al: Two dosages of imipramine in hospitalized endogenous and neurotic depressives. Arch Gen Psychiatry 33:1093–1102, 1976

Singer I: Lithium and the kidney. Kidney Int 19:374–387, 1981

Singer I, Rotenberg D, Puschett JB: Lithium-induced nephrogenic diabetes insipidus: in vivo and in vitro studies. J Clin Invest 51:1081–1091, 1972

Singh L, Lewis AS, Field MJ, et al: Evidence for an involvement of the brain cholecystokinin B receptor in anxiety. Proc Natl Acad Sci U S A 88:1130–1133, 1991

Sitaram N, Weingartner H, Gillin J: Human serial learning: enhancement with arecoline and choline, and impairment with scopolamine. Science 201:274–276, 1978

Sitaram N, Nurnberger JI, Gershon ES: Faster cholinergic REM sleep induction in euthymic patients with primary affective illness. Science 208:200–201, 1980

Sitaram N, Nurnberger JJ, Gershon ES, et al: Cholinergic regulation of mood and REM sleep: potential marker of vulnerability to affective disorder. Am J Psychiatry 139:571–576, 1982

Sitaram N, Dube S, Keshavan M, et al: The association of supersensitive cholinergic REM induction and affective illness within pedigrees. J Psychiatr Res 21:487–497, 1987

Sitland-Marken PA, Wells BG, Froemming JH, et al: Psychiatric applications of bromocriptine therapy. J Clin Psychiatry 51:68–82, 1990

Sitsen JMA, Zivkov M, Dieterle D: Wirksamkeit and Vertragliehkeit von Org 3770 bei Patienten mit ciner Major Depression. Eine vergleichende Studie gegen Amitriptyline und Plazebo. Psycopharmakotherapie 2:68–71, 1995

Sivam SP, Strunk C, Smith DR, et al: Proenkephalin-A gene regulation in the rat striatum: influence of lithium and haloperidol. Mol Pharmacol 30:186–191, 1986

Sivam SP, Takeuchi K, Li S, et al: Lithium increases dynorphin A(1–8) and prodynorphin mRNA levels in the basal ganglia of rats. Brain Res 427:155–163, 1988

Sivam SP, Krause JE, Takeuchi K, et al: Lithium increases rat striatal beta- and gamma-preprotachykinin messenger RNAs. J Pharmacol Exp Ther 248:1297–1301, 1989

Sizer AR, Long SK, Roberts MHT: A modulatory function of 5-hydroxytryptamine in the central nervous system, in Serotonin, CNS Receptors and Brain Function (Advances in the Biosciences, Vol 85). Edited by Bradley PB, Handley SL, Cooper SJ, et al. Oxford, England, Pergamon, 1992, pp 135–146

Skett P: Biochemical basis of sex differences in drug metabolism. Pharmacol Ther 38:269–304, 1988

Skuster DZ, Digre KB, Corbett JJ: Neurologic conditions presenting as psychiatric disorders. Psychiatr Clin North Am 15:311–333, 1992

Skutella T, Criswell H, Moy S, et al: Corticotropin-releasing hormone (CRH) antisense oligodeoxynucleotide induces anxiolytic effects in rat. Neuroreport 5:2181–2185, 1994

Slobodyansky E, Berkovich A, Bovolin P, et al: The endogenous allosteric modulation of GABA-A receptor subtypes: a role for the neuronal posttranslational processing products of rat brain DBI, in GABA and Benzodiazepine Receptor Subtypes. Edited by Biggio G, Costa E. New York, Raven, 1990, p 52

Small DH, Nurcombe V, Moir R: Association and release of the amyloid protein precursor of Alzheimer's disease from chick brain extracellular matrix. J Neurosci 12:4143–4150, 1992

Small GW, Propper MW, Randolph ET, et al: Mass hysteria among student performers: social relationship as a symptom predictor. Am J Psychiatry 9:1200–1205, 1991

Small IF, Milstein V, Miller MJ, et al: Electroconvulsive treatment—indications, benefits, and limitations. Am J Psychother 40:343–356, 1986

Small JG, Klapper MH, Kellams JJ, et al: Electroconvulsive therapy compared with lithium in the management of manic states. Arch Gen Psychiatry 45:727–732, 1988

Small JG, Klapper MH, Milstein V, et al: Carbamazepine compared with lithium in the treatment of mania. Arch Gen Psychiatry 48:915–921, 1991

Smeyne RJ, Klein R, Schnapp A, et al: Severe sensory and sympathetic neuropathies in mice carrying a disrupted Trk/NGF receptor gene. Nature 368:246–249, 1994

Smith CD, Carney JM, Starke-Reed PE: Excess brain protein oxidation and enzyme dysfunction in normal aging and in Alzheimer's disease. Proc Natl Acad Sci U S A 85:10540–10543, 1991

Smith DF: Lithium attenuates clonidine-induced hypoactivity: further studies in inbred mouse strains. Psychopharmacology 94:428–430, 1988

Smith DF, Amdisen A: Lithium distribution in rat brain after long-term central administration by minipump. J Pharm Pharmacol 33:805–806, 1981

Smith J, Williams K, Birkett S, et al: Neuroendocrine and clinical effects of electroconvulsive therapy and their relationship to treatment outcome. Psychol Med 24:547–555, 1994

Smith MA, Davidson J, Ritchie JC, et al: The corticotropin-releasing hormone test in patients with post-traumatic stress order. Biol Psychiatry 26:349–355, 1989

Smith MA, Makino S, Kvetnansky R, et al: Stress and glucocorticoids affect the expression of brain-derived neurotrophic factor and neurotrophin-3 mRNAs in the hippocampus. J Neurosci 15:1768–1777, 1995

Smith RB, Divoll M, Gillespie WR, et al: Effect of subject age and gender on the pharmacokinetics of oral triazolam and temazepam. J Clin Psychopharmacol 3:172–176, 1983

Snidman N, Kagan J, Riordan L, et al: Cardiac function and behavioral reactivity during infancy. Psychophysiology 32:199–207, 1995

Snodgrass J, Corwin J: Pragmatics of recognition memory: application to dementia and amnesia. J Exp Psychol Gen 117:34–50, 1988

Snyder F: The dynamic aspects of sleep disturbances in relation to mental illness. Biol Psychiatry 1:119–130, 1969

Snyder FR, Henningfield JE: Effects of nicotine administration following 12 hours of tobacco deprivation: assessment on computerized performance tasks. Psychopharmacology 97:17–22, 1989

Sobin C, Sackeim HA, Prudic J, et al: Predictors of retrograde amnesia following ECT. Am J Psychiatry 152:995–1001, 1995

Søgaard U, Michalow J, Butler B, et al: A tolerance study of single and multiple dosing of the selective dopamine uptake inhibitor GBR 12909 in healthy subjects. Int Clin Psychopharmacol 5:237–251, 1990

Soldatos CR: Computerized sleep EEG (CSEEG) in psychiatry and psychopharmacology, in Biological Psychiatry Today. Edited by Obiolo J, Ballus C, Monclus EG, et al. Amsterdam, Elsevier, 1979

Soldatos CR: Insomnia in relation to depression and anxiety: epidemiologic considerations. J Psychosom Res 38 (suppl 1):3–8, 1994

Soldatos CR, Paparrigopoulos TJ: Sleep patterns in depression, in WPA Teaching Bulletin on Depression. November (issue 11), 1995

Soldatos CR, Vela-Bueno A, Kales A: Sleep in psychiatric disorders. Psychiatric Medicine 4(2):119–132, 1987

Soldatos CR, Stefanis CN, Bergiannaki JD, et al: An experimental antidepressant increases REM sleep. Prog Neuropsychopharmacol Biol Psychiatry 12:899–907, 1988

Soldatos CR, Sakkas P, Bergiannaki JD, et al: Sleep laboratory studies in the evaluation of antidepressants: methodological considerations, in Psychiatry: A World Perspective, Vol 2: Neuroscience in Psychiatry: Biological Correlates of Mental Disorders. Edited by Stefanis CN, Soldatos CR, Rabavilas AD. New York, Excerpta Medica, 1990, pp 636–642

Solomon I, Williamson P: Verapamil in bipolar illness. Can J Psychiatry 31:442–444, 1986

Solyom L, Heseltine G, McClure D, et al: Behavior therapy vs drug therapy in the treatment of phobic neurosis. Canadian Psychiatric Association Journal 18:25–31, 1973

Song F, Freemantle N, Sheldon TA: Selective serotonin reuptake inhibitors: meta-analysis of efficacy and acceptability. BMJ 306(6879):683–687, 1993

Song L, Jope R: Chronic lithium treatment impairs phosphatidylinositol hydrolysis in membranes from rat brain regions. J Neurochem 58:2200–2206, 1992

Souza FG, Mander AJ, Goodwin GM: The efficacy of lithium in prophylaxis of unipolar depression: evidenced from its discontinuation. Br J Psychiatry 157:718–722, 1990

Spagnoli A, Lucca U, Menasce G: Long-term acetyl-L-carnitine treatment in Alzheimer's disease. Neurology 41:1726–1732, 1991

Spengler D, Rupprecht R, Phi Van L, et al: Identification and characterization of a 3',5'-cylic adenosine monophosphate-responsive element in the human corticotropin-releasing hormone gene promoter. Mol Endocrinol 6:1931–1941, 1992

Spengler RN, Hollingsworth PJ, Smith CB: Effects of long-term lithium and desipramine treatment upon clonidine-induced inhibition of ^{3}H-norpinephrine release from rat hippocampal slices. Federation Proceedings 45:681, 1986

Spiegel R: The NOSGER (Nurses' Observation Scale for Geriatric Patients). Basel, Switzerland, August 1989 (distributed by the author)

Spier SA, Tesar GE, Rosenbaum JF, et al: Treatment of panic disorder and agoraphobia with clonazepam. J Clin Psychiatry 47:238–242, 1986

Spiker DG, Weiss JC, Dealy RS, et al: The pharmacological treatment of delusional depression. Am J Psychiatry 142:430–436, 1985

Spillich GJ, June L, Renner J: Cigarette smoking and cognitive performance. British Journal of Addiction 87:1313–1326, 1992

Spirtes MA: Lithium levels in monkey and human brain after chronic, therapeutic, oral dosage. Pharmacol Biochem Behav 5:143–147, 1976

Spitzer RL, Endicott J: The Schedule for Affective Disorders and Schizophrenia—Change Version, 3rd Edition. New York, New York State Psychiatric Institute, Biometrics Research, 1978

Spitzer RL, Endicott J, Robins E: Research Diagnostic Criteria (RDC) for a Selected Group of Functional Disorders. New York, New York State Psychiatric Institute, 1985

Sprouse JS, Wilkinson LO: Innovative therapeutic actions by targeting serotonin 1A receptors selectively. International Review of Psychiatry 7:5–15, 1995

Squillace K, Post R, Savard R, et al: Life charting of the longitudinal course of recurrent affective illness, in Neurobiology of Mood Disorders, Vol 1. Edited by Post RM, Ballenger JC. Baltimore, MD, Williams & Wilkins, 1984, pp 38–59

Squires RF, Braestrup C: Benzodiazepine receptors in rat brain. Nature 266:732–734, 1977

Stabel S, Parker PJ: Protein kinase C. Pharmacol Ther 51:71–95, 1991

Stagno SJ, Smith ML, Hassenbusch SJ: Reconsidering "psychosurgery": issues of informed consent and physician responsibility. J Clin Ethics 5:217–223, 1994

Stahl SM: Is serotonin receptor down regulation linked to the mechanism of action of antidepressant drugs? Psychopharmacol Bull 30:39–43, 1994

Stahl SM: Mixed anxiety and depression: serotonin 1A receptors as a common pharmacological link. J Clin Psychiatry (in press)

Stallone F, Shelley E, Mendlewicz J, et al: The use of lithium in affective disorders, III: a double-blind study of prophylaxis in bipolar illness. Am J Psychiatry 130:1006–1010, 1973

Stam CJ, Visser SL, Op de Coul AAW, et al: Disturbed frontal regulation of attention in Parkinson's disease. Brain 116:1139–1158, 1993

Stamenkovic M, Aschauer H, Kasper S: Risperidone for Tourette's syndrome. Lancet 344:1577–1578, 1994

Stanley BG, Leibowitz SF: Neuropeptide Y injected in the paraventricular hypothalamus: A powerful stimulant of feeding behavior. Proc Natl Acad Sci U S A 82:3940–3943, 1985

Stanley MA, Turner SM: Current status of pharmacological and behavioral treatment of obsessive-compulsive disorder. Behav Ther 26:162–186, 1995

Starkman MN, Schteingart DE, Schork MA: Depressed mood and other psychiatric manifestations of Cushing's syndrome: relationship to hormone levels. Psychosom Med 43:3–18, 1981

Starkman MN, Schteingart DE, Schurtt AM: Cushing's syndrome after treatment: changes in cortisol and ACTH levels and amelioration of the depressive syndrome. Psychiatry Res 19:177–188, 1985

Starkstein SE, Mayberg HS, Berthier ML, et al: Mania after brain injury: neuroradiological and metabolic findings. Ann Neurol 27:652–659, 1990

Starkstein SE, Fedoroff P, Berthier ML, et al: Manic-depressive and pure manic states after brain lesions. Biol Psychiatry 29:149–158, 1991

Stassen HH, Delini-Stula A, Angst J: Time course of improvement under antidepressant treatment: a survival-analytical approach. Eur Neuropsychopharmacol 3:127–135, 1993

Stassen HH, Angst J, Delini-Stula A: Severity of baseline and onset of improvement in depression: metanalysis of imipramine and moclobemide versus placebo. European Psychiatry 9 (suppl 3):129–136, 1994

Staubli U, Xu FB: Effects of 5-HT$_3$ receptor antagonism on hippocampal theta rhythm, memory and LTP induction in the freely moving rat. J Neurosci 15:2445–2452, 1995

Staunton DA, Magistretti PJ, Shoemaker WJ, et al: Effects of chronic lithium treatment on dopamine receptors in the rat corpus striatum, I: locomotor activity and behavioral supersensitivity. Brain Res 232:391–400, 1982a

Staunton DA, Magistretti PJ, Shoemaker WJ, et al: Effects of chronic lithium treatment on dopamine receptors in the rat corpus striatum, II: no effect on denervation or neuroleptic-induced supersensitivity. Brain Res 232:401–412, 1982b

Steardo L, Barone P, Hunnicutt E: Carbamazepine lowering effect on CSF somatostatin-like immunoreactivity in temporal lobe epilepsy. Acta Neurol Scand 74:140–144, 1986

Steiger A, Holsboer F, Benkert O: Long-term studies on the effect of tricyclic antidepressants and selective MAO-A-inhibitors on sleep, nocturnal penile tumescence and hormonal secretion in normal controls, in Sleep '86. Edited by Koella WP. Stuttgart, Fischer Verlag, 1988, pp 335–337

Steiger A, von Bardeleben U, Herth T, et al: Sleep EEG and nocturnal secretion of cortisol and growth hormone in male patients with endogenous depression before treatment and after recovery. J Affect Disord 16:189–195, 1989

Steiger A, Trachsel AL, Guldner J, et al: Neurosteroid pregenolone induces sleep EEG changes in man compatible with inverse agonistic GABAa receptor modulation. Brain Res 615:267–274, 1993

Stein MB, Millar TW, Larsen DK, et al: Irregular breathing during sleep in patients with panic disorder. Am J Psychiatry 152:1168–1173, 1995

Steiner M, Oakes R, Gergel IP, et al: Predictors of response to paroxetine therapy in OCD. Paper presented at the annual meeting of the American Psychiatric Association, Philadelphia, PA, May 25, 1994

Steiner W, Fontaine R: Toxic reaction following the combined administration of fluoxetine and L-tryptophan: five case reports. Biol Psychiatry 21:1067–1071, 1986

Steingard S, Chengappa KNR, Baker RW, et al: Clozapine, obsessive symptoms, and serotonergic mechanisms (letter). Am J Psychiatry 150:1435, 1993

Stengaard-Pedersen K, Larsson LI, Fredens K, et al: Modulation of cholecystokinin concentrations in the rat hippocampus by chelation of heavy metals. Proc Natl Acad Sci U S A 81:5876–5880, 1984

Stenzel-Poore MP, Heinrichs SC, Rivest S, et al: Overproduction of corticotropin-releasing factor in transgenic mice: a genetic model of anxiogenic behavior. J Neurosci 14:2579–2584, 1994

Stephens DN, Schneider HH, Kehr W, et al: Abecarnil, a metabolically stable anxio-selective beta carboline acting at benzodiazepine receptors. J Pharmacol Exp Ther 253:334–343, 1990

Stephens DN, Turski L, Jones GH, et al: Abecarnil: a novel anxiolytic with mixed full agonist/partial agonist properties in animal models of anxiety and sedation, in Anxiolytic Beta-Carbolines: From Molecular Biology to the Clinic. Edited by Stephens DN. Berlin, Springer-Verlag, 1993, p 79

Stern M, Fram DH, Wyatt R, et al: All-night sleep studies of acute schizophrenics. Arch Gen Psychiatry 20:470–477, 1969

Stern RA, Nevels CT, Shelhorse ME, et al: Antidepressant and memory effects of combined thyroid hormone treatment and electroconvulsive therapy: preliminary findings. Biol Psychiatry 30:623–627, 1991

Stern TA, Jenike MA: Treatment of obsessive-compulsive disorder with lithium carbonate. Psychosomatics 24:671–673, 1983

Sternbach H: Fluoxetine treatment of social phobia. J Clin Psychopharmacol 10:230–231, 1990

Stevens DA, Resnick O, Krus DM: The effects of p-chlorophenylalanine, a depleter of brain serotonin, on behaviour, I: facilitation of discrimination learning. Life Sci 6:2215–2220, 1967

Stewart SH, Knize K, Pihl RO: Anxiety sensitivity and dependency in clinical and non-clinical panickers and controls. J Anxiety Disord 6:119–131, 1992

Stewart WF, Kawas C, Corrada M, et al: Risk of Alzheimer's disease and duration of NSAID use. Neurology 48:626–632, 1997

Stock G, Klimpel L, Sturm V, et al: Resistance to tonic clonic seizures after amygdaloid kindling in cats. Exp Neurol 69:239–246, 1980

Stoehr GP, Kroboth PD, Juhl RP, et al: Effect of oral contraceptives on triazolam, temazepam, alprazolam, and lorazepam kinetics. Clin Pharmacol Ther 36:683–690, 1984

Stokes PE, Shamoian CA, Stoll PM, et al: Efficacy of lithium as acute treatment of manic-depressive illness. Lancet 1:1319–1325, 1971

Stokes PE, Pick GR, Stoll PM, et al: Pituitary adrenal function in depressed patients: resistance to dexamethasone suppression. J Psychiatr Res 12:271–281, 1975

Stoll AL, Cohen BM, Snyder MB, et al: Erythrocyte choline concentration in bipolar disorder: a predictor of clinical course and medication response. Biol Psychiatry 29:1171–1180, 1991

Stoll AL, Banov M, Kolbrener M, et al: Neurological factors predict a favorable valproate response in bipolar and schizoaffective disorders. J Clin Psychopharmacol 14:311–313, 1994

Stoll KD, Bisson HE, Fischer E, et al: Carbamazepine versus haloperidol in manic syndromes—first report of a multicentric study in Germany, in Biological Psychiatry 1985. Edited by Shagass C, Joiassen RC, Bridger WH, et al. Amsterdam, Elsevier, 1986, pp 332–334

Strakowski SM, Tohen M, Stoll AL, et al: Comorbidity in psychosis at first hospitalization. Am J Psychiatry 150:752–757, 1993a

Strakowski SM, Wilson DR, Tohen M, et al: Structural brain abnormalities in first-episode mania. Biol Psychiatry 33:602–609, 1993b

Strand M, Hetta J, Rosen A, et al: A double-blind, controlled trial in primary care patients with generalised anxiety: a comparison between buspirone and oxazepam. J Clin Psychiatry 51 (suppl):40–45, 1990

Study RE, Barker JL: Diazepam and pentobarbital: fluctuation analysis reveals different mechanisms for potentiation of gabaaminobutyric acid responses in cultured central neurons. Proc Natl Acad Sci U S A 78:7180–7184, 1981

Stumpo DJ, Bock CB, Tuttle JS, et al: MARCKS deficiency in mice leads to abnormal brain development and perinatal death. Proc Natl Acad Sci U S A 92:944–948, 1995

Sugrue MF: The inability of chronic mianserin to block central α_2-adrenoceptors. Eur J Pharmacol 69:377–380, 1980

Suhara T, Nakayama K, Inoue O: D_1 dopamine receptor binding in mood disorders measured by positron emission tomography. Psychopharmacology 106:14–18, 1992

Sulser F: Antidepressant treatment and regulation of norepinephrine-receptor-coupled adenylyl cyclase systems in brain. Adv Biochem Psychopharmacol 39:249–261, 1984

Sulser F, Vetulani J, Mobley PL: Mode of action of antidepressant drugs. Biochem Pharmacol 27:257–271, 1978

Summers WK, Majowski LV, Marsh GM, et al: Oral tetrahydroaminoacridine in long-term treatment of senile dementia, Alzheimer-type. N Engl J Med 315:1241–1245, 1986

Sunderland T, Tariot P, Murphy DL, et al: Scopolamine challenges in Alzheimer's disease. Psychopharmacology 87:247–249, 1985

Sunderland T, Tariot, P, Weingartner H, et al: Pharmacologic modelling of Alzheimer's disease. Prog Neuropsychopharmacol Biol Psychiatr 10:599–610, 1986

Sunderland T, Tariot P, Newhouse PA: Differential responsivity of mood, behavior, and cognition to cholinergic agents in elderly neuropsychiatric populations. Brain Res Rev 13:371–389, 1988

Suomi SJ: Factors affecting responses to social separation in rhesus monkeys, in Animal Models in Human Psychobiology. Edited by Serban G, Kling A. New York, Plenum, 1976, pp 9–26

Suomi SJ: Abnormal behavior in nonhuman primates, in Primate Behavior. Edited by Fobes JL, King JE. New York, Academic Press, 1982, pp 171–215

Suomi SJ, Seaman SF, Lewis JK, et al: Effects of imipramine treatment of separation-induced social disorder in rhesus monkeys. Arch Gen Psychiatry 35:321–325, 1978

Suppes T, Baldessarini RJ, Faedda GL, et al: Risk of recurrence following discontinuation of lithium treatment in bipolar disorder. Arch Gen Psychiatry 48:1082–1088, 1991

Suppes T, McElroy SL, Gilbert J, et al: Clozapine in the treatment of dysphoric mania. Biol Psychiatry 32:270–280, 1992

Susdak PD, Schwartz RD, Scolnick P, et al: Ethanol stimulates gamma-aminobutyric acid receptor–mediated chloride transport in rat brain synaptoneurosomes. Proc Natl Acad Sci U S A 83:4071–4075, 1986

Sussman EJ, Chrousos GP: Negative affect and hormone levels in young adolescents: concurrent and predictive perspectives. Journal of Youth and Adolescence 20:185–190, 1991

Sussman N: The uses of buspirone in psychiatry. J Clin Psychiatry Monograph 12:3–19, 1994

Svestka J, Nahunek K, Ceskova E, et al: Carbamazepine prophylaxis of affective psychoses (intraindividual comparison with lithium carbonate). Activ Nerv Sup 27:261–262, 1985

Swann AC: Norepinephrine and (Na^+, K^+)-ATPase: evidence for stabilization by lithium or imipramine. Neuropharmacology 27:261–267, 1988

Swann AC, Koslow SH, Katz MM, et al: Lithium carbonate treatment of mania. Arch Gen Psychiatry 44:345–354, 1987

Swartz CM, Abrams R: Prolactin levels after bilateral and unilateral ECT. Br J Psychiatry 144:643–645, 1984

Swartz CM, Lewis RK: Theophylline reversal of electroconvulsive therapy (ECT) seizure inhibition. Psychosomatics 32:47–51, 1991

Swayze VW, Andreasen NC, Alliger RJ, et al: Structural brain abnormalities in bipolar affective disorder. Arch Gen Psychiatry 47:1054–1059, 1990

Swayze VW, Andreasen NC, Alliger RJ, et al: Subcortical and temporal structures in affective disorder and schizophrenia: a magnetic resonance imaging study. Biol Psychiatry 31:221–240, 1992

Swedo SE, Rapoport JL, Cheslow DL, et al: High prevalence of obsessive-compulsive symptoms in patients with Sydenham's chorea. Am J Psychiatry 146:246–249, 1989

Swedo SE, Leonard HL, Kiessling LS: Speculations on antineuronal antibody-mediated neuropsychiatric disorders of childhood. Pediatrics 93:323–326, 1994

Swerdlow NR, Andia AM: Trazodone-fluoxetine combination for treatment of obsessive-compulsive disorder. Am J Psychiatry 146:1637, 1989

Swerdlow NR, Britton KT: Alphaxalone, a steroid anesthetic, inhibits the startle-enhancing effects of corticotropin releasing factor, but not strychnine. Psychopharmacology 115(1–2):141–146, 1994

Swerdlow NR, Britton KT, Koob GF: Potentiation of acoustic startle by corticotropin-releasing factor (CRF) and by fear are both reversed by α-helical CRF (9–41). Neuropsychopharmacology 2:285–292, 1989

Swierczynski SL, Siddhanti SR, Tuttle JS, et al: Nonmyristoylated MARCKS complements some but not all of the developmental defects associated with MARCKS deficiency in mice. Dev Biol 179:135–147, 1996

Swinson RP, Joffe RT: Biological challenges in obsessive compulsive disorder. Prog Neuropsychopharmacol Biol Psychiatry 12:369–375, 1988

Szostak C, Tipper SP, Stuss DT: Aging-associated changes in selective attention: examination of negative priming, interference, and response inhibition effects, 1995 (submitted for publication)

Takahashi R, Sakuma A, Itoh K, et al: Comparison of efficacy of lithium carbonate and chlorpromazine in mania: report of collaborative study group on treatment of mania in Japan. Arch Gen Psychiatry 32:1310–1318, 1975

Takahashi Y, Kato K, Hayashizaki Y, et al: Molecular cloning of the human cholecystokinin gene by use of a synthetic probe containing deoxyinosine. Proc Natl Acad Sci U S A 82:1931–1935, 1985

Talalaenko AN, Abramets IA, Stakhovskii YuV, et al: The role of dopaminergic mechanisms on the brain in various models of anxious states. Neurosci Behav Physiol 24:284–288, 1994

Tamimi RR, Mavissakalian MR: Are effective antiobsessional drugs interchangeable? (letter). Arch Gen Psychiatry 48:857–858, 1991

Tan CH, Javors MA, Seleshi E, et al: Effects of lithium on platelet ionic intracellular calcium concentration in patients with bipolar (manic-depressive) disorder and healthy controls. Life Sci 46:1175–1180, 1990

Tanda G, Carboni E, Frau R, et al: Increase of extracellular dopamine in the prefrontal cortex: a trait of drugs with antidepressant potential. Psychopharmacology 115:285–288, 1994

Tandon R, Shipley J, Eiser AS, et al: Association between abnormal REM sleep and negative symptoms in schizophrenia. Psychiatry Res 27:359–361, 1988

Tang L, Todd RD, O'Malley KL: Dopamine D_2 and D_3 receptors inhibit dopamine release. J Pharmacol Exp Ther 270:475–479, 1994

Taniguti K: Experimental study on the effects of intraventricularly injected noradrenaline, acetylcholine, dopamine and serotonin on memory and learning in the rat. Nichidai Igaku Zasshi 39:663–672, 1980

Tanimoto K, Maeda K, Terada T: Inhibitory effect of lithium on neuroleptic and serotonin receptors in rat brain. Brain Res 256:148–151, 1983

Tanquary J, Masand P: Paradoxical reaction to buspirone augmentation of fluoxetine (letter). J Clin Psychopharmacol 10:377, 1990

Targum SD, Marshall LE: Fenfluramine provocation of anxiety in patients with panic disorder. Psychiatry Res 28:295–306, 1989

Targum SD, Rosen LN, DeLisi LE, et al: Cerebral ventricular size in major depressive disorder: association with delusional symptoms. Biol Psychiatry 18:329–336, 1983

Targum SD, Greenberg RD, Harmon RL, et al: Thyroid hormone and the TRH stimulation test in refractory depression. J Clin Psychiatry 45:345–346, 1984

Tariot PN, Cohen RM, Sunderland T: L-Deprenyl in Alzheimer's disease. Arch Gen Psychiatry 44:427–433, 1987

Tariot PN, Cohen RM, Welkowitz JA, et al: Multiple-dose arecoline infusions in Alzheimer's disease. Arch Gen Psychiatry 45:901–905, 1988

Taylor AE, Saint-Cyr JA, Lang AE: Frontal lobe dysfunction in Parkinson's disease: the cortical focus of neostriatal outflow. Brain 109:845–883, 1986

Taylor DP, Smith DW, Hyslop DK, et al: Receptor binding and atypical antidepressant drug discovery, in Receptor Binding in Drug Research. Edited by O'Brien RA. New York, Marcel Dekker, 1986, pp 151–165

Tejedor-Real P, Mico JA, Maldonado R, et al: Effect of mixed (RB 38A) and selective (RB 38B) inhibitors of enkephalin degrading enzymes on a model of depression in the rat. Biol Psychiatry 34:100–107, 1993

Terry AV, Buccafusco JJ, Prendergast MA, et al: The 5-HT$_3$ receptor antagonist, RS-56812, enhances delayed matching performance in monkeys. Neuroreport 20:49–54, 1996

Terry JB, Padzernik TL, Nelson SR: Effect of LiCl pretreatment on cholinomimetic-induced seizures and seizure-induced brain edema in rats. Neurosci Lett 114:123–127, 1990

Terry RD: Alzheimer's disease, in Textbook of Neuropathology. Edited by Davis RL, Robertson DM. Baltimore, MD, Williams & Wilkins, 1985, pp 824–841

Tesar GE, Rosenbaum JF: Recognition and management of panic disorder. Adv Intern Med 28:123–149, 1993

Thakore JH, Dinan TG: Cortisol synthesis inhibition: a new treatment strategy for the clinical and endocrine manifestations of depression. Biol Psychiatry 37:364–368, 1995

Thakur AK, Remillard AJ, Meldrum LH, et al: Intravenous clomipramine and obsessive-compulsive disorder. Can J Psychiatry 36:521–524, 1991

Thal L: Clinical trials in Alzheimer disease, in Alzheimer Disease. Edited by Terry RD, Katzman R, Bick K. New York, Raven, 1994, pp 431–444

Thase ME: Relapse and recurrence in unipolar major depression: short-term and long-term approaches. J Clin Psychiatry 51 (suppl): 51–59, 1990

Thase ME, Rush AJ: When at first you don't succeed: sequential strategies for antidepressant nonresponders. J Clin Psychiatry 58 (suppl 13):23–29, 1997

Thase ME, Kupfer DJ, Spiker DG: Electroencephalographic sleep in secondary depression: a revisit. Biol Psychiatry 19:805–814, 1984

Thellier M, Wissocq JC, Heurteaux C: Quantitative microlocation of lithium in the brain by a (n, α) nuclear reaction. Nature 283:299–302, 1980

Thiebot MH, Martin P, Puech AJ: Animal behavioral studies in the evaluation of antidepressant drugs. Br J Psychiatry 160 (suppl 15):44–50, 1992

Thiele EA, Eipper BA: Effect of secretogogues on components of the secretory system in AtT-20 cells. Endocrinology 126:809–817, 1990

Thigore JH, Dinan TG: Cortisol synthesis inhibition: a new treatment strategy for the clinical and endocrine manifestations of depression. Biol Psychiatry 37:364–368, 1995

Thoenen H: Neurotrophins and neuronal plasticity. Science 270:593–598, 1995

Thompson D: Repeated acquisition as a behavioral base line for studying drug effects. J Pharmacol Exp Ther 184:506–514, 1973

Thompson JW, Weiner RD, Myers CP: Use of ECT in the United States in 1975, 1980, and 1986. Am J Psychiatry 151:1657–1661, 1994

Thoren P, Asberg M, Gronholm B, et al: CMI treatment of OCD. A controlled clinical trial. Arch Gen Psychiatry 37:1281–85, 1980

Thorne RG, Perfetti PA, Emory CR, et al: Quantitative assessment of transneuronal transport to the rat olfactory bulb following intranasal administration of wheat germ agglutinin-horseradish peroxidase. Neurobiol Aging 13 (suppl 1) 132–133, 1992

Thyrer BA, Parrish RT, Himle J, et al: Alcohol abuse among clinically anxious patients. Behav Res Ther 24:357–359, 1986

Tignol J, Stoker MJ, Dunbar GC: Paroxetine in the treatment of melancholia and severe depression. Int Clin Psychopharmacol 7:91–94, 1992

Tilders FJH, Schmidt ED, Van Dijken HH, et al: Adaptive changes in hypothalamic CRH-neurons in experimental animals and man (abstract). American College of Neuropsychopharmacology Annual Meeting, San Juan, Puerto Rico, December 1994

Tohgi H, Abe T, Takahashi S, et al: Indoleamine concentrations in cerebrospinal fluid from patients with Alzheimer type and Binswanger type dementias before and after administration of citalopram, a synthetic serotonin uptake inhibitor. J Neural Transm 9:121–131, 1995

Tollefson G: Alprazolam in the treatment of obsessive symptoms. J Clin Psychopharmacol 5:39–42, 1985

Tollefson GD, Senogles S: A cholinergic role in the mechanism of lithium in mania. Biol Psychiatry 18:467–479, 1982

Tollefson GD, Rampey AH Jr, Potvin JH, et al: A multicenter investigation of fixed-dose fluoxetine in the treatment of obsessive-compulsive disorder. Arch Gen Psychiatry 51:559–567, 1994

Tome de la Granja MB, Harte R, Holland C, et al: Paroxetine and pindolol: a randomised trial of serotonergic antireceptor blockade in the reduction of antidepressant latency. Int Clin Psychopharmacol 12:81–90, 1997

Torok TL: Neurochemical transmission and the sodium pump. Prog Neurobiol 32:11–76, 1989

Tortella FC, Cowan A: Studies on opioid peptides as endogenous anticonvulsants. Life Sci 31:2225–2228, 1982

Trapp T, Holsboer F: Heterodimerization between mineralocorticoid and glucocorticoid receptor increases the functional diversity of corticosteroid action. Trends Pharmacol Sci 17:145–149, 1996

Trapp T, Rupprecht R, Castrén M, et al: Heterodimerization between mineralocorticoid and glucocorticoid receptor: a new principle of glucocorticoid action in the central nervous system. Neuron 13:1–6, 1994

Treiser S, Kellar KJ: Lithium effects on adrenergic receptor supersensitivity in rat brain. Eur J Pharmacol 58:85–86, 1979

Treiser S, Kellar KJ: Lithium: effects on serotonin receptors in rat brain. Eur J Pharmacol 64:183–185, 1980

Treiser SL, Cascio CS, O'Donohue TL, et al: Lithium increases serotonin release and decreases serotonin receptors in the hippocampus. Science 213:1529–1531, 1981

Tricklebank M, Forler C, Fozard J: The involvement of subtypes of the 5-HT1 receptor and of catecholaminergic systems in the behavioural response to 8-hydroxy-2-(di-n-propylamino) tetralin in the rat. Eur J Pharmacol 106:271–282, 1984

Tricklebank MD, Singh L, Jackson A, et al: Evidence that a proconvulsant action of lithium is mediated by inhibition of myo-inositol phosphatase in mouse brain. Brain Res 558:145–148, 1991

Triggle DJ: Biochemical and pharmacologic differences among calcium channel antagonists: clinical implications, in Calcium Antagonists in Clinical Medicine. Edited by Epstein M. Philadelphia, PA, Hanley and Belfus, 1992, pp 1–27

Triggs W, Cros D, Macdonell RA, et al: Cortical and spinal motor excitability during the transcranial magnetic stimulation silent period in humans. Brain Res 628:39–48, 1993

Trousseau A: Clinique Medicale de l'Hotel-Dieu de Paris, 3rd Edition. Paris, France, Bailliere, 1868

Trullas R, Skolnick P: Functional antagonists at the NMDA receptor complex exhibit antidepressant actions. Eur J Pharmacol 185:1–10, 1990

Tseng FY, Pasquali D, Field JB: Effects of lithium on stimulated metabolic parameters in dog thyroid slices. Acta Endocrinol 121:615–620, 1989

Tseng WS, Asai M, Kitanshi K, et al: Diagnostic patterns of social phobia: comparison in Tokyo and Hawaii. J Nerv Ment Dis 180:380–385, 1992

Tsuang MT, Lyons MJ, Faraone SV: Heterogeneity of schizophrenia. Conceptual models and analytic strategies. Br J Psychiatry 156:17–26, 1990

Tsuji K, Nakamura Y, Ogata Y, et al: Rapid decrease in ATP content without recovery phase during glutamate-induced cell-death in cultured spinal neurons. Brain Res 662:289–292, 1994

Tucker DM, Leckman JF, Scahill L, et al: A putative poststreptococcal case of OCD with chronic tic disorder, not otherwise specified [see comments]. J Am Acad Child Adolesc Psychiatry 35:1684–1691, 1996

Turner DM, Ransom RW, Yang JS-J, et al: Steroid anesthetics and naturally occurring analogs modulate the gamma-aminobutyric acid receptor complex at a site distinct from barbiturates. J Pharmacol Exp Ther 248:960–966, 1989

Turner SM, Beidel D, Jacob RG: Social phobia: a comparison of behavior therapy and atenolol. J Consult Clin Psychol 62:350–358, 1994

Tyrer P, Candy J, Kelly D: A study of the clinical effects of phenelzine and placebo in the treatment of phobic anxiety. Psychopharmacology 32:237–254, 1973

Uchiumi M, Susuki M, Ishigooka J, et al: Effects of DN-2327, new anxiolytic, on daytime sleepiness. Clin Neuropharmacol 15 (suppl 1 part B):541B, 1992

Udassin R, Ariel I, Haskel Y, et al: Salicylate as an in vivo free radical trap: studies on ischemic insult to the rat intestine. Free Radic Biol Med 10:1–6, 1991

Ueda S, Aikawa M, Kawata M, et al: Neuro-glial neurotrophic interaction in the S-100 beta retarded mutant mouse (Polydactyly Nagoya), III: transplantation study. Brain Res 738:15–23, 1996

Uhde TW, Roy-Byrne P, Gillin JC, et al: The sleep of patients with panic disorders: a preliminary report. Psychiatry Res 12:251–259, 1984

Uhde TW, Tancer ME, Rubinow DR, et al: Evidence for hypothalamo-growth hormone dysfunction in panic disorder: profile of growth hormone response to clonidine, yohimbine, caffeine, glucose, TRF and TRH in panic disorder patients versus healthy volunteers. Neuropsychopharmacology 6:101–118, 1992

Uhde T, Terril DR, Chambless DL, et al: Pentagastrin model of anxiety in humans, in Abstracts of Panels and Posters of the 32nd Annual Meeting of American College of Neuropsychopharmacology, Honolulu, HI, 1993, p 59

Ui M: Pertussis toxin as a valuable probe for G protein involvement in signal transduction, in ADP-Ribosylation Toxins and G Proteins. Edited by Moss J, Vaughn M. Washington, DC, American Society for Microbiology, 1990, pp 45–79

Uncini A, Treviso M, Di-Muzio A, et al: Physiological basis of voluntary activity inhibition induced by transcranial cortical stimulation. Electroencephalogr Clin Neurophysiol 89:211–220, 1993

Uney JB, Marchbanks RM, Marsh A: The effect of lithium on choline transport in human erythrocytes. J Neurol Neurosurg Psychiatry 48:229–233, 1985

Ungerer A, Mathis C, Mélan C, et al: The NMDA receptor, CPP and g-L-glutamyl-L-aspartate, selectively block post-training improvement of performance in a Y-maze avoidance learning task. Brain Res 549:59–65, 1991

Urabe M, Hershman JM, Pang XP, et al: Effect of lithium on function and growth of thyroid cells in vitro. Endocrinology 129:807–814, 1991

Ure A: Researches on gout. Medical Times 11:145, 1844/1845

Uvnäs-Moberg K, Arn I, Theorell T, et al: Personality traits in a group of individuals with functional disorders of the gastrointestinal tract and their correlation with gastrin, somatostatin and oxytocin levels. J Psychosom Res 35:515–523, 1991

Uvnäs-Moberg K, Arn I, Jonsson CO, et al: The relationships between personality traits and plasma gastrin, cholecystokinin, somatostatin, insulin, and oxytocin levels in healthy women. J Psychosom Res 37:581–588, 1993

Uvnäs-Moberg K, Ahlenius S, Hillegaart V, et al: High doses of oxytocin cause sedation and low doses cause an anxiolytic-like effect in male rats. Pharmacol Biochem Behav 49:101–106, 1994

Vaccarino FJ: Nucleus accumbens dopamine-CCK interactions in psychostimulant reward and related behaviours. Neurosci Biobehav Rev 18:207–214, 1994

Vadnal R, Parthasarathy R: Myo-inositol monophosphatase: diverse effects of lithium, carbamazepine, and valproate. Neuropsychopharmacology 12:277–285, 1995

Vale W, Spiess J, Rivier C, et al: Characterization of a 41 residue ovine hypothalamic peptide that stimulates secretion of corticotropin of β-endorphin. Science 213:1394–1397, 1981

Vallejo J, Olivares J, Marcos T, et al: Clomipramine versus phenelzine in obsessive-compulsive disorder: a controlled clinical trial. Br J Psychiatry 161:665–670, 1992

Valls-Sole J, Pascual-Leone A, Wassermann EM, et al: Human motor evoked responses to paired transcranial magnetic stimuli. Electroencephalogr Clin Neurophysiol 85:355–364, 1992

Valzania F, Quatrale R, Strafella AP, et al: Pattern of motor evoked response to repetitive transcranial magnetic stimulation. Electroencephalogr Clin Neurophysiol 93:312–317, 1994

Van Ameringen M, Mancini C, Streiner DL: Fluoxetine efficacy in social phobia. J Clin Psychiatry 54:27–32, 1993

van Balkom AJLM, van Oppen P, Vermeulen AWA, et al: A meta-analysis on the treatment of obsessive-compulsive disorder: a comparison of antidepressants, behavior, and cognitive therapy. Clin Psychol Rev 14(5):359–381, 1994

van Bemmel AL (ed): Sleep, Depression and Antidepressants. Maastricht, The Netherlands, CIP-Gegevens KoninklijkeBibliotheek, 1993

van Bemmel AL, Mevius GJ, van Diest R: EEG power density of NREM sleep in depression during treatment with trazodone. J Sleep Res 1(1):238, 1992a

van Bemmel AL, Havermans AG, van Diest R: Effects of trazodone on EEG sleep and clinical state in major depression. Psychopharmacology 107:569–574, 1992b van Bemmel AL, Beersma DGM, van den Hoofdakker RH: Changes in EEG power density of NREM sleep in depressed patients during treatment with citalopram. J Sleep Res 2:156–162, 1993a

van Bemmel AL, Hoofdakker van den RH, Beersma DGM, et al: Changes in sleep polygraphic variables and clinical state in depressed patients during treatment with citalopram, in Sleep, Depression and Antidepressants. Edited by Van Bemmel AL. Maastricht, The Netherlands, 1993b, pp 67–81

van den Burg W, van den Hoofdakker RH: Total sleep deprivation on endogenous depression. Arch Gen Psychiatry 32:1121–1125, 1975

van der Linden C, Bruggeman R, Van Woerkom T: Serotonin-dopamine antagonist and Gilles de La Tourette's syndrome: an open pilot dose-titration study with risperidone (letter). Mov Disord 9:687–688, 1994

Van Dijk A, Richards JG, Trzeciak A, et al: Cholecystokinin receptors: biochemical demonstration and autoradiographical localization in rat brain and pancreas using [3H] cholecystokinin 8 as radioligand. J Neurosci 4:1021–1033, 1984

Van Duijn CM, Havekes LM, Van Broeckhoven C, et al: Apolipoprotein E genotype and association between smoking and early onset Alzheimer's disease. BMJ 310:627–631, 1995

Van Harten J: Clinical pharmacokinetics of selective serotonin reuptake inhibitors. Clin Pharmacokinet 24:203–230, 1993

Van Kammen DP, Docherty JP, Marder SR, et al: Lithium attenuates the activation-euphoria but not the psychosis induced by d-amphetamine in schizophrenia. Psychopharmacology 87:111–115, 1985

van Megen HJM, den Boer JA, Westenberg HGM: Single blind dose response study with cholecystokinin in panic disorder. Clin Neuropharmacol 15 (suppl 1):532B, 1992

van Megen H, Westenberg H, den Boer J: Effect of the selective serotonin reuptake inhibitor (SSRI) fluvoxamine on CCK-4 induced panic attacks (abstract). Neuropsychopharmacology 10:270S, 1994a

van Megen HJGM, Westenberg HGM, Denboer JA, et al: Pentagastrin induced panic attacks—enhanced sensitivity in panic disorder patients. Psychopharmacology 114:449–455, 1994b

van Megen HJGM, Westenberg HGM, den Boer JA, et al: The panic-inducing properties of the cholecystokinin tetrapeptide CCK4 in patients with panic disorder. Eur Neuropsychopharmacol 6(3):187–194, 1996

van Megen HJ, Westenberg HG, den Boer JA, et al: Effect of the selective serotonin reuptake inhibitor fluvoxamine on CCK-4 induced panic attacks. Psychopharmacology 129(4):357–364, 1997

van Moffaert M, Pregaldien JL, Von Frenckell R, et al: A double-blind comparison of nefazadone and imipramine in the treatment of depressed patients. New Trends Exp Clin Psychiatry 10:85–87, 1994 van Moffaert M, De Wilde J, Vereecken A, et al: Mirtazapine is more effective than trazodone: a double-blind controlled study in hospitalized patients with major depression. Int Clin Psychopharmacol 10:3–10, 1995

Van Praag HM: Diagnosing depression. Looking backward into the future. Psychiatric Developments 7:375–394, 1989

Van Praag HM: Two-tier diagnosing in psychiatry. Psychiatry Res 34:1–11, 1990

Van Praag HM: Make Believes in Psychiatry or The Perils of Progress. New York, Brunner/Mazel, 1992a

Van Praag HM: Reconquest of the subjective: against the waning of psychiatric diagnosing. Br J Psychiatry 160:266–271, 1992b

Van Praag HM: Comorbidity (psycho) analysed [review]. Br J Psychiatry 30 (suppl):129–134, 1996

Van Praag HM, Leijnse B: Neubewertung des Syndroms. Skizze einer funktonellen Pathologie. Psychiatria, Neurologia, Neurochirurgia 68:50–66, 1965

Van Praag HM, Korf J, Lakke JPWF, et al: Dopamine metabolism in depression, psychoses and Parkinson's disease: the problem of the specificity of biological variables in behaviour disorders. Psychol Med 5:138–146, 1975

Van Praag HM, Kahn R, Asnis GM, et al: Denosologization of biological psychiatry, or the specificity of 5-HT disturbances in psychiatric disorders. J Affect Disord 13:1–8, 1987

Van Praag HM, Asnis GM, Kahn RS, et al: Monoamines and abnormal behavior: a multi-aminergic perspective. Br J Psychiatry 157:723–734, 1990

van Valkenburg C, Akiskal HS, Puzantian V, et al: Anxious depression: clinical, family history and naturalistic outcome—comparison with panic and major depressive disorders. J Affect Disord 6:67–82, 1984

van Veldhuizen MJA, Feenstra MGP, Heinsbroek RPW, et al: In vivo microdialysis of noradrenaline overflow: effects of-adrenoceptor agonists and antagonists measured by cumulative concentration-response curves. Br J Pharmacol 109:655–660, 1993

Van Vliet IM, Westenberg HGM, den Boer JA: MAO-inhibitors in panic disorder: clinical effects of treatment with brofaromine. Psychopharmacology 112:483–489, 1993

Van Vliet I, Den Boer JA, Westenberg HGM: A double-blind comparative study of brofaromine and fluvoxamine in outpatients with panic disorder. J Clin Psychopharmacol 16:299–306, 1996a

Van Vliet IM, Westenberg HGM, den Boer JA: Effects of the 5-HT$_{1A}$ receptor agonist flesinoxan in panic disorder. Psychopharmacology 127:174–180, 1996b

Vanderhaeghen J, Crawley J: Neuronal cholecystokinin. Ann N Y Acad Sci 448:1–697, 1985

Varney MA, Godfrey PP, Drummond AH, et al: Chronic lithium treatment inhibits basal and agonist-stimulated responses in rat cerebral cortex and GH$_3$ pituitary cells. Mol Pharmacol 4:671–678, 1992

Varney MA, Galione A, Watson SP: Lithium-induced decrease in spontaneous Ca^{2+} oscillations in single GH3 rat pituitary cells. Br J Pharmacol 112:390–395, 1994

Vasar EE, Otter MY, Ryago LK: Intracerebroventricular administration of cholecystokinin inhibits the activity of the dopaminergic and serotoninergic systems of the brain. Neurosci Behav Physiol 15:232–236, 1985

Vasar E, Peuranen E, Ööpik T, et al: Ondansetron, and antagonist of 5HT3 receptors, antagonizes the anti-exploratory effect of caerulein, an agonist of CCK receptors, in the elevated plus maze. 110:213–218, 1993a

Vasar E, Peuranen E, Harro J, et al: Social isolation of rats increases the density of cholecystokinin receptors in the frontal cortex and abolishes the anti-exploratory effect of caerulein. Naunyn Schmiedebergs Arch Pharmacol 348:96–101, 1993b

Vassout A, Bruinink A, Krauss J, et al: Regulation of dopamine receptors by bupropion: comparison with antidepressants and CNS stimulants. Journal of Receptor Research 13:341–354, 1993

Vaughan J, Donaldson C, Bittencourt J, et al: Urocortin, a mammalian neuropeptide related to fish urotensin I and to corticotropin-releasing factor. Nature 378:287–292, 1995

Vazquez-Rodriguez AM, Arranz-Pena M, López-Ibor J, et al: Clomipramine test: serum level determination in three groups of psychiatric patients. J Pharm Biomed Anal 9(10–12):949–952, 1991

Vecsei L, Widerlov E: Effects of intracerebroventricularly administered somatostatin on passive avoidance, shuttle-box and openfield activity in rats. Neuropeptides 12:237–242, 1988

Velez CN, Johnson J, Cohen P: A longitudinal analysis of select risk factors for childhood psychopathology. J Am Acad Child Adolesc Psychiatry 28:861–864, 1989

Venter JC, DiPorzio U, Robinson DA, et al: Evolution of neurotransmitter receptor systems. Prog Neurobiol 30:105–169, 1988

Verdoorn TA, Draguhn A, Ymer S, et al: Functional properties of recombinant rat GABAa receptors depend on subunit composition. Neuron 4:919–928, 1990

Verge D, Daval G, Marcinkiewicz M, et al: Quantitative autoradiography of multiple 5-HT1 receptor subtypes in the brain of control or 5,7-dihydroxytryptamine-treated rats. J Neurosci 6:3474–3482, 1986

Verimer T, Goodale DB, Long JP, et al: Lithium effects on haloperidol-induced pre- and postsynaptic dopamine receptor supersensitivity. J Pharm Pharmacol 32:665–666, 1980

Versiani M, Mundim FD, Nardi AE, et al: Tranylcypromine in social phobia. J Clin Psychopharmacol 8:279–282, 1988

Versiani M, Nardi AE, Mundim FD: Fobia social. Jornal Brasileiro de Psiquiatria 38:251–263, 1989

Versiani M, Nardi AE, Mundim FD, et al: Pharmacotherapy of social phobia. Br J Psychiatry 161:353–360, 1992

Vezzani A, Wu HQ, Stasi MA, et al: Effect of various calcium channel blockers on three different models of limbic seizures in rats. Neuropharmacology 27:451–458, 1988

Vidal C: The functional role of nicotinic receptors in the rat prefrontal cortex: electrophysiological, biochemical, and behavioral characterizations, in Effects of Nicotine on Biological Systems II. Edited by Clarke PBS, Quick M, Thuran K, et al. Boston, MA, Birkhäuser, 1994a, p 70

Vidal C: Nicotinic potentiation of glutamatergic synapses in the prefrontal cortex: new insight into the analysis of the role of nicotinic receptors in cognitive functions. Drug Dev Res 31:120–126, 1994b

Vinar O, Klein DF, Potter WZ, et al: A survey of psychotropic medications not available in the United States. Neuropsychopharmacology 5:201–217, 1991

Vitiello B, Spreat S, Behar D: Obsessive-compulsive disorder in mentally retarded patients. J Nerv Ment Dis 177:232–236, 1989

Vitiello B, Shimon H, Behar D, et al: Platelet imipramine binding and serotonin uptake in OCD patients. Acta Psychiatr Scand 84:29–32, 1991

Vizi ES, Harsing LG, Zsilla G: Evidence of the modulatory role of serotonin in acetylcholine release from striatal interneurones. Brain Res 212:89–99, 1981

Vogel GW: A review of REM sleep deprivation. Arch Gen Psychiatry 32:749–761, 1975

Vogel GW: Evidence for REM sleep deprivation as the mechanism of action of antidepressant drugs. Prog Neuropsychopharmacol Biol Psychiatry 1:343–349, 1983

Vogel GW, Thurmond A, Gibbons P, et al: REM sleep reduction effects on depression syndromes. Arch Gen Psychiatry 32:765–777, 1975

Vogel GW, McAbee R, Barker K, et al: Endogenous depression improvement and REM pressure. Arch Gen Psychiatry 34:96–97, 1977

Vogel GW, Vogel F, McAbee RS, et al: Improvement of depression by REM sleep deprivation, new findings and a theory. Arch Gen Psychiatry 37:247–253, 1980

Vogel GW, Buffenstein A, Minter K, et al: Drug effects on REM sleep and on endogenous depression. Neurosci Biobehav Rev 14:49–63, 1990

Vogel JR, Beer B, Clody DE: A simple and reliable conflict procedure for testing antianxiety agents. Psychopharmacology 21:1–7, 1971

Volavka J, Neziroglu F, Yaryura JA: CMI and imipramine in OCD. Psychiatry Res 14:85–93, 1985

Volrath M, Angst J: Outcome of panic and depression in a seven-year follow-up: results of the Zurich Study. Acta Psychiatr Scand 80:591–596, 1989

von Bardeleben U, Holsboer F: Cortisol response to a combined dexamethasone-h-CRH challenge in patients with depression. J Neuroendocrinol 1:485–488, 1989

von Bardeleben U, Holsboer F, Stalla GK, et al: Combined administration of human corticotropin-releasing factor and lysine vasopressin induces cortisol escape from dexamethasone suppression in healthy subjects. Life Sci 37:1613–1618, 1985

Vorhees CV, Brunner RL, Butcher RE: Psychotropic drugs as behavioral teratogens. Science 205:1220–1225, 1979

Wade AG, Lepola U, Koponen HJ, et al: The effect of citalopram in panic disorder. Br J Psychiatry 170:549–553, 1997

Waeber C, Hoyer D, Palacios JM: 5-HT$_3$ receptors in the human brain: audioradiographic visualization. Neuroscience 31:393–400, 1989

Wafford KA: Ethanol sensitivity of the GABA A receptor expressed in Xenopus oocytes requires 8 amino acids contained in the gamma2L subunit. Neuron 7:27–33, 1991

Wafford KA, Burnett D, Harris RA, Whiting PJ: GABA A receptor subunit expression and sensitivity to ethanol, in Advances in Biomedical Alcoholism Research. Edited by Taberner PV, Badawy AA. Oxford, England, Pergamon, 1993, pp 327–330

Wagner HR, Reches A, Yablonskaya E, et al: Clonazepam-induced up-regulation of serotonin-1 and serotonin-2 binding sites in rat frontal cortex. Adv Neurol 43:645–651, 1986

Wahlestedt C, Reis DJ: Neuropeptide Y-related peptides and their receptors—are the receptors potential therapeutic drug targets? Annu Rev Pharmacol Toxicol 32:309–352, 1993

Wahlestedt C, Pich EM, Koob GF, et al: Modulation of anxiety and neuropeptide Y-Y1 receptors by antisense oligodeoxynucleotides. Science 259:528–531, 1993

Waka T, Fukada N: Pharmacologic profile of a new anxiolytic, DN 2327: effect of RO15–1788 and interaction with diazepam in rodents. Psychopharmacology 103:314–322, 1991

Wakelin JS: The role of serotonin in depression and suicide: do serotonin reuptake inhibitors provide a key? Recent Advances in Biological Psychiatry 17:70–83, 1988

Walden J, Grunze H, Bingmann D: Calcium antagonistic effects of carbamazepine as a mechanism of action in neuropsychiatric disorders: studies in calcium dependent model epilepsies. Eur Neuropsychopharmacol 2:455–462, 1992

Walden J, Fritze J, Van Calker D, et al: A calcium antagonist for the treatment of depressive episodes: single case reports. J Psychiatr Res 29:71–76, 1995a

Walden J, Wegerer JV, Roed I, et al: Effects of the serotonin-1A agonists buspirone and ipsapirone on field potentials in the hippocampus slice: comparison with carbamazepine and verapamil. Eur Neuropsychopharmacol 5:57–61, 1995b

Waldmeier PC: Is there a common denominator for the antimanic effect of lithium and anticonvulsants? Pharmacopsychiatry 20:37–47, 1987

Walsh BT, Goetz R, Roose SP, et al: EEG-monitored sleep in anorexia nervosa and bulimia. Biol Psychiatry 20:947–956, 1985

Walsh BT, Giardina E, Sloan RP, et al: Effects of desipramine on autonomic control of the heart. J Am Acad Child Adolesc Psychiatry 33:191–197, 1995

Walton SA, Berk M, Brook S: Superiority of lithium over verapamil in mania: a randomized, controlled, single-blind trial. J Clin Psychiatry 57:543–546, 1996

Wang HY, Friedman E: Chronic lithium: desensitization of autoreceptors mediating serotonin release. Psychopharmacology 94:312–314, 1988

Wang HY, Friedman E: Lithium inhibition of protein kinase C activation-induced serotonin release. Psychopharmacology 99:213–218, 1989

Wank SA, Pisegna JR, de Weerth A: Brain and gastrointestinal cholecystokinin receptor family: structure and functional expression. Proc Natl Acad Sci U S A 89:8691–8695, 1992

Warburton DM, Rusted JM: Cholinergic control of cognitive resources. Neuropsychobiology 28:43–46, 1993

Ware JC: Increased deep sleep after trazodone use: a double-blind placebo-controlled study in healthy young adults. J Clin Psychiatry 519 (suppl):18–22, 1990

Ware JC, Brown FW, Morad PJ, et al: Effects on sleep: a double blind study comparing trimipramine to imipramine in depressed insomniac patients. Sleep 12:537–549, 1989

Warneke LB: Intravenous chlorimipramine therapy in obsessive-compulsive disorder. Can J Psychiatry 34:853–859, 1989

Warner V, Mufson L, Weissman MM: Offspring at low and high risk for depression and anxiety: mechanisms of psychiatric disorder. J Am Acad Child Adolesc Psychiatry 34:786–797, 1995

Warrington SJ: Clinical implications of the pharmacology of sertraline. Int Clin Psychopharmacol 6:11–21, 1991

Wassermann EM, Pascual-Leone A, Valls-Sole J, et al: Topography of the inhibitory and excitatory responses to transcranial magnetic stimulation in a hand muscle. Electroencephalogr Clin Neurophysiol 89:424–433, 1993

Watkins PB: Drug metabolism by cytochrome P450 in the liver and small bowel. Gastrointestinal Pharmacology 21(3):511–526, 1992

Watkins SE, Callender K, Thomas DR, et al: The effect of carbamazepine and lithium on remission from affective illness. Br J Psychiatry 150:180–182, 1987

Watson DG, Lenox RH: Chronic lithium-induced down-regulation of MARCKS in immortalized hippocampal cells: potentiation by muscarinic receptor activation. J Neurochem 67:767–777, 1996

Watson DG, Wainer BH, Lenox RH: Phorbol ester- and retinoic acid-induced regulation of the PKC substrate MARCKS in immortalized hippocampal cells. J Neurochem 63:1666–1674, 1994

Watson DG, Watterson JM, Lenox RH. Sodium valproate down-regulates the myristoylated alanine-rich C kinase substrate (MARCKS) in immortalized hippocampal cells: a property unique to PKC-mediated mood stabilization J Pharmacol Exp Ther 285:307–316, 1998

Watson M, Roeske WR, Yamamura HI: Cholinergic receptor heterogeneity, in Psychopharmacology: The Third Generation of Progress. Edited by Meltzer HY. New York, Raven, 1987, pp 241–248

Watson SP, Shipman L, Godfrey PP: Lithium potentiates agonist formation of [3h]CDP-diacylglycerol in human platelets. Eur J Pharmacol 188:273–276, 1990

Watterson D: The effect of age, head resistance, and other physical factors on the stimulus threshold of electrically induced convulsions. J Neurol Neurosurg Psychiatry 8:121–125, 1945

Wedmann B, Schmidt G, Wegener M: Effects of age and gender on fat-induced gallbladder contraction and gastric emptying of a caloric liquid meal: a sonographic study. Am J Gastroenterol 86:1765–1770, 1991

Wedzony K, Gofembiowska K: Concomitant administration of MK-801 and desipramine enhances extracellular concentration of dopamine in the rat prefrontal cortex. Neuroreport 5:75–77, 1993

Wehr TA: Phase and biorhythm studies in affective illness. Ann Intern Med 87:319–335, 1977

Wehr TA: Effects of wakefulness and sleep on depression and mania, in Sleep and Biological Rhythms: Basic Mechanisms and Applications to Psychiatry. Edited by Montplaisir J, Godbout R. New York, Oxford University Press, 1990, pp 42–86

Wehr TA, Rosenthal NE, Sack DA, et al: Antidepressant effects of sleep deprivation in bright and dim light. Acta Psychiatr Scand 72:161–165, 1985

Weilburg JB, Rosenbaum JF, Biedereman J, et al: Fluoxetine added to non-MAOI antidepressants converts nonresponders to responders: a preliminary report. J Clin Psychiatry 50:447–449, 1989

Weinberger DR, Gallhoffer B: Cognitive function in schizophrenia. Int Clin Psychopharmacol 12:S29–S36, 1997

Weiner ED, Kalaaspudi VD, Papolos DF, et al: Lithium augments pilocarpine-induced fos gene expression in brain. Brain Res 553:117–122, 1991

Weiner RD: ECT and seizure threshold: effects of stimulus wave form and electrode placement. Biol Psychiatry 15:225–241, 1980

Weiner RD, Rogers HJ, Davidson JRT, et al: Effects of stimulus parameters on cognitive side effects. Ann N Y Acad Sci 462:315–325, 1986

Weingartner H, Rudorfer MV, Buchsbaum MS, et al: Effects of serotonin on memory impairments produced by ethanol. Science 221:472–474, 1983

Weisler R, Risner ME, Ascher J, et al: Use of lamotrigine in the treatment of bipolar disorder. Paper presented at the annual meeting of the American Psychiatric Association, Philadelphia, PA, May 21–26, 1994

Weiss JM, Stout JC, Aaron MF, et al: Depression and anxiety: role of the locus coeruleus and corticotropin-releasing factor. Brain Res Bull 35(5–6):561–572, 1994

Weiss SRB, Post RM, Sohn E, et al: Cross tolerance between carbamazepine and valproate on amygdala-kindled seizures. Epilepsy Res 16:37–44, 1993

Weiss SRB, Clark M, Rosen JB, et al: Contingent tolerance to the anticonvulsant effects of carbamazepine: relationship to loss of endogenous adaptive mechanisms. Brain Res Brain Res Rev 20:305–325, 1995

Weissman MM: Panic disorder: impact on the quality of life. J Clin Psychiatry 52 (suppl):6–8, 1991

Weissman MM: Epidemiology of major depression in women. Paper presented at the annual meeting of the American Psychiatric Association, New York, May 4, 1996

Weissman MM, Leckman JF, Merikangas KR, et al: Depression and anxiety disorders in parents and children: results from the Yale Family Study. Arch Gen Psychiatry 41:845–852, 1984

Weissman MM, Bruce ML, Leaf PJ, et al: Affective disorders, in Psychiatric Disorders in America. Edited by Robins LN, Regier DA. New York, Free Press, 1991, pp 53–80

Weissman MM, Wickramaratne P, Adams PB, et al: The relationship between panic disorder and major depression: a new family study. Arch Gen Psychiatry 50:767–780, 1993

Weissman MM, Bland RC, Canino GJ, et al: The cross national epidemiology of OCD. J Clin Psychiatry 55:5–10s, 1994

Weizman A, Carmi M, Hermesh H, et al: High affinity imipramine binding and serotonin uptake in platelets of 8 adolescent and 10 adult OCD patients. Am J Psychiatry 143:335–339, 1986

Wells KB, Stewart A, Hays RD, et al: The functioning and well-being of depressed patients: results from the Medical Outcome Study. JAMA 262:914–919, 1989

Wells KB, Burnam A, Rogers W, et al: The course of depression in adult outpatients. Results from the Medical Outcomes study. Arch Gen Psychiatry 49:788–801, 1992

Welsh GS: MMPI profiles and factors A and R. J Clin Psychol 21:43–47, 1965

Wenzel K, Meinhold H, Ruffenberg M: Classification of hypothyroidism in evaluating patients after radioiodine therapy by serum cholesterol, T_3 uptake, total T_4, F T_4 index, total T_3, basal TSH and TRH test. Eur J Clin Invest 4:141, 1974

Wernicke JF: The side effect profile and safety of fluoxetine. J Clin Psychiatry 46 (3 sec 2):59–67, 1985

Wernicke JF, Dunlop SR, Dornscif BE, et al: Fixed-dose fluoxetine therapy for depression. Psychopharmacol Bull 23:164–168, 1987

Wernicke JF, Dunlop SR, Dornscif BE, et al: Low dose fluoxetine therapy for depression. Psychopharmacol Bull 24:183–188, 1988

Wesnes K, Revell A: The separate and combined effects of scopolamine and nicotine on human information processing. Psychopharmacology 84:5–11, 1984

Wesnes K, Warburton D: Smoking, nicotine, and human performance. Pharmacol Ther 21:189–208, 1983

Wesnes K, Warburton D: Effects of scopolamine and nicotine on human performance. Psychopharmacology 82:147–150, 1985

West SA, Keck PE Jr, McElroy SL, et al: Open trial of valproate in the treatment of adolescent mania. J Child Adolesc Psychopharmacol 4:263–267, 1994

Westenberg HGM, De Leeuw AS, Den Boer JA: Serotonin reuptake blockers in OCD. Paper presented at the 18th CINP Congress, Nice, France, 1992

Wetzel W, Getsova VM, Jork R, et al: Effect of serotonin on Y-maze retention and hippocampal protein synthesis in rats. Pharmacol Biochem Behav 12:319–322, 1980

Wheadon DE, Bushnell WD, Steiner M: A fixed dose comparison of 20, 40, or 60 mg paroxetine to placebo in the treatment of obsessive-compulsive disorder (abstract). Paper presented at the annual meeting of the American College of Neuropsychopharmacology, Honolulu, HI, December 1993

Wheatley D: Trazodone in depression. International Pharmacopsychiatry 15:240–246, 1980

Whitaker-Azmitia PM, Azmitia EC: Serotonin trophic factors in development, plasticity and aging, in Serotonin, Molecular Biology, Receptors and Functional Effects. Edited by Fozard JR, Saxena PR. Basel, Switzerland, Birkhauser Verlag, 1991, pp 43–49

Whitaker-Azmitia PM, Murphy R, Azmitia EC: S-100 protein is released from astroglial cells by stimulation of 5-HT$_{1A}$ receptors and regulates development of serotonin neurons. Brain Res 528:155–158, 1990

White P, Hiley C, Goodhardt MJ, et al: Neocortical cholinergic neurons in elderly people. Lancet 1:668–670, 1977

Whitehouse PJ, Price DL, Clark AW, et al: Alzheimer disease: evidence for selective loss of cholinergic neurons in the nucleus basalis. Ann Neurol 10:122–126, 1981

Whitehouse PJ, Price DL, Struble RG, et al: Alzheimer's disease and senile dementia—loss of neurons in the basal forebrain. Science 215:1237–1239, 1982

Whitehouse PJ, Hedreen JC, White CL, et al: Basal forebrain neurons in dementia of Parkinson's disease. Ann Neurol 13:243–248, 1983

Whitehouse P, Martino A, Antuono P, et al: Nicotinic acetylcholine binding sites in Alzheimer's disease. Brain Res 371:146–151, 1986

Whitehouse PJ, Martino AM, Marcus KA, et al: Reductions in acetylcholine and nicotine binding in several degenerative diseases. Arch Neurol 45:722–724, 1988

Whitton PS, Sarna GS, O'Connell MT: The effect of the novel antidepressant tianeptine on the concentration of 5-hydroxytryptamine in rat hippocampal diasylates in vivo. Neuropharmacology 39:1–4, 1991

Whitworth P, Kendall DA: Lithium selectively inhibits muscarinic receptor-stimulated inositol tetrakisphosphate accumulation in mouse cerebral cortex slices. J Neurochem 51:258–265, 1988

Whitworth P, Kendall DA: Effects of lithium on inositol phospholipid hydrolysis and inhibition of dopamine D$_1$ receptor-mediated cyclic AMP formation by carbachol in rat brain slices. J Neurochem 53:536–541, 1989

Whybrow PC: The therapeutic use of triiodothyronine and high dose thyroxine in psychiatric disorder. Acta Med Austriaca 21:44–47, 1994

Whybrow PC: Update on thyroid axis approaches to treatment of rapid cycling bipolar disorder. Paper presented at the annual meeting of the New Clinical Drug Evaluations Unit (NCDEU), Boca Raton, FL, May 30, 1996

Whyte S, Beyrether K, Masters C: Rational therapeutic strategies for Alzheimer's disease, in Neurodegenerative Diseases. Edited by Calne DB. Philadelphia, PA, WB Saunders, 1994

Widerlöv E, Kalivas PW, Abelson JL, et al: Influence of cholecystokinin on central monoaminergic pathways. Regul Pept 6:99–109, 1983

Widerlöv E, Lindstrom LH, Wahlestedt C, et al: Neuropeptide Y and peptide YY as possible cerebrospinal markers for major depression and schizophrenia, respectively. J Psychiatr Res 22:69–79, 1988

Wieck A, Kumar P, Hirst AD, et al: Increased sensitivity of dopamine receptors and recurrence of affective psychosis after childbirth. BMJ 303:613–616, 1991

Wiegand M, Berger M, Zulley J, et al: The effect of trimipramine on sleep in patients with major depressive disorder. Pharmacopsychiatry 19:198–199, 1986

Wieland S, Lan NC, Mirasedeghi S, et al: Anxiolitic activity of the progesterone metabolite 5a-pregnan-3a-ol-20-one. Brain Res 565:263–268, 1991

Wiesbader H, Kurzrok R: Menopause consideration of symptoms, etiology, and treatment by means of estrogens. Endocrinology 23:32–38, 1938

Wiesenfeld-Hallin Z, Xu XJ, Langel U, et al: Galanin-mediated control of pain: enhanced role after nerve injury. Proc Natl Acad Sci U S A 89:3334–3337, 1992

Wilcock GK, Surmon DJ, Scott M, et al: An evaluation of the efficacy and safety of tetrahydroaminoacridine (THA) without lecithin in the treatment of Alzheimer's disease. Age Ageing 22:316–324, 1993

Wilde MJ, Benfield P: Tianeptine—a review of its pharmacodynamic and pharmacokinetic properties and therapeutic efficacy in depression and coexisting anxiety and depression. Drugs 49:411–439, 1995

Wilde ML, Plosker GL, Benfield P: Fluvoxamine: an updated review of its pharmacology and therapeutic use in depressive illness. Drugs 45:895–924, 1993

Williams JMG, Watts FM, MacLeod C, et al: Cognitive Psychology and Emotional Disorders. Chichester, England, Wiley, 1988

Williams K, Smith J, Glue P, et al: The effects of electroconvulsive therapy on plasma insulin and glucose in depression. Br J Psychiatry 161:94–98, 1992

Williams M, Sullivan JP, Arneric SP: Neuronal nicotinic acetylcholine receptors. Drug News and Perspective 7:403–443, 1993

Willner P: Animal models as simulations of depression. Trends Pharmacol Sci 12:131–136, 1991

Willner P: Dopaminergic mechanisms in depression and mania, in Psychopharmacology: The Fourth Generation of Progress. Edited by Bloom FE, Kupfer DJ. New York, Raven, 1995, pp 921–931

Willner P, Scheel-Krüger J (eds): The Mesolimbic Dopamine System: From Motivation to Action. New York, Wiley, 1991

Willner P, Muscat R, Papp M: Chronic mild stress-induced anhedonia: a realistic animal model of depression. Neurosci Biobehav Rev 16:525–534, 1992

Wilson AL, Langley LK, Monley J, et al: Nicotine patches in Alzheimer's disease: pilot study on learning, memory, and safety. Pharmacol Biochem Behav 51:509–514, 1995

Wilson CL, Babb TL, Halgren E, et al: Habituation of human limbic neuronal response to sensory stimulation. Exp Neurol 84:74–97, 1984

Wilson K: Sex-related differences in drug disposition in man. Clin Pharmacokinet 9:189–202, 1984

Wilson MA, Roy EJ: Pharmacokinetics of imipramine are affected by age and sex in rats. Clin Pharmacokinet 9:189–202, 1984

Wilson MA, Roy EJ: Pharmacokinetics of imipramine are affected by age and sex in rats. Life Sci 38:711–718, 1986

Wilson MA, Dwyer KD, Roy EJ: Direct effects of ovarian hormones on antidepressant binding sites. Brain Res Bull 22:181–185, 1989

Winblad B, Adolfsson R, Carlsson A, et al: Biogenic amines in brains with Alzheimer's disease, in Alzheimer's Disease: A Report of Progress (Ageing, Vol 19). Edited by Corkin S, Davis KL, Growdon JH, et al. New York, Raven, 1982, pp 25–33

Winker MA: Tacrine for Alzheimer's disease. Which patient, what dose? JAMA 271:1023–1024, 1994

Winokur A, Amsterdam JD, Oler J, et al: Multiple hormonal responses to TRH administration in depressed patients and healthy volunteers. Arch Gen Psychiatry 40:525–531, 1983

Winokur A, Amsterdam J, Berwish N, et al: The relationship between the change in thyrotropin response to TRH and therapeutic response to DMI in depressed patients. Proceedings of the 44th Annual Society of Biological Psychiatry Meeting, San Francisco, CA, May 1989

Winter JC, Petti DT: The effects of 8-hydroxy-2-di-n-propylaminotetralin and other serotonergic agonists on performance in a radial maze: a possible role for 5-HT_{1A} receptors in memory. Pharmacol Biochem Behav 27:625–628, 1987

Wise SP, Rapoport JL: Obsessive compulsive disorder: is it basal ganglia dysfunction? in Obsessive-Compulsive Disorder in Children and Adolescents. Edited by Rapoport JL. Washington, DC, American Psychiatric Press, 1989, pp 327–344

Witte EA, Davidson MC, Marrocco RT: Effects of altering brain cholinergic activity on covert orienting of attention: comparison of monkey and human performance. Psychopharmacology 132:324–334, 1997

Wolfe N, Katz DI, Albert ML, et al: Neuropsychological profile linked to low dopamine: in Alzheimer's disease, major depression, and Parkinson's disease. J Neurol Neurosurg Psychiatry 53:915–917, 1990

Wolkowitz OM: Hormones as psychotropic medications: the HPA system. Paper presented at the 10th World Congress of Psychiatry, Madrid, Spain, August 1996

Wolkowitz OM, Doran A, Breier A, et al: Specificity of HVA response to dexamethasone in psychotic depression. Psychiatry Res 29:177–186, 1989

Wolkowitz OM, Bartko JJ, Pickar D: Drug trials and heterogeneity in schizophrenia: the mean is not the end. Biol Psychiatry 28:1021–1025, 1990

Wolkowitz OM, Reus VI, Manfredi F, et al: Ketoconazole administration in hypercortisolemic depression. Am J Psychiatry 150:810–812, 1993

Wolkowitz OM, Reus VI, Chan T, et al: Antiglucocorticoids in depression and schizophrenia. Paper presented at the annual meeting of the American Psychiatric Association, New York, 1996a

Wolkowitz OM, Reus VI, Chan T, et al: Dexamethasone for depression (letter). Am J Psychiatry 153:1112, 1996b

Wolkowitz OM, Reus VI, Roberts E, et al: Dehydroepiandrosterone (DHEA) treatment of depression. Biol Psychiatry 41:311–318, 1997

Wong DF, Wagner HN, Pearlson G: Dopamine receptor binding of ^{11}C-3-N-methylspirone in the caudate in schizophrenia and bipolar disorder: a preliminary report. Psychopharmacol Bull 21:595–598, 1985

Wong DT, Bymaster FP: Effect of nisoxetine on uptake of catecholamines in synaptosomes isolated from discrete regions of rat brain. Biochem Pharmacol 25:1979–1983, 1976

Wonnacott S: The paradox of nicotinic acetylcholine receptor upregulation by nicotine. Trends Pharmacol Sci 11:216–219, 1990

Wonnacott S, Irons J, Rapier C, et al: Presynaptic modulation of transmitter release by nicotinic receptors, in Progress in Brain Research. Edited by Nordberg A, Fuxe K, Holmstedt B, et al. Amsterdam, Elsevier, 1990, pp 157–163

Wood A: Pharmacotherapy of bulimia nervosa—experience with fluoxetine. Int Clin Psychopharmacol 8:295—301, 1993

Wood AJ, Elphick M, Aronson JK, et al: The effect of lithium on cation transport measured in vivo in patients suffering from bipolar affective illness. Br J Psychiatry 155:504–510, 1989

Wood K, Coppen A: Prophylactic lithium treatment of patients with affective disorder is associated with decreased platelet ^{3}H-dihydroergocryptine binding. J Affect Disord 5:253–258, 1983

Woodruff GN, Hughes J: Cholecystokinin antagonists. Annu Rev Pharmacol Toxicol 31:469–501, 1991

Woods SW, Black D, Brown S, et al: Fluvoxamine in the treatment of panic disorder in outpatients: a double-blind, placebo-controlled study. Neuropsychopharmacology 10:103S, 1994

World Health Organization: ICD-10 Classification of Mental and Behavioural Disorders. Clinical description and diagnostic guidelines. Geneva, Switzerland, World Health Organization, 1992

Wragg RE, Jeste DV: Overview of depression and psychosis in Alzheimer's disease. Am J Psychiatry 146:577–587, 1989

Wright MJ, Burns RJ, Geffen GM, et al: Covert orienting of visual attention in Parkinson's disease: an impairment in the maintenance of attention. Neuropsychologia 28:151–159, 1990

Wu FS, Gibbs TT, Farb DH: Pregnenolone sulfate: a possible allosteric modulator at the N-methyl-D-aspartate receptor. Mol Pharmacol 40:333–336, 1991

Wurpel JN, Iyer SN: Calcium channel blockers verapamil and nimodipine inhibit kindling in adult and immature rats. Epilepsia 35:443–449, 1994

Wyatt RJ, Fram DH, Kupfer DJ, et al: Total prolonged drug-induced REM sleep suppression in anxious-depressed patients. Arch Gen Psychiatry 24:145–155, 1971

Yamamoto T, Hirano A: Nucleus raphe dorsalis in Alzheimer's disease: neurofibrillary tangles and loss of large neurons. Ann Neurol 17:573–577, 1985

Yaryura-Tobias JA, Neziroglu FA, McKay DR: The action of venlafaxine on obsessive-compulsive disorder. Abstract 441. Proceedings of Society of Biological Psychiatry 35:737, 1994

Yatham LN, Barry S, Dinan TG, et al: Which patients will respond to ECT? Br J Psychiatry 154:879–880, 1989

Yehuda R, Boisoneau D, Lowy MT, et al: Dose-response changes in plasma cortisol and lymphocyte glucocorticoid receptors following dexamethasone administration in combat veterans with and without posttraumatic stress disorder. Arch Gen Psychiatry 52:583–593, 1995

Yellowlees PM, Alpers JH, Bowden JJ, et al: Psychiatric morbidity in patients with chronic airflow obstruction. Med J Aust 146:305–307, 1987

Yeragani VK, Pohl R, Berger R, et al: Decreased heart rate variability in panic disorder: a study of power-spectral analysis of heart rate. Psychiatry Res 46:89–103, 1993

Yocca FD, Iben L, Meller E: Lack of apparent receptor reserve at postsynaptic 5-hydroxytryptamine 1A receptors negatively coupled to adenyl cyclase activity in rat hippocampal membranes. Mol Pharmacol 41:1066–1072, 1992

Yoney TH, Pigott TA, L'Heureux F, et al. Seasonal variation in obsessive-compulsive disorder: preliminary experience with light treatment. Am J Psychiatry 148:1727–1729, 1991

Yonkers KA, Hamilton JA: Psychotropic medications: issues for use in women, in American Psychiatric Press Review of Psychiatry, Vol 14. Edited by Weissman MM, Riba M. Washington, DC, American Psychiatric Press, 1995, pp 147–178

Yonkers KA, Hamilton JA: Sex differences in pharmacokinetics of psychotropic medications, part II: effects on selected psychotropics, in Psychopharmacology of Women: Sex, Gender and Hormonal Considerations, Vol 1. Edited by Jensvold MJ, Halbreich U, Hamilton JA. Washington, DC, American Psychiatric Press, 1996

Yonkers KA, Kando JC, Cole JO, et al: Gender differences in pharmacokinetics and pharmacodynamics of psychotropic medication. Am J Psychiatry 149:587–595, 1992

Yoshikai S, Sasaki H, Doh-ura K, et al: Genomic organization of the human amyloid beta-protein precursor gene. Gene 87:257–263, 1990

Young CR, Bostic JQ, McDanald CL: Clozapine and refractory obsessive-compulsive disorder: a case report. J Clin Psychopharmacol 14:3, 209–210, 1994

Young LT, Li PP, Kish JS, et al: Postmortem cerebral cortex $G_s\alpha$-subunit levels are elevated in bipolar affective disorder. Brain Res 553:323–326, 1991

Young RC, Biggs JT, Ziegler VE, et al: A rating scale for mania: reliability, validity, and sensitivity. Br J Psychiatry 133:429–435, 1978

Young S, Parker PJ, Ullrich A, et al: Down regulation of protein kinase C is due to an increased rate of degradation. Biochem J 24:775–779, 1987

Yuan PX, Chen G, Manji HK: Lithium stimulates gene expression through the AP-1 transcription factor pathway. Mol Brain Res 58:225–230, 1998

Zarcone VP, Benson KL, Berger PA: Abnormal rapid eye movement latencies in schizophrenia. Arch Gen Psychiatry 44:45–48, 1987

Zatz M, Reisine TD: Lithium induces corticotropin secretion and desensitization in cultured anterior pituitary cells. Proc Natl Acad Sci U S A 82:1286–1290, 1985

Zebrowska-Lupina I, Ossowska G, Klenk-Majewska B: The influence of antidepressants on aggressive behaviour in stressed rats: the role of dopamine. Polish Journal of Pharmacology and Pharmacy 44:325–335, 1992

Zhang SJ, Jackson MB: Neuroactive steroids modulate GABAa receptors in peptidergic nerve terminals. J Neuroendocrinol 6:533–538, 1994

Zhou FC, Azmitia EC: A neurotrophic factor—SNTF—for serotonergic neurons, in Serotonin, Molecular Biology, Receptors and Functional Effects. Edited by Fozard JR, Saxena PR. Basel, Switzerland, Birkhauser Verlag, 1991, pp 50–68

Ziegler VE, Biggs JT: Tricyclic plasma levels: effects of age, race, sex, and smoking. JAMA 238:2167–2169, 1977

Zielinski RJ, Roose SP, Devanand DP, et al: Cardiovascular complications of ECT in depressed patients with cardiac disease. Am J Psychiatry 150:904–909, 1993

Zimmerberg B, Farley MJ: Sex differences in anxiety behavior in rats: role of gonadal hormones. Physiol Behav 54:1119–1124, 1993

Zimmerberg B, Brunelli SA, Hofer MA: Reduction of rat pup ultrasonic vocalizations by the neuroactive steroid allopregnanolone. Pharmacol Biochem Behav 47:735–738, 1994

Zis AP, Goodwin FK: Major affective disorders as a recurrent illness: a critical review. Arch Gen Psychiatry 36:835–839, 1979

Zis AP, Grof P, Webster M, et al: The cyclicity of affective disorders and its modifications by drugs. Psychopharmacol Bull 16:47–49, 1980

Zis AP, McGarvey KA, Clark CM, et al: Effect of stimulus energy on electroconvulsive therapy-induced prolactin release. Convulsive Therapy 9:23–27, 1993

Zitrin CM, Klein DF, Woerner MG, et al: Treatment of phobias, I: comparison of imipramine hydrochloride and placebo. Arch Gen Psychiatry 40:125–138, 1983

Zivkov M, De Jongh GD: Org 3770 versus amitriptyline: a 6-week randomized double-blind multicentre trial in hospitalized depressed patients. Human Psychopharmacology 3–180, 1995

Zivkovic B, Morel E, Joly D, et al: Pharmacological and behavioral profile of alpidem as an anxiolytic. Pharmacopsychiatry 23:108, 1990

Zivkovic B, et al: Alpidem, an omega-1 receptor-selective agonist: a new approach to anxiety treatment. Eur Neuropsychopharmacol 1:202, 1991

Zohar J, Insel T: OCD: Psychobiological approaches to diagnosis, treatment and pathophysiology. Biol Psychiatry 22:667–687, 1987

Zohar J, Mueller EA, Insel TE, et al: Serotonergic responsivity in obsessive-compulsive disorder: comparison of patients and healthy controls. Arch Gen Psychiatry 44:946–951, 1987

Zohar J, Insel TR, Zohar-Kadouch R, et al: Serotonergic responsivity in obsessive compulsive disorder: effects of chronic clomipramine treatment. Arch Gen Psychiatry 45:167–172, 1988a

Zohar J, Insel TR, Zohar-Kadouch RC, et al: Serotonergic role in OCD, in Progress in Catecholamine Research, Part C: Clinical Aspects. New York, Alan R Liss, 1988b, pp 385–391

Zohar J, Insel TR, Zohar-Kadouch RC, et al: Serotonergic responsivity in OCD: effects on CMI treatment. Arch Gen Psychiatry 45:167–172, 1988c

Zohar J on behalf of the Study Group: A double-blind study to assess the efficacy and tolerance of paroxetine compared with CMI and placebo in OCD patients. Paper presented at the AEP Congress, Copenhagen, 1994

Zorilla R, Simard J, Rheaume E, et al: Multihormonal control of pre-pro-somatostatin mRNA levels in the periventricular nucleus of the male and female rat hypothalamus. Neuroendocrinology 52:527–536, 1990

Zornberg GL, Pope HG Jr: Treatment of depression in bipolar disorder: new directions for research. J Clin Psychopharmacol 13:397–408, 1993

Zornetzer SF: Catecholamine system involvement in age-related memory dysfunction. Ann N Y Acad Sci 444:242–254, 1985

Zung WWK: Effect of antidepressant drugs on sleeping and dreaming, III: on the depressed patient. Biol Psychiatry 1:283–287, 1969

Zyss T: Deep magnetic brain stimulation—the end of psychiatric electroshock therapy. Med Hypotheses 43:69–74, 1994

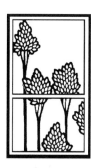

INDEX

Page numbers printed in **boldface** *type refer to tables or figures.*